C

Obstetrics & Gynecology

Fred Foshee

CORE TEXTBOOK OF

Obstetrics & Gynecology

JOHN H. MATTOX, M.D.

Professor
Clinical Obstetrics, Gynecology, Family and
Community Medicine
University of Arizona Health Sciences Center
Tucson, Arizona;
Chairman
Department of Obstetrics and Gynecology
Good Samaritan Regional Medical Center
Phoenix, Arizona

with 191 *illustrations*

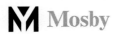 Mosby

St. Louis Baltimore Boston
Carlsbad Chicago Naples New York Philadelphia Portland
London Madrid Mexico City Singapore Sydney Tokyo Toronto Wiesbaden

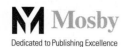

Mosby

Dedicated to Publishing Excellence

A Times Mirror Company

Editor: Susie H. Baxter
Developmental Editor: Anne Gunter
Project Manager: Linda Clarke
Production Editor: Kathleen Hillock
Designer: Carolyn O'Brien
Manufacturing Manager: William A. Winneberger, Jr.

Printed in the United States of America
Composition by Graphic World, Inc.
Printing/binding by R.R. Donnelley & Sons Co.

Mosby–Year Book, Inc.
11830 Westline Industrial Drive
St. Louis, Missouri 63146

Library of Congress Cataloging in Publication Data

Core textbook of obstetrics and gynecology / [edited by] John H.
  Mattox.
     p.   cm.
    Includes index.
    ISBN 0-8151-6035-6
    1. Gynecology 2. Obstetrics.   I. Mattox, John H.
    [DNLM: 1. Obstetrics. 2. Genital Diseases, Female.
  3. Reproduction.   WQ 100 C797 1997]
  RG101.C67   1997
  618—dc21
  DNLM/DLC
  for Library of Congress   96-49800
                                                    CIP

98 99 00 01 02 / 9 8 7 6 5 4 3 2 1

Contributors

Joseph B. Buxer, M.D.
Clinical Associate Professor
Department of Obstetrics and Gynecology
University of Arizona Health Sciences Center
Tucson, Arizona;
Medical Director
Women's Health Service
Good Samaritan Regional Medical Center
Phoenix, Arizona

Joanna M. Cain, M.D.
Professor and Chair
Department of Obstetrics and Gynecology
Pennsylvania State University
Milton S. Hershey Medical Center
Hershey, Pennsylvania

William H. Clewell, M.D.
Clinical Professor
Department of Obstetrics and Gynecology
University of Arizona Health Sciences Center
Tucson, Arizona;
Chief of Service
Department of Obstetrics and Gynecology
Good Samaritan Regional Medical Center
Phoenix, Arizona

P. Coney, M.D.
Professor and Chair
Department of Obstetrics and Gynecology
Southern Illinois University School of Medicine
Springfield, Illinois

John P. Elliott, M.D.
Clinical Professor
Department of Obstetrics and Gynecology
University of Arizona Health Sciences Center
Tucson, Arizona;
Co-Director
Division of Maternal-Fetal Medicine
Department of Obstetrics and Gynecology
Good Samaritan Regional Medical Center
Phoenix, Arizona

Lisa M. Fromm, Ph.D.
Assistant Professor
Department of Psychiatry
University of New Mexico Health Sciences Center
Albuquerque, New Mexico

Robert L. Johnson, M.D.
Phoenix Perinatal Associates
Mesa, Arizona

Dorothy Kammerer-Doak, M.D.
Assistant Professor
Department of Obstetrics and Gynecology
University of New Mexico Health Sciences Center
Albuquerque, New Mexico

Michael F. Koszalka, Jr., M.D.
Division of Maternal-Fetal Medicine
Department of Obstetrics and Gynecology
Marshfield Clinic
Marshfield, Wisconsin

Teresita A. McCarty, M.D.
Associate Professor
Department of Psychiatry
University of New Mexico Health Sciences Center
Albuquerque, New Mexico

Marlin D. Mills, M.D.
Phoenix Perinatal Associates
Phoenix, Arizona

Daniel F. O'Keeffe, Jr., M.D.
Co-Director
Division of Maternal-Fetal Medicine
Department of Obstetrics and Gynecology
Good Samaritan Regional Medical Center
Phoenix, Arizona

Jordan H. Perlow, M.D.
Phoenix Perinatal Associates
Mesa, Arizona

Sharon T. Phelan, M.D.
Associate Professor and Clerkship Director
Department of Obstetrics and Gynecology
University of Alabama—Birmingham
School of Medicine
Birmingham, Alabama

Laura Weiss Roberts, M.D.
Assistant Professor
Department of Psychiatry
University of New Mexico Health Sciences Center
Albuquerque, New Mexico

Philip A. Rosenfeld, M.D.
Clinical Professor
Department of Obstetrics and Gynecology
University of Arizona Health Sciences Center
Tucson, Arizona;
Assistant Chair
Department of Obstetrics and Gynecology
Good Samaritan Regional Medical Center
Phoenix, Arizona

Shirley K. Sawai, M.D.
Phoenix Perinatal Associates
Phoenix, Arizona

Melissa Schiff, M.D.
Assistant Professor
Department of Obstetrics and Gynecology
University of New Mexico Health Sciences Center
Albuquerque, New Mexico

Thomas H. Strong, Jr., M.D.
Clinical Assistant Professor
Department of Obstetrics and Gynecology
University of Arizona Health Sciences Center
Tucson, Arizona;
Phoenix Perinatal Associates
Phoenix, Arizona

To my dear friends and colleagues,
Drs. J. Robert Willson and
Elsie Reid Carrington, in recognition of
their effort to educate medical students

Preface

Men learn as they teach
Seneca, circa AD 1

Faculty have realized for a long time that the great attraction and benefit in academic medicine is teaching while learning simultaneously. That theme is underscored in this textbook. The book is written for medical students taking their clerkship in obstetrics and gynecology. It is designed around the *Medical Student Educational Objectives* published by the Association of Professors of Gynecology and Obstetrics (APGO). The focus is on what the student needs to know. Each chapter begins with a rationale and a listing of the APGO learning objectives. The listing of critical points and self-assessment questions at the end of each chapter are intended to help students gauge their progress and review for board examinations. A glossary of terms completes the text.

The faculty represented in this text are a special group for me. They are all successful practitioners—from seasoned senior "traditional" faculty to physicians who are available to students and residents 24 hours a day, 365 days a year. I had to resist my strong inclination to over editorialize to retain the originality that each author brought to the text. Each practitioner's contribution was gratefully received and speaks for itself. I also wish to thank everyone including the editors.

My fellow authors and I enjoyed the learning, and we sincerely hope the readers of this book will enjoy being taught.

John H. Mattox

Contents

Approach to the patient

History

APGO LEARNING OBJECTIVE #1

John H. Mattox

An annual gynecologic evaluation is an important part of primary health care and preventive medicine for women. A gynecologic assessment should be part of every woman's general medical history and physical examination. Certain questions must be asked of every woman, whereas other questions are specific to particular problems. To accomplish these objectives, optimal communication must be achieved between patient and physician.

The student will demonstrate a knowledge of the following skills:

A. Performing a thorough obstetric-gynecologic history as part of a general medical history, including the following:
   1. Chief complaint
   2. Present illness
   3. Menstrual history
   4. Obstetric history
   5. Gynecologic history
   6. Contraceptive history
   7. Sexual history
   8. Family history
   9. Social history

B. Communicating with the patient to gain her confidence and cooperation, including developing an appreciation of the effects of her age, racial and cultural background, personality, mental state, and economic status

C. Communicating the results of the obstetric-gynecologic and general medical history by well-organized written and oral reports with the relevant and necessary components

The Oslerian admonition to "Listen to the patient" is no less applicable today, despite the advancement of medical technology. An accurate medical history, accompanied by a complete physical examination, is as important for the obstetric or gynecologic patient as for patients with other medical or surgical disorders. Although they function as specialists for patients with unique problems who are referred from physicians of other disciplines, obstetrician-gynecologists also act as the primary care providers for many of the women in their practices. Therefore an evaluation may be problem-oriented, relying on the required history and physical exam to address a specific problem (e.g., infertility), or it may be a general assessment of the healthy patient, a periodic health screen, or an *annual examination*.

EVALUATION

Taking the patient's history is a two-part process. A written data inquiry form covers the medical history. It should also include areas or issues the patient may wish to discuss. When that is complete, the patient is encouraged to tell her story in her own words, at her own pace. Omitted details can be filled in with strategically placed prompts. Questions should be phrased in ordinary language, not medical jargon; too many patients answer "No" to questions they cannot understand, rather than display what they presume to be their ignorance. Although this chapter's purpose is not to discuss in detail every segment of a thorough history, a suggested outline can be seen in Fig. 1-1. Physicians, attired appropriately, should always introduce themselves to a patient and address her by her title and last name, until subsequent visits warrant closer rapport. While taking a medical history, physicians should observe a patient's demeanor. She may wish to discuss serious problems such as weight loss or gain; alcohol, substance, or sexual abuse; or issues relating to domestic violence. She must be made

to feel secure so that she is willing to discuss these difficult issues. Indeed, she may require gentle and sensitive probing to uncover some problems, with inquiries such as, "During the course of this visit I noticed that you seem worried. Is there anything else you wish to discuss?" Open-ended but leading questions can uncover sensitive problems.

Chief complaint

The chief complaint is the primary reason the patient gives for coming to see the physician. Her chief complaint may be the occurrence of inappropriate vaginal bleeding or an unexpected discomfort, or it may be routine: a periodic health examination, Pap test, or other routine screening test along with a prescription refill for medicine, such as birth control pills. Occasionally the patient may start by describing something minor while she gains the assurance she needs to disclose some intimate, perhaps socially distressing, problem. Whatever her reason, the patient must be allowed time to express herself, without interruption. If questions need to be asked, they should be open-ended when possible. The physician should sit at the patient's level, without furniture in-between, and should maintain eye contact and allow his or her facial expression to show sincere interest in what the patient is saying. While the patient is talking the physician should avoid reading the chart or writing in it. Consultation time is the patient's time.

Present illness

A chronologic account is the most useful way to learn about the complaint. The account should integrate information concerning any testing or therapy, even though the patient may not remember all of the medical terms. Pertinent data from any of the categories in Fig. 1-1 should be incorporated into this section. At the end of the interview, the physician should ask if the patient wishes to include any additional information.

I. Identifying information
A. Age
B. Parity
C. Marital status
D. Current contraceptive
E. Last menstrual period
F. Last Pap smear
G. Breast self-examination

II. Chief complaint(s)
A. List in order
B. Duration
C. Characterization
1. Location
2. Self-administered remedies
3. Prior episodes
4. Prior testing
5. Relation to menses

III. Menstrual history
A. Pubertal sequence
B. Menarche
C. Periodicity
D. Duration flow
E. Pain
F. Abnormal bleeding
G. Perimenstrual symptoms

IV. Obstetric data
A. Pregnancies
B. Outcome
C. Complications

V. Gynecologic data
A. Contraceptives
B. Surgery

C. Sexual history (including potential for physical and verbal abuse)
D. Prior lower or upper genital tract infections
E. Pelvic pain
F. Vaginal drainage

VI. Significant past history
A. Serious medical illness and sequelae
B. Surgical procedures
C. Hospitalizations

VII. Personal data
A. Occupation
B. Weight change
C. Medications
D. Smoking
E. Drug use
F. Alcohol intake
G. Allergies or drug sensitivities
H. Exercise

VIII. Family history
A. Health problems of first-degree relatives
B. Problems with diabetes mellitus, heart attack at an earlier age, breast cancer
C. Birth defects, mental retardation, pregnancy losses

IX. Review of systems (special emphasis)
A. Genitourinary
B. Gastrointestinal
C. Musculoskeletal
D. Bleeding disorders
E. Psychiatric

Fig. 1-1. Topic outline for history. Information can be obtained in any sequence; some headings may necessitate in-depth questioning.

Menstrual history

The menstrual history should include the age at which the patient's periods began and the type of flow at onset, as well as the interval (regular or irregular) of periods, the patient's educational preparation for menstruation, and her reaction to its onset. One should ask about the frequency and duration of periods and the amount of bleeding (number of well-saturated or stained pads, clots, color), the pain (type, when it begins, how long it lasts, how much it interferes with her activity, what medications are required for relief),

and the date of onset of the last normal menstrual period. Any abnormal bleeding should be identified.

Obstetric history

Each pregnancy should be listed chronologically, with information concerning prenatal complications, duration of pregnancy, outcome, and complications of labor or the puerperium; the history should include the sex and weight of the infants and their subsequent development, as well as the patient's reactions to her pregnancies.

Gynecologic history

The gynecologic history is taken in addition to the menstrual and sexual histories. Information concerning vaginal discharge, pelvic pain, infertility, congenital anomalies, and abnormal uterine bleeding is required. Information concerning vaginal discharge should include how long it has been present; its relation to menses, coitus, or other stimuli; whether there is bleeding, irritation, or odor; and whether there have been any previous diagnoses and treatments. If there has been pelvic pain, the physician should ask if it was acute, periodically recurrent, or chronic. Follow-up questions should be asked about its location, what makes it better, what makes it worse, and what the previous diagnoses and treatments were.

The gynecologic history will determine if infertility is primary or secondary, what work-ups have been done, what diagnoses have been made, and which treatments have been successful and which unsuccessful. Congenital anomalies, such as imperforate hymen or vaginal septa, may have been previously diagnosed and treated. Regularly recurring yet abnormal bleeding may include too much bleeding *(hypermenorrhea)*, too little bleeding *(hypomenorrhea)*, too frequent bleeding *(polymenorrhea)*, or infrequent bleeding *(oligomenorrhea)*. Intermenstrual bleeding may occur in addition to regular menses *(metrorrhagia)* or without demonstrable periodicity, suggesting a disorder of ovulation. Each abnormality can be determined by history, even though the patient will refer to all of her bleeding as menses.

Contraceptive history

The contraceptive history determines whether the patient currently uses, or has ever used, any method to prevent or to space pregnancies. If so, which methods has she tried? Which methods have worked well for her? Which have not? Which one was used properly yet failed, resulting in an unwanted pregnancy? The physician may ask if the patient wishes to become pregnant, and she may say "No," she is not trying to become pregnant. Yet when she is asked what she does to keep from getting pregnant, the patient may well say "Nothing; we're just not trying to get pregnant." This not unusual response may demonstrate a problem of which the patient is unaware, such as ineffective coitus or perhaps reproductive compromise of one or both partners. The question, "When was your last episode of unprotected intercourse?" may help the patient obtain insight about the use of postcoital contraception, the prevention of sexually transmitted diseases, and the need for a reliable method of birth control.

Sexual and marital history

Sexual and marital history are important topics covered in greater detail in other chapters. For a general history one may ask the patient if she is married and, if so, for how long. If she is not married one may ask if she is sexually active and, if so, with one steady partner or more than one. These questions will provide some understanding of the patient's risk for sexually transmitted disease and her need for more frequent evaluation. She should be asked whether she wishes to be pregnant. If she does not, what does she do to prevent pregnancy? Her sexual history may indicate how to help her with issues she may not have been able to otherwise discuss. If done properly, only a rare individual will be offended by such an inquiry. The more usual patient is relieved to speak with a knowledgeable professional who is willing and able to give appropriate answers to her questions. Optimally, the physician should gain comfort and experience dealing with sensitive issues, that is, orgasm, masturbation, and symptoms of sexual dysfunction. Remember, the prevalence of sexual problems at some time in a person's life approaches 100%.

Family history

The Human Genome Project, mapping the genetic structure of *Homo sapiens,* promises a succession of answers to intriguing medical questions. If answers are in the genes, they may well be in the family, making a family history critical. For such an inquiry, preprinted question forms are most helpful. A completed form reviewed before consultation will give the physician knowledge of the patient's health risks, as well as information about family illnesses, longevity, and reproductive results. Answers, whether positive or negative, will make the physician's counsel more meaningful.

Social history

Although it is difficult to deal with, or to even ask about, problems of alcohol and illicit drug use, the physician must learn what he or she can about the burdens the patient carries. There must be questions about tobacco use, alcohol use and abuse, and drugs, whether prescription or not. Inquiries about physical and sexual abuse should be made at the first interview, perhaps after the physical examination. They are made again at later meetings because those who suffer the "shame" of physical or sexual abuse may be reticent to reveal it until comfort and confidence are established. An appropriate setting for these discussions would be after the physical examination, in the privacy of the consultation room, with the patient fully clothed and composed. That is also a good time and place for the physician to review physical findings, assess the patient's condition, and outline a proposal for its management. As uncomfortable as these questions may be for the physician to ask, patients are uniformly pleased to be asked, to be given an opportunity to express any anxieties, or to simply smile and say, "I'm OK."

Communicating with the patient is essential to gain her confidence and cooperation. No therapy can be effective if she refuses it. The physician's goal is to establish a sound, mutually agreeable therapeutic contract with the patient, and for her to "sign on" she must trust the physician. Giving her a fair hearing, listening to her complaints and her fears, and trying to gently educate her about the misinformation given to her by well-meaning friends will gain the physician the patient's trust. Words and demeanor will demonstrate an appreciation for the patient's individuality as it relates to her age, her racial and cultural background, her personality, her mental state, and her economic status.

Unfortunately, though good communication with a patient may achieve an exceptionally valuable verbal history, the effort is wasted if the information is not immediately written down or dictated while it is still fresh. The physician may encourage his or her patient to make notes concerning the discussion or to write down questions as they arise. A document or a written history is necessary for the physician's work, to refresh his or her memory and to present to consultants and to appropriate colleagues. It is not by chance that a documented, complete history is mandatory within 24 hours of the hospital admission of a medical patient, and before any surgery for a surgical patient. Everyone who cares for a patient must have ready access to an excellent, well-organized history, containing every relevant and necessary component.

CRITICAL POINTS

- There is no substitute for a thorough history.
- A previsit questionnaire completed by the patient can increase the information and identify areas the patient wishes to discuss.
- Asking open-ended, nonjudgmental questions is a key to obtaining the "best" history.
- The most conscientious providers spend their professional lives honing their communication skills.

Questions

1. The most important reason to use a pre-office visit questionnaire is to:
   A. Obtain the necessary background demographic information
   B. Identify the insurance coverage for the office visit
   C. Encourage the patient to spend more time recalling her family history
   D. Be a thorough physician
   E. Encourage the patient to list areas of concern she would like to discuss during the office visit

2. When conducting a problem-oriented history in a 68-year-old woman, the least important issue is:
   A. Sexual history
   B. Contraceptive history
   C. Social history
   D. Life-style history
   E. Past obstetric history

Answers

1. E
2. B

Examination

APGO LEARNING OBJECTIVE #2

John H. Mattox

> *An accurate examination complements the history, provides additional information, and helps guide diagnosis and management. It also provides an opportunity to educate and reassure the patient.*

The student will demonstrate a knowledge of the following skills:

A. Communicating with the patient to gain her confidence and cooperation, including demonstrating an appreciation of her comfort and modesty

B. Performing a thorough obstetric-gynecologic examination as part of a woman's general medical examination, including these areas:
   1. Breasts
   2. Abdomen
   3. Pelvis, including rectovaginal examination

C. Communicating the relevant results of the examination in well-organized written and oral reports

D. Incorporating patient education in the examination, including the following:
   1. Breast self-examination
   2. External genital examination

A complete general physical examination should be performed on all new patients, with perhaps the exception of those referred from other physicians for a targeted gynecologic evaluation. The basic gynecologic examination includes the recording of weight and blood pressure, the complete examination of the breasts, and the complete examination of the abdomen, pelvis, and rectum. Proper hand washing by the physician before and following the examination should be part of the routine.

A comfortable milieu should be maintained for the patient. The ambient temperature in the examination room must be neither too hot nor too cold for a patient who has disrobed. The patient must not be left alone in that strange room, for a prolonged period of time, wearing nothing but an examination gown. The room itself should be tidy and cheerful, and the physician must appear relaxed and unharried during the examination. The impression created during the examination must be that the physician is not only competent but also sensitive to the patient's needs.

BREAST EXAMINATION

Breast examination is discussed in detail in Chapter 37, Disorders of the Breasts.

ABDOMINAL EXAMINATION

In most instances abdominal tenderness that is caused by painful lesions of the pelvic structures is located low in the abdomen. Tenderness in the upper abdomen—near the umbilicus, in the region of the cecum, or along the course of the descending colon—is less characteristic of disease of the pelvic organs. Sometimes the warmed, flat surface of the stethoscope can be used in conjunction with palpating the abdominal wall and listening to bowel sounds.

PELVIC EXAMINATION

The pelvic examination is customarily performed with the patient in lithotomy position, suitably draped with a sheet, her feet in stirrups or leg rests, and her buttocks extending just over the lower end of the table. Unless the physician wishes to obtain a specimen of urine by catheter or to check for urinary control, the patient should be asked to void immediately before the examination because a full bladder may make it impossible to feel small pelvic structures.

Abdominal and pelvic muscle relaxation are also essential for a meaningful examination, but the anxious patient may not be able to achieve the required muscle relaxation without help. Being told, step by step, what to anticipate during the examination often helps the patient to relax.

After the physician has gloved *both* hands, and with a female chaperone present to assist, the patient's external genitalia are carefully inspected using a good light source. The external genitalia are then palpated. Note should be made of developmental anomalies, hair distribution, clitoral size, skin changes, discharge, irritation, new growths, and enlargement of either of the Bartholin gland ducts.

A single digit is placed inside the introitus, and gentle pressure is applied to the posterior perineal muscles. This provides the examiner some insight into the patient's comfort with the process, as well as what size speculum should be used (Fig. 2-1). Different sizes of specula will be used depending on the patient's age, parity, and the size of the vaginal introitus.

The labia minora and majora are separated with the thumb and the index finger to expose the introitus. A warmed speculum moistened with warm water is gently inserted into the vagina to expose the cervix. Lubricating jelly will interfere with the accurate evaluation of vaginal and cervical secretions, as well as with the Pap smear. As the tip of the speculum is inserted into the vaginal opening, downward pressure is exerted posteriorly to expand the size of the introitus enough to admit the speculum with a minimum of discomfort. The *urethral meatus* is the most sensitive structure in the area, so every precaution must be taken to protect it. The examiner must be gentle and move slowly because pain produced by the speculum will make the rest of the examination more difficult. Finally, material is collected from the cervix for cytologic examination, and, when indicated, an endocervical sample is obtained for culture.

The exposed cervix should be wiped clean with a dry cotton swab. The color, size, and configuration of the cervix should be noted. Any obvious lesions are described in detail, and as the speculum is slowly withdrawn, the vaginal walls are inspected. One or two fingers, usually of the examiner's left hand, are then inserted into the vagina to depress the posterior wall as the patient is requested to bear down. If the muscular and connective tissue support of the bladder and rectum

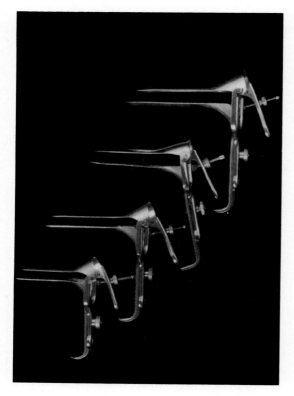

Fig. 2-1. Metal specula vary from small size for young females to larger size for obese, parous women.

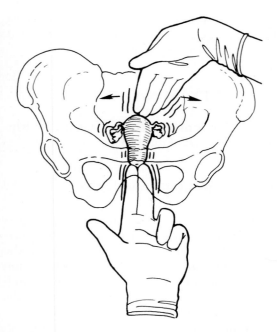

Fig. 2-2. Bimanual palpation of uterus. Hands are moved to right or left to palpate adnexa.

have been damaged, these structures will bulge through the open introitus as intraabdominal pressure is increased. The bulging-through of the anterior wall of the vagina is called *cystocele*. The bulging-through of the posterior wall of the vagina is called *rectocele*. The uterus also may be forced downward if its supporting structures have been weakened. This is called uterine *descensus* or *prolapse*. Asking the patient to contract her pelvic muscles *(pubococcygeus)* around the examining fingers provides some insight to the strength of her pelvic support.

Although it is not possible to visualize the body of the uterus and the adnexal structures, their size, shape, position, mobility, and sensitivity can usually be determined by bimanual examination (Figs. 2-2 and 2-3), in which a well-lubricated index finger alone or the index and second finger of one hand are inserted into the vagina while those of the other hand palpate through the abdominal wall. The accuracy with which bimanual examination can be performed is determined by the thickness of the abdominal wall, the patient's ability to relax her voluntary muscles, and whether a painful lesion is present. Nothing can be done about obesity, but it is possible to perform pelvic examinations on most women, even virgins, without causing undue pain. Two fingers can usually be inserted into the vagina of most multiparous women, but this is not often possible when the hymen is intact. If one learns to perform pelvic examination using only the index finger, one can examine almost anyone without causing pain. If the practitioner believes the examination is not satisfactory, some diagnostic imaging procedure, usually *pelvic ultrasound,* should be considered.

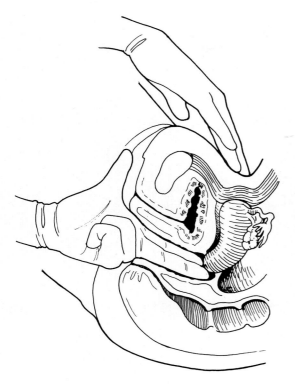

Fig. 2-3. Bimanual palpation of uterus.

Excellent technique includes appropriate handling of biologic materials, as well as proper disposal of the materials used for the examination, that is, gown, gloves, drapes, and exam table paper. There are federal requirements designed by the Occupational Safety and Health Administration that must be fulfilled to ensure patient and provider safety.

The consistency of the cervix and the direction in which it points are determined by the examiner, and he or she gently pushes the cervix and uterus upward and tilts the cervix from side to side to determine whether the structures are mobile or fixed and if motion of the cervix produces pain. The location of the body of the uterus and its size, shape, and consistency are determined by palpating the uterus between the fingers in the vagina

and by gently pushing the abdominal wall structures inward with the flat of the hand. The examiner attempts to touch the hands with the uterus between them.

The uterine corpus normally weighs about 60 to 100 g and is usually palpable in one of three positions: *anteflexed* (tipped forward), in the axis of the vagina, or *retroflexed* (tipped backward) (Fig. 2-4). An attempt is then made to feel the tube and ovary on each side, the adnexal area, between the fingertips of the practitioner's hands. The right adnexum can be outlined most accurately with the fingers of the right hand in the vagina and with the fingers of the left hand palpating abdominally. The left adnexum can be felt best with the fingers of the left hand in the vagina. Normal tubes cannot be felt as distinct structures, and it may be difficult to feel normal ovaries unless the patient is very thin or the abdominal wall is relaxed; she may experience momentary discomfort as the ovary is squeezed between the tips of the palpating fingers. Adnexal masses can usually be felt if the patient can relax her abdominal muscles and if she is not obese. For the woman who is obese or who has a rigid abdomen, pelvic ultrasound may be needed to assess the pelvic structures.

The posterior surfaces of the uterus and broad ligaments, the uterosacral ligaments, the posterior cul-de-sac, and the structures on the lateral pelvic sidewalls can be felt more accurately by rectovaginal examination than by vaginal palpation. Rectocele and other lower bowel lesions such as polyps and carcinoma can also be felt. A rectal or rectovaginal examination should be done, or at least attempted, as part of every pelvic examination. Many patients will refuse this examination, and they have a right to do so. The physician must not force it, but should encourage it because unexpected findings on rectal examination can be lifesaving. Above the age of 35 the risks of polyps and malignancy increase; thus the rectal examination is critical. Stool obtained on the examining glove can be examined for occult blood. This may provide some useful information

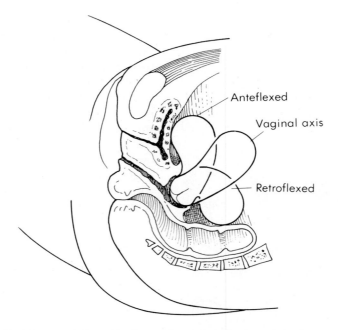

Fig. 2-4. Retroflexed corpus is found in about 15% to 20% of women. It is abnormal if it is tender or nonmobile.

on the day of the visit; however, this does not constitute an adequate screen for colon cancer. Any expected discomfort may be avoided by the use of adequate amounts of lubricating jelly around and within the anus and by encouraging the patient to "bear down" as the examining finger is inserted.

The physical examination offers a unique opportunity for patient education. As the physician does the breast exam, he or she should teach the patient how to do breast self-examination by simply guiding her hands over her breasts with the motion the physician prefers but can only describe verbally in any other setting. Some women have never looked at their genitals because they think they are not supposed to or because they just cannot bend enough to do so. A large mirror held by the chaperone will show the patient what the physician is trying to describe about her vulvar lesion, where it is, what it looks like, how to watch

for recurrence, and how and where to apply medication. These brief diversions take very little time but give much information, as well as reassurance, and are greatly appreciated by patients. They are definitely cost-effective.

After the exam is completed, the thoughtful examiner will offer the patient a moist disposable towel or soft facial tissue to wipe away the lubricating jelly. The examiner then will leave the room, allowing the patient adequate time to dress and compose herself before discussing any findings in the privacy of the consultation room. Questions posed by the examination but not covered during the history session are discussed. Pertinent physical findings, with their implications, are also discussed. Perhaps a working diagnosis can be made, confirmatory laboratory studies ordered, and a therapeutic plan agreed upon with the patient. Finally, a return appointment must be made so the patient can learn the results of her laboratory work and the physician can learn the results of the therapy. The patient should be encouraged to ask questions or even take notes to improve information retention.

Verbally reporting the results of the physical examination to the patient, however, is only the first step in documentation. Before details of the encounter are forgotten, the physician should dictate the complete physical examination into the patient's chart, so that when referring to it in the future the physician will know it is accurate. If the physician waits until the end of the day, or the end of the week, the intervening dozen examinations will blur his or her memory. One should get it down while it is still fresh. A seasoned dictator can record a complete physical in less than a minute, but it takes practice. The charted physical examination will be shared with all consultants in the future and with a partner or covering physician when the examining physician is unavailable for his or her patient, so the record should be clear and complete. Unfortunately, medicolegally, if the examination is not on the chart, it was not done. If it is on the chart when a legal issue arises, everyone will read it, and the examiner will want to be proud of his or her work.

CRITICAL POINTS

- A complete general physical examination, including the gynecologic component, is recommended for all new patients; only the gynecologic examination is performed when the physician has been consulted for a specific issue.
- The key components for conducting the most successful and productive examination are maintaining a comfortable examination room setting, paying attention to the temperature and the cheerfulness of the examination room, warming the instruments, and having the appropriately attired professional present a soft, quiet demeanor. The provider should develop a methodic sequence of performing the pelvic examination to ensure that no area is overlooked. For patients in whom the bimanual examination is unsatisfactory or in whom an abnormality is found, pelvic ultrasound should be considered.

Question

1. The following statements are valid concerning the physical examination *except:*
   A. The examination room atmosphere is important to conduct the most productive examination.
   B. An abbreviated examination (breasts, abdomen, pelvis) should only be conducted as part of a problem-specific consultation.
   C. An anterior vaginal wall bulge, produced with the patient straining, is called a cystocele.
   D. A speculum moistened with warm water will not interfere with obtaining a satisfactory Pap smear.
   E. Following the rectovaginal examination, stool tested for occult blood, when evaluated annually, is the recommended screen for colon cancer.

Answer

1. E

3

Pap smear and cultures

APGO LEARNING OBJECTIVE #3

John H. Mattox

The Pap smear is one of many screening methods used in medicine. Proper technique in perform-ing the Pap smear or obtaining specimens for micro-biologic culture will improve its accuracy and use-fulness.

The student will demonstrate a knowledge of the following skills:

A. Performing an adequate Pap smear
B. Obtaining specimens for cultures to detect sexually transmitted diseases
C. Proper handling of specimens to improve di-agnostic accuracy
D. Providing an explanation to the patient re-garding the purpose of these tests

Screening for female genital cancer is a major endeavor for physicians providing periodic health examinations for women. Cytologic screening of various tissues in the body is conducted using a basic technique originally described by Papani-colaou. The focus of this chapter emphasizes the examination of exfoliated cells to diagnose cervical cancer, although it is recognized that this screening technique is advantageous in other sites of the body as well. Some of the common benign cervical lesions look much like cancer on gross inspection but can be differentiated by this special test. Cervical specimens must be properly collected and handled to provide accu-rate information.

PAP SMEAR

A cytologist can detect abnormal cervical cells in specially prepared and stained specimens ob-tained from the cervix. The most accurate results are obtained when the material is collected from the endocervical canal and the junction of the squamous and columnar epithelium (Fig. 3-1). This junction is the area at which squamous can-cer cells usually originate. Material from the

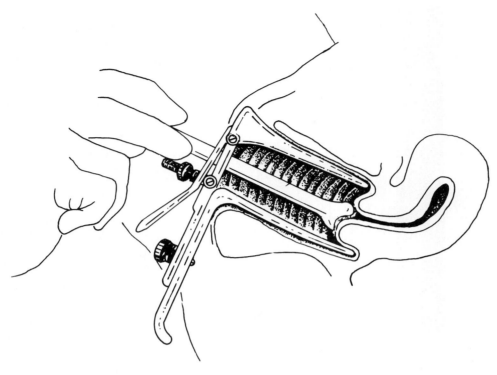

Fig. 3-1. Cytologic examination. Material obtained by rotational scrape of squamocolumnar junction.

squamocolumnar junction is collected by scraping the area with a special spatula and transferring the material to a clean glass slide, to which a fixative is applied. The endocervical sample is obtained by rotating a brush in the cervical canal. The material is processed in a similar fashion (Fig. 3-2). To ensure the greatest accuracy the fixative must be applied within 10 to 15 seconds. If the material is allowed to dry on the slide, so much artifact is introduced as to make the slide useless.

The cells are then sent to the cytologic laboratory, where they are stained and evaluated. The reports are returned to the clinician using standardized criteria called the *Bethesda system* (Table 3-1).

The management of atypical squamous cells of undetermined significance (ASCUS) is controversial because many of these lesions will clear with-

out further diagnosis or therapy. In general the recommendation is to examine the cervix for any obvious signs of infection and, following therapy, to repeat the smear in 3 to 6 months. Low-grade squamous intraepithelial lesions necessitate further evaluation, as do high-grade squamous intraepithelial lesions. The generally accepted approach is to form a colposcopically directed biopsy, along with an endocervical curettage. Because adenocarcinoma of the cervix seems to be increasing, it is important that the endocervical cells be identified in the sample. The cytologic examination is of less value in screening for endometrial cells; however, exfoliated endometrial cancer cells can sometimes be detected when sampling the endocervical canal.

The colposcope is a binocular magnifying instrument through which one can detect epithelial

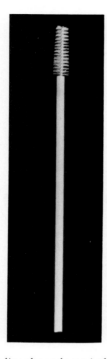

Fig. 3-2. By abrading the endocervical canal and transferring the material to a slide, the optimum sample can be obtained.

Table 3-1. The Bethesda system (modified)
I. Adequacy of sample
A. Satisfactory for evaluation
B. Satisfactory for evaluation, but limited
C. Unsatisfactory
II. Descriptive diagnosis
A. Normal
B. Benign cellular changes
C. Epithelial cell abnormalities
1. Atypical squamous cells of undetermined significance
2. Low-grade squamous intraepithelial lesion
3. High-grade squamous intraepithelial lesion
D. Glandular cell abnormalities

changes that are not visible by gross inspection. The cervix is initially prepared with 6% acetic acid, which allows the cervical and endocervical epithelium to be more prominent. It is beyond the scope of this chapter to describe in detail the colposcopic findings. The experienced colposcopist knows to biopsy any suspicious area, which would include abnormalities of the transformation zone, white patches of epithelium, and abnormal vascular patterns seen on the cervix (specifically, mosaicism).

The frequency of Pap smears is controversial. If a woman is at low risk for cervical neoplasia and has had three consecutive normal Pap smears, some authors would recommend that the Pap can be done at a minimum of 2-year intervals. In the United States, many patients have identified their Pap smear as part of their annual examination. The concern is that if patients are led to believe they can come in less frequently, they might forego their annual examinations, which would include the screening of such important general health concerns as blood pressure, breast examination, the assessment of health risks, and immunizations. In the current environment, the frequency of the Pap smear assessment is often determined by practice care guidelines provided by managed care organizations.

OBTAINING CULTURES TO DETECT SEXUALLY TRANSMITTED DISEASE

The topic of sexually transmitted disease is discussed in more detail in Chapter 32. However, it is imperative for the provider to understand that properly obtaining material for office or laboratory examination is critical to the accuracy of the diagnosis, as well as to the formulation of a logical management plan. The physician should know the optimum way to collect the material to screen for gonorrhea, chlamydia, herpes simplex, syphilis, human papillomavirus, and human immunodeficiency virus, as well as the common organisms responsible for vulvovaginitis. The predominant difficulty in ambulatory settings is maintaining an adequate supply of cultures or transfer media and making sure that the media are not outdated. Following the acquisition of the biologic material it is critical to identify the source accurately, as well as to include a way to identify the patient on the laboratory requisition. Maintaining patient confidentiality can be an issue, and all attempts must be made to do so. The second most difficult problem is to ensure the timely transfer of the material to the laboratory setting. Finally, the provider must have a thorough understanding of the pathogenesis and sequelae to be able to sit down and counsel the patient appropriately about therapy and follow-up. It cannot be too strongly emphasized that counseling must take place using concepts and words that the patient can easily understand.

CRITICAL POINTS

- Obtaining a Pap smear to screen for cervical neoplasia is a fundamental skill that all providers examining women should possess.
- The most important component of obtaining the Pap smear is having an adequate sample of the squamocolumnar junction, as well as the endocervical canal. This requires the use of a spatula and an endocervical brush. After the specimen is applied to the glass slide, a cytologic fixative must be used promptly to minimize artifact caused by drying.
- The current laboratory reports reflect the universal application of the Bethesda system. Abnormalities and cervical cytology, depending upon their severity, are usually more definitely assessed by a colposcopically directed biopsy and endocervical curettage.
- To adequately assess sexually transmitted disease, cervical material obtained must be transferred to the appropriate culture media, which are then sent to the laboratory in a timely fashion.
- Discussing the findings and the management, including follow-up, with the patient should be conducted in terms that are easy for the patient to understand.

Questions

1. To obtain adequate cervical cytologic material for a Pap smear, one must not:
   A. Lubricate the speculum with water-soluble lubricant to facilitate insertion.
   B. Obtain cells from the squamocolumnar junction with a spatula.
   C. Obtain cells from the endocervical canal with a cytologic brush.
   D. Obtain samples when there is no menstrual bleeding or cervical infection.
   E. Allow more than 10 to 15 seconds following the deposition of material before the fixative is applied.
2. The Bethesda system is a nationally recognized method of describing the material

obtained from the cervix on a Pap smear. The report should include information about all of the following *except:*

A. The adequacy of the sample
B. A comment about the presence or absence of endocervical cells
C. Cytologic changes compatible with human papillomavirus infection
D. A grouping of the significant abnormalities into low-grade or high-grade lesions
E. Cytologic information about the presence or absence of gonococcal infection

Answers

1. A
2. E

Diagnosis and management plan

John H. Mattox

> *Accurately identifying problems and selecting the most likely diagnosis lead to effective management plans.*

After completing the history and physical examination, the student will demonstrate a knowledge of the following skills:

A. Generating a problem list
B. Forming diagnostic impressions
C. Developing a management plan, including the following:
    1. Laboratory and diagnostic studies
    2. Treatment
    3. Patient education
    4. Plans for continuing care of the patient
    5. Economic considerations
    6. Assessment of patient values

GENERATING A PROBLEM LIST

A problem list is generated by the patient's history, starting with the chief complaint; it is augmented by abnormal findings during the physical examination. Listed problems are conditions that cause an unwanted alteration in life-style and activity.

They are signs and symptoms portending future morbidity, perhaps early mortality. They are items that will alter a management plan, items not to be forgotten. A problem list is a separate piece of paper usually found at the front of a medical record and designed to remind the physician that there remain unresolved or ongoing issues. It is headed by drug allergies and sensitivities and any idiosyncratic drug interactions. Then follows a simple numbered list including an entry date, the problem and its resolution, and the dates of onset and resolution. A single page is used to avoid errors. A prenatal record often includes a problem list that specifically deals with medical issues related to the pregnancy.

FORMING DIAGNOSTIC IMPRESSIONS

The history and physical examination invariably create a diagnostic impression. It is necessary, however, to resist the assumption that the first impression is the correct one. Instead, a differential diagnosis should be created. It will list entities that may reasonably be thought to cause the history and physical findings. Its primary purpose is to remind the physician to consider alternate possibilities. Secondarily, it will be a list for reconsideration should the presumptive diagnosis be wrong. The diagnostic list should reflect prioritization, enumerating the most to the least likely explanations.

DEVELOPING A MANAGEMENT PLAN

A plan of action evolves from the history, the physical examination, and the appropriate laboratory and imaging studies. It is then presented to the patient for her consideration. There may be several reasonable methods of management of the presumptive diagnosis, and these methods should be carefully explained to the patient, including their risks and benefits. The patient may have concerns about the plan's impact on her value system. It may adversely affect her cultural comfort. Economic considerations necessitate discussion as well. Likewise, the patient must be helped to understand the results of no treatment, of no plan. This is an educational dialogue and forms the basis of an informed consent agreement. The conversation should be supplemented with other educational materials, that is, handouts, videos, and reference lists to help the patient formulate the best possible decision.

Diagnostic tests

For many women the information obtained from the history and the physical examination is enough to indicate what treatment, if any, is required. For others, further study is necessary before a treatment plan can be developed. Most organic gynecologic disorders are caused by infection, endocrine dysfunction, tumor growth, and the late effects of childbirth injury; of these,

the last can usually be diagnosed without difficulty by physical examination alone, but it is necessary to perform certain laboratory studies to identify a type of tumor, infecting organism, or hormone disorder. Many diagnostic tests are simple, can be performed in the physician's office, and necessitate little equipment other than a microscope and stains for bacteria. Some tests can be done only in elaborate and specialized laboratories.

A hemoglobin should be performed periodically because iron deficiency is common, particularly during pregnancy and in patients with abnormal uterine bleeding. In cases of suspected intraperitoneal bleeding, serial hemoglobin or hematocrit levels can document blood loss. Leukocyte counts are helpful if infection is suspected, and they can assist in the differentiation between a tubal pregnancy and acute salpingo-oophoritis. A cleanly voided urine sample can be tested in the office with a test strip for glucose, protein, blood, acetone, and leukocyte esterase. If any of the tests are positive, appropriate follow-up is required.

TESTS FOR PELVIC INFECTIONS. The physician should try to identify the organisms responsible for the various types of pelvic infections. Delineating between infections of the lower genital tract (cervix, vagina, vulva) and the upper genital tract (endometrium, tubes, ovaries) is helpful; the specific diagnoses and therapies of these entities are covered in later chapters. In some instances diagnosis of the lower genital infections can be made by the physician by examining a wet smear. A culture may be taken and sent to a laboratory. Special precautions are necessary when anaerobic infections are suspected.

WET SMEAR. A small amount of vaginal discharge is obtained. In a small tube the discharge is diluted with about 1 ml of normal saline at body temperature and then shaken; a drop of the suspension is placed on a clean glass slide, covered with a coverslip, and examined under a microscope at 400×. Trichomonads may be identified because they are motile and somewhat larger than a leukocyte. If one to two drops of 10% aqueous potassium hydroxide are added to another slide preparation, mycelia with spores signify the presence of candidiasis. If the discharge has a strong fishy odor and large, stippled epithelial cells, the "clue cells," the most likely diagnosis is bacterial vaginosis.

Bacterial cultures are more informative for diagnosing vulvar or vaginal ulcers and gonorrhea. Besides obtaining a culture, ulcerations—particularly painless ones—should prompt the physician to obtain a dark field examination for syphilis and a screening serology.

Gonorrhea can be diagnosed more accurately by culture of cervical and urethral secretions than by clinical examination or by stained smear. However, a Gram stain of cervical or vaginal secretions may sometimes provide information necessary to initiate appropriate treatment while awaiting the reports of bacterial cultures. This is particularly important in the treatment of septic abortions and suspected streptococcal, clostridial, and other serious acute infections.

HORMONE ASSAYS. Disturbances in production and metabolism of reproductive hormones may be important as causes of menstrual abnormalities and infertility. Because, in a sense, the patient is herself a bioassay of specific hormonal activity, one can determine if the ovary is producing estrogen or if a woman is ovulating through the use of simple, inexpensive tests that can be done in the office. Specific assays are required when more precise information concerning hormonal production is necessary. Examples of conditions for which accurate assay is essential are the follow-up of patients who have been treated for hydatidiform mole, the evaluation of women suspected of having anterior pituitary dysfunction, and the evaluation of women with amenorrhea, infertility, or hirsutism.

Measuring reproductive hormonal function is different from measuring activity of other endocrine organs. Thyroid function, for example, varies little from day to day, and one can usually assess thyroid activity reasonably accurately with an ultrasensitive thyroid-stimulating hormone

performed on one occasion. This is not true of ovarian function, which changes from day to day throughout the menstrual cycle. It is easy to get a false impression of reproductive endocrine function if one fails to relate the results of the test to the day of the cycle or if one accepts a single study as representative of a constantly changing production of hormones. The frequency and the pulse amplitude of follicle-stimulating hormone (FSH) and luteinizing hormone (LH) are often more important than a random level of either hormone.

In short, endocrine assays are expensive, and they provide little useful information if they are ordered indiscriminately and unless they are performed in a laboratory in which the techniques are well designed and carefully controlled. Before an assay is ordered, one should decide whether it will provide the information needed and also whether equally satisfactory information can be obtained by a simpler and less expensive method.

TESTS FOR ESTROGEN

VAGINAL CYTOLOGY. Among other functions, estrogen stimulates the growth of vaginal epithelial cells. The basal and parabasal cells respond to this hormone by proliferating and becoming cornified. During periods of low estrogen production, before puberty, and after menopause, the vaginal epithelium is thin and made up almost entirely of basal and parabasal cells. The cells contain little or no glycogen. Estrogen produced by the active ovaries of mature women stimulates epithelial cell growth. These changes can be demonstrated by examining stained spreads of exfoliated cells in vaginal secretions. The presence of systemic estrogen activity may be assumed when a smear of cellular material collected from the upper vagina and stained by the Papanicolaou technique reveals cornified or precornified cells (Fig. 4-1).

CERVICAL MUCUS. Papanicolaou described an interesting pattern of arborization, or *ferning,* in cervical mucus spread on a clean glass slide and allowed to dry. The intensity of ferning is determined by the concentration of sodium chloride and other electrolytes in the cervical secretion,

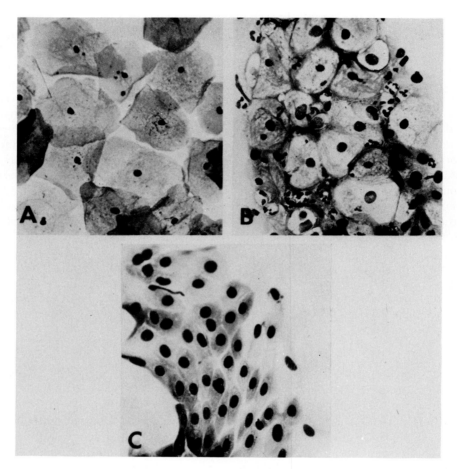

Fig. 4-1. Estrogen-induced changes in vaginal epithelial cells. **A,** Cornified (superficial) cells, strong estrogen effect. **B,** Intermediate cells and parabasal cells, smaller rounder cells with large nuclei, progesterone effect. **C,** Clump of basal cells, vaguely outlined with large nuclei, indicating lack of estrogen. *(From Riley G: Clin Obstet Gynecol 7:432, 1964.)*

which is stimulated by estradiol (E_2). The greater the amount, the more pronounced the ferning (Fig. 4-2).

Ferning is absent immediately after menstruation, when estrogen is low. It increases progressively to the maximum at the time of ovulation, when the estrogen concentration peaks.

Ferning is inhibited by progesterone; hence the pattern is not present during the postovulatory phase of the normal menstrual cycle and during pregnancy.

To obtain mucus, an unlubricated speculum is inserted into the vagina, exposing the cervix, from which the visible discharge is wiped. A cotton-tipped applicator is gently inserted into the cervical canal and rotated. The mucus that adheres to the cotton swab is spread on a clean slide and allowed to dry at room temperature. The dried, unstained spread is scanned under the low power of the microscope. A slightly different technique is used to examine cervical mucus after intercourse for a postcoital exam.

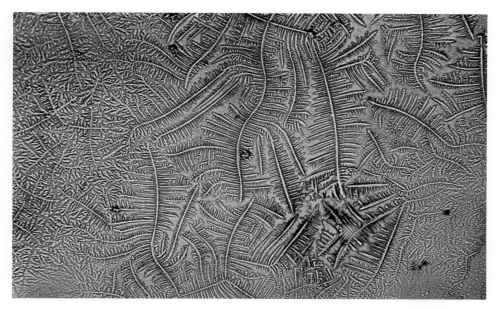

Fig. 4-2. Complete arborization of cervical mucus seen in midcycle peak of unopposed estrogen activity. (× 164.)

ESTRADIOL ASSAY. The technique for the measurement of plasma E_2 enables one to determine quantities of these compounds in serum. The plasma concentrations of E_2 during the early follicular phase of the normal menstrual cycle are in the range of 40 to 75 pg/ml, and during the midcycle phase about 200 to 400 pg/ml. During the luteal phase the concentrations fall to a level of 100 to 300 pg/ml for E_2. In postmenopausal women the concentrations of this hormone are as low as 5 to 25 pg/ml.

TESTS FOR PROGESTERONE. Progesterone activity can be detected by simple tests; a precise measurement necessitates a complicated assay.

BASAL BODY TEMPERATURE CHARTS. Because progesterone has a thermogenic property, a sustained rise in the basal body temperature during the latter half of the menstrual cycle is presumptive evidence of progesterone activity. A monophasic curve is suggestive of absent or deficient progesterone secretion. Daily record-ing by the patient is required to detect the 0.4 to 0.6° F increase following ovulation; the actual event of ovulation probably occurs 1 to 2 days earlier (Fig. 4-3).

PROGESTERONE ASSAY. Immunoassay proce-dures are used for the determination of plasma progesterone levels, which increase from low fol-licular phase levels to significantly elevated con-centrations (3 to 20 ng/ml) during the luteal phase. These luteal phase progesterone levels drop before the onset of the next menstruation or rise sharply in early pregnancy under the stimulus of human chorionic gonadotropin (HCG) on the corpus luteum. Plasma progesterone con-centration increases throughout the course of pregnancy.

TESTS FOR GONADOTROPINS. Con-centrations of anterior pituitary gonadotropins in peripheral blood can be determined by radioim-munoassay, which not only distinguishes between FSH and LH, but also measures minute amounts of the hormones in small volumes of serum. The

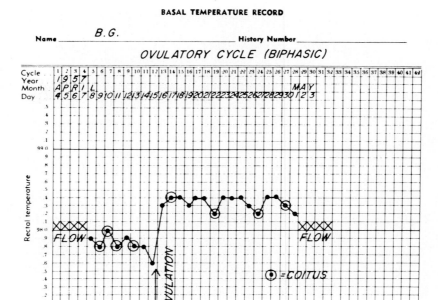

Fig. 4-3. Basal body temperature chart showing biphasic curve indicative of ovulatory cycle. Note drop and sharp rise at time of ovulation. Anovulatory cycle produces monophasic pattern. If temperature is elevated for greater than 16 days in luteal phase, pregnancy should be considered.

pattern of FSH and LH secretion during a normal menstrual cycle is described in Chapter 42, Normal and Abnormal Uterine Bleeding. Follicular phase FSH concentration varies from 5 to 20 mIU/ml, whereas LH concentrations in the serum range from 5 to 25 mIU/ml; the value more than doubles around the time of the LH surge.

TESTS FOR ANDROGENS. Radioimmunoassay procedures are available for the measurement of testosterone and dehydroepiandrosterone sulfate in serum. During the normal menstrual cycle, the plasma testosterone level is 0.2 to 0.8 ng/ml.

TESTS FOR OVULATION. Without ovulation, reproduction is impossible. This makes it important not only to be able to detect ovulation, but also to time its occurrence with some degree of accuracy. The only certain method to document ovulation is to recover an ovum—which, while possible, is clinically impractical—or by the initiation of pregnancy. However, a number of fairly

reliable indirect indexes that ovulation has occurred may be used to determine and to time this event. The indirect tests depend predominantly on the presence of progesterone. Some of these tests have been discussed previously.

ENDOMETRIAL BIOPSY. Histologic examination of endometrium removed either by curettage or by biopsy 3 to 5 days before the onset of a normal menstrual period should demonstrate a late secretory endometrium. The limitations of this method are that it indicates only what has happened in one isolated cycle and that the expense and discomfort involved make it impractical to repeat the test during several cycles.

That the risk of interrupting pregnancy is not great is suggested by the experience of Rosenfeld and Garcia. They obtained endometrial biopsies during the cycles in which 18 infertile patients conceived; 14 delivered normal infants at term, one delivered prematurely, one aborted, and two were lost to follow-up. A pregnancy can be de-

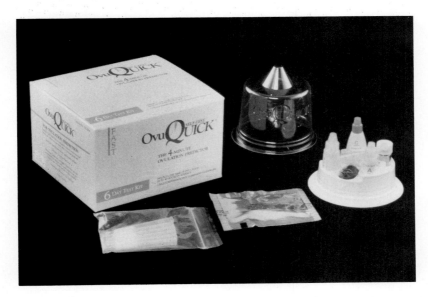

Fig. 4-4. Urinary luteinizing hormone predictor kits are expensive, vary in reliability from brand to brand, and require patient to perform simple laboratory test.

tected as early as 10 days gestation with the current serologic test.

Examination of temperature curves, endometrial biopsy, and progesterone assay usually indicates that ovulation has occurred or at least that progesterone is being secreted. None of these tests, however, is of value in determining the time of ovulation. It may be possible to anticipate ovulation by the use of rapid urinary LH assay to detect the LH surge. Over-the-counter test kits are available for the patient to use at home. Fertility testing and coital timing can be facilitated if the woman can use the kit (Fig. 4-4).

ULTRASOUND. Monitoring follicle growth for 2 to 4 days with ultrasound to look for the formation of a dominant follicle (DF) is a reliable way of assessing ovulation. A DF in a spontaneous cycle ranges from 18 to 22 mm in mean diameter (Fig. 4-5). The collapse of the follicle is thought to correlate with ovum release.

TESTS FOR CHORIONIC GONADO-TROPIN. Soon after the ovum is fertilized and implantation occurs, the trophoblast begins to secrete HCG. The detection of this hormone in serum or urine is the basis of all pregnancy tests. It can be detected as early as 7 to 9 days after fertilization by the highly sensitive techniques of β-subunit immunoassay. The production of HCG increases rapidly; the serum concentration doubles about every 48 hours during the early weeks of pregnancy. Serum levels and urinary excretion of HCG rise to a peak at about the sixtieth or seventieth day after conception and then decline toward a lower plateau, which is maintained throughout the second and third trimesters. Pregnancy tests generally remain positive throughout gestation or as long as viable trophoblastic tissue is in contact with the maternal circulation.

The half-life of HCG is approximately 36 hours. The rate of disappearance is contingent on the level of circulating HCG, which can be significantly elevated in patients with gestational trophoblastic disease and those having functioning residual trophoblastic tissue, as occurs following pregnancy termination. Typically, HCG levels return to normal after 10 to 14 days following delivery. Serial hormone levels are often needed in the clinical setting to monitor the disappearance of HCG.

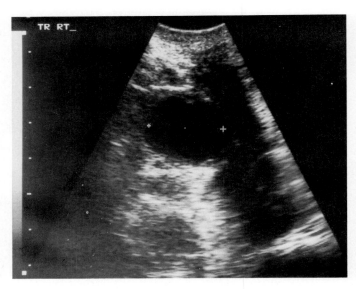

Fig. 4-5. Dominant follicle, mean diameter 20 mm, is seen in sonogram obtained from region of right adnexa by using 5-MHz endovaginal probe.

A highly sensitive enzyme-linked immunoabsorbent assay designed to detect concentrations of HCG as low as 25 mIU/ml in urine is available. Monoclonal antibodies that react to different areas, the α-subunits and β-subunits of the HCG molecule, can be produced. The first antibodies immobilize HCG molecules on a membrane; the second antibodies, combined with an enzyme that produces a color change, attach to the captured HCG molecules. If HCG is present, a characteristic color appears on the membrane. If there is no HCG, the color of the membrane is unchanged. The necessary materials are supplied in kit form, and tests can be run in 10 to 20 minutes. A monoclonal antibody test is far more sensitive than an ordinary immunologic test and can be used to detect HCG soon after implantation and in women suspected of having ectopic pregnancies. The test depends on an immunologic reaction that results in a colorimetric response, thereby eliminating the precautions and equipment required to perform the radioimmunoassay. This test is an example of a qualitative pregnancy test.

Although the α-subunits of HCG and LH are identical chemically, the β-subunits are different. Thus one can prepare a specific antibody against the β-subunit of HCG that will not react with LH. β-Subunit radioimmunoassay on serum is highly sensitive and quantitative but is not practical for rapid use as a pregnancy test. The assay is more expensive and takes several hours to run. Most large metropolitan hospitals offer this test on a daily basis; it is more difficult to have access to this quantitative assay on a 24-hour basis in smaller institutions. The detection level is 5 mIU/ml.

Diagnostic imaging

Diagnostic imaging techniques offer significant potential in the evaluation of the obstetric or gynecologic patient. Table 4-1 presents a list of studies and their applications. With the possible exception of ultrasound, there should always be some reluctance about ordering these procedures during pregnancy. This hesitation is stimulated mostly by the lack of information concerning possible deleterious effects on the embryo or fetus.

Table 4-1. Imaging procedures in obstetrics and gynecology

Study	Assessment
Hysterosalpingography	Uterine cavity contour and tubal patency
Ultrasonography	Pregnancy diagnosis and dating; fetal studies including
1. Abdominal	growth evaluation and to exclude anomalies; pelvic
2. Transvaginal	masses
Mammography	Early detection of malignancy
1. Xeromammography	
2. "Low dose" screen film mammography	
Computed tomography	Pituitary tumor; adrenal tumor
Bone densitometry (DEXA)	Osteoporosis
Magnetic resonance imaging	Abdominal, pelvic, pituitary tumor

---

X-RAY. An important use of x-ray film examination in gynecology is for hysterosalpingography, by which small intracavitary uterine lesions, as well as abnormalities in the tubes, can be detected.

Radiologic studies are used infrequently during pregnancy. X-ray film studies during the first few weeks of pregnancy are more likely to disturb fetal growth than are those during the second and third trimesters, when the organs are reasonably well formed. The tissues are particularly susceptible from the second to the sixth week after conception, when it may be difficult to diagnose pregnancy. After the primary organ systems have developed and the embryonic cells are transformed into those with adult characteristics, it is less likely that ordinary diagnostic procedures will influence fetal development.

Radiographic studies should be ordered when the patient is in her follicular phase if possible; the newer, more sensitive HCG determination provides greater but not total assurance that an intrauterine gestation is not present when x-rays are needed in the luteal phase.

ULTRASOUND. Ultrasound is useful in diagnosing both normal and abnormal pregnancy during the early weeks, in identifying multifetal pregnancy and fetal anomalies, in differentiating hydatidiform moles from normal pregnancy, in

diagnosing missed abortion and intrauterine fetal death, as an aid in diagnosing ectopic pregnancy, in identifying abnormalities in amniotic fluid volume, in measuring the biparietal diameter of the fetal skull, in assessing fetal size and the rate of fetal growth, for placental localization, and in the differential diagnosis of various uterine and ovarian enlargements. These are discussed in detail in the appropriate sections of the book. Diagnostic sound waves appear to have no deleterious effect on maternal or fetal tissues. The acquisition of the endovaginal probe has enhanced the diagnostic and therapeutic potential of this modality.

A pelvic ultrasound should be obtained for every gynecology patient who has significant abnormalities detected on bimanual examination or if the initial exam is unsatisfactory. The size of uterine myoma or an adnexal mass can be measured, thereby increasing the accuracy and the quality of the information obtained from the more subjective bimanual exam.

MAGNETIC RESONANCE IMAGING. Magnetic resonance imaging (MRI) is based on the principle that nuclei of certain atoms possess the property of angular momentum, or spin, which makes them function as magnets. In a magnetic field the atoms assume positions either parallel to or opposite from the direction of the field. The tissue images provided by this technique

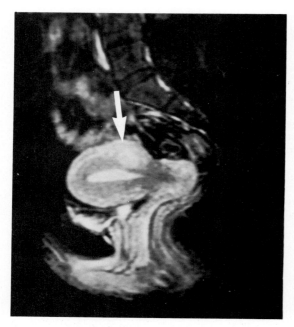

Fig. 4-6. Intramural leiomyoma, 2-cm posterior, in sagittal view obtained with 1.5 Tesla magnet enhanced with gadolinium.

are far superior to those of ultrasound and eliminate the potential dangers from radiation associated with computed tomography (CT) scans. Because there are no known ill effects on tissue, MRI has an important potential for use in obstetrics and gynecology; but it is too early to evaluate its contribution (Fig. 4-6).

BONE DENSITOMETRY. There are a group of studies that attempt to assess bone density to determine which patients are at greater risk to develop osteoporosis and possible fracture. Single-photon beam densitometry evaluates changes predominantly in cortical bone of the distal forearm; dual-photon beam densitometry measures bone thickness of the thoracolumbar spine and/or femoral neck. Quantitative CT also examines the spine. Currently there is controversy concerning the clinical use of these studies. The current method, dual-energy x-ray absorptiometry (DEXA), is preferred because the spine and the femoral neck can be evaluated.

The results from each method relate solely to that particular technique and cannot be compared with those of a different technique. Serial studies prove more useful than one determination because the physician is attempting to detect relatively small losses in bone density, that is, 1% to 3% annually. Bone densitometry studies should not, at the present time, be used as a routine screen in perimenopausal women. Ideally, each institution should develop its own normative data with clinical correlation over a period of time.

LAPAROSCOPY. The development of high-intensity, fiberoptic light sources has led to a reevaluation of an old method of examining the peritoneal cavity. With the laparoscope, which is inserted through a subumbilical incision after pneumoperitoneum with carbon dioxide has been established, it is possible to inspect the contents of both the pelvis and the upper abdomen. The view of the pelvic organs is usually excellent; one looks down from above and can see the bladder, the anterior surface of the uterus, the adnexa, and the posterior cul-de-sac.

The principal indications for laparoscopy are the evaluation of pelvic pain, the inspection of uterine or ovarian masses, infertility, endocrinopathies, amenorrhea, congenital anomalies, and sterilization. The serious complications are hemorrhage from punctured blood vessels and perforation of a hollow viscus.

Laparoscopy can be classified as diagnostic or operative. The latter term applies when electrocautery, laser, or special instruments facilitate the removal of adhesions, biopsy of a pelvic structure, or incision of a fallopian tube with evacuation of an ectopic pregnancy.

HYSTEROSCOPY. The advantages of diagnosing intrauterine disease by direct inspection rather than by indirect exploration of the cavity with a curet are obvious. Hysteroscopy was first described in 1869. Improved optics, lighting sources, and operating instruments have been designed, and hysteroscopy is becoming an important tool.

Lysis of intrauterine adhesions, polyp or intra-uterine device removal, and resection of a septum are the major operative procedures for which hysteroscopy is used. Because the cavity must be distended to permit visualization, carbon dioxide (for diagnostic study) and glycine or saline (for surgery) are required. In spite of its simplicity, there is potential for serious complications with hysteroscopy.

AMNIOCENTESIS. A variety of examinations can be performed on amniotic fluid. Almost all tests performed during early pregnancy are to diagnose genetic defects. The majority performed during the third trimester are to obtain fluid to assess fetal maturity.

The aim of genetic amniocentesis is to detect fetal chromosomal and biochemical abnormalities during early pregnancy so that parents may either obtain an abortion or plan for the care of the child if a defect is present. Fetal cells in amniotic fluid are cultured for karyotyping, identification of certain enzymatic deficiencies, and determination of fetal sex. The fluid can also be assayed for its α-fetoprotein, which may indicate open neural tube defects.

The majority of amniocenteses are performed to detect chromosomal abnormalities, which increase with maternal age. Some abnormalities of carbohydrate, lipid, and protein metabolism can be diagnosed by studying cultured or uncultured cells. The determination of fetal sex is important in considering the possible outcome of sex-linked genetic disorders.

Genetic amniocentesis is usually performed at about 14 to 16 weeks' gestation. Before this there may be too little amniotic fluid and too few shed cells to ensure a successful result. If done much later, the pregnancy may be so far advanced when the results are available that the possibility of abortion is eliminated. Genetic amniocentesis is an outpatient procedure performed with local infiltration anesthesia and ultrasound guidance.

The principal indications for genetic amniocentesis are as follows:

1. Maternal age of 35 years or more (at the time of delivery)
2. Chromosomal abnormality in a previous child
3. Known chromosomal abnormality in either parent
4. Metabolic disorder in a previous child
5. History of a sex-linked genetic disorder
6. Family history of chromosomal, enzymatic, or metabolic abnormality or of neural tube defects

The potential complications are infection of either mother or fetus, injury to the fetus, feto-maternal transfusion with possible Rh allo-immunization if a placental blood vessel is punctured, and abortion. Infection can be kept at a minimum by using meticulous, sterile technique. One can usually avoid injuring the placenta by identifying its position with ultrasound and selecting a puncture site beyond its edge. Genetic amniocentesis does not increase the rates of abortion, preterm delivery, fetal or neonatal death, or neonatal complications. It is estimated that fetal death within 3 weeks of midtrimester amniocentesis occurs in about 0.5% of cases when experienced operators perform the procedure.

ADDITIONAL PRENATAL DIAGNOSTIC STUDIES. Discussing new prenatal diagnostic developments in detail is beyond the scope of this text. However, an explosion of scientific knowledge has permitted greater study of the intrauterine environment in early pregnancy. Improved optic systems, advances in ultrasound imaging and recognition of anomalies, and molecular genetic techniques form the foundation of this technology.

CHORIONIC VILLUS SAMPLING. Chorionic villus sampling can be performed at about the eighth to tenth week of pregnancy either transabdominally or transvaginally with ultrasound guidance.

Cells can be analyzed for biochemical markers and karyotype, and deoxyribonucleic acid probes can examine portions of the genome of the fetus. As experience grows, the risk of infection and spontaneous abortion diminishes; currently the risk is about 1% to 2%.

CRITICAL POINTS

- A problem list, usually maintained in the front of the patient's inpatient or ambulatory record, will provide a systematized, chronologic list of the patient's most important medical problems. The list should be easily identifiable in the record and contain the date the problem was identified, as well as the date it was resolved. Some conditions will be ongoing. This important document serves to remind the clinician not only of what the current medical issues are, but also of any past medical conditions that might impact on the present illness.
- With few exceptions, following a thorough history and physical examination the provider has a strong sense of the patient's medical problems. Clinicians should train themselves to list the possibilities in a logical and prioritized fashion. Although the final diagnosis is often strongly suspected, it can only be confirmed with the acquisition of diagnostic studies that could include laboratory or radiographic information.
- As part of the management plan, it is important to involve the patient in any decisions concerning therapy. This occurs not only by direct discussion, but also by supplementing the visit with other educational materials that help the patient formulate the best clinical decision.
- When ordering laboratory tests it is important to distinguish between those tests that might be interesting and help to confirm a diagnosis and those that are essential and will affect the decision-making process.
- A commonly performed and clinically useful test is the wet smear. All providers dealing in the care of women should be familiar with the advantages and disadvantages of this test as a cornerstone to treat vulvovaginitis.
- When ordering hormone tests that assess the hypothalamic-pituitary-ovarian axis, it is critical that the physician know where the patient is in the menstrual cycle to produce the optimum interpretation of the results. This is because many of the tests fluctuate substantially even in women who are oligoovulatory.
- Most tests that assess ovulation are indirectly assessing the effects on the female body of serum progesterone, which occurs following ovulation. The tests include a basal body temperature determination, changes in vaginal cytology and cervical mucus, and a timed endometrial biopsy in secretory phase. The direct measurement of serum progesterone can also be helpful to determine if ovulation has occurred.
- Serum E_2 levels are ordered infrequently unless the provider practices in a setting where there is a large infertility practice.
- The serum HCG is one of the most accurate and specific laboratory tests available. A pregnancy can be diagnosed at 9 to 10 days' gestation. An accurate HCG determination is essential to the management of ectopic pregnancies and gestational trophoblastic disease.
- Of all of the diagnostic imaging studies the abdominal ultrasound and pelvic ultrasound are the most useful both for obstetric and gynecologic patients.
- Although the current technology for assessing bone density, DEXA, is commonly available, it should not be used routinely as a screen in perimenopausal patients; it is too costly.
- Genetic amniocentesis is readily available. The clinician must decide whether the value of the test is sufficient to warrant the risk of doing the procedure. While the risk is low, it is important that the patient understand there is some risk involved, and the genetic amniocentesis should be performed under ultrasound guidance.

Questions

1. The following statements concerning the problem list are valid *except:*
   A. The problem list is constructed immediately after a thorough history is performed.
   B. The problem list represents a chronologic list of the patient's serious medical problems.
   C. The problem list should be headed by any drug allergies or sensitivities.
   D. The problem list is usually placed in an easily identifiable place in the patient's medical record.
   E. The entry information on the problem list includes the problem, its date of onset, and date of resolution.
2. The most sensitive test to determine the estrogen status in a woman is:
   A. Serum E_2 level
   B. Monitoring the changes in cervical mucus and examining for ferning
   C. Vaginal cytology
   D. Serum FSH level
   E. Use of an over-the-counter urinary LH detection kit
3. The following tests are strongly suggestive of ovulation having occurred *except:*
   A. Biphasic basal body temperature graph
   B. Serum progesterone greater than 10 ng/ml
   C. Secretory endometrium obtained on an endometrial biopsy
   D. Positive pregnancy test
   E. Cloudy, thick cervical mucus that does not fern

Answers

1. A
2. C
3. E

Obstetrics

5

Maternal-Fetal physiology

APGO LEARNING OBJECTIVE #5

Sharon T. Phelan

Understanding physiologic adaptations to pregnancy will allow the student to know more completely the principles of antepartum, intrapartum, and postpartum care, as well as the abnormalities that may occur at these times in pregnancy.

The student will demonstrate a knowledge of the following:

A. Maternal physiologic changes associated with pregnancy
B. Physiologic functions of the placenta and fetus
C. Effect of pregnancy on common diagnostic studies

Profound local and systemic changes in maternal physiology are initiated by conception and continue throughout pregnancy (Table 5-1). With delivery many of these changes are rapidly reversed, yet others take longer. It is important to realize that the effects of pregnancy are not fully reversed until at least 6 weeks after the baby is born.

GENERAL CHANGES

Abdominal walls

Tension and stretching of the anterior abdominal wall and the tissues over the outer aspects of the thighs frequently cause changes in the collagen and elastic fibers of the skin, producing reddish irregular lines called the *striae gravidarum*. After delivery the discoloration gradually fades, but the scarred lines do not disappear.

In the latter part of pregnancy, the rectus abdominis muscles are under considerable strain, and their tone is reduced. Wide separation of the muscles *(diastasis recti)* develops when the linea alba gives way to the stress and permits abdominal contents to protrude in the midline.

Table 5-1. Summary of physiologic changes associated with pregnancy

	Increased	Decreased
Skin	Pigmentation	
Breast	Glandular size	
	Colostrum	
	Areolar size	
CV	Plasma volume	Serum protein concentration
	Red blood cell mass	Blood pressure
	Vasodilatation	
	Cardiac output	
Respiratory	Vital capacity	Residual volume
	Tidal volume	Pulmonary resistance
	Respiratory rate	
Renal	Glomerular filtration	Peristalsis of ureter
	Renal plasma flow	Serum urea
		Serum creatinine
		Sensitivity to angiotensin II
GI	Constipation	Gastric motility
	Biliary stasis	Albumen production
	Cholesterol concentration	
Endocrine	TBG	TSH free T_3
	Total T_3 and T_4	T_4 unchanged
Metabolism	Insulin resistance	
	Free fatty acids	
	Demand for iron and folic acid	
Gynecologic organs	Uterine volume and blood flow	Connective tissue in vagina
	Ovarian enlargement	
Placental-fetal unit hormonally	Estriol	
	HCG	
	HPL	
	Progesterone	

CV, Cardiovascular; *GI,* gastrointestinal; *TBG,* thyroxine-binding globulin; *T_3,* triiodothyronine; *T_4,* thyroxine; *TSH,* thyroid-stimulating hormone; *HCG,* human chorionic gonadotropin; *HPL,* human placental lactogen.

Breasts

The breasts become enlarged and sensitive by the eighth week of pregnancy. The areola deepens in color, and the sebaceous glands located in the areola undergo hypertrophy, forming *Montgomery's tubercles.*

Estrogen stimulates proliferation of the ducts; progesterone causes proliferation of the lobular-alveolar tissue. As the breasts enlarge the vascular supply is increased, engorged veins are frequently visible beneath the surface of the skin, and striae may appear over the outer aspects.

Colostrum can be expressed from the nipples after about the tenth week, but lactation is inhibited by the high estrogen-progesterone levels. After delivery the drop in estrogen and progesterone allows the prolactin from the anterior pituitary to stimulate synthesis of milk. The release of oxytocin created by suckling promotes the ejection of the milk.

Skin

Pigmentation of the skin in areas other than the breasts is common. The *linea nigra,* a brown-black streak down the midline of the abdomen, is especially prominent in brunettes. Occasionally pigmentation occurs in a characteristic distribution over the face, forming the "mask of pregnancy," or *chloasma,* which may persist for months after delivery. The external genitals are similarly affected.

Palmar erythema and spider nevi or telangiectases sometimes appear over the face and upper trunk and are related to the increased concentration of estrogen.

There are significant changes in hair growth during pregnancy. A greater portion of the hair follicles are in the anagen (synthesis) phase relative to the telogen (resting) phase. This probably is due to the higher estrogen and androgen levels during pregnancy since this change can also be seen with some hormonal contraceptives. The patient perceives the change as thicker, fuller hair. Postpartum, with the marked drop in hormones, the ratio reverses—causing an increased number of hair follicles to enter telogen. These hairs then undergo normal shedding in approximately 2 to 3 months. This loss can be fairly pronounced (telogen effluvium) but is self-limiting and reversible. There may also be mild hirsutism during pregnancy, but severe changes necessitate further evaluation.

CIRCULATORY SYSTEM

Vast alterations in the vascular system occur as a result of (1) the increased metabolic demands of new tissue growth, (2) the expansion of vascular channels, and (3) the increase in steroid hormones, which exert a positive effect on sodium and water balance.

Blood

The total blood volume increases approximately 30% to 40% (Fig. 5-1). Although the red cell volume and the total hemoglobin increase during pregnancy, the expansion of plasma volume is approximately 3 times greater than that of the red cell mass. Studies indicate an average increase in red cell mass of 500 ml at term and calculate the concomitant whole blood rise at 1800 ml. If dietary iron supplements are withheld, the expected red cell increase is lessened by as much as 30% to 40%.

The disparity between the increase in fluid and cellular elements is reflected in the peripheral blood count as an apparent or dilution anemia, which becomes more pronounced in the third trimester. The average reduction is a 3% decrease in the hematocrit or 1 g/dl of hemoglobin. If the hematocrit is less than 32% or the hemoglobin less than 11 g/dl, true anemia should be considered.

The plasma volume begins to increase during the first trimester, reaches a peak approximately 40% above normal at 32 to 34 weeks' gestation, and remains elevated to term. During and immediately after the third stage of labor there is a sharp temporary rise in plasma volume, followed by a rapid drop toward the normal nonpregnancy range, although the original level is not actually reached until 3 or 4 weeks postpartum. On the contrary, in the presence of adequate iron, the red cell mass continues to rise until the end of pregnancy and does not decline to its original level until 8 weeks postpartum.

Most of the increase in plasma volume occurs between the sixth and the twenty-fourth weeks of gestation. These findings parallel the curve of increases in cardiac output. Thus maximal risk for the patient with heart disease is reached earlier in pregnancy than previously thought and persists throughout gestation.

The bone marrow is hyperplastic throughout pregnancy and remains so for about 2 months after delivery. The white cells and the erythrocytes

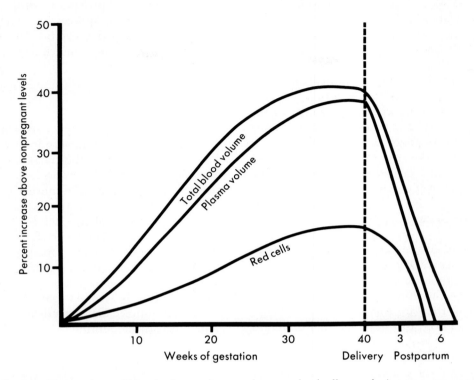

Fig. 5-1. Changes in total blood volume, plasma volume, and red cell mass during pregnancy and puerperium, based on compilation of reported data.

are increased. A leukocytosis in the range of 10,000 to 12,000 is normal in gravid women.

Serum protein concentrations are approximately 1 to 1.5 g/dl lower in pregnant than in nonpregnant women. It is not unusual to obtain values of 5.5 to 6 g/dl. The colloid osmotic pressure of the plasma is thereby reduced by about 20%.

Total serum lipid increases by 46% during the latter part of pregnancy. There is a marked increase in triglycerides, resulting primarily from a rise in the very-low-density lipoproteins. Total cholesterol and free fatty acids are also increased.

Fibrinogen concentration increases progressively to term from 300 mg/dl to 400-600 mg/dl.

Pregnancy is often thought to be a state of a relative suppression of the immune system, to avoid "rejection" of the foreign body (the fetus). It appears that activity of the leukocytes is depressed through the second and third trimester and may account for some of the apparent increase in infections, as well as the improvement of some autoimmune diseases. Humoral antibody titers may decrease during pregnancy, but this appears to be only a dilutional effect from the vasoexpansion that occurs in pregnancy.

Heart

Serial studies at various stages of pregnancy reveal an actual alteration in position and apparent increase in size of the cardiac silhouette. The heart is rotated slightly anteriorly and displaced upward and to the left. An electrocardiogram will show a 15-degree left axis deviation. The factors responsible for these alterations are controversial, although recognized changes in the chest wall doubtless play an important role. The rib cage is flared out so that its circumference is increased at the base. The diaphragm is pushed up as the uterus enlarges.

In addition to the altered appearance of the heart on the x-ray film, functional changes must be recognized. A soft systolic (ejection) murmur at the base or over the precordium is demonstrable in more than 50% of patients. Extrasystoles are common, and the pulse rate is slightly increased.

Blood pressure

Arterial blood pressure does not increase in normal pregnancy. The level may decrease during the second trimester and return to the normal range during the third trimester. The increased sensitivity of the baroreflex center in the aortic arch causes a decreased heart rate and promotes the peripheral vasodilatation (initiated by progesterone) despite the decreased blood pressure. In other words, the system resets so that a lower blood pressure is seen as normal. Venous pressure measured in the antecubital region remains constant and normal. Femoral venous pressure rises 10 to 15 cm water above normal in the upright or supine position as a result of increasing pressure by the enlarging uterus on the pelvic veins, a factor that contributes to the development of ankle edema and varicose veins. Femoral pressure is normal in the lateral recumbent position. There is an increased venous capacity that is due to the vasodilatation effects of progesterone and the shunting mechanism of the placental circulation.

Late in pregnancy, patients often complain of feeling faint in the supine position, when venous pressure may rise to at least 20 cm of water. The syncope is attributed to the vena cava syndrome. When the heavy uterus falls back on the inferior vena cava, venous return to the heart is sufficiently impeded to cause a precipitous drop in blood pressure. The patient appears pale, tachycardic, diaphoretic, and apprehensive, but if she can turn on her side, the symptoms disappear almost immediately.

Cardiac output

Increased tissue demands for oxygen may be met by an increase in cardiac output of oxygenated blood and/or an increased extraction of oxygen from the blood at the capillary level. Measurements of cardiac output during normal pregnancy indicate a rise, primarily in stroke volume, with a maximal increase of about 30% to 35% at the twenty-eighth week. The heart rate follows the same general course, but with a much lower increment of rise. Cardiac output is increased slightly during the first stage of labor and appreciably increased during the second stage with the bearing down efforts. Immediately after delivery there is a sudden increase amounting to about 29% as the uterus contracts and forces a large volume of blood into the circulation. During these periods the patient with a diseased heart experiences further increased cardiac strain.

RESPIRATORY SYSTEM

Anatomic changes become evident as the intraabdominal pressure increases from the advancing gestation. The lower half of the thoracic cage is pushed upward and widened, and the diaphragm is accordingly elevated. However, the diaphragmatic excursion is the same or even increased. The vital capacity remains unchanged or undergoes a slight increase, although the residual volume is decreased because of the elevated diaphragm. A decrease in vital capacity should always be considered significant.

The respiratory rate is slightly increased, and tidal volume rises by up to 50%. This is due to decreased residual volume and decreased pulmonary resistance. These changes may increase the margin of safety for the fetus. Hyperventilation (probably mediated centrally by progesterone) lowers the carbon dioxide content of alveolar air, and, in turn, reduced carbon dioxide tension favors diffusion of carbon dioxide from fetal to maternal circulation. Thus all changes in the respiratory system during pregnancy are well compensated, and pulmonary function is not impaired in normal patients.

URINARY SYSTEM

Pregnancy exerts a profound influence on the entire urinary tract. The major effect is a dilatation of the ureter and renal pelvis, resulting in hydronephrosis. The capacity of a dilated kidney, pelvis, and ureter increases from an original of 10-15 ml to 60 ml. These changes appear early and are progressive until the last month or two of a pregnancy. The ureter is elongated, widened, curved, and tortuous. The dilatation is frequently more prominent on the right side, probably because of the cushioning effect of the rectosigmoid and the dextrorotation of the uterus. The flow of urine is reduced because ureteral peristalsis and tone are diminished, primarily caused by progesterone effect on the smooth muscles.

Renal function changes in a predictable fashion. Effective renal plasma flow increases approximately 25% for the first two trimesters. The glomerular filtration increases by about 50%, and the filtration fraction is increased to 40% by the third trimester. The alterations in renal function are most probably a result of increased maternal and chorionic hormonal secretions. These changes have important clinical implications. Glycosuria is common because of the increase in glomerular filtration. Amino acids are excreted in larger amounts during pregnancy. Serum concentrations of urea, uric acid, and creatinine are lowered as a result of increased clearance rates. Allowances must be made for

changes in the urinary system in the interpretation of renal function tests. In the normal gravid patient, clearance rates range between 130 and 160 ml/min.

The activity of renin, produced largely by the kidney, is increased during normal pregnancy. Renin acts on angiotensinogen to form angiotensin. Vascular reactivity to angiotensin II is reduced during pregnancy, so that elevation of blood pressure does not normally occur with the increased levels of this substance. In pregnancies complicated by preeclampsia, this relative resistance to angiotensin is lost. Angiotensin II is a major stimulus for adrenocortical secretion of aldosterone, which promotes salt and water retention during pregnancy.

GASTROINTESTINAL TRACT

Gastric motility is somewhat diminished through pregnancy, particularly during labor. For this reason anesthesiologists will treat all laboring patients as if they have a full stomach. The nausea and vomiting of early pregnancy may well be influenced by these functional alterations. Reduced peristaltic activity and diminished tone are evident in bowel function as well. These effects primarily are due to progesterone effect. Constipation usually results, although the condition is undoubtedly aggravated by vitamins containing iron and by pressure of the uterus on the rectosigmoid. This constipation contributes to the development of hemorrhoids antenatally. These can be exacerbated by the elevated pressure in the veins below the level of the enlarged uterus.

During the last half of pregnancy, the stomach is gradually pushed upward into the left dome of the diaphragm. Hormonal effects may cause relaxation or dilatation of the hiatus and predispose to the development of hiatal hernia. The patient will experience "heartburn" due to the reflux of acidic secretions into the lower esophagus. The cecum also undergoes a progressive upward displacement, beginning during the third month and continuing until term, when the appendix is located out toward the right flank above the level of the iliac crest. This is important to remember when evaluating a pregnant woman for possible appendicitis.

Gallbladder emptying time is increased during pregnancy. Serum cholinesterase activity is reduced by about 25%. Relative biliary stasis and increased cholesterol levels may contribute to the formation of biliary calculi in gravid women.

There is increased hepatic production of various hormone-binding globulins and decreased albumen production. This has a major impact on dosages of certain medications and on the interpretation of many hormone assays.

During pregnancy the gums may become swollen and bleed easily when traumatized (i.e., brushing). This does not always mean periodontal disease, but a patient should be encouraged to perform good dental hygiene, including flossing and regularly visiting the dentist.

ENDOCRINE SYSTEM

Thyroid

The thyroid undergoes a diffuse hyperplasia of glandular elements, new follicle formation, and increased vascularity. Thyroid function is greatly affected by the elevated estrogen levels of pregnancy. Estrogens increase the response of pituitary thyroid-stimulating hormone (TSH) to thyrotropin-releasing hormone and also cause significant increases in thyroxine-binding globulin (TBG). Thus the total thyroxine (T_4) and triiodothyronine (T_3) are increased, but the TBG is also increased. The free T_4 and free T_3 are unchanged. Thus the most useful means of evaluating thyroid function during pregnancy is by direct assay for T_4 and TSH.

Pituitary gland

The anterior lobe of the pituitary gland increases 20% to 40% in size during pregnancy. This increase is largely in cells containing prolactin. Prolactin levels rise steadily from 10 ng/ml at onset of pregnancy to 200 ng/ml at term. Despite the high levels of prolactin, lactation does not occur before delivery probably because the high levels of placental steroids inhibit the secretory activity of the breast by blocking the peripheral action of prolactin on the breast.

Adrenal gland

During pregnancy there is little anatomic change of the adrenal gland. There are notable changes in hormone levels that are not well understood. Cortisol levels increase apparently because of decreased clearance. Aldosterone levels are also increased. This may be to provide protection from the natriuretic effect of high levels of progesterone.

METABOLISM

There is an increase (20% by term) of the basal metabolic rate, which probably represents fetal and placental metabolic activity. The increase, along with progesterone activity, causes pregnant women to have elevated basal body temperatures.

Proteins

A positive nitrogen balance increases progressively through the pregnancy as the fetal requirements increase. This nitrogen accumulation exceeds the demands of the fetus to be prepared for the postpartum demands of blood loss, lactation, and involutional changes in the uterus and other tissues. To meet these needs the maternal protein intake should be at least 65 g/day throughout the pregnancy. Amino acids are freely transported to the fetus. The decreased albumen fraction will cause decreased colloid osmotic pressure, contributing to edema.

Carbohydrates

A maternal glucose sparing effect noted in the pregnancy is related to the demands of the fetus. The fetus uses glucose almost exclusively as its metabolic energy source. Glucose crosses the placenta by facilitated diffusion. Although secretion of insulin during pregnancy is increased, resistance to insulin by elevated free fatty acids (FFAs) and destruction of insulin by the placenta are also increased. Chorionic human placental lactogen (HPL) is greatly elevated and is probably responsible for the elevated FFAs by promoting lipolysis. This gives the woman an alternative fuel source. The FFAs also contribute to the increased insulin resistance.

Fats

Fat metabolism is altered during pregnancy in concert with the changes in carbohydrate metabolism. These alterations include an increase in maternal use of fat stores and a related increase in insulin resistance. The HPL plays an important role in mobilization of FFAs. The elevated level of FFAs exerts an antiinsulin effect by interfering with peripheral use of glucose. Oxidation of fats provides an alternate maternal source of energy, and glucose sparing ensures that the critical needs of the fetus for this energy source are met.

Minerals and vitamins

Demands for inorganic substances necessary for growth rise sharply at the second trimester. Requirements for calcium and phosphorus are double during pregnancy. These demands are met by an intake of 1.5 g of calcium per day. The total serum calcium levels fall in the last half of pregnancy as a result of the decrease in serum albumen

that binds the calcium. However, the free ionized calcium level remains within the normal range.

The demand for iron is increased, especially in the last trimester because fetal absorption is the greatest then. Many women in an apparently good nutritional state have less than the normal amount of iron in available storage. Therefore most women require iron supplementation during pregnancy of 30 to 60 mg/day of elemental iron.

Folic acid demand increases during pregnancy because of rapid tissue growth of trophoblastic, maternal, and fetal origins. The daily requirement of folic acid during pregnancy is about 300 to 500 μg. Green vegetables, some fruits, liver, and kidney are the principal sources. Since preconceptional supplementation of folic acid appears to decrease the occurrence (recurrence) of neural tube defects, many women planning a pregnancy are encouraged to start prenatal vitamins with folic acid before conception.

MUSCULOSKELETAL SYSTEM

The primary musculoskeletal change is a progressive lordosis to compensate for the enlarging uterus. This change—along with the hormonally induced increased mobility of the sacroiliac, sacrococcygeal, and pubic joints—can cause a fair amount of lower back and pelvic discomfort in the latter stages of a pregnancy. This relaxation of the pelvic girdle joints may increase the obstetric diameters for delivery.

GYNECOLOGIC ORGANS

The uterine weight undergoes a twentyfold increase (from 50 to 1000 g), and the capacity increases 1000-fold (from 4 to 4000 ml). This growth is almost entirely by hypertrophy of the muscle cells (Fig. 5-2). In addition, an increase in the amount of elastic connective tissue adds consid-

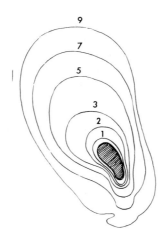

Fig. 5-2. Growth of uterus during successive months of pregnancy.

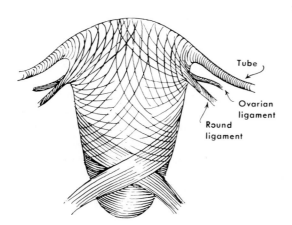

Fig. 5-3. Diagram showing interwoven pattern of uterine muscle fibers.

erably to the strength of the uterine wall, and an increase in the size and number of blood vessels meets the demands for oxygen and nutrients. The blood flow to the uterus changes from 50 ml/min to 500 ml/min at term.

The initial stimulus to uterine enlargement is hormonal. Thus at 6 weeks' gestation the enlarge-

ment occurs, even if the pregnancy is extrauterine. Afterward, the enlargement depends on the size of the conceptus and the actual growth of the muscle fibers. The uterus differentiates into an upper and lower segment. The contractile fibers are concentrated in concentric circles in the upper segment (Fig. 5-3).

Changes in the cervix are apparent by the sixth week. Softening and congestion are a result of increased vascularity. The glands hypertrophy; mucus secretion is greatly increased, and the consistency is altered by steroid hormonal activity. This results in the formation of the thick mucus plug, which acts as a barrier protecting the conceptus against mechanical or bacterial invasion throughout pregnancy.

Because of the increased vascularity, both ovaries become somewhat enlarged and elongated. The enlargement is more pronounced in the ovary containing the corpus luteum during the third month. Ovulation is suspended during pregnancy because of pituitary inhibition.

The vagina becomes deeply congested and cyanotic (Chadwick's sign) because of the greatly increased vascularity. In preparation for the great distention that the vagina must undergo during delivery, the mucosa thickens, the connective tissue becomes less dense, and the muscular coat hypertrophies to such an extent that the vault is lengthened.

PLACENTAL-FETAL UNIT

Many of the changes already described, as well as the maintenance of the pregnancy, are dependent on hormones secreted by the placenta or fetus. The first hormone necessary is human chorionic gonadotropin (HCG). This is a glycoprotein that is necessary to prevent involution of the corpus luteum before the placental-fetal unit achieves adequate progesterone and estrogen production on its own. Also, the peak HCG levels occur around the time of fetal testicular differentiation. The HCG acts as luteinizing hormone, thus stimulating the fetal Leydig's cells to produce testosterone and the fetus to undergo male phenotypic differentiation.

The fetus and the placenta must be present for the production of the large quantities of estrogen normally found in a pregnant woman. The placenta aromatizes the androgens produced by the fetus—dehydroepiandrosterone, androstenedione, and testosterone—to estrogens. This process takes place in the placental microsomes. The synthesis of estrogen is known to be stimulated by HCG and HPL; thus the placenta may regulate its own estrogen synthesis. The estrogen seems to stimulate growth of the uterus and the breasts. The secreted estrogens in the urine are estriol (80%), estrone (15%), and estradiol (5%). The production of estriol requires one step (16 α-hydroxylation) to convert the fetal dehydroepiandrosterone sulfate (originating in the fetal adrenal gland) to precursors that the placenta can then convert to estriol. Thus the fetus is the source of 90% of the precursor for estriol production in pregnancy.

Progesterone is also synthesized in large amounts by the placenta, using maternal blood cholesterol as the principal substrate with the fetus contributing very little. Progesterone has all the effects previously alluded to in the maternal system.

There are more than 16 other hormones produced by the placenta to facilitate fine tuning the maternal adaptations necessary for pregnancy.

FETAL PHYSIOLOGY

Placenta

The human placenta is not only an endocrine organ, but it serves both as the source of nutrients and as a vehicle to eliminate wastes. The chorionic villi, which contain fetal capillaries, are effectively suspended in the intervillous space that is filled with circulating maternal blood. Up to 700 ml/min of maternal blood goes to the placental bed at term.

Throughout the pregnancy the syncytiotrophoblast of the placenta participates in the transfer of substance to and from the fetus. The rate and direction of transfer will vary if the substance has a large molecular weight, is bound to carrier protein, is ionized, has an active or passive transport system, or has a high concentration and rate of blood flow. If less than 500 d, molecules will diffuse easily (e.g., water, carbon dioxide, oxygen, and most electrolytes). This still results in a partial pressure of oxygen (pO_2) that is relatively low but well tolerated by the fetus because of higher cardiac output and fetal hemoglobin that has an increased oxygen carrying ability.

There is active transport across the placenta of many sugars, iron, amino acids, immunoglobulin G, iodine, calcium, and vitamins A, D, and C. Glucose, the main energy source for the fetus, is transported with facilitated diffusion.

Fetal circulation

Just like the adult lung has low pO_2 in the arterial side and high pO_2 in the venous side, so too does the umbilical cord, with the placenta serving as "lungs" (or, better yet, "gills"). The fetal circulation allows the oxygenated blood to go through the liver and to the right atrium (Fig. 5-4). There it passes through the foramen ovale into the left atrium, thus bypassing the uninflated lungs. The oxygenated blood then goes through the left ventricle and out the aorta. The venous return to the right side of the heart mainly bypasses the lungs by going through the patent ductus arteriosus. It should be noted that this poorly oxygenated blood mixes with the oxygen-rich blood after the branching of the brachial arteries, thereby protecting the developing brain's oxygen supply.

With birth the expansion of the lungs lowers the vascular bed resistance, thus shunting more blood through the lungs. This decreases right-side pressures in the heart while increasing left-side pressures, thus closing the foramen ovale. The ductus arteriosus closes in response to higher pO_2 levels. These steps occur over a short time as the

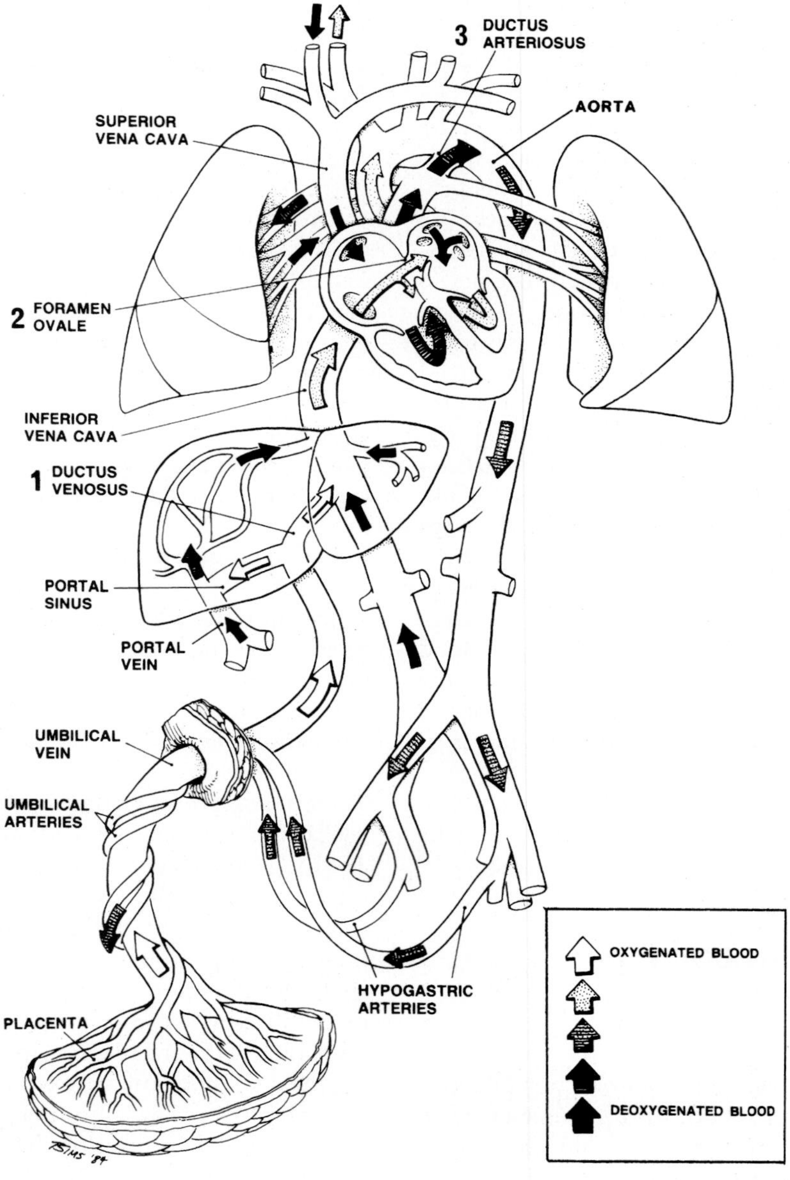

Fig. 5-4. Fetal circulation with notations regarding oxygenation of blood. *(From Cunningham FG et al: Williams Obstetrics, ed 20, Norwalk, Conn, 1997, Appleton & Lange.)*

fetus goes from a water environment to the air, achieving the normal circulatory pattern.

Gastrointestinal system

The fetus swallows throughout much of the pregnancy. This is a crucial control in maintaining a normal volume of amniotic fluid in the latter part of the pregnancy. The debris from the amniotic fluid that is swallowed, along with the excretions of the gastrointestinal tract, make up the meconium that comprises the first bowel movements.

The fetal liver has difficulty converting free bilirubin to a conjugated form. This can pose a problem if the infant is born preterm (a more immature liver) or has an event that causes hemolysis (i.e., Rh incompatibility). The levels of free bilirubin increase and the infant may get kernicterus, which can cause brain damage.

Renal system

The kidneys and urinary system are not only functional but are crucial in controlling the volume and composition of amniotic fluid in the pregnancy because much of the fluid is composed of urine later in the pregnancy. A blockage in the urethra or absent kidneys will cause decreased amniotic fluid (oligohydramnios).

Respiratory system

The lungs tend to be the last organ system to develop. The gasping efforts of the fetus throughout pregnancy encourage the branching and maturation of the alveolar morphology. The production of surfactant is the final step in lung maturation. This can be evaluated in the amniotic fluid in a number of ways: L/S ratios, PG, FLM. (See Chapter 19, Preterm Labor.)

Reproductive systems

Gonadal differentiation to testes occurs by 6 to 7 weeks' gestation, with the influence of testes determining factor (TDF) from the Y chromosome. The gonad is stimulated by the high levels of HCG to produce testosterone, create the male phenotype, and develop the wolffian ductal sys-

CRITICAL POINTS

- The typical cardiovascular changes are designed to respond to the increased blood volume necessitated by the large placental shunt. The changes include increases in plasma volume, red cell mass (to carry oxygen), cardiac output, and increased venous capacity. In addition, there is a decrease in the blood pressure.
- Despite increased abdominal pressure the vital capacity remains unchanged during pregnancy, and tidal volume and respiratory rate increase.
- Owing to progesterone effects and the marked increase of blood volume, there is dilatation of the entire renal collection system and marked increase in the glomerular filtration rate.
- The metabolic rate increases with the marked increase in the need for protein. Also, pregnancy is a diabetogenic state, with increased FFA production for a maternal energy source; thus the glucose is reserved for fetal needs.
- The uterus undergoes massive enlargement while maintaining the ability to actively contract and force expulsion of the fetus in labor. The cervix and vagina undergo changes to protect the fetus from outside effects, as well as to be able to stretch during the delivery.

tem into epididymis and vas deferens. The testes also produce müllerian inhibitor factor, which causes müllerian regression. In the absence of TDF the müllerian system will develop, forming the uterus, tubes, and vagina. In cases of gonadal dysgenesis the infant will be phenotypically female regardless of chromosomal sex. Abnormalities in genitalia at birth can be the result of a gonadal or hormonal (e.g., androgens from the adrenal) problem.

CONCLUSION

The normal physiologic changes in a woman during pregnancy may cause some concern to a couple. More important, these changes may cause the presentation of other diseases to be more frequent or varied in symptoms. Failure for certain changes to occur may predict development of certain complications of pregnancy. Finally, therapies for illnesses may be varied due to changes in the woman's physiology.

Questions

1. Which of the following statements is the most accurate regarding the normal changes in the cardiovascular system at term?
   A. The total volume increases by 20%, with the red blood cell mass increase exceeding the plasma volume increase.
   B. The total volume increases by 20%, with the plasma volume increase exceeding the red blood cell mass increase.
   C. The total volume increases by 40%, with the red blood cell mass increase exceeding the plasma volume increase.
   D. The total volume increases by 40%, with the plasma volume increase exceeding the red blood cell mass increase.
   E. The total blood volume does not appreciably change.

2. Which of the following is *not* a true statement regarding carbohydrate fat metabolism in a pregnant woman?
   A. The secretion of insulin is decreased in pregnancy.
   B. There is increased destruction of insulin by the placenta.
   C. Chorionic HPL promotes the elevation of FFAs.
   D. The FFAs contribute to the increased insulin resistance.
   E. The fetus primarily uses glucose as its metabolic fuel.

3. The respiratory system response to pregnancy includes all of the following *except:*
   A. The diaphragm is elevated but has at least the same excursion.
   B. The vital capacity is decreased.
   C. The thoracic cage is pushed up and widened.
   D. The residual volume decreases.
   E. There is a respiratory alkalosis.

4. Changes in the urinary system include all of the following *except:*
   A. There is a marked increase in the glomerular filtration rate.
   B. Glycosuria is common because the tubular reabsorption capacity is exceeded.
   C. Serum concentrations of uric acid and creatinine are higher as a result of the presence of the fetus.
   D. Vascular reactivity to angiotensin II is reduced in pregnancy.
   E. There is dilatation of the ureters and renal pelvis.

Answers

1. D
2. A
3. B
4. C

6

Preconception and antepartum care

APGO LEARNING OBJECTIVE #6

Sharon T. Phelan

> *The proven benefits of good health before conception include a significant reduction in maternal and fetal morbidity and mortality. Antepartum care promotes patient education and facilitates ongoing risk assessment and the development of an individualized patient management plan.*

The student will demonstrate a knowledge of the following:

A. Conditions that warrant preconception counseling, including such medical conditions as diabetes, chronic hypertensive vascular disease and heart disease, recurrent pregnancy loss, history of genetic abnormalities, maternal age over 35, substance abuse, and nutrition

B. Methods to diagnose pregnancy; assess gestational age; identify an at-risk pregnancy; and assess fetal growth, well-being, and maturity

C. Appropriate diagnostic studies and patient education programs

D. Nutritional needs of pregnant women and adverse effects of drugs and environmental factors

PRECONCEPTIONAL CARE AND COUNSELING

To optimize each pregnancy, greater emphasis is placed on reducing risks before conception. A number of different aspects of a woman's health may be noted (Table 6-1). An obvious consideration is to optimize the status of other health concerns. The more out of control a diabetic patient is at conception, the greater her risk for fetal anomalies. The hypertensive patient may benefit from medication changes to products less likely to affect the fetus. The patient with heart disease may need surgical intervention before conceiving or even strong counseling about risks of morbidity and mortality in pregnancy (such as a patient with pulmonary hypertension).

A patient who has experienced recurrent pregnancy losses may have an anatomic problem (incompetent cervix or müllerian anomaly) that would respond to evaluation and/or surgery before conception. There may be a hormonal disorder that would benefit from supplementation. Also, one or both parents might carry a genetic flaw that could necessitate early amniocentesis or even a gamete donor. This type of genetic work-up may be indicated for a couple with a previously affected pregnancy or child. The risk of certain genetic complications are age-related, and women 35 years old or older may prefer counseling regarding their risk before conception.

Some prescription drugs carry a risk of fetal anomalies; use of other substances such as alcohol, cocaine, opiates, cigarettes, and so on may involve a greater risk for poor outcome. Folic acid supplementation before conception appears to decrease the risk of neural tube defect.

For these reasons every woman who is contemplating a pregnancy needs a detailed personal and family medical history, a complete physical examination, and appropriate laboratory tests.

PREGNANCY DIAGNOSIS

Because of the ready availability of very accurate and inexpensive urine pregnancy tests, subjective and objective findings are used more often to prompt the ordering of a pregnancy test than to diagnose pregnancy.

Subjective signs

Subjective symptoms are inconsistent and have low sensitivity and specificity for pregnancy diagnosis. The most common one is amenorrhea. However, amenorrhea has many causes other than pregnancy, and not uncommonly a pregnant woman will have vaginal bleeding ("a period") while pregnant.

"Morning sickness" is the nausea and some vomiting commonly (up to 50% of pregnancies) experienced in the first trimester. This usually appears at the fifth or sixth week of pregnancy and continues until the twelfth to fourteenth. Its severity varies from mild nausea easily relieved by ingesting food to persistent vomiting that depletes fluid and electrolytes. Morning sickness may occur primarily at a certain time of day or throughout the day. Although this is bothersome for the woman, as long as it does not cause dehydration it is not dangerous for the patient or the fetus. In fact, nausea may be a marker for elevated human chorionic gonadotropin (HCG) levels, which in turn may suggest a better gestation or in some cases twinning.

The woman may complain of urinary frequency, probably caused by pressure on the bladder from the enlarging uterus. Also, enlargement, tingling, or actual discomfort in the breast commonly results from hormonal stimulation of alveolar and ductal structures.

Quickening is a term that indicates the perception of fetal movement by the mother. Multiparas first feel movement about the sixteenth week,

---

Table 6-1. Preconceptional counseling: issues to be addressed

Optimize medical status: control diabetes, cardiac function, asthma.

Review prior pregnancies: reason for recurrent losses, second trimester deliveries, anomalous fetus.

Review prescribed medications and use of alcohol, tobacco, and other substances that affect the fetus.

Discuss termination of current contraception.

Evaluate nutritional status-habits: plan treatment for obesity and eating disorders; prescribe folate and, if needed, iron supplements.

whereas primigravidas experience this around the twentieth week. The timing of quickening can be affected by maternal weight, placental location, amount of amniotic fluid, activity of the infant, and the psychologic state of the mother. It is not rare for a patient to deliver a term infant while denying that she ever knew she was pregnant. At the other extreme, some women with pseudocyesis will claim to have quickening.

Objective signs

Objective signs require an examiner who is familiar with maternal physiology. The vaginal wall becomes cyanotic and congested (Chadwick's sign). The isthmus of the uterus is soft at 6 to 8 weeks (Hegar's sign) (Fig. 6-1). However, after a few weeks the entire cervix and corpus become much softer, and this difference can no longer be

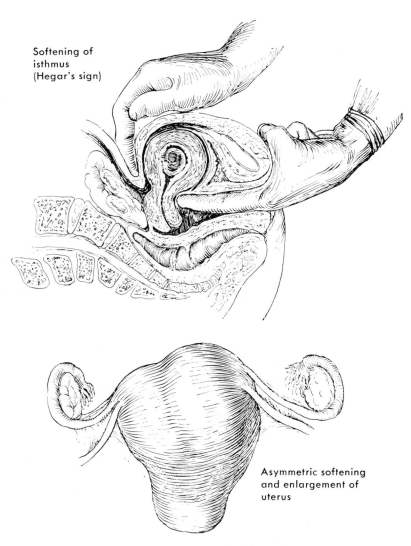

Softening of isthmus (Hegar's sign)

Asymmetric softening and enlargement of uterus

Fig. 6-1. Uterine changes in early pregnancy.

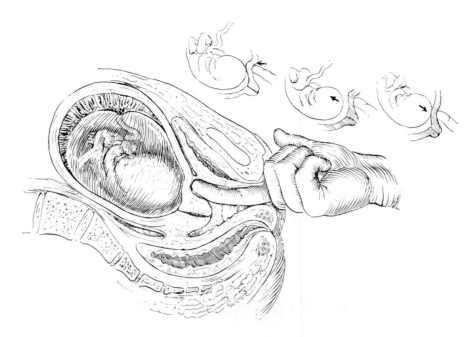

Fig. 6-2. Ballottement of fetus.

detected. There is also a progressive increase in uterine size.

Changes in the uterus and cervix can occur without an actual pregnancy. The detection of a fetus is the definite indication of pregnancy. This can be done by ballottement of the fetus on bimanual exam (Fig. 6-2); the examiner feels fetal movement and detects fetal heart tones. Again, maternal obesity, very early gestation, excessive amniotic fluid, anterior placenta, or abdominal pain will interfere with detection of these signs. Doppler apparatus now makes it possible to detect fetal heart tones and frequently to confirm fetal heart rate as early as 10 weeks' menstrual age. Fetal heart rate is easily differentiated from maternal because typically it is twice as fast (normal range 120 to 160 beats/min).

Pregnancy can be confirmed much earlier by sonography than by physical examination. A gestational sac usually can be identified at 5 to 6 weeks' menstrual age. A fetal pole can be identified approximately 1 to 2 weeks later, and fetal cardiac activity usually can be verified. Embryonic structures can be detected earlier with an endovaginal ultrasound probe than with an abdominal transducer.

Pregnancy tests

Pregnancy tests are based on the identification of the beta chain of HCG. Because HCG can be produced by certain teratomas of the ovary and testes, choriocarcinoma, and hydatiform mole, as well as by a normal placenta, a positive HCG test does not necessarily indicate a normal intrauterine pregnancy. Current urine tests are sensitive to approximately 50 mIU/ml, which is the level present at the time of the first missed menses. Serum HCG tests are more sensitive and allow quantification of concentrations. However, in most situations the increased costs and time to do the test are not indicated clinically.

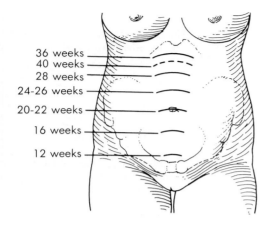

36 weeks
40 weeks
28 weeks
24-26 weeks
20-22 weeks
16 weeks
12 weeks

Fig. 6-3. Height of uterus above pubis at various weeks of pregnancy.

ASSESSMENT OF GESTATIONAL AGE

The first question asked after the diagnosis of pregnancy is, "When is the due date?" The classic determination of expected date of confinement (EDC) is based on a 280-day gestation from the first day of the last normal menstrual period (LMP), assuming 28-day cycles. This is 40 weeks.

The accuracy of this estimate can be further supported by a comparison of the clinical examination early in pregnancy to the EDC determined by LMP. The fundus is felt above the upper border of the pubis at 12 weeks. By 16 weeks it is halfway to the umbilicus. At 20 weeks the fundus is level with the umbilicus. From 20 to approximately 34 to 36 weeks the fundal height in centimeters from the pubic symphysis is the same as the weeks' gestation (Fig. 6-3). However, the later in a pregnancy one makes the initial determination of EDC, the more inaccurate it will be.

Although the physical exam will give an indication of dating, it is reassuring to confirm your estimate by another objective piece of data. Pelvic ultrasounds are commonly used to clarify dating questions. During the first trimester, fetal age can be estimated with reasonable accuracy (± 1 week) by measuring the crown-to-rump length of the fetus. Starting in the second trimester, measurements of the biparietal diameter of the fetal skull and femur length are used to determine estimated gestational age. The further along the pregnancy, the more inaccurate the dating (approximately ± 2 weeks in the second trimester and ± 3 weeks in the third trimester). For this reason if a sonar study is to be used for determining gestation dating, the earlier it is obtained the better. Subsequent ultrasound reports should *not* be used to readjust the initial dating.

DISTINGUISHING AN AT-RISK PREGNANCY

The recognition of high-risk patients or pregnancies at the initial prenatal care visit may allow tailoring of prenatal care to prevent or minimize adverse effects on the pregnancy. For this reason the first prenatal care visit should occur in the first trimester, with a complete baseline medical, social, and family history that emphasizes the conditions noted in Table 6-2. In addition, baseline blood pressure, weight, fundal size, gestation age and EDC, and baseline laboratory tests should be obtained. If problems are identified, additional testing, a modified schedule of prenatal visits, or referral to a specialist in high-risk pregnancies may be indicated.

One should record the date of onset and the duration of at least the last normal menstrual period. One also should record which contraceptive method the patient was using before conception because ovulation often is delayed for some time after oral contraceptive pills are discontinued.

Since history tends to repeat itself, a very important risk factor is the occurrence of obstetric complications in a previous pregnancy. Information concerning earlier pregnancies should include their duration at delivery; the length of labor; the type of delivery; and the size, condition, and subsequent development of the infant. For those who have delivered by cesarean section, it is

Table 6-2. Distinguishing an at-risk pregnancy

I. Sociodemographic risks

    A. Age and parity
1. Maternal age of <16 yr
2. Maternal age of ≥35 yr
3. Birth order 1 or ≥5

    B. Lowest social classes

    C. Mother will be a single parent

II. Medical-obstetric risks

    A. Previous multiple spontaneous abortions, ectopic pregnancy, fetal death, neonatal death, or congenital anomaly

    B. Previous low birth–weight infant (<2500 g)

    C. Less than 1 yr since termination of last pregnancy

    D. Difficulty in conceiving

    E. Chronic cardiovascular, renal, endocrine, or collagen diseases

    F. Diabetes mellitus

    G. Malnutrition and/or anemia

    H. Chronic or recurrent urinary tract infections

    I. Seizure disorder, especially if on medications

    J. Congenital malformation of reproductive organs

    K. Sexually transmitted diseases, including syphilis, gonorrhea, chlamydia, papilloma virus, and human immunodeficiency virus

    L. Tuberculosis

    M. Chronic active hepatitis

    N. Substance abuse, including alcohol, cigarettes, cocaine, or other drugs

    O. Uterine or ovarian neoplasms

Table 6-3. Possible strategies for monitoring fetal well-being in at-risk pregnancies

6 + weeks	Fetal cardiac activity by ultrasound
14-20 weeks	MSAFP and/or genetic amniocentesis
16 + weeks	Baseline ultrasound for dating and major anomalies
22-36 weeks	Fundal height compared with dates
34 + weeks	Fetal movement counts NST and/or CST Serial ultrasound for growth (every 3-4 wk) and/or amniotic fluid (every wk) Biophysical profile

MSAFP, Maternal serum α-fetoprotein; *NST*, nonstress test; *CST*, contraction stress test.

A general medical and gynecologic exam is done to evaluate any medical problems, as well as to date the pregnancy. Both basic laboratory tests and any other indicated tests should be obtained.

ASSESSMENT OF FETAL GROWTH, WELL-BEING, AND MATURITY

After the initial prenatal assessment, the remainder of the routine prenatal care approach is designed to identify problems in fetal well-being or developing complications for the mother. Serial assessments must be made of the mother and, indirectly, the fetus. These should be recorded in a fashion that allows ready comparison of findings over successive visits (Table 6-3). For this reason most providers of obstetric care use a flow sheet format for recording the information. The American College of Obstetricians and Gynecologists (ACOG) has developed one such prototype.

important to obtain a copy of the operative note to identify the reason and the type of uterine incision. Such previous pregnancy failures as abortion, ectopic pregnancy, and fetal and neonatal deaths should be recorded.

In an anticipated uncomplicated pregnancy, the frequency of visits is determined by the gestational age. Traditionally visits are every 4 weeks until 28 weeks; then, every 2 weeks until 36 weeks; followed by weekly visits for the remainder of the pregnancy.

Fundal height relative to gestational dating should be compared at each visit. A 2-cm to 3-cm discrepancy may represent normal variations in fetal lie, amount of amniotic fluid, maternal habitus, and measurement technique. Consistent serial growth is reassuring of normal progression. Arrest of fundal growth or a precipitate increase should prompt further evaluations (Fig. 6-3).

Fetal heart rate should be in the 120 to 160 range. Marked irregularity, sustained tachycardia, or spontaneous deceleration of heart rate below 100 may indicate a problem and necessitates further testing.

Fetal motion as reported by the mother and perceived by the examiner can be an indicator of fetal well-being. Many infants who experience chronic compromise will have decreased fetal movement that is reported by the mother before heart rate changes are noted.

Symptoms of increased vaginal discharge, pelvic pressure, cramping, or vaginal bleeding might precede the onset of preterm labor. The sensitivity and specificity of these questions can be poor, but it is still probably worthwhile to inquire about such problems.

Fetal lie during the third trimester should be determined. A patient who demonstrates persistent breech presentation may be a candidate for external version before labor.

Maternal weight gain is an indicator of nutritional status, as well as fluid retention. The weight gain during the first trimester is 1 to 3 lb. During the last two trimesters the gain is usually steady at a rate of less than 1 lb/wk. An increase of about 9 kg (20 lb) can be accounted for by the products of conception and physiologic changes in the mother (Table 6-4). The expected rate of weight gain varies according to the initial body mass index of the patient when she starts the pregnancy.

Table 6-4. Sources of maternal weight gain in pregnancy

Source	Grams	Pounds
Fetus	3600	7.5
Placenta	720	1.5
Amniotic fluid	960	2
Uterus	960	2
Breasts	480	1
Plasma volume	1440	3
Extracellular fluid	1440	3

Excessive gain or lack of weight gain may suggest nutrition problems that are due to finances, lack of knowledge of proper diet, or cultural factors. An abrupt weight gain in the third trimester commonly represents fluid retention, which may be one of the first signs of developing pregnancy-induced hypertension.

Maternal blood pressure is followed throughout the pregnancy to determine both the baseline (first trimester) blood pressure and the physiologic response to pregnancy (normally a decrease in blood pressure during the second trimester). Preeclampsia is still a major cause of maternal and fetal morbidity and mortality. The earlier it is diagnosed, the more effective will be the intervention to prevent or minimize complications.

Presence of edema is noted. Although pedal edema is common in pregnancy, facial or hand edema may represent developing hypertension.

Cervical examination for dilatation, effacement, and station is not usually done unless such information will change management.

APPROPRIATE DIAGNOSTIC STUDIES DURING PREGNANCY

Many laboratory and imaging studies are currently available. However, the cost-effectiveness of performing all available tests on each pregnancy is

Table 6-5. Laboratory evaluations during prenatal care

	Basic	Optional (depending on patient risks or community prevalence)
Initial visit	Hematocrit-hemoglobin	Chlamydia culture
	Syphilis screen	Sickle cell screen
	Offer HIV screen	Gonorrhea
	Hepatitis B screen	TB
	Pap (if not done in past 6 mo)	
	Urine analysis and infectious screen	
	Blood type and Rh	
	Antibody screen	
	Rubella antibody titer	
Each visit	Urine protein and glucose	
Approximately 16 wk	Offer MSAFP	Ultrasound baseline
		Genetic evaluation and amniocentesis
		Multiple marker screen (HCG, MSAFP, E$_2$)
Approximately 24 wk	Blood sugar screen for diabetes	Hematocrit-hemoglobin if anemic
Approximately 28 wk		If Rh-negative repeat antibody screen and administer RhoGAM
Approximately 32 wk	Repeat hematocrit-hemoglobin	Gonorrhea
		Chlamydia
		Pap
		Syphilis screen

MSAFP, Maternal serum α-fetoprotein; *HIV,* human immunodeficiency virus; *TB,* tuberculosis; *HCG,* human chorionic gonadotropin; *E$_2$,* estradiol.

questionable. Certain standard tests should be done on each gravida, but most others are done only in selected situations or are offered electively to patients (Table 6-5).

Baseline testing

Baseline diagnostic testing should include blood studies for determination of the hemoglobin level or hematocrit, blood type, and Rh; a serologic test for hepatitis B and syphilis; urine tests for protein, sugar, and asymptomatic bacteriuria; and a screening cytologic examination for cervical abnormalities. A screening antibody test and rubella antibody titer also should be obtained.

Depending on the background incidence in the population being cared for, chlamydia, gonorrhea, and tuberculosis screening can be done. African-American patients should have been screened for sickle cell trait. Given the advances in prevention of maternal transmission to the fetus, screening for human immunodeficiency virus should be offered to all pregnant women.

Serial testing

Serial testing includes urine dipstick for glucose and protein monitoring for diabetes or preeclampsia. Hematocrit (or hemoglobin) testing late in the second trimester will show the maternal response. In fact, absence of a typical 3% drop in hematocrit may identify a group of patients who are not experiencing the normal increase in plasma volume and hence may be at increased risk for pregnancy-induced hypertension.

If the patient is Rh-negative, a repeat antibody screen should be done at 28 weeks before administration of Rh immunoglobulin.

Interval testing

Currently most women are screened for gestational diabetes in the late second trimester, either by universal screening using a 50-g glucose challenge or by a history screening for risks followed by a 3-hour glucose tolerance test for patients found to be at high risk. The suggested timing is to allow maximum human placental lactogen (HPL) effect to unmask gestational diabetes but early enough to permit intervention to minimize macrosomia and potential fetal-maternal morbidity.

Maternal serum α-fetoprotein (MSAFP) screening should be offered at around 16 weeks. Since the normal levels vary depending on the laboratory, the gestational age and maternal weight results are reported as multiples of the mean (MOM). Elevated results may indicate neural tube defect, misdated pregnancy, multiple gestation, fetal death, abdominal wall defects, and other anomalies (Table 6-6). Sonography is used to evaluate a single elevated MSAFP screen. It has also been noted that very low values indicate an increased risk of genetic anomalies, particularly trisomy 21. This screening examination has been refined by adding levels of estradiol and HCG to the calculations.

Genetic amniocentesis is recommended for women at risk for a fetus affected by a disease that can be identified by amniotic fluid testing. Common examples include advanced maternal age (35 years old or older at projected birth), prior affected infant, or unexplained elevated or depressed MSAFP test. Because a genetic amniocentesis cannot guarantee a normal infant and the procedure

Table 6-6. Conditions associated with abnormal maternal alpha-fetoprotein levels
ELEVATED
Neural tube defects
Multiple gestations
Fetal death
Abdominal wall defects: omphalocele and gastroschisis
Esophageal and duodenal atresia
Congenital nephrosis
Cystic hygroma
Subsequent intrauterine growth retardation and poor fetal outcome
Renal anomalies
Sacrococcygeal teratoma
Underestimation of fetal age
LOW
Chromosomal abnormalities, especially trisomies
Fetal death
Subsequent poor fetal outcome
Overestimation of gestational age

carries a risk (albeit a small one) of miscarriage, it is not recommended as a routine screening test.

Obstetric ultrasound is a commonly used diagnostic test. Currently there is debate as to whether this should be done routinely during pregnancy. Since there appears to be no risk to the fetus, arguments center around cost-effectiveness. An ultrasound clearly improves accuracy of dating if done early, but the only demonstrated advantage of this is to decrease the number of "postdate" pregnancies. Prospective studies have not demonstrated either cost-effectiveness or clinically significant findings that routine ultrasounds modify care in an otherwise uncomplicated pregnancy. A compromise used by many is to do a single dating scan at around 16 weeks, when the scan is accurate for dating but the fetus is also large enough to evaluate for such major anomalies as ventral wall defects, signifi-

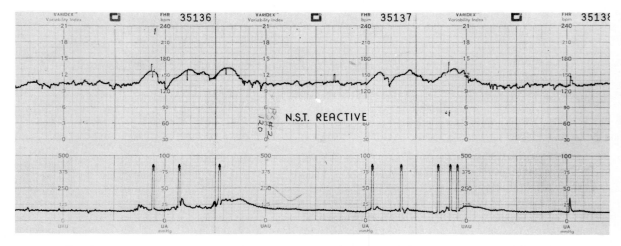

Fig. 6-4. Reactive nonstress test *(NST)*. Arrows on lower panel document timing of fetal movement. Strip has 12 minutes of observation, and accelerations are clearly evident.

cant cardiac defects, anencephaly, and twinning. Any other scan is done for a medical indication. Determination of fetal sex is not a medical indication.

Serial sonographic measurements of the biparietal diameter and body size should be obtained at regular intervals whenever fetal growth retardation is suspected. Comparison of body measurements against standard tables of growth will help differentiate between asymmetric and symmetric growth retardation.

Counting fetal movements

Fetal movements can be quantified by the mother. She is instructed to recline comfortably after a meal and then count the number of "kicks" that occur during a specified period. The patient is given "alarm" values that tell her to contact the clinic or the labor and delivery unit for further instructions. Many protocols have been described in the literature, and no ideal one has yet been determined. Generally, fetal movements decline rapidly over a day or two and are then absent for another 1 to 2 days before intrauterine death occurs. If a woman in the third trimester complains of decreased fetal movement, further biophysical testing should be considered.

Nonstress test

The nonstress test (NST) is designed to evaluate the reactivity of the fetus during the antepartum period. The NSTs are appropriate for women suspected of having placental dysfunction or insufficiency: for example, those with chronic hypertension or diabetes or with fetuses suspected of growth retardation or postmaturity. This test is based on the principle that a noncompromised fetus will demonstrate a heart rate acceleration when it moves. This reactivity is believed to be a good indicator of fetal autonomic function. Although the most common reason for loss of this reactivity is a fetal sleep cycle, the loss may result from any cause of central nervous system depression, including fetal acidosis.

A normal reaction to fetal movement is an acceleration in fetal heart rate of 15 beats/min over the baseline and lasting 15 seconds. The most common definition for a reactive NST (normal) is two or more accelerations within a 20-minute period (Fig. 6-4).

If only one or no accelerations occur during a 20-minute period, the fetus may be unhealthy or simply resting. If no accelerations occur during an additional 20-minute observation period, further testing should be done, such as a contraction stress test (CST). An NST is intended to evaluate for placental insufficiency. An acute event such as nuchal cord is not predicted by an NST. Figure 6-5 shows the result of fortunate timing of the test, not the predictive ability of NST.

Contraction stress test

The CST is designed to stress the fetoplacental unit and to test the reserve of the fetus. Contractions are induced by nipple stimulation or oxytocin, and the fetal heart rate response is monitored until there are at least three contractions of 40 seconds' duration in a 10-minute span.

The interpretation of the CST is categorized as follows by the ACOG technical bulletin:

Negative: No late decelerations (Fig. 6-6)

Positive: Late decelerations following 50% or more of contractions, even if the contraction frequency is less than three in 10 minutes

Suspicious (equivocal): Intermittent late or significant variable decelerations

Unsatisfactory: Fewer than three contractions per 10 minutes or poor-quality tracing, such as hyperstimulation

A positive CST in this setting is very worrisome, and delivery often is warranted. Nearly half of women with a positive CST will go through labor without late decelerations.

Biophysical profile

The fetus is evaluated sonographically for fetal breathing movements, gross body movements, muscle tone, and the quantity of amniotic fluid; and an NST is performed. The score categorizes the fetus as normal, equivocal test, or abnormal.

PATIENT EDUCATION

Patient education should be part of prenatal care. A patient should be given essential information concerning reproduction, motherhood, nutrition, and general health. This can be done in small groups where patients are encouraged to ask questions. Instructions about what is permitted and what should be avoided during pregnancy should be covered. Individual counseling sessions can be arranged for patients who need them. A normal individual does not need to alter her activities much simply because she is pregnant.

Exercise

The amount of physical activity permitted is determined by the tolerance of the individual patient, what she is used to doing, and whether she has a complication that would ordinarily necessitate rest rather than activity. Although uterine blood flow is decreased and maternal temperature is increased during strenuous activity, there is no evidence to suggest that maternal exercise (within the tolerance of the individual) has a deleterious effect on the fetus.

Work

Pregnant women can continue working until term if the pregnancy is normal and if the job environment and the physical activity involved pose no threat to the fetus or to the pregnancy.

Travel

The only danger in travel for the normal patient is that she may develop an acute complication, abort, or go into labor while away from home. Wearing seat belts should be routine. The belt should encircle the bony pelvis, not the abdomen, to reduce the possibility of injury to the fetus in an accident.

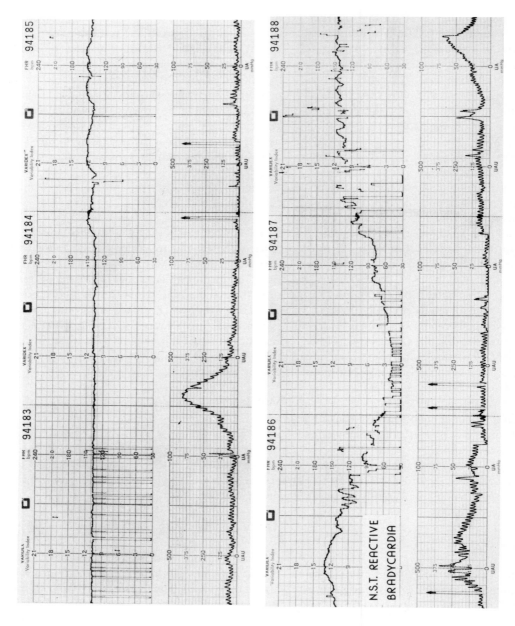

Fig. 6-5. Reactive nonstress test (*NST*) involving prolonged bradycardia (i.e., more than 5 minutes). Patient who was beyond term was immediately transferred to labor and delivery area, where a carefully monitored induction was performed. Another prolonged bradycardia occurred, emergency cesarean section was performed, and an infant with tight nuchal cord and thick meconium was delivered. Infant was resuscitated at birth and had an uncomplicated course after birth.

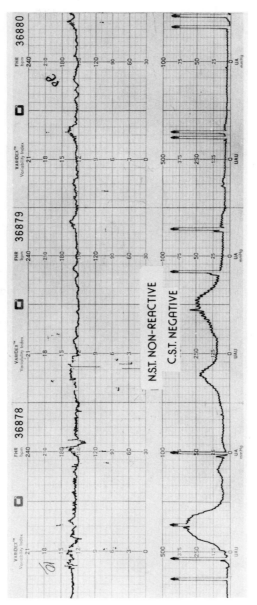

Fig. 6-6. Normal contraction stress test (CST). No decelerations are seen.

Intercourse

Women with uncomplicated pregnancies can continue intercourse without fear of injury or infection.

NUTRITIONAL NEEDS OF PREGNANT WOMEN

The caloric content of the diet influences fetal growth. Excessive weight gain in the mother increases the risk of a macrosomic infant. Poor weight gain tends to result in a smaller infant.

If the necessary ingredients for fetal growth and development are not supplied in the mother's diet, the fetus will obtain them at the expense of maternal tissues. The daily dietary requirements for mature women and the additions necessary during pregnancy and lactation are listed in Table 6-7.

Multivitamins with folate are traditionally given, although it is unclear whether most women need them. Iron supplementation probably is wise because most reproductive-age women are iron-deficient. Others recommend folate supplementation before conception and for the first trimester to reduce the risk of neural tube defects.

ADVERSE EFFECTS OF SUBSTANCE ABUSE

Alcohol

Fetal alcohol syndrome has been described in the offspring of alcoholics. Affected infants may

Table 6-7. Recommended daily dietary allowances for mature women with added allowances for pregnancy and lactation

	Recommended daily allowances for nonpregnant women	Recommended daily allowances added for pregnancy	Recommended daily allowances added for lactation
Calories (kcal)	2200	300	400
Protein (g)	50	10	15
Vitamin A (RE)	800	0	500
Vitamin D (μg)	10	0	0
Vitamin E (mg equiv)	8	2	4
Ascorbic acid (mg)	60	10	35
Folate (μg)	180	220	100
Niacin (mg equiv)	15	2	5
Riboflavin (mg)	1.3	0.3	0.5
Thiamine (mg)	1.1	0.4	0.5
Vitamin B_6 (mg)	1.6	0.6	0.5
Vitamin B_{12} (μg)	2	0.2	0.5
Calcium (g)	1200	0	0
Phosphorus (g)	1200	0	0
Iodine (μg)	150	25	50
Iron (mg)	15	15	0
Magnesium (mg)	280	20	75
Zinc (mg)	12	3	7

Based on data from *Recommended dietary allowances*, ed 10, Washington, DC, 1989, National Academy of Sciences.

have a variety of craniofacial, limb, and neurologic anomalies. They are below normal intelligence and may develop behavioral problems. The effects of high alcohol levels may be enhanced by excessive smoking, drug use, and malnutrition, all of which can accompany alcoholism.

Tobacco

The babies of women who smoke heavily are smaller than those of nonsmokers. The newborns are at greater risk of respiratory problems. The perinatal death rates among infants born to smoking mothers also are increased. Recent studies indicate that these children are more likely to smoke during their teen years than are children not exposed to smoke interutero.

Other drugs

Recreational drugs such as cocaine, heroin, and others may lead to a multitude of disorders depending on the timing, frequency, and intensity of the drug exposure. Also, the lifestyle that often accompanies the use of illegal drugs compromises prenatal care and nutrition and increases exposure to infectious agents. These infants may experience growth retardation, delayed mental development, placental abruption, preterm delivery, and even fetal death.

CRITICAL POINTS

- Every woman contemplating pregnancy should be examined before conception in order to optimize the status of preexisting health concerns, to improve nutrition, and to modify current medications as needed.
- Pregnancy diagnosis consists of subjective findings of amenorrhea, nausea, breast tenderness, urinary frequency, and quickening.
- Objective clinical findings consist of Chadwick's sign, Hegar's sign, and uterine enlargement with confirmation by auscultation of fetal heart tones or palpation of the infant.
- Diagnostic tests include β-HCG and pelvic ultrasound.
- Dating of a pregnancy is based on a typical gestation of 280 days from the first day of the last menstrual period. This can be confirmed or modified by clinical sizing and ultrasound measurements.
- Routine prenatal care is designed to effectively identify problems in fetal well-being or developing complications for the mother that may affect the fetus adversely. The determination of problems necessitates serial assessments of the mother and, indirectly, the fetus.
- The cost-effectiveness of performing *all* available tests on each pregnancy has been questioned. Certain standard tests should be done on each pregnancy, but most others are done only in selected situations or are offered electively to patients.
- Patient education is a major component of prenatal care. This includes discussion about exercise, work, travel, coitus, and nutrition.
- If the necessary ingredients for fetal growth and development are not supplied in the mother's diet, the fetus will obtain them at the expense of maternal tissues.

SUMMARY

Early diagnosis and initiation of care may improve the medical, nutritional, and psychologic status of the pregnant woman. Prenatal care is designed to identify developing complications early so that intervention can be done, which will help reduce perinatal and maternal morbidity-mortality.

Questions

1. Which of the following is *not* an objective finding consistent with a pregnancy?
   A. Ballottement of the fetus
   B. Chadwick's sign
   C. Fetal heart tones auscultated
   D. Obstetric ultrasound
   E. Quickening
2. The most accurate means of dating a pregnancy involves:
   A. Calculations based on first day of reported last menstrual period
   B. Auscultation of fetal heart tones with a fetoscope
   C. First trimester pelvic ultrasound
   D. Time of quickening
   E. Fundal height in early third trimester
3. Data points that should be ascertained at each prenatal visit include each of the following *except:*
   A. Blood pressure
   B. Cervical dilatation
   C. Fundal height in cm
   D. Fetal heart tones
   E. Maternal weight
4. Which of the following accounts for the greatest amount of maternal weight gain?
   A. Amniotic fluid
   B. Breasts
   C. Placenta
   D. Plasma volume
   E. Uterus
5. Patient education during an uncomplicated pregnancy should include the following *except:*
   A. Exercise is acceptable.
   B. Working up to term is acceptable if the job environment and physical activities pose no threat to the fetus.
   C. Intercourse is acceptable up to term.
   D. Seat belts should not be worn since they will injure the fetus.
   E. Dental work may be done during pregnancy, including extractions.

Answers

1. E
2. C
3. B
4. D
5. D

7

Intrapartum care

APGO LEARNING OBJECTIVE #7

Sharon T. Phelan

Understanding the process of normal labor and delivery allows optimal care and reassurance for the parturient and timely recognition of abnormal events.

The student will demonstrate a knowledge of the following:

A. Characteristics of true and false labor
B. Initial assessment of the laboring patient
C. Stages and mechanism of normal labor
D. Techniques to evaluate the progress of labor
E. Pain management during labor
F. Methods of monitoring the mother and fetus
G. Management of normal delivery and episiotomy repair
H. Indications for operative delivery
I. Immediate postpartum care of the mother

Labor is the mechanism by which the products of conception are expelled from the uterus and vagina. This is accomplished almost entirely by the activity of the uterine muscles.

Certain definitions essential to an understanding of labor and delivery are based on the typical duration of a pregnancy. Pregnancies are dated from the first day of the last normal menstrual period, even though classically fertilization does not occur until 2 weeks later. Delivery before 22 weeks' gestation is referred to as an *abortion.* Delivery between the beginning of the twenty-third week and the end of the thirty-sixth week is called *premature delivery. Delivery* at term occurs between the beginning of the thirty-seventh week and the completion of the forty-second week. *Postterm delivery* occurs after the forty-second week.

A woman is a *parturient* when she is in labor and a *puerpera* after delivery. The term *gravida* refers to the total number of pregnancies, regardless of their type, location, and time or method of termination-delivery. For example, a woman who has had two normal intrauterine pregnancies, one ectopic pregnancy, one abortion, and one hydatidiform mole is a gravida 5. A *primigravida* is pregnant for the first time, and a *nulligravida* has never been pregnant.

P = # of deliveries > 22 wks

G_3 P_2 2 0 0 1
term premature abort living

(Parity) refers to the number of deliveries of viable infants. A fetus weighing 500 g (22 weeks) theoretically can live an independent existence. *Para* therefore indicates the number of pregnancies, regardless of the methods of delivery or number of fetuses, that terminate after the twenty-second week. A *nullipara* has never carried a pregnancy beyond the twenty-second week, a *primipara* has carried one pregnancy beyond the twenty-second week, and a *multipara* has carried more than one. A more complete description of past pregnancies can be indicated by summarizing their outcomes by a series of numbers indicating (in order) term deliveries, premature deliveries, abortions, and presently living children. For example, 4-2-0-5 means four term deliveries, two premature deliveries, no abortions, and five living children.

CHARACTERISTICS OF UTERINE CONTRACTIONS AND LABOR

Certain changes take place in the uterus during pregnancy. These consist of the demarcation of the uterus into two separate divisions: the *upper uterine segment,* which is composed of the active contracting muscle tissue that supplies the force necessary to complete delivery; and the thin passive *lower uterine segment,* through which the presenting part passes into the pelvic cavity.

The lower uterine segment is derived principally from the isthmus of the uterus—the area just above the internal cervical os. The muscle tissue of the isthmus is indistinguishable from that of the rest of the body of the uterus. In contrast, the stroma of the cervix contains fibrous connective tissue with some elastic tissue and only a few smooth muscle cells. Until about the sixteenth week of pregnancy, identifying the isthmus as a distinct entity is almost impossible. At this time the isthmus lengthens to accommodate the rapidly growing fetus.

Uterine muscle fibers have certain characteristics that are essential for normal pregnancy and

successful delivery. They must be able gradually to elongate to permit the progressive increase in uterine size necessary to accommodate the growing fetus. As pregnancy advances, the length of individual muscle cells increases from an original 50 μm to about 500 μm. They must be elastic so they can return to their normal length after periods of uterine distention. Because labor and delivery are accomplished by the force generated by uterine muscle activity, the muscles must be able to contract and force the products of conception from the uterus. It is evident that unless the uterus remains closely approximated to the fetus while the fetus is gradually expelled from the cavity, the effect of each successive contraction will be diminished. As labor advances and the fetus descends through the birth canal, the uterine cavity gradually becomes smaller, so that effective force is maintained. This is accomplished by *brachystasis,* the unique ability of uterine muscle fibers to become progressively shorter and thicker while they retain their power to contract forcibly.

Uterine activity increases during the last 8 to 10 weeks of pregnancy. The Braxton Hicks contractions gradually become stronger. This increased muscle activity is responsible for the characteristic prelabor changes in the uterine corpus and cervix.

Because the fibers in the active upper segment shorten during each contraction, it is obvious that this portion of the uterine wall must become shorter and thicker during the period of muscle activity. In response to the contractions, the relatively passive fibers in the wall of the isthmus elongate as they are pulled upward, while the relatively firm cervix remains closed. This defines the more passive thinner lower uterine segment.

The cervix remains closed until the last 2 to 3 weeks, and in many cases remains closed until labor begins. As the isthmus is stretched by the contraction and retraction of the muscle fibers in the active segment, the internal cervical os begins to open, being gradually pulled upward around the membranes and the presenting part and incorporated with the isthmus in the lower segment. This process continues as the cervix *effaces.* These changes are usually well established in a term pregnancy of a nulliparous woman before the onset of true labor. This may happen early in labor with a multiparous patient.

Since this process is a continuum, it is often difficult for the woman and her care provider to distinguish between false and true labor. The contractions of true labor produce progress with thinning of the cervix, dilatation of the cervical opening, or descent of the presenting part. The principal criterion necessary for the diagnosis and evaluation of labor therefore is progress, not the character of the contractions. Many providers also have difficulty differentiating between latent phase labor and active labor. Traditionally, once a woman is contracting "regularly" and has dilated to 4 cm or more, she is considered to be in active labor. This differentiation is important when one interprets labor curves.

FORCES AND MECHANISMS IN LABOR

Labor occurs as a result of the force of muscular contractions, both primary (involuntary uterine contractions) and secondary (voluntary increases in intraabdominal pressure). The secondary forces are really only effective after complete cervical dilatation.

Uterine contractions during labor are presumed to be initiated by one of two pacemakers situated in the cornual areas of the fundus. One predominates, and during normal labor each contraction is initiated by a single pacemaker. The contraction mechanism is so well coordinated that the peak of contraction is reached in all parts of the uterus simultaneously. This means that the systolic phase of the contraction is longest in the region of the pacemaker and that it becomes progressively shorter in areas more distant from the fundus of the uterus. There is more muscle in the fundus than in the lower part of the uterus; hence the intensity of the contraction in this area is approximately twice that in the isthmus. At

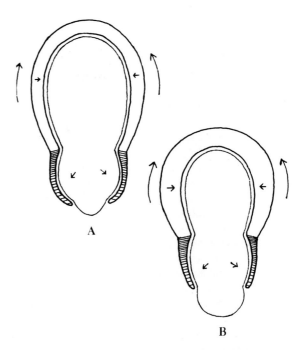

Fig. 7-1. A, Cervix is partially dilated and has not yet retracted around presenting part. **B,** Cervical dilatation is complete, and cervix is being pulled upward as presenting part descends.

their peak, contractions generate 35 to 60 mm Hg over the baseline of 4 to 12 mm Hg. This process is called fundal dominance. The force generated by each contraction is applied to the amniotic fluid and directly against the pole of the infant that occupies the upper segment of the uterus. Therefore, each time the muscle contracts the uterine cavity becomes smaller and the presenting part of the infant or the forebag of waters lying ahead of it is pushed downward into the cervix. This tends to force the cervix open or to dilate.

A more potent factor in cervical dilatation is the retraction of the upper segment. As the fundal portion of the uterus becomes shorter and thicker it pulls the lower segment and the dilating cervix upward around the presenting part at the same time that the uterus contracting directly against the infant tends to push it through the cervical opening (Fig. 7-1).

The secondary force of voluntary contractions of the abdominal muscles, with the diaphragm fixed, increases intraabdominal pressure and in turn intrauterine pressure. The secondary forces have no effect on cervical dilatation, but they are of considerable importance in aiding the expulsion of the infant from the uterus and vagina after the cervix is completely dilated.

The *mechanism of labor* is a term applied to the series of changes in the attitude and position of the fetus that permits it to progress through the irregularly shaped pelvic cavity. The steps in the mechanism of labor for the occiput positions are *descent, flexion, internal rotation, extension, restitution, and external rotation.* These do not occur as separate processes but are combined. For example, descent through the pelvis; flexion; and internal rotation all may occur more or less simultaneously.

The progress of labor is the result of the tendency for each uterine contraction to push the fetus downward through the pelvis; of the resistance of the soft tissue and the bony pelvis to its descent; and of the shape of the fetal head, which must conform to the different shapes of the pelvic cavity at its various levels. The infant itself is entirely passive. With each uterine contraction the fetus is pushed lower into the pelvic cavity and its position gradually is altered to accommodate it to the shape of the part of the pelvis through which it must pass.

Descent

In occiput positions, the longest diameter of the infant's head (the anteroposterior) enters the normal pelvis in the longest diameter of the inlet (the transverse) in almost every instance. If the sagittal suture is equidistant from the symphysis and the sacral promontory, the head is said to be entering the inlet in a synclitic manner (Fig. 7-2, *B*). Some degree of asynclitism generally is present at this point of labor (Fig. 7-2, *A* and *C*). The head descends through the inlet with its biparietal diameter approximately parallel to the plane of the inlet.

Generally, some degree of molding of the fetal head is correlated with descent through the inlet. The term *molding* describes the changes in the shape of the head necessary to permit it to adapt itself to the size and shape of the maternal pelvis. Molding is accomplished by gradual elevation or depression of the parietal, frontal, and occipital skull plates made possible by the mobility of these bones (which are not yet fused to each other). Molding is a dynamic process: the shape of the head changes constantly throughout labor. Little molding is necessary to permit a normal-size fetus to pass through a normal pelvis; however, if pelvic diameters are reduced, considerable change in the shape of the head may be necessary to permit vaginal delivery.

The head is said to be *engaged* after the widest transverse diameter, the biparietal, has passed the plane of the inlet. In the normal *unmolded* head the distance between the occiput and the plane of the biparietal diameter is less than the distance between the ischial spines and the inlet.

Descent can be delayed by an incompletely dilated cervix; resistant soft tissues; disproportion between the size of the head and the size or shape of the pelvic cavity; and weak, ineffective uterine contractions. Descent usually occurs more gradually in primigravidas than in multiparas because the cervix dilates more slowly and the soft tissue resistance is greater.

The degree of descent is gauged by the *station* of the presenting part (Fig. 7-3), which is its relationship to the plane of the ischial spines. If the lowest point of the presenting part is at the level of the spines, it is at station 0; if it is one third of the distance between the spines and the pelvic inlet, it is at station −1; if it is two thirds of the distance to the inlet, it is at station −2; and if it is at the inlet, it is at station −3. If the lowest level of the presenting part is above the plane of the pelvic inlet, it is said to be *floating.* The distance between the plane of the ischial spines and the pelvic floor is also divided into thirds. A station +1 therefore indicates that the lowest level of the head is one third of the distance between the spines and the pelvic

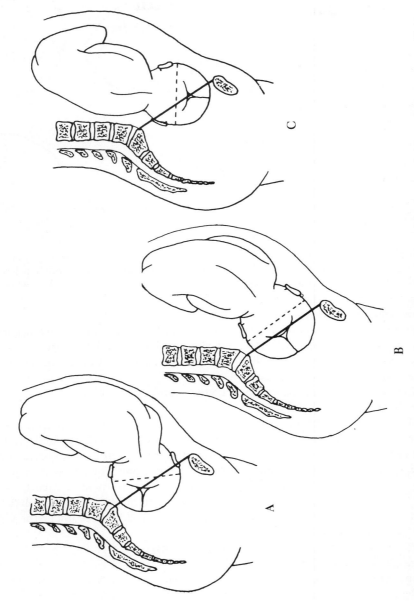

Fig. 7-2. Descent through inlet. **A,** Anterior parietal bone presentation. Sagittal suture is in posterior segment of inlet. **B,** Synclitism. Sagittal suture is equidistant from sacrum and pubis. **C,** Posterior parietal bone presentation. Sagittal suture is in anterior segment of inlet.

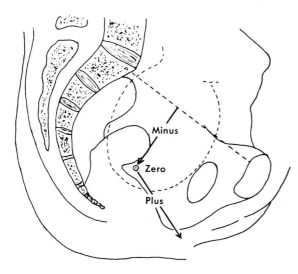

Fig. 7-3. Stations of birth canal. Presenting part *(dotted lines)* is just below station 0. Biparietal diameter has passed plane of inlet.

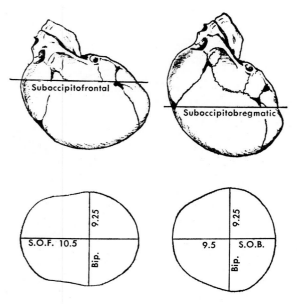

Fig. 7-4. As flexion increases, anteroposterior diameter of head, which must pass through pelvis, becomes shorter. *(From Beck AC:* Obstetrical practice, *Baltimore, 1955, Williams & Wilkins.)*

floor. When the presenting part reaches station +3, it usually has just reached the pelvic floor. Some use a five-point scale that measures in cm from the reference point of the spines.

FLEXION. During late pregnancy the fetal head usually lies in the pelvic inlet in a partially flexed attitude. The degree of flexion increases during descent owing to resistance of maternal bone and soft tissue. The purpose of the flexion is to substitute the suboccipitobregmatic diameter of 9.5 cm for the occipitofrontal diameter, which measures 10.5 to 11 cm (Fig. 7-4). Descent of the head through the inlet and upper pelvis is illustrated in Fig. 7-5.

Internal rotation

Rotation of the long axis of the fetal head from the transverse diameter in which it descended through the upper pelvis to the anteroposterior diameter at the outlet is essential. The transverse diameters of the normal middle and lower pelvis are too short to permit the head of a normal-size infant to descend farther without rotating. Rotation begins at the level of the ischial spines, but it

is not completed until the presenting part reaches the lower pelvis. Both the levator muscles and the bony pelvis are important for anterior rotation.

Extension

The upper half of the pelvic canal is directed posteriorly toward the sacrum and the lower half anteriorly, making the canal a curved tube rather than a straight one. The course of descent of the presenting part must therefore change to conform to the pelvic architecture. This involves some deflexion as the head passes under the symphysis.

Restitution

After the head is free from the introitus, it rotates 45 degrees to the right or left of the midline to assume its normal relationship to the back and shoulders. If the fetal back is on the left, the occiput rotates in that direction; if on the right, it rotates to that side.

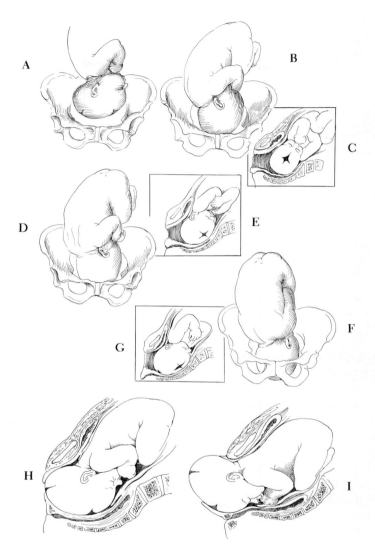

Fig. 7-5. A, Position of head in inlet when labor begins. **B,** Flexion as head descends. **C,** Head descends to mid-pelvis in transverse position. **D** and **E,** Partial anterior rotation as head passes spines. **F** and **G,** Further anterior rotation as occiput reaches lower pelvis. **H** and **I,** Complete anterior rotation and extension of head.

External rotation

As the shoulders descend and rotate within the pelvis, the occiput rotates farther externally; thus external rotation of the head actually indicates a change in position of the undelivered body of the fetus. With some mild downward pressure the anterior shoulder is delivered, followed by the posterior shoulder (Fig. 7-6). Many attendants promote the delivery of the anterior shoulder before complete restitution to minimize the risk of shoulder dystocia.

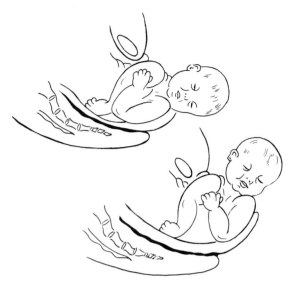

Fig. 7-6. Anterior shoulder remains beneath pubic arch, as posterior shoulder is forced anteriorly over distended perineum.

TECHNIQUES TO EVALUATE THE PROGRESS OF LABOR

One of the most critical variables influencing the calculated length of labor is the decision as to when labor began. The progression of uterine activity from prelabor to real labor, when recognizable changes in the cervix occur, is difficult to pinpoint. At the time of admission to the labor and delivery unit, the admitting provider should decide what time will be considered the start of labor for further evaluations. Once a patient is determined to be in labor, the first stage of labor usually is described in two phases: (1) a *latent* phase, during which effacement is completed and cervical dilatation begins; and (2) an *active* phase, during which cervical dilatation is completed. The duration of labor in any individual is determined by parity, the size and position of the fetus, the shape and capacity of the pelvis, the consistency of the cervix, and the efficiency of the uterine contraction. A typical labor curve is shown in Fig. 7-7. The maximum slope will vary from a nullipara to a multipara. The second stage of labor from complete dilatation to delivery of the infant also follows a typical pattern, with completion usually in under 2 hours. A second stage of labor longer than that necessitates evaluation for dystocia.

PAIN MANAGEMENT DURING LABOR

The act of normal labor and delivery is a painful and often long process. Over the years multiple approaches have been used to provide analgesia or anesthesia for this process. Many advocate prepared childbirth, which promotes the concept that an educated woman armed with techniques of patterned breathing can manage the pain more effectively and without pharmacologic assistance. This works well in a motivated patient, particularly a parous individual.

Many drugs have been given to make labor and delivery less painful, but unfortunately all have disadvantages that limit their usefulness. The "perfect" agent must provide relief from pain while it neither interferes with the progress of labor nor adds to the risk for the mother or fetus. Such an agent has not yet been discovered.

Systemic analgesia

The use of parenteral narcotic agents is limited by their effects on the newly born infant. Because these drugs cross the placenta, they exert a cerebral depressant effect on the fetus as well as on the mother.

Systemic analgesics should be used to reduce the discomfort to a tolerable level and to relax the patient enough to permit her to rest during the pain-free intervals between contractions. They are not intended to eliminate pain completely.

Regional analgesia-anesthesia

The transmission of pain impulses can be controlled by nerve block. With this type of analgesia,

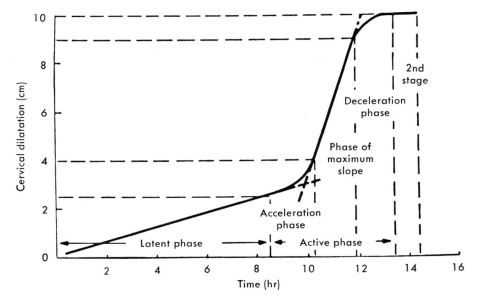

Fig. 7-7. Phases of labor in primigravida. *(From Friedman EA: A graphicostatistical analysis,* Obstet Gynecol *6:567, 1955.)*

the mother is awake and comfortable and the baby rarely is depressed.

Pain sensations from the uterus, the cervix, and the upper vagina are transmitted to ganglia just lateral to the cervix; then through the inferior and superior hypogastric plexuses; and, by way of the lumbar and lower thoracic sympathetic chains, to the spinal cord through nerves arising from T10, T11, T12, and L1.

The major pain sensations from the lower vagina and posterior vulva and perineum, which are the principal sources of discomfort while the presenting part distends the lower vagina and delivers, are transmitted through the pudendal nerves. These nerves are derived from the ventral branches of S2, S3, and S4.

Epidural block

The injection of an anesthetic drug into the extradural space controls pain by blocking the transmission of painful stimuli without interfering with the muscular activity of the uterus.

The most serious complications are massive spinal anesthesia following the inadvertent injection of the agent into the subarachnoid space, meningitis, epidural abscess, intravenous injection, and breakage of the needle or catheter. Because sympathetic block is a common complication of any type of regional anesthesia, several measures aimed at reducing its incidence are appropriate, including administration of a fluid bolus before placement of the block, left uterine displacement, and prophylactic administration of ephedrine.

Peripheral nerve block

Local injection of anesthetic agents to block the peripheral nerve endings affords some relief; but these drugs are less effective than nerve root blocks, which commonly involve simple infiltration of the perineal body for episiotomy or its repair.

Pudendal nerve block by injection of up to 10 ml of 1% lidocaine around each perineal nerve

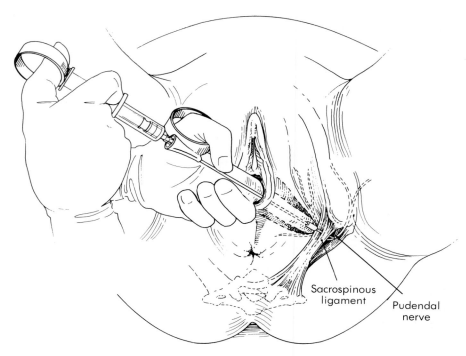

Fig. 7-8. Pudendal nerve block. Needle point is directed behind inferior tip of ischial spine by fingertip.

trunk as it passes behind the ischial spine can provide excellent pelvic anesthesia for normal or low forceps delivery and episiotomy (Fig. 7-8).

METHODS OF MONITORING THE MOTHER AND FETUS

Multiple methods of monitoring are used to determine how well patients tolerate labor and its progression as plotted on a labor curve.

Fetal heart rate

Fetal heart rate is an index of the condition of the fetus and should be counted and recorded at least every 15 to 30 minutes during first stage and every 5 to 15 minutes in second stage, with the timing of auscultation being the first 30 seconds after a contraction. Since this is relatively labor intensive for nursing staff, many labor and delivery units use continuous electronic fetal heart rate monitoring with either an external or internal electrode. The interpretation of fetal heart rate tracing is described in Chapter 21, Intrapartum Fetal Distress.

Maternal blood pressure should be recorded every 30 minutes because it may rise to dangerous levels during labor or may drop if there is unappreciated bleeding or an anesthesia complication.

Contractions—including their length, frequency, and intensity—are recorded either at 30-minute intervals or continuously by external toco- or internal pressure catheter. Any fetal heart deviations from normal must be linked to the contractions for proper interpretation. For this reason, many delivery units commonly do continuous monitoring. Continuous monitoring in an uncomplicated labor is "standard," but it has not been proved to change outcome except to decrease the already low incidence of intrapartum fetal death. There are also concerns that continuous fetal monitoring may lead to increased operative intervention, including cesarean sections.

Maternal temperature should be taken every 4 hours. Elevation in maternal temperature may be the first indication of chorioamnionitis. This complication should be aggressively managed with intrapartum antibiotics, and the pediatric staff must be notified of probable infectious problems.

Urinary protein should be assessed periodically, particularly in any woman with elevated blood pressure.

Vaginal examination

Vaginal examinations are used to determine cervical dilatation, fetal stations, and general progress of labor. However, cervical exams carry a risk of infection. For this reason as few exams as possible should be done. Each vaginal exam should include cervical dilatation, station, and position of the presenting part.

During labor a lateral position is often the most comfortable for the patient. It also prevents vena cava compression with resultant hypotension. Patients should not eat because there is delayed emptying of the stomach in labor. Whether a patient may have clear liquids depends on the preference of the anesthetist and the obstetric attendant. Care must be taken to ensure that the bladder remains empty. A full bladder may interfere with normal descent of the fetus.

Intrapartum fetal heart rate monitoring

The fetus in utero is entirely dependent on the mother for its supply of oxygen and the other nutrients it obtains from the maternal blood in the placental sinuses. Circulation of the blood through the sinuses is regulated by the mother's arterial blood pressure and by the activity of the uterine muscle.

The pressure within the intervillous space is about the same as or slightly higher than the amniotic fluid pressure, being about 5 to 10 mm Hg when the uterus is at rest and 55 mm Hg or more at the peak of a contraction. The intervillous pressure rises during a contraction because the veins are nicked and compressed by the uterine muscle fibers before the caliber of the more resistant arterioles is affected. Thus blood continues to flow into the spaces for some time after its means of egress are closed.

The fetal oxygen supply can be reduced by any of the following:

1. *Reduction in blood flow through the maternal vessels.* The caliber of the arteries may be reduced by spasm in women with hypertensive complications of pregnancy, thus limiting blood flow. It is estimated that arterial blood flow can be reduced by as much as 50% in women with hypertensive disease. The flow of blood will also be impaired whenever the maternal systolic blood pressure is lower than the amniotic fluid pressure. Fetal hypoxia is likely to develop when maternal systolic blood pressure levels fall below 60 mm Hg.

2. *Reduction in blood flow through the uterine sinuses.* Blood flow through the intervillous space will be reduced if the veins or arterioles are compressed over long periods by forceful, rapidly recurring, or prolonged tetanic uterine contractions. A reduction in maternal blood pressure will have the same result.

3. *Reduction of the oxygen content of maternal blood.* The available circulating maternal hemoglobin can be reduced by profound chronic anemia or hemorrhage, thereby reducing the total oxygen capacity.

4. *Alterations in fetal circulation.* The circulation of blood through the vessels of the infant's body and the placenta is maintained by the fetal heart. Anything that alters normal cardiac function will impair the circulation, as

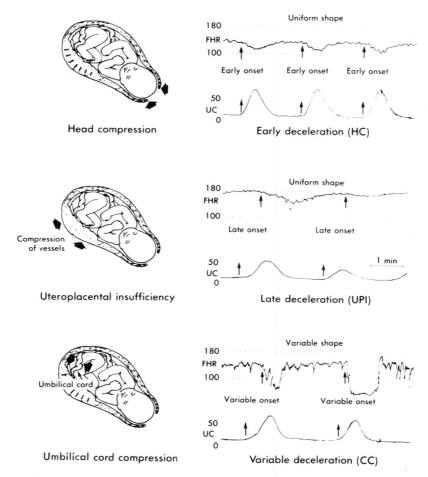

Fig. 7-9. Changes in fetal heart rate patterns related to various causes. *(From Hon EH: An atlas of fetal heart rate patterns, New Haven, Conn, 1968, Harty Press.)*

will compression of the umbilical cord. Placental infarction or separation will decrease the total area available for oxygen transfer from the maternal blood; if a considerable portion of placenta is involved, the infant cannot survive.

Accurate assessment of fetal well-being during labor depends on an understanding of the physiology of the fetal heart rate tracing so that proper interpretation can be made. Periodic changes in fetal heart rate during labor have been classified according to their relationship to uterine contractions. In *early decelerations* the onset of the decrease in rate begins with the onset of the contraction, and normal rate resumes as the uterus relaxes; in *variable decelerations* there is no constant relationship of the deceleration to contractions; and *late decelerations* begin after the contractions start and recovery is prolonged (Fig. 7-9).

Early decelerations are reflex, are related to pressure on the fetal head, and are mediated by the vagus. They are not associated with a poor out-

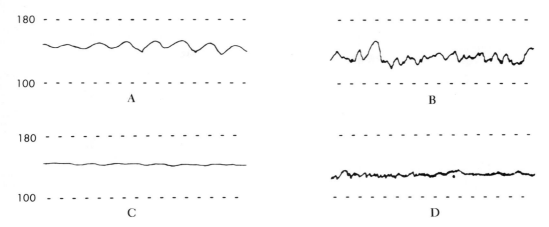

180 - - - - - - - - - - - - -

100 - - - - - - - - - - - - -
A

180 - - - - - - - - - - - - -

100 - - - - - - - - - - - - -
C

- - - - - - - - - - - - -

B

- - - - - - - - - - - - -

D

Fig. 7-10. Variability differences observed with fetal scalp electrode. **A,** Long-term variability only. **B,** Both long- and short-term variability. **C,** Neither long- nor short-term variability. **D,** Short-term variability only. *(From Zanini B, Paul RH, Huey JR: Intrapartum fetal heart rate: Correlation with scalp pH in the preterm labor,* Am J Obstet Gynecol *136:43, 1980.)*

come. *Variable decelerations* are caused by cord compression. They are reflex changes characterized by a sudden drop in the fetal heart rate and a rapid return to normal. Whether this will cause a problem for the fetus depends on the length of time the circulation is disturbed and the reserve of the fetus. *Late decelerations* are a sign of uteroplacental insufficiency.

Probably the most important point in the evaluation of the health of the intrauterine passenger is the presence or absence of *beat-to-beat variability of the fetal heart rate* (Fig. 7-10). Good beat-to-beat variability indicates good fetal reserve. Poor beat-to-beat variability may indicate either fetal intolerance of labor or changes caused by exogenous medications such as meperidine given to the mother during labor. To differentiate between these two options, a review of the timing of the decreased beat-to-beat variability in relationship to doses given the mother; use of fetal scalp stimulation to cause fetal heart rate acceleration; or fetal scalp blood sampling should be done. This last test was thought to hold great promise. A low pH is evidence of anaerobic tissue metabolism. The normal pH of fetal scalp blood is above 7.25. Testing shows that pH probably needs to be

less than 7.0 before significant fetal morbidity or mortality is likely. However, because of the difficulty in obtaining the sample, in addition to the cost and inconsistent results (e.g., a large caput may yield a falsely low pH value), many institutions no longer use this test.

As noted in the American College of Obstetricians and Gynecologists (ACOG) technical bulletin #207, specific fetal heart rate patterns have been reported to be associated with an increased incidence of fetal compromise:

1. Severe bradycardia
2. Repetitive late decelerations
3. Undulating baseline, a pattern of rapid change between tachycardia and bradycardia
4. Any nonreassuring pattern associated with unexplained poor or absent baseline variability

Other nonreassuring patterns and combinations of patterns may be associated with fetal deterioration as labor progresses, and these should be followed closely. Management can be directed to correcting the possible insult by changing maternal position; stopping oxytocin; increasing intravenous fluids; correcting hypotension; giving oxygen by mask; or, in cases of potential cord compression without prolapse, amnioinfusion.

No benefit for continuous fetal heart rate monitoring in uncomplicated normal pregnancy and labor has been proved. Most reports find no difference in neonatal morbidity with respect to Apgar scores, cord blood gases, or the need for neonatal resuscitation and intensive care. There is no correlation between adverse neurologic outcome and various heart rate patterns. When infants are stressed by pregnancy complications or abnormal labor the benefits of continuous monitoring are much clearer. However, there is a significant increase in maternal morbidity owing to increased operative deliveries when continuous fetal heart monitoring is done. In most studies the incidence of cesarean delivery also was increased.

All patients in labor should have some type of fetal heart rate assessment throughout. Depending on the antenatal care, progression of labor, and staffing on the delivery unit, this may be done by intermittent auscultation (as outlined by the ACOG) or by continuous electronic fetal heart rate monitoring.

MANAGEMENT OF NORMAL DELIVERY AND EPISIOTOMY REPAIR

Patient positioning during delivery is often the dorsal lithotomy position. This probably is simplest for the attendant and provides the best exposure of the perineum, but it may not be the best for the patient. The Sims' position is an alternative, where the patient lies on her side with the upper leg supported by an attendant. This is often more difficult if an episiotomy is needed.

After the perineum and inner thighs are prepped with an antiseptic solution, the patient is draped in a sterile fashion. Any necessary episiotomy is performed after the perineum has been flattened by the crowning fetal head. The incision

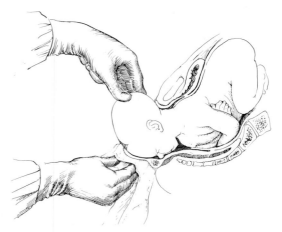

Fig. 7-11. Modified Ritgen's maneuver.

should be deep enough to sever the fascia covering the lower surface of the levator muscles. A midline episiotomy is the most common. There is some controversy about the potential long-term benefits of episiotomy versus the increased risk of extension into the rectal sphincter and anal mucus when a midline episiotomy is used. A mediolateral episiotomy is an alternative; but it carries a number of potential complications, including more bleeding and subsequent dyspareunia.

With each contraction, the infant's head will extend, and more of the scalp will be visible through the dilated introitus. Delivery of the head can be controlled by *Ritgen's maneuver* (Fig. 7-11). Upward pressure is applied through a sterile towel with the thumb and forefinger of the pronated right hand, or with the first and second fingers with the hand supinated first to the supraorbital ridges and later to the chin through the distended perineal body. The upward pressure, which increases extension and prevents the head from slipping back between contractions, is counteracted by downward pressure on the occiput with the fingertips of the other hand. This tends to prevent extension. With this maneuver, the delivery of the head can be readily controlled; and its

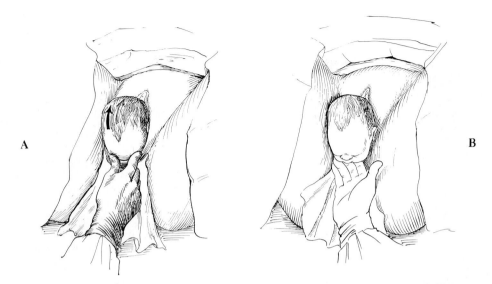

Fig. 7-12. Completion of delivery of head. **A,** Forehead is supported to maintain extension. **B,** Face is freed from perineum.

rapid expulsion, which causes perineal tearing, can be prevented. As the head descends farther, the perineum is pushed back over the face and chin (Fig. 7-12).

As soon as the head is delivered, the attendant feels along the infant's neck for any signs of a nuchal cord. If one is felt and it is loose, it may be slipped over the infant's head or over the shoulders as they deliver. Very tight and/or multiple loops of cord may necessitate double clamping and cutting (between the clamps) the cord. If there is no nuchal cord, the attendant should proceed immediately with the delivery of the anterior shoulder after delivery of the fetal head *before* restitution and external rotation. This allows the shoulders to be delivered before impingement under the pubic symphysis. Many believe that this may help avoid a shoulder dystocia. After the delivery of the anterior shoulder, the infant's airway should be suctioned before delivery of the rest of the body.

After the delivery of the anterior shoulder, the head is elevated toward the ceiling and traction is applied to deliver the posterior shoulder over the perineum (Fig. 7-13). Then the remainder of the body is slowly extracted by traction on the shoulders (Fig. 7-14).

If the cord has not already been clamped and cut, there is some debate about the best timing of clamping the cord and the position of the infant. If the newborn is held below the level of the introitus, blood will be infused from the placental vessels to the baby. The amount is determined by the time interval between delivery and cord clamping, but as much as a 75- to 100-ml increase in blood volume can be anticipated. Conversely, there is no transfer of blood if the infant is held above the level of the mother's abdomen.

The infant is placed in a heated crib with its head slightly lower than its body. The head-down position should not be too deep; nor should the infant be held upside down for any length of time because the pressure of the abdominal viscera against the diaphragm interferes with normal respiratory efforts.

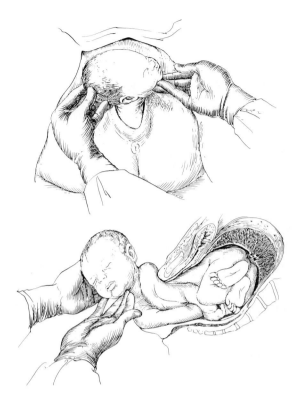

Fig. 7-13. Delivery of posterior shoulder.

Third stage

The interval between the delivery of the infant and the delivery of the placenta is the third stage and the most dangerous for the mother. Abnormalities of placental separation and expulsion often are accompanied by profuse bleeding that may cause maternal death.

Under normal circumstances the placenta is relatively noncontractile and has only limited ability to alter its size and shape to compensate for changes in the area of the uterine wall over which it is attached. As the uterus becomes smaller during expulsion of the infant, the surface area of its cavity must diminish. As the area of the placental site is reduced, the placenta thickens, and its diameter decreases. Because the size of the placenta cannot be altered enough to equal the change in the muscular uterine wall beneath it, the placenta is at least partially sheared off (Fig. 7-15).

The separation occurs in the spongy portion of the decidua basalis: a thin layer of decidua remains on the uterine wall, and the remainder covers the cotyledons of the maternal surface of the placenta.

After the birth of the infant, the uterus continues to contract regularly, sometimes even more actively than during late labor. The placenta, al-

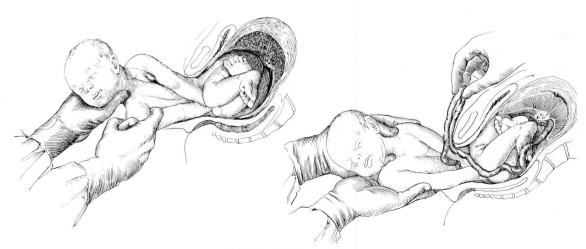

Fig. 7-14. Delivery of body.

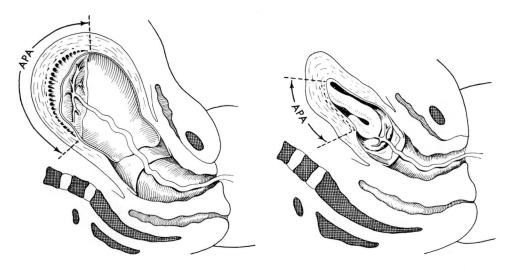

Fig. 7-15. Reduction in size of area of placental attachment *(APA)* as upper segment contracts, separates placenta, and expels it into lower uterine segment.

though separating, will continue to remain in the upper part of the uterine cavity. Continued uterine contractions complete the separation of the placenta and force it downward into the flaccid, distended lower segment. Ultimately the placenta is forced from the lower segment and vagina by voluntary bearing-down efforts by the mother; or, as is more often the case, it is expressed by the attendant. The duration of the third stage will be from 15 to 30 minutes, or even longer if the physician waits for the mother to expel the placenta herself.

Control of bleeding

The branches of the uterine arteries wind between the interlacing smooth muscle bundles as they traverse the uterine wall, and they eventually open into the large sinuses in the decidua basalis at the placental site. *The source of the blood loss after delivery, except that caused by soft-tissue injury, is from sinuses left open by separation of the placenta.* Excess bleeding is prevented by firm contraction of the uterine muscle bundles, which kink and compress the vessels passing between them. This is followed by clot formation and retraction in the sinuses, the

usual method by which bleeding from open vessels is controlled.

Placental expulsion

The so-called signs of separation of the placenta are more accurately evidences of its expulsion from the firmly contracted uterine fundus into the lower segment and vagina, indicating that it can be delivered. The signs are as follows:

1. *A show of blood* appears as the uterus contracts and the placenta is forced downward.
2. *The cord advances.* The length of cord visible outside the introitus increases as the placenta descends into the lower segment and vagina.
3. *The shape of the uterus changes.* The uterus becomes globular rather than wide and flat after the placenta has been expelled into the lower segment.
4. *Nontransmission of impulse occurs.* As slight traction is made on the cord while the uterus is pushed downward by pressure on the fundus, the amount of cord outside the vagina increases. If the placenta is still in the upper segment, the cord is withdrawn

into the vagina when the suprapubic pressure is released and the uterus is allowed to rise. If the placenta is detached and in the lower segment, the cord retracts very little when the uterus rises.

As the fundus becomes firm and globular, placenta expulsion may be aided by downward pressure over the superior surface of the uterus with the palmar surfaces of the fingers; it should not be squeezed (Fig. 7-16).

With the delivery of the placenta, the attendant should massage the uterus to verify that spontaneous contractions are continuing that will control bleeding. Some attendants massage only the abdomen; others do a bimanual massage that also will assess for uterine inversion. During the same interval the placenta should be inspected to make certain it is intact and that none of the cotyledons has been left in the uterine cavity. During the inspection, ascertain that none of the fetal vessels extend to the edge of the membranes and then end abruptly—which may indicate a retained accessory lobe of the placenta. At this time an oxytocic drug usually is given to stimulate uterine muscle contractions.

Uterotonic (oxytocic) drugs stimulate firm uterine contraction and, when properly used, will reduce the blood loss accompanying placental separation and delivery.

The synthetic ergot derivative *methylergonovine maleate (Methergine),* when administered intramuscularly in 0.1- to 0.2-mg doses, produces a sustained tetanic contraction of the uterine muscles that reduces the blood loss from the vessels at the placental site.

Methylergonovine maleate may produce vasoconstriction and an alarming rise in blood pressure in susceptible women. It should not be given to women with hypertension or to those with labile blood pressures.

Oxytocin from which almost all the vasopressor factor has been removed can be administered instead of ergot preparations as an aid in managing the third stage. It is preferred over methyler-gonovine maleate for women with hypertensive disorders because it is less likely to produce alarming blood pressure elevations. The dose is 0.5 ml (5 U) intramuscularly, or 2 ml (20 U) dissolved in 1000 ml of 5% dextrose solution as an intravenous drip. The latter method is preferred if an intravenous infusion already is running. One potentially serious but rare side effect of oxytocin may be a profound decrease in blood pressure after administering the drug.

When oxytocin does not work, another therapy—especially in hypertensive women—is prostaglandin $F_{2\alpha}$. The initial suggested dose is 250 µg intramuscularly and is repeated in 15 minutes. This medication is contraindicated in asthmatic patients.

Episiotomy repair

If an episiotomy has been cut, the repair can be done in many ways as long as each provides hemostasis, reapproximates the tissue properly in layers, and uses meticulous surgical technique. Adequate anesthesia must be ensured. The epidural anesthesia used for labor often will suffice. Otherwise a pudendal block or local infiltration is effective. The episiotomy needs to be explored carefully to rule out compromise of the rectal sphincter (third degree) or rectal mucosa (fourth degree). If these are not repaired correctly the patient may experience a rectal-vagina fistula or fecal incontinence. For a standard second-degree episiotomy the following principles should be followed. The vaginal mucosa is closed with a running stitch that starts approximately 1 cm above the apex of the vaginal incision to the hymenal ring. This layer should include vaginal fascia for support. Using deep interrupted stitches the perineal body, including the levator ani, should be reapproximated. One should not attempt to stitch the actual muscles but the fascia around them. Then the transverse perineal muscles are approximated. The skin is closed with a continuous subcuticular stitch. Sutures should approximate, *not* strangulate, the tissue because this causes ischemia and

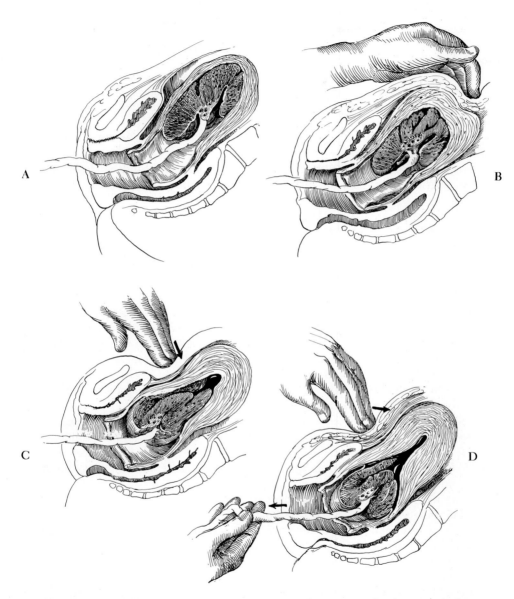

Fig. 7-16. A, Uterus before placenta is expelled. **B,** Manual pressure on fundus as uterus begins to contract aids expulsion of placenta into lower segment **(C),** from where it can be expressed by upward pressure on contracted fundus and tension on cord **(D).**

poor healing. Once the closure is done, many recommend performing a rectal exam to ensure that no stitch has extended through the rectal mucosa.

Operative delivery

When the mother is unsuccessful in accomplishing a spontaneous vaginal delivery or when severe fetal compromise is suspected and vaginal delivery is not imminent, an operative delivery may be needed. This may include a forceps or vacuum extraction for ineffective maternal pushing (exhaustion or anesthesia), or malpre-

sentation, occiput posterior for moderate fetal distress with delivery imminent. A cesarean section may be necessary for many indications. Fetal malpresentation (transverse or footling breech), cephalopelvic disproportion (fetal macrosomia, abnormal position, or contracted bony pelvis), failure to progress (ineffective labor despite oxytocin), marked fetal distress, placenta previa, and cord prolapse are a few such indications.

Immediate postpartum care of mother

The patient should be closely supervised for at least 1 hour after delivery. During this time

CRITICAL POINTS

- Uterine muscle fibers must be able to elongate; remain elastic; and, while contracting, become progressively shorter to allow effective transmission of the force of labor to the presenting part. This is called brachystasis and allows fundal dominance during labor.
- The lower uterine segment and the cervix are stretched gradually during pregnancy and eventually are retracted-effaced during labor to allow the passage of the fetus.
- True labor is contractions that produce progress, such as thinning of the cervix, dilatation of the cervix, or descent of the presenting part. The principal criterion for the diagnosis of labor is progress, not the character of the contractions.
- The steps in the mechanism of labor for the occiput positions are descent, flexion, internal rotation, extension, restitution, and external rotation.
- The duration of labor in any individual is determined by parity, the size and position of the fetus, the shape and capacity of the pelvis, the consistency of the cervix, and the efficiency of the uterine contractions.
- The use of narcotic agents in labor is limited by their cerebral depressant effects on the newborn and depression on the respiratory centers.
- Multiple methods of monitoring may be used to determine how the mother and fetus are tolerating labor and its progression as plotted on a labor curve. These include maternal and fetal heart rates, maternal blood pressure, temperature, assessment of contraction timing and intensity, vaginal examinations, and urinary evaluations for protein and glucose.
- The interval between the delivery of the infant and the placenta is the most dangerous stage for the mother, with abnormalities of placental separation and expulsion being associated with profuse bleeding that may be life threatening. Excessive bleeding is prevented by firm contraction of the uterine muscle, constricting the vessels as they pass through the myometrium to the placental bed, not by clot formation.
- If an episiotomy is cut, the repair must direct attention to providing hemostasis, reapproximating tissues properly in layers, and using meticulous surgical technique.

her pulse and blood pressure should be checked every 15 minutes. The uterus should be palpated frequently to make certain that it remains well contracted, and the vulvar pad should be inspected for evidence of excess bleeding. The attendant should not have to manipulate and massage the uterus to prevent relaxation; if this is necessary, something is wrong.

Questions

1. The following are steps in the mechanism of labor for occiput presentation *except:*
   A. Descent
   B. Effacement
   C. Extension
   D. Internal rotation
   E. Restitution
2. The primary mode of hemostasis at the end of the third stage of labor is:
   A. Clot formation and retraction
   B. Myometrial contraction compressing vessels to placenta bed
   C. Placenta site involution
   D. Decidual and trophoblastic patch
3. The principles of episiotomy repair include the following *except:*
   A. Achieving hemostasis.
   B. Reapproximating layers.
   C. Reinforcing fascial layers.
   D. Tight repair will promote vaginal tone and healing.
   E. Minimizing the amount of suture material.
4. Fundal dominance is essential for effective labor and delivery. Factors that promote fundal dominance include the following *except:*
   A. Uterine isthmus elongates and retracts in labor.
   B. Muscle fibers are concentrated in the fundal portion of the uterus.
   C. Uterine pacemakers are fundally placed, with one dominating.
   D. Peak of the contraction is reached in all parts of the uterus simultaneously.
   E. There is maternal effort with voluntary contractions of the abdominal wall.
5. The following are standards for monitoring a mother and fetus in labor *except:*
   A. Fetal heart rate for the first 30 seconds after uterine contractions
   B. Maternal heart rate
   C. Pelvic ultrasound for position and estimated fetal weight
   D. Urine for protein
   E. Maternal temperature

Answers

1. B
2. B
3. D
4. E
5. C

8

Immediate care of the newborn

APGO LEARNING OBJECTIVE #8

Sharon T. Phelan

Assessment of the newborn allows recognition of abnormalities necessitating intervention.

The student will demonstrate a knowledge of the following:

A. Techniques for assessing newborn status
B. Immediate care of the normal newborn
C. Situations necessitating immediate intervention in newborn care

Most infants make the change from intrauterine to extrauterine existence without difficulty, but some need the help of the physician and all should be observed closely during the immediate postnatal period. The normal infant cries and begins to breathe well within 1 minute of its birth without artificial stimulation. Mucus and blood should be aspirated from the mouth and nasopharynx after the head is born or soon after completion of the delivery. To minimize evaporative heat loss and subsequent cold stress, the infant should be dried with a warmed towel or blanket and placed under a radiant heat source with the head down. In an emergency out-of-hospital delivery and in some birthing room environments, the mother's chest is used as an alternative to the warmer. The infant is placed on the bare chest and then covered with a wrap, one that is warmed if possible. The skin-to-skin contact prevents cold stress. The main problem with this method is that the infant must be uncovered to be monitored.

A standardized method for the assessment of the newborn was proposed by Dr. Virginia Apgar. It evaluates the condition of the infant at 1 and 5 minutes after birth on the basis of five objective signs. Each is scored as 0, 1, or 2 (Table 8-1). The highest possible score is 10, with most normal infants scoring between 7 and 10. The lower scores indicate increasing degrees of infant compromise and depression and a need for treatment. Infants who are moderately affected usually have scores between 4 and 6. Muscle tone is somewhat reduced, and the infant is cyanotic; the heart rate is 100 beats/min or more. The infant usually responds to stimulation and can be resuscitated without difficulty. Those with scores below 4 are severely compromised and must be treated immediately.

Table 8-1. Signs for determining condition of newborn infant

Sign	0	1	2
Heart rate	Absent	Below 100	Over 100
Respiratory effort	Absent	Slow, irregular	Good, crying
Response to catheter in nostril	None	Grimace	Cough or sneeze
Muscle tone	Limp	Some flexion of extremities	Active motion
Color	Blue, pale	Body pink, extremities blue	Completely pink

It must be stressed that Apgar scores are only an indication of the effectiveness of the infant's transition from intrauterine to extrauterine life and have little long-term predictive value. These scores are very poor predictors of cerebral paralyses, and they have little value in the evaluation of the appropriateness of labor management. However, some have tried to use these scores as long-term predictors of infant outcome.

INTRAUTERINE HYPOXIA

The more depressed an infant is at birth, the more intervention will be necessary. Any interference with the supply of oxygenated blood to the fetus may cause intrauterine hypoxia. The most frequent causes are maternal hypotension, placental abnormalities, abruptio placenta, and cord compression. Most intrapartum causes of respiratory acidosis are transient, with minimal effect on Apgar score or transition to extrauterine life. Causes may include rapid second stage, nuchal cord, and placental accidents. Some authorities encourage obtaining cord blood samples for venous blood gas testing. This may help in distinguishing respiratory (acute) from metabolic (more chronic) hypoxic situations.

Among the factors making up the Apgar scores, the heart rate is the most sensitive indicator of the infant's oxygenation. A sustained rate of over 100 beats/min is the goal of any resuscitative effort.

APNEA

Infants may fail to breathe initially. Besides intrauterine hypoxia, this may be caused by narcosis from drugs administered to the mother, especially anesthetic agents. Malformations such as diaphragmatic hernia or tracheal atresia also may cause immediate respiratory difficulties.

RESUSCITATION

The important steps in resuscitating depressed infants are establishment of an airway, delivery of oxygen, and establishment of ventilation. Usually the heart rate is adequate or responds to ventilation. If it doesn't, cardiac massage may be indicated. In short, the same ABC's of resuscitation principles that apply to an adult are relevant to neonatal resuscitation.

Airway

Initially the nasopharynx and, if necessary, the trachea are aspirated. This can be done with a bulb suction or catheter with a secretions trap (DeLee suction). This is particularly important if the delivery has been complicated by thick meconium. In this situation many advocate aggressive suctioning of the nasopharynx once the head is delivered and before delivery of the thorax. The concern is that if the respiratory passages contain thick meconium it will be drawn into the lungs on the first breath (or ventilation), where it can cause an intense reaction. It should be noted that active suction at delivery will not necessarily prevent the syndrome of meconium aspiration, since this may occur intrautero and not just at the first breath.

Ventilation

Although the most efficient means of artificial ventilation for newborn infants is the bag-to-endotracheal tube method, bag-to-mask ventilation is most often used for initial resuscitation efforts. A self-inflating bag that has a pressure control to avoid excessive inflation pressures should be used. The compression rate should be 30 to 40 times per minute. If the infant does not respond quickly to this, placement of an endotracheal tube should be considered if the attendant is trained in tube placement. Otherwise, mask-assisted ventilation should be continued. Bradycardia and failure to initiate spontaneous breathing will necessitate further procedures, such as cardiac massage.

All resuscitative maneuvers should be performed gently. There is no place for rough and potentially traumatic procedures, such as holding the baby upside down and slapping it.

Stimulant drugs are not indicated in the resuscitation of the newborn. If the infant's depression may have been caused by the administration of narcotics to the mother, naloxone (Narcan), 0.1 mg/kg, should be injected intramuscularly (IM) or into the umbilical vein. If narcotics have caused the neonatal depression, there should be a response in 30 to 60 seconds after naloxone administration.

SUMMARY

Although in many larger hospitals a neonatal nurse or physician is present or readily available for each delivery, the obstetric attendant may assume responsibility for both the newborn infant and the mother during the immediate neonatal period. The ability to assess the infant objectively and determine when resuscitative measures are needed may be critical to the outcome of a pregnancy. In cases where fetal compromise is suspected, it is often wise to request a pediatric attendant be present for the delivery.

CRITICAL POINTS

- Apgar scores are extremely useful as an indicator of the success of the transition from an intrauterine to extrauterine environment and the potential need for resuscitation. They do *not* predict long-term outcomes effectively.
- Initial neonatal care involves drying the infant, keeping the infant warm, and careful observation for signs of compromise. This should not keep the mother from bonding with the infant.
- Neonatal resuscitation efforts should be first to clear the airway, then to ventilate, and last to perform cardiac massage.
- In cases where the mother has received narcotics, administration of naloxone to the infant can reverse the respiratory suppressant effect.

Questions

1. After the appropriate steps have been taken, the infant is assessed as follows at 5 minutes. The heart rate is 140 beats/min. The child is crying with some grimacing to suctioning efforts. The extremities, although still blue, show active motion. The Apgar score at this time is:
   A. 6
   B. 7
   C. 8
   D. 9
   E. 10
2. Resuscitation efforts should include all of the following *except:*
   A. Adrenaline IM
   B. Ensuring clear airway
   C. Warming
   D. Use of self-inflating bag for ventilation
   E. Cardiac massage if no response to ventilation
3. A term newborn is noted at 1 minute to have a heart rate of 90, and irregular respiratory efforts, and to be limp with no response to catheter suctioning. The body is cyanotic. The Apgar score is:
   A. 1
   B. 2
   C. 3
   D. 4
   E. 5

Answers

1. C
2. A
3. B

9

Postpartum care

APGO LEARNING OBJECTIVE #9

Sharon T. Phelan

Knowledge of normal postpartum events allows appropriate care, reassurance, and early recognition of abnormal events.

The student will demonstrate a knowledge of the following:
A. Normal maternal physiologic changes of the postpartum period
B. Normal postpartum care
C. Appropriate postpartum patient counseling

The postpartum period, often called the puerperium, is the period from 6 to 8 weeks after delivery during which the physiologic changes produced by pregnancy regress.

NORMAL PHYSIOLOGIC CHANGES

Uterus

The uterus, which at term weighs about 1000 g, returns to its nonpregnant weight of 60 to 80 g by a process known as involution. During involution the excess protein in the uterine muscle cells is either broken down by autolysis and excreted in the urine; or it is used, at least partially, if the patient is lactating. *The number of muscle cells does not change during involution but rather the size of each individual cell decreases by about 90%.*

After the lower segment has regained its tone during the first few hours after delivery, the superior surface of the fundus can be felt below the umbilicus. The size of the uterus decreases rapidly, so that at the tenth to twelfth day it is at the level of the upper border of the pubis, and by the sixth week it usually has returned to normal size. The more superficial layers of the decidua become necrotic and slough, but the bases of the glands that dip into the muscularis remain intact and active. The new endometrium, which eventually will line the entire cavity, regenerates from the remaining glandular epithelium.

The placental site is reduced to about half its predelivery size as the uterus contracts after expelling the placenta. It becomes progressively smaller, measuring only about 3 cm by 4 cm at the end of the second week. Immediate control of bleeding from the open choriodecidual sinuses is obtained by compression and kinking of the blood vessels leading to them. This is followed by clot formation in the open vessels. The remaining decidual and trophoblastic tissue at the placental site, the thrombosed choriodecidual sinuses and blood vessels, and a superficial layer of myometrium beneath the placental site are infiltrated with leukocytes; and tissue necrosis begins by the second day. Eventually the crust, composed of decidua, thrombosed vessels, endometrial glands, and myometrium, separates from the normal uterine wall beneath. This permits healing without significant scarring.

Regeneration of the endometrium from the remaining glandular tissue begins on the third day and progresses rapidly. The entire uterine cavity, except for the placental site, is covered by endometrium by the end of the third week. The placental site is reepithelialized within another 2 to 3 weeks by endometrium growing in from the edges and from the glands beneath the remaining crust.

The discharge from the uterus, which is made up of blood from the vessels of the placental site and debris from decidual necrosis, is called *lochia.* The discharge of pure blood from the open vessels soon changes to the *lochia rubra,* which is made up of necrotic decidua and blood. It gradually becomes less red as the vessels thrombose, but bloody discharge often persists for 4 to 5 weeks. This gradually changes into the white or yellow *lochia alba.* Bloody discharge may persist if placental fragments remain in the uterus or if for some reason involution does not proceed at its usual rate.

Cervix

Immediately after delivery the cervix is relaxed and gaping, but it regains its tone fairly rapidly. Within a few days the canal reforms as both the internal and the external os contract; after 10 to 14 days, the canal is well formed and narrow.

Vagina

The vagina never returns completely to the pregravid state, and sometimes there may even be some relaxation after primary cesarean sections.

Urinary tract

The bladder may be edematous and hyperemic, and there may even be areas of submucosal hemorrhage from the trauma of delivery. The hydronephrosis and hydroureter regress rapidly if the urinary tract is normal and within 3 weeks may have disappeared completely.

A marked diuresis begins within the first few hours after delivery in normal women; this is the mechanism by which excess tissue fluid is eliminated. Naturally, the diuresis is more pronounced in women who have been edematous than in those with normal fluid retention.

Breasts

During pregnancy the glandular and ductal tissues of the breasts are stimulated by rising concentrations of estrogen, progesterone, human placental lactogen, prolactin, cortisol, and insulin. The concentration of these hormones decreases promptly after delivery, and the time required for them to return to prepregnancy levels is determined in part by whether the mother nurses her infant. Prolactin concentrations rise abruptly but temporarily as a result of the stimulus of sucking. Although prolactin stimulation is essential for initiation of milk production, there is no direct relationship between the level of prolactin secretion and maintenance of an adequate milk supply. Women without anterior pituitary function do not lactate (e.g., Sheehan's syndrome).

Colostrum, a thin yellow alkaline fluid, is secreted by the glandular tissue of the breasts during late pregnancy and the first few days after delivery. Colostrum contains more protein than does milk, but less fat and sugar. The con-

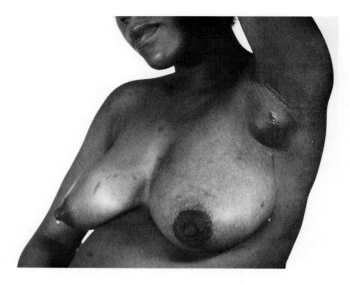

Fig. 9-1. Secretion from axillary breast tissue.

centration of globulin is greater than that of albumin.

On the third or fourth day after delivery, the breasts become *engorged* and are distended, firm, tender, and warm, and milk can be expressed from the nipples. Engorgement may involve axillary breast tissue or even that in other accessory nipples along the milk line (Fig. 9-1). Breast distention is primarily the result of engorgement of blood vessels and lymphatics, not from an accumulation of milk.

There is no large supply of ready-made milk; much of it is produced in response to the stimulus of nursing. The activity of suckling initiates a stimulus from the nipple that releases oxytocin from the posterior lobe of the pituitary gland. Oxytocin stimulates the myoepithelial cells surrounding the mammary glands to contract and force the milk into the ducts and from the nipples. This is called *milk ejection*, or *"let down."* In some instances the sight of the baby or even the thought of nursing will initiate the reflex.

Vital signs

There should be no great change in body temperature during the puerperium. A rise usually indicates infection. The pulse rate often is low. A rapid pulse should suggest the possibility of undue blood loss. Blood pressure should be altered only slightly in normal women.

Blood

The white blood cell count increases during labor and in the early puerperium. It may reach 20,000 to 30,000 if the labor has been prolonged. The rise is almost entirely the result of an increase in granulocytes. The count usually returns to normal within a few days.

As the plasma volume diminishes during the puerperium, the hemoglobin reading and the red blood cell count rise. The patient who has had an adequate iron intake during pregnancy and who has not bled excessively at delivery should not be anemic.

Body weight

An immediate weight loss of 4.8 to 5.8 kg (10 to 12 lb) occurs at delivery. During the first few days of the puerperium, the mother's body weight will decrease by 1.9 to 2.4 kg (4 or 5 lb) more as excess tissue fluid is eliminated. If the patient has been edematous, the loss will be greater. A further decrease will occur as the uterus involutes and plasma volume contracts.

Endocrine status

The major sources of hormone production during pregnancy are the placenta and the adrenal, thyroid, and anterior pituitary glands. Hormone secretion changes considerably after delivery of the infant and the placenta. The levels of estrogen and progesterone reach the nonpregnant range within the week.

Adrenal function is increased during pregnancy and returns to normal rather rapidly after delivery. Aldosterone production decreases promptly after delivery and the excretion of corticoids returns to normal levels within the first week.

Pituitary function, except for the production of prolactin and oxytocin, which are increased by suckling, appears to be unchanged by delivery. The production of anterior pituitary gonadotropic hormones is gradually resumed.

Ovarian function

The anterior pituitary inhibiting effect of estrogen and progesterone are removed when the placenta is delivered, and follicle-stimulating hormone (FSH) and luteinizing hormone (LH) secretions gradually rise, but the levels are lower than those noted during menstrual cycles. The time required for return of normal ovarian function is governed by the rapidity with which both hypothalamic-pituitary activity and ovarian response are restored. This is determined principally by whether the mother is nursing her infant.

Even though FSH and LH levels are well above those during the early puerperium, the high levels of prolactin inhibit the ovarian response to gonadotropin stimulation. Estrogen and progesterone concentrations in lactating mothers are comparable to those found in women with hyperprolactinemic amenorrhea.

Most women who do not nurse their babies will have a period of bleeding within 4 to 6 weeks of the baby's birth; whereas those who are lactating are often, but not invariably, amenorrheic as long as they nurse. Reports show the return to menstrual function in 91% of nonlactating multiparas and in one third of lactating primiparas within 3 months after delivery. Multiparas more often start to menstruate earlier, even though lactating. The first period of bleeding may be heavier than a normal menstrual period, and often but not always is ovulatory. If postdelivery endometrial biopsies are done, secretory endometrium is first noted at the forty-fourth postpartum day.

Ovulation can occur in women who are lactating, even though menstruation has not been reestablished. One study reported that ovulation occurred in 14% of women who were on a full nursing schedule and in 29% of those nursing partially. The earliest ovulation occurred on day 36 and the latest on day 422. These figures indicate the need for contraception in all recently delivered women.

CARE AFTER DELIVERY

Puerperal care is directed toward returning the patient to normal as rapidly as possible. In general, these patients are not ill and are treated like those who have undergone major surgical procedures. Ambulation should resume as soon as possible. A regular diet can be ordered immediately postpartum from a vaginal delivery.

Bladder care

The renal excretion of urine is increased during the early puerperium, but the patient may have difficulty in voiding because of perineal pain or local edema from trauma. The bladder may be atonic and can become remarkably distended without producing discomfort. If the patient voids spontaneously after delivery, no particular care is necessary except to check for the adequacy of urinary output and to palpate the abdomen frequently to make certain the bladder is not distended.

The patient who has not voided during the first 6 hours after delivery should be strongly encouraged to try. If she is unsuccessful, she should be catheterized. An indwelling catheter can be left in place for 24 to 48 hours if it is necessary to empty the bladder more than 2 times.

Perineal care

The patient needs to cleanse the vulva after each voiding and bowel movement with soft tissue and soap and water. The perineum should be wiped from its anterior aspect toward the anus. Tenderness in the episiotomy is usually caused by edema from too much suture material or sutures that have been tied too tightly. An ice pack will reduce swelling and should be used for the first 6 to 8 hours after delivery. The discomfort can be relieved by the use of a heat lamp for 20 to 30 minutes 3 times daily or by the administration of aspirin and codeine or nonsteroidal antiinflammatory drugs. Hot sitz baths can be taken as soon as the patient can get into the tub.

Postpartum patients may shower whenever they are strong enough. Tub bathing may be resumed when the patient can get into and out of the tub comfortably.

Afterpains

Multiparas often are troubled by painful uterine contractions during the first 48 hours after delivery. These usually are stronger while the baby is nursing. The pain can be relieved with aspirin and codeine or a prostaglandin synthesis inhibitor.

Lactation

Breast milk is clean, inexpensive, and readily available; and mothers should be encouraged to nurse their babies. It is well known that nursing infants develop passive immunity against certain infectious diseases from maternal antibodies that cross the placenta and that are present in colostrum and milk.

Maternal immunoglobulin (Ig) antibodies are transferred to the fetus across the placenta before birth. The predominant Ig in human milk is secretory IgA, which provides protection within the infant's gastrointestinal tract. The IgA contains antibodies against certain bacteria (e.g., *E. coli,* to which the infant is regularly exposed and against which it has little or no immunity).

The normal baby may be allowed to nurse before leaving the delivery room if the mother wishes. Babies and mothers, particularly primiparas, must be taught the techniques of nursing; consequently, the first attempts should be supervised by an experienced observer. She can show the mother how to hold the infant and help it grasp the nipple.

Breast engorgement is temporary; the acute symptoms last only a day or two. The discomfort is mostly caused by lymphatic and venous engorgement rather than by distention with milk; pumping the breast may not be particularly helpful and may even increase the symptoms after relieving them temporarily. In most women the discomfort can be controlled with a tight, supporting binder; ice; and simple analgesics. This will often happen after discharge from the hospital, so the mother needs to be warned about what to expect. Pharmaceutical methods to prevent engorgement are no longer encouraged.

Since drugs and medications can be excreted in the milk, the woman should be educated to only use drugs that are necessary and known to be innocuous to the infant. Concentrations of drugs in milk usually are no greater than in maternal serum. Even then, the immature digestive tract of the infant often prevents much of this from being absorbed. It is particularly important that the woman avoid the use of such substances as alcohol, heroin, cocaine, and methadone.

Contraception

Most women will already have resumed intercourse before the first postpartum examination, and some of those who use no contraception will have conceived. Breast-feeding provides some protection against pregnancy because prolactin appears to reduce ovarian response to gonadotropins. However, the contraceptive effect of suckling cannot be relied on, particularly when the interval between nursings is increased to several hours. Ovulation may occur before the first period of uterine bleeding in both nursing and nonnursing mothers. Pregnancy spacing should be discussed with the patient before she leaves the hospital, and a suitable and reliable method of contraception should be prescribed.

Low-dose oral contraceptives can be started soon after delivery, even though the infant is being breast-fed. If combined oral contraceptives are contraindicated, progesterone-only methods, condoms, or spermicidal agents should be suggested. *Diaphragms cannot be fitted or intrauterine devices inserted safely until the reproductive organs have involuted completely.* Intercourse can be resumed when the episiotomy is healed and coitus is comfortable.

DISCHARGE FROM THE HOSPITAL

Most women who have had normal pregnancies and labors are often discharged on the first or second postpartum day. Before the patient is discharged the breasts, abdomen, perineum, and uterus should be inspected and palpated. The provider should be sure that the patient is voiding normally, that her blood pressure has stabilized, and that she is physically able to cope with her responsibilities at home. Each patient should be instructed specifically as to what she may and may not do after leaving the hospital. It is preferable that she limit her activity for a week or two after delivery, but this may be impossible if she has no help.

She should be given specific instructions on symptoms-signs of endometritis, infection of the episiotomy, complications of contraceptive methods, when to resume activities (especially coitus), a schedule of follow-up visits for her and the infant, and signs of feeding problems with the infant. The last issue is particularly important for women who are breast-feeding and are being discharged before effective initiation of lactation.

Subsequent examination

Normal patients return to the office for examination when the infant is 4 to 6 weeks old. Those with abnormalities must be seen earlier. At the first visit the patient is weighed; her blood pressure is recorded; and the breasts, abdomen, and pelvis are examined. A clean-voided urine specimen should be examined. A follow-up hematocrit should be done. This is also a good time to obtain material for a cervical cytologic examination.

The patient should be evaluated for how effectively she is adjusting to her role as a parent and whether she has any questions regarding infant care. One should ascertain that she is keeping the appointments for the infant. If the patient has the infant with her, one can observe how she interacts with her child.

Follow-up on contraceptive methods or preferences should be done. Inquiries whether coitus has resumed and whether there are any problems should be made, especially in the breast-feeding woman who is more likely to have difficulty with dyspareunia. The possible presence of postpartum anxiety or depression should be ruled out or addressed as needed. If involution is complete, and the woman is normal physically and appears to be adjusting well to parenthood, she can be instructed to return in a year for her annual care.

POSTPARTUM COMPLICATIONS

A number of complications can affect the postpartum course. A quick outline of a few common ones and their management follows.

Hemorrhoids

During labor and delivery, pressure from the presenting part impedes the flow of blood through the hemorrhoidal veins, and the resultant distention of the vessels may produce permanent injury to their walls. The hemorrhoids usually decrease in size rapidly and cause little discomfort, but some may produce severe pain, particularly if they thrombose.

The local application of witch hazel packs or Anusol suppositories reduces the distention and relieves discomfort. The clot should be removed from hemorrhoids that thrombose. Hot sitz baths also may be ordered.

Pubic separation

The symphysis may be unusually mobile and there may be considerable separation of the pubic bones. This causes severe pain when the patient attempts to walk. The area is tender to palpation and the defect may be palpated. The only treatment necessary is a tight supporting garment to immobilize the pelvic girdle, and bed rest. Recovery usually is rapid.

Subinvolution

Involution of the uterus may be delayed by endometritis, inadequate uterine drainage, retention of placental fragments, uterine fibroids, and other less obvious causes. It occurs most often in multiparas. With delayed involution, bloody discharge is more profuse and lasts longer than usual. The uterus is large, soft, and boggy. Generally it is freely movable and there is no evidence of infection.

Normal involution can be aided by promoting adequate drainage during the early puerperium.

CRITICAL POINTS

- Most pregnancy-related changes have virtually reversed themselves at 2 weeks postpartum. By 6 weeks the maternal physiology has returned to its normal nonpregnant state.
- Lactation is dependent on the interaction of many hormones, but particularly estrogen for ductal priming, progesterone for alveolar maturation, prolactin for lactogenesis, and oxytocin for milk ejection.
- Return of ovulation may take 6 or more weeks but often occurs before the first menses. Therefore a woman needs to use an effective form of contraception even if breast-feeding.
- Postpartum care is directed to the mother's physical needs as her body recovers from the demands and changes created by pregnancy and delivery; toward education of the parent(s) regarding the expected medical changes and needs; and toward emotional needs as the woman redefines herself now that she is a parent.

This is best accomplished by ambulation. The course of involution is influenced only slightly by oxytocic drugs, and ordinarily they need not be prescribed during the puerperium.

Amenorrhea

Return of menstruation may be delayed after delivery because of minor and easily correctable endocrine dysfunctions. Other disorders such as anterior pituitary necrosis (Sheehan's syndrome) are more difficult to treat. The galactorrhea-amenorrhea syndrome, which is characterized by amenorrhea and persistent lactation, is discussed in Chapter 40, Amenorrhea.

SUMMARY

Not only the physical health of the postpartum woman is important; psychologic and social issues should be explored and optimized. The birth of a child is a window of opportunity to improve the health of the entire family unit.

Questions

1. The hormone most responsible for the production of milk is:
   A. Estriol
   B. Progesterone
   C. Aldosterone
   D. Oxytocin
   E. Prolactin
2. The process of uterine involution involves all of the following *except:*
   A. Autolysis of uterine muscle cells
   B. Decreased number of uterine muscle cells
   C. Decrease in size of the uterine muscle cells
   D. Return to normal size by 6 weeks postpartum
   E. Lactation and breast-feeding
3. The following contraceptive methods can be initiated within the first week postpartum in non–breast-feeding women *except:*
   A. Oral contraceptive pills
   B. Condoms
   C. Contraceptive foam
   D. Depo-Provera
   E. Intrauterine device

Answers

1. E
2. B
3. E

Ectopic pregnancy

APGO LEARNING OBJECTIVE #10

Philip A. Rosenfeld

Ectopic pregnancy is the leading cause of maternal morbidity and mortality in the United States. Early diagnosis and management not only save lives but also may preserve future fertility.

The student will demonstrate a knowledge of the following:

A. Differential diagnosis of first trimester bleeding
B. Risk factors predisposing to ectopic pregnancy
C. Symptoms and physical findings suggestive of ectopic pregnancy
D. Methods used to confirm the diagnosis of ectopic pregnancy
E. Treatment options

In their October 14, 1993, review article in the *New England Journal of Medicine,* Carsen and Buster wrote that "ectopic pregnancy may be the only life-threatening disease in which the prevalence has increased as the mortality has decreased." There are 40 to 50 deaths from ectopic pregnancy annually in this country.

According to the authors, the most logical explanation for the decrease in mortality despite the increased incidence is the improved technologic skill of the practicing physician and the ability to use ancillary tests to make a diagnosis before a life-threatening rupture occurs. About 88,000 ectopic pregnancies were diagnosed in the United States in 1989.

Implantation sites of ectopic pregnancies, in order of the frequency, are as follows:

1. Tubal (97% of all ectopic pregnancies) (Fig. 10-1)
   a. Ampullar
   b. Isthmic
   c. Fimbrial
2. Ovarian
3. Abdominal
4. Uterine
   a. Cornual
   b. Cervical

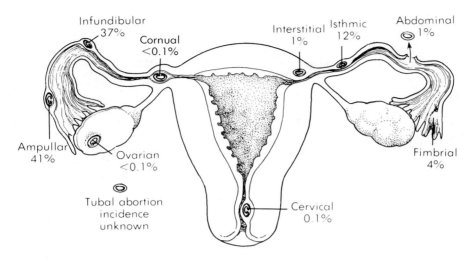

Fig. 10-1. More than 97% of ectopic pregnancies are located in fallopian tube.

Although every pregnant woman is at risk for an ectopic pregnancy, certain phenomena—such as sexually transmitted diseases leading to pelvic inflammatory disease, tubal reconstruction, artificial reproductive techniques and intrauterine devices, and other conditions that render the fimbria and/or the tubal structures functioning less than normally—generally precede the catastrophic event.

When a patient originally sees the physician (usually in the first trimester of the pregnancy) a gestation in an ectopic position must always be considered. The word *ectopic* means "out of the ordinary location" and refers in this case to a pregnancy outside the uterus. Most of these (41%) occur in the ampulla of the tube, with the second most common occurrence in the isthmus. Lesser percentages are found in the interstitial or cornual portions and still fewer in the ovary, cervix, and elsewhere in the abdomen.

While only 1.4% of all pregnancies were ectopic in location in 1986, ectopic pregnancy accounted for 13% of all maternal deaths, according to Lawson in the *MMWR. Morbidity and Mortality Weekly Report* (38:1-10, 1989). Those re-ported deaths ordinarily involved individuals who either sought no medical attention or reached the physician very late. It is now possible to make the diagnosis early, and it is important that this be done. Procedures that ultimately will save the tube for further fertility are best performed *without* the massive destruction of tubal epithelium and surrounding tissues that precede rupture. The physician can reassure the patient that nearly 50% of all patients with a prior ectopic pregnancy become pregnant again, but must also caution that approximately 16% will have another ectopic pregnancy.

EARLY DIAGNOSIS

Not long ago, when human chorionic gonadotropin (HCG) levels were difficult to obtain and were nonspecific and time consuming, the diagnosis of ectopic pregnancy too often was made only upon rupture of the tube. This condition obviously was immediately life-threatening. Today, HCG levels are confined to the more specific diagnostic beta level; and studies can be obtained as accurately on urine as on blood. Levels are now read down to less than 5 mIU quickly and with ease. The rise, fall, or plateauing of HCG levels becomes the basis for all early diagnoses. This gold standard of an HCG level taken early and followed repeatedly over days is today accompanied by the liberal use of the ultrasound.

As technical skills in ultrasound have improved, abdominal ultrasound has largely been replaced by vaginal ultrasonography, which has made early discovery or exclusion of ectopic pregnancy much easier than previously.

Until recently, this diagnosis was most often made by exclusion—that is, by the absence of an intrauterine pregnancy (IUP) with an HCG titer of 6000 mIU or more. With today's technical skills and vaginal ultrasound, the absence of an IUP with a level of approximately 1500 HCG units leads to suspicion of an ectopic pregnancy. Because of the improved definition of ultrasound, the ectopic pregnancy itself may well be found in its usual adnexal position.

The former triad of a delayed period, pain, and menstrual spotting must still be considered by the student; but because of the new accuracy of HCG findings an ectopic pregnancy sometimes is suspected when the menstrual period has barely been missed.

Reviewing repeated HCG studies, many authors have reported that a normal pregnancy will double its HCG level in about 60 hours. Abnormal pregnancies, including ectopic pregnancies, do *not* routinely double their HCG levels in this time. Some normal pregnancies, however, have shown a much slower than average rise. This factor alone, therefore, should not be used to establish the diagnosis of ectopic pregnancy except when HCG levels are followed over a longer period of time (approximately 2 weeks).

Pelvic pain is a symptom that always should be considered. The student should avoid the obvious maneuver of rapidly moving the cervix back and forth to recreate the pain during a pelvic exam. This could create confusion with the possible diagnosis of pelvic inflammatory disease. If the examiner pushes the cervix gently off to one side (3 o'clock or 9 o'clock), putting the mesosalpinx on stretch, the ectopic pregnancy and its location may more easily be found. The isthmus of the uterus acts as the fulcrum, and, in effect, the cervix points "to the side of the ectopic."

Intermenstrual bleeding is still a prominent sign and is due to a partial slough of the decidual reaction in the uterus to the ectopic pregnancy and its fluctuating hormone levels. Culdocentesis, the insertion of a needle into the posterior cul-de-sac of Douglas, will reveal nonclotting or, more properly, previously clotted blood in a large percentage of leaking ectopic pregnancies (Fig. 10-2). This test itself, however, is not absolutely diagnostic of an ectopic pregnancy, but rather suggests that there has been defibrogenated bleeding from some source in the pelvis. DeCherney pointed out that 65% of patients with an unruptured ectopic pregnancy can have a positive culdocentesis. Culdocentesis is used less frequently today because of previously mentioned diagnostic modalities and the discomfort caused by the procedure.

Another method of making an early diagnosis involves obtaining a single sample to test the level of serum progesterone. The finding of less than 10 ng/ml would indicate that the pregnancy is not normal. Some investigators suggest a level of less than 5. This too will not distinguish an ectopic pregnancy from another type of abnormal pregnancy, but will put the physician on alert.

Some of the less commonly used diagnostic indicators include curettage (done only in individuals who do not desire the pregnancy) and the flotation in saline of the material obtained at curettage to determine the presence or absence of chorionic villi. The Arias-Stella histologic reaction described originally in 1954 showed endometrial changes that pathologists thought were typical of a pregnancy outside of the uterus. This test is not truly specific.

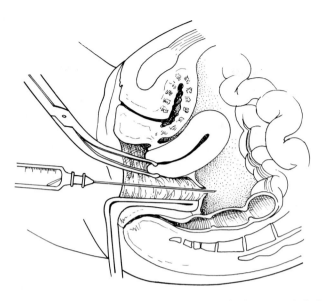

Fig. 10-2. Culdocentesis. Eighteen-gauge needle, with attached syringe, is being inserted into cul-de-sac.

Another method for diagnosis is laparoscopy. This test obviously may be used when HCG levels are abnormal, and with questionable ultrasonographic results or positive culdocentesis. Because ectopic pregnancy is now diagnosed earlier, the laparoscope is sometimes inserted when the ectopic pregnancy cannot be definitely localized to one side or another. When inserting the laparoscope, the gynecologist should be prepared to correct the ectopic pregnancy surgically through the instrument rather than simply making the diagnosis and "backing out."

TUBAL STERILIZATION AND SUBSEQUENT ECTOPIC PREGNANCY

Case-controlled studies—including those of Holt, Chu, and Daling from the University of Washington—indicate that women who have "undergone sterilization actually have a lower rate of ectopic pregnancies compared with either all women who have not undergone sterilization or women using no contraception." When compared directly, however, "women who had undergone interval sterilization (between pregnancies) had 3.2 times the ectopic pregnancy risk of women who underwent postpartum sterilization."

PATHOGENESIS

DeCherney has reported that the pathogenesis of ectopic pregnancy varies with its location. Ectopic pregnancies in the ampulla represent "a different anatomical entity from isthmic ectopic pregnancies. This is apparently based on the characterization of the muscularis of the two portions of the fallopian tube." Ectopic pregnancies in the ampulla develop in looser adventitious tissue, and there is less tubal luminal destruction. This is not true with ectopic pregnancies in the isthmus, when muscularis involvement leads to much more destruction of the lumen, necessitating segmental resection.

TREATMENT

In the past, ectopic pregnancies were radically excised. A laparotomy incision was made, usually vertically if the patient was hematologically unstable, and the entire affected tube was removed. At that time some recommended that the ipsilateral ovary, although it appeared perfectly normal, be removed. This was considered therapeutic because of the suspicion that if the ipsilateral ovary were not removed, a subsequent pregnancy might involve transabdominal fertilization. The development of a fertilized ovum too large to transport down the remaining fallopian tube could then occur, an "ideal" set-up for another ectopic pregnancy.

The standard of care today is operative laparoscopy, performed in the hope of finding an unruptured, early ampullar ectopic pregnancy. A linear salpingostomy is performed through additional laparoscopic openings, and trophoblastic material is removed from the tube—which one hopes is left undamaged. Hemostasis is achieved at the point of this incision (usually antimesenteric), and the tube is left open to close by secondary intention.

After such conservative therapy is done, serial HCG studies must be ordered to ensure that no actively growing trophoblastic material remains. Tubal patency following this less radical operative procedure remains high, in the 75% to 80% range. As previously indicated, 50% of these women become pregnant again. Probably one reason that this figure is not higher is because the other tube also may be abnormal, especially when a pelvic inflammatory process has been involved—usually a bilateral condition.

Today, if a decision for surgery is made, the location of the ectopic pregnancy is confirmed by laparoscopy. If the pregnancy is interstitial or cornual the salpingostomy described above is not appropriate, and more radical excision of the cornual portion of the tube must be done via a laparotomy with careful hemostasis. If the ectopic pregnancy is aborting out the fimbria, careful milking of the end of the tube can be accomplished. Such "milking" is not recommended with isthmic and ampullary ectopic pregnancies because the technique destroys endothelial mucosa, and because the procedure ordinarily cannot be done via a laparoscope.

A segmental resection generally is performed if the ectopic pregnancy is in the isthmus. This will, however, necessitate a second operation to anastomose the surgically shortened tube to preserve fertility through that tube. About 5 cm of normal tube ideally has to remain to allow such an anastomosis.

Newer techniques involving medical therapy are tried if, following laparoscopic surgery, trophoblastic elements remain and if the HCG levels do not quickly revert to negative or are rising.

Methotrexate therapy

Methotrexate therapy involves single or multiple dose methotrexate by mouth or intramuscularly or the insertion of methotrexate directly into the tube.

Methotrexate can be given in a 1 mg/kg intravenous or intramuscular dose on 4 alternate days, using 0.1 mg/kg of leucovorin rescue factor on the intervening days. It also can be given on a 1-time basis (50 mg), with the dose being determined by the patient's body area in m^2. Methotrexate is a folinic acid antagonist and has been used in the treatment of gestational trophoblastic disease. It interferes with the deoxyribonucleic acid (DNA) of the abnormal pregnancy and has been quite successful. Its use should be limited to ectopic pregnancies less than 3.5 cm and in those with HCG levels less than 5000 IU. The drug should not be used in ectopic pregnancies with known or impending rupture.

Tubal patency as demonstrated post–methotrexate treatment runs as high as 80%. However, one is not sure that the tube is functional as well as patent. Side effects of the drug, including local Stevens-Johnson syndrome, have been reported only occasionally; but the patient must be frequently assessed for glossitis, swollen lips, and other side effects.

One of the most difficult clinical decisions to be made before beginning methotrexate therapy involves the patient with pelvic pain that might well represent a rupture or leak, contraindicating the use of methotrexate. Some clinicians use methotrexate primarily *without* laparoscopic confirmation or linear salpingostomy for small early ectopic pregnancies. Some successful use of this drug in patients whose ectopic pregnancy has advanced to the stage of fetal cardiac activity has been reported.

Other therapies

Other treatment modalities should be considered by the student. Autotransfusion, Cell Saver, and other treatments have been suggested and used in the past. These probably are not justified at the present time. The Cell Saver may well keep the patient from donor transfusion and the risk of human immunodeficiency virus (HIV) transmission. One hopes that the correct diagnosis will be made before such a catastrophic event.

Concomitant intrauterine and extrauterine pregnancies, known as *heterotopic pregnancies,* traditionally were reported as 1 in 30,000. It is now believed that these are much more common, and the figures now quoted range between 1 in 4000 down to 1 in 2600. This may confuse the patient's postoperative course but must be accounted for, especially when reproductive assistance has been provided.

In addition, because of the potential of a fetal-maternal bleed, even with an early ectopic pregnancy, the Rh status of the mother should be determined. If she is Rh-negative, the patient must be given RhoGAM for later protection. The amount of blood loss is immaterial, and the student must always remember this step.

SUMMARY

Ectopic pregnancy diagnoses are best made early. Ultrasound, repeated HCG studies, and laparoscopy all contribute to diagnosis *before* rupture. Preceding conditions to be considered include sexually transmitted diseases (STDs), pelvic inflammatory disease (PID), tubal surgery, and use of intrauterine devices (IUDs).

"Think ectopic" when pain, missed menses, and a positive HCG are noted.

Rupture of an ectopic pregnancy is one of the few truly life-threatening events in gynecology. We cannot miss an opportunity to save such patients.

CRITICAL POINTS

- Although the incidence of ectopic pregnancies has increased, the mortality has decreased. This is due to increased sensitivity of β-HCGs, pelvic ultrasonography, and laparoscopy.
- Treatment is now done via a laparoscope, with less normal tissue removed than in the past.
- Preceding conditions to be considered include history of STD, previous tubal surgery, PID, and IUDs.

Questions

1. What is the relationship between the number of ectopic pregnancies and the mortality rate?
   A. Number is increasing while mortality is decreasing
   B. Number is decreasing while mortality is increasing
   C. Both are remaining steady
2. The majority of ectopic pregnancies occur in:
   A. The cornua
   B. The ampulla
   C. The isthmus
   D. The cervix
3. Early diagnosis is now easier because of:
   A. Culdocentesis
   B. β-HCG levels
   C. Early recognition of pain
   D. Ultrasound (abdominal and vaginal)
4. Recommended therapy for an unruptured ectopic pregnancy in the ampulla with an HCG greater than 5000 IU is:
   A. Laparotomy and salpingoophorectomy
   B. Segmental resection of the tube
   C. Methotrexate with rescue factor
   D. Salpingostomy and follow-up of HCGs

Answers

1. A
2. B
3. B
4. D

11

Spontaneous abortion

APGO LEARNING OBJECTIVE #11

John H. Mattox

Bleeding is a common complaint in early pregnancy. A logical approach to its evaluation may not only affect the outcome of the pregnancy, but also will help to reassure the patient.

The student will demonstrate a knowledge of the following:
A. Differential diagnosis of first trimester bleeding
B. Clinical differentiation of incomplete and threatened abortion
C. Definition of recurrent abortion
D. Signs of missed abortion
E. Complications of spontaneous abortion
F. Causes and complications of septic abortion

Abortion is the expulsion of the products of conception before the end of the twentieth week, when the fetus weighs less than 500 g. Abortions that occur during the first 12 weeks are *first trimester abortions;* those that occur from the thirteenth through the twentieth week are *second trimester abortions*. Abortions that occur because of some maternal, genetic, or embryonic defect are termed *spontaneous,* whereas those that are produced in-

tentionally are said to be *induced. Elective abortion,* a legal procedure in the United States, can be performed in a suitable facility by a qualified provider adhering to the statutes in each state and based on the request of the patient. *Therapeutic abortion* denotes a procedure to interrupt the pregnancy that is performed to maintain the health of the mother, a concept that includes her psychosocial well-being. Abortions that are accompanied by infection are termed *septic*. There are significant religious, ethical, and societal issues involved with the elective termination of a pregnancy that are not addressed in this chapter.

Early spontaneous abortions are estimated to occur in 15% of clinically recognized pregnancies, but the actual rate is higher. Some occur after a slight delay in the onset of menstruation and cause so few symptoms that medical aid is not sought. About 40% of implanted fertilized eggs die spontaneously, and most are not recognized clinically.

ETIOLOGY

The causes of spontaneous abortion are multiple and include fetal, maternal, and probably paternal factors. A definite reason for a specific spontaneous abortion cannot always be established because a complete analysis of all causative factors is impossible.

Genetic factors

Many early abortions of so-called *blighted ova* are actually a result of chromosomal aberrations. Boué, Boué, and Lazar—studying tissue from 1500 spontaneous abortions—identified chromosomal anomalies in 61%. On the basis of their material, they estimate that 150 of every 1000 pregnancies will terminate in recognizable spontaneous abortion. Banding techniques have shown that about 52% are autosomal trisomies; the next most common cause is monosomy 45 X, at about 20%. The remainder will demonstrate a mixture of karyotypic abnormalities.

Late abortions more often are associated with defective placental implantations than with defects in the embryo. However, Haxton and Bell—in a detailed study that included karyotyping of abortuses at 12 to 26 weeks—found major somatic anomalies in 20% and minor abnormalities in 14%.

Maternal factors

The maternal factors that may be responsible for abortion include both local and systemic conditions.

INFECTION. Acute serious febrile illness may be responsible for death of the embryo and abortion, whereas tuberculosis and other chronic diseases generally do not disturb pregnancy. Syphilis may cause fetal death but rarely causes abortion. Generalized peritonitis, appendiceal and pelvic abscesses, and other serious local infections often but not invariably cause abortion.

GENITAL TRACT ABNORMALITIES. *Cervical lacerations* that extend through the internal os may be responsible for repeated second trimester abortion and early labor. As pregnancy advances, the support provided by an intact cervix is lacking; the internal os dilates and retracts, the membranes rupture, and labor begins.

Developmental abnormalities of the uterus, especially the more advanced duplication defects, increase the premature delivery rate. The septate uterus can be responsible for spontaneous abortions.

The incidence of abortion associated with *uterine leiomyoma* also is increased if submucous tumors distort the uterine cavity and reduce the area in which normal placental implantation and growth can take place. Subserous and intramural tumors are less likely to interfere with the progression of the pregnancy. An increased incidence of spontaneous abortion has been postulated in women with *endometriosis*.

ENDOCRINE FACTORS. Disturbances in the secretions of reproductive hormones undoubtedly are responsible for some abortions, but probably are less important than previously thought. Reduced hormone secretion may be a result of abnormal trophoblastic secretion rather than a primary factor in abortion.

If the ovum is fertilized, human chorionic gonadotropin (HCG) from the trophoblast stimulates the corpus luteum to continue to produce estrogen and progesterone rather than to regress as it does during the normal menstrual cycle.

If the secretion of progesterone by the corpus luteum is inadequate, the endometrium may be so poorly prepared for nidation and for support of the fertilized egg that early abortion may result. It has been postulated that corpus luteum regression may be a result of defects in the trophoblast. If the trophoblast fails to develop normally—e.g., when the embryo is defective—the secretion of HCG may be too low to support the corpus luteum, and production of estrogen and progesterone is inadequate to maintainnormal decidua.

After the *tenth gestational week,* the trophoblast usually provides enough estrogen and progesterone to maintain pregnancy.

Normal function of other endocrine glands (e.g., adrenal, thyroid, pancreas) is important for maintenance of a healthy gestation. However, it appears that only when there is a clinically serious dysfunction could one ascribe the pregnancy loss to an endocrine abnormality.

PHYSICAL TRAUMA. Surgical removal of the corpus luteum or direct uterine trauma before 6 weeks' gestation increases the chances of spontaneous abortion significantly. If pelvic surgery is necessary, it should be postponed until early in the second trimester if medically feasible. Abdominal trauma rarely interrupts a normally implanted pregnancy. In many instances, pregnancy has continued despite fractures or crushing injuries to the pelvic girdle. Although a minor bump or fall can almost always be remembered by the patient to have preceded an abortion, it seems highly unlikely that injury is often a responsible factor.

MISCELLANEOUS CAUSES. Many of the miscellaneous causes for abortion are even less well understood than those already listed. Advanced maternal age, poor socioeconomic status and/or malnutrition, infertility, and ABO blood type incompatibility probably result in a hostile environment for an early pregnancy. The male contribution to abortion has been inadequately explored, but it may account for some instances of pregnancy failure. Daughters of women exposed to diethylstilbestrol run an increased risk of abortion.

Many studies suggest that *cigarette smoking* is responsible for a variety of reproductive failures, one of which may be abortion. Kline and colleagues reported that 41% of 574 women who aborted spontaneously were smokers, compared with 28% of 320 whose pregnancies continued for at least 28 weeks. *Excessive alcohol consumption* and *cocaine abuse* also have been implicated in an increased incidence of spontaneous abortion.

MECHANISM

The precipitating cause of most abortions is death of the embryo or its failure to develop normally. The demise usually occurs an average of 6 weeks before expulsion. The loss of the stimulus of the growing embryo results in a gradual diminution in trophoblastic production of HCG and, subsequently, ovarian estrogen and progesterone. This is followed by spasm of the spiral arterioles, ischemic necrosis of the decidua, and bleeding into the decidua vera and the choriodecidual space. The accumulation of blood separates the placental tissue at least partially from its attachment to the decidua basalis. Uterine contractions, which are induced by increasing prostaglandin synthesis in the disintegrating decidua, complete the placental separation and expel the ovum completely or in part.

CLINICAL STAGES AND TYPES

As an abortion progresses, it advances through a series of fairly characteristic stages that usually can be recognized clinically. These are classified as *threatened, inevitable, incomplete,* and *complete* (Figs. 11-1 and 11-2). Abortion also may be *missed* or *recurrent.*

Threatened abortion

During early pregnancy, usually after having missed one or two periods, the patient becomes aware of bleeding, which is slight and usually consists of the spotting of bright blood or of dark brown discharge. She also may experience mild cramping pain. The symptoms may subside within a day or two, but in about half of the cases both the cramps and the amount of bleeding increase. The eventual outcome is uncertain, and pregnancy may continue uneventfully. No change is observed in the cervix during this stage.

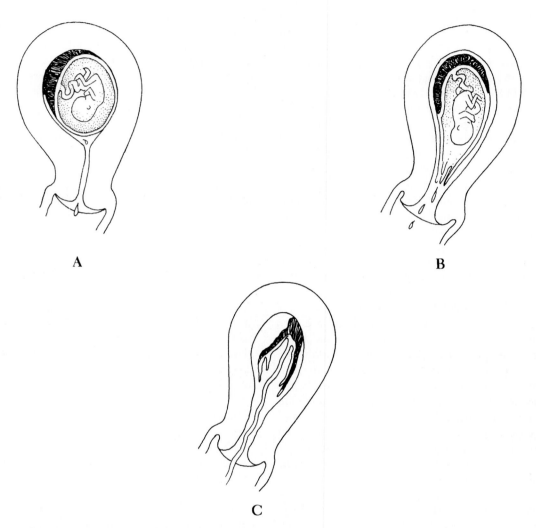

Fig. 11-1. A, Threatened abortion. Edge of placenta has separated but cervix is closed. **B,** Inevitable abortion. Placenta has separated, cervix is effaced and partially dilated, and membranes may be ruptured. **C,** Incomplete abortion. Fetus and part of placenta have been expelled.

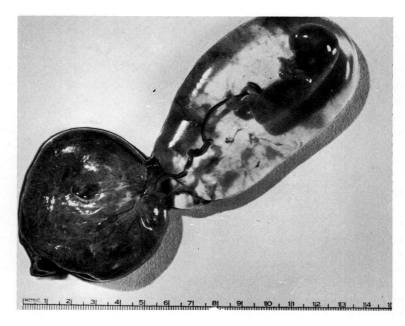

Fig. 11-2. Complete abortion. Entire products of conception have been expelled.

Inevitable abortion

If the cramps become more severe, the cervix begins to dilate; the placenta is separated from the uterine wall. The bleeding increases and often is accompanied by the passage of clots. The term *inevitable abortion* means that the cervical changes are irreversible and that any attempt to maintain pregnancy is useless. Progesterone therapy is futile at this time.

Incomplete abortion

In most spontaneous abortions, except those that occur before 8 weeks, varying amounts of placental tissue may remain within the uterus, either attached to the wall or lying free in the cavity. The patient usually reports the passage of some type of tissue, but rarely observes the fetus because it either has never developed or has degenerated some time before the contractions began. Pain associated with the cramps is severe; and the

amount of bleeding in some instances may be sufficient to produce profound anemia, hypovolemia, shock, and even death. The bleeding will continue until the remaining tissue has been removed or expelled, because only then can the uterine muscle contract to compress the bleeding vessels and control the hemorrhage.

Complete abortion

A complete abortion is one in which the uterus empties itself completely of the fetus and its membranes, the placenta, and the decidual lining. This usually occurs during the first 8 weeks after the last menstrual period.

Missed abortion

Occasionally, the products of conception are retained within the uterus long after the fetus has died. Because fetal death occurs some time before the products are expelled in the usual abortion, it has been suggested that the term *missed abortion* should not be applied unless the products are retained for at least 8 weeks. The cause for the delay is unknown, but spontaneous evacuation almost always occurs. Because of the increased sensitivity of the current pregnancy test measuring the specific amount of circulating β-HCG and the widespread use of transvaginal ultrasound, the diagnosis of missed abortion is infrequent.

Habitual abortion

Although isolated instances of spontaneous abortion are fairly common and abortions do not necessarily recur in subsequent pregnancies, repeated abortions may be the result of a permanent maternal or paternal defect. The term *habitual abortion* is pejorative and should be eliminated. *Recurrent pregnancy loss* is a more useful clinical term. This category is reserved for patients who have lost three or more consecutive first trimester pregnancies. In terms of clinical practicality, patients often are evaluated to some degree after they have lost two first trimester pregnancies.

MANAGEMENT

Because the treatment of each of the various uterine stages and types of abortion is different, an accurate evaluation must be made before treatment can be planned. A properly performed pelvic examination does not adversely influence the course of the abortion and is necessary to establish the presence of a pregnancy, to eliminate tubal pregnancy as a cause of the symptoms, and to determine how far the abortive process may have advanced. The examination should include visual examination and a gentle digital exam of the cervix and bimanual palpation of the uterus and adnexa. The degree of cervical effacement and dilatation can be determined by palpation. Because pathogenic organisms may be carried directly to the placental site—possibly in-creasing the risk of infection—gloves, instruments, and materials used in the examination must be sterile.

Patients threatening to abort experience a small amount of bright red bleeding after a period is missed; when the fertilized ovum is actively invading the uterine epithelium, bleeding can occur. This type of bleeding usually is of short duration and does not recur; but occasionally it becomes progressively more severe, particularly if caused by separation of a placenta implanted low in the uterine cavity. Such benign lesions of the cervix as polyps and cervicitis may be a source of bright red bleeding, as can invasive cancer. Such lesions can be detected by visual examination of the cervix.

Many women want to go to bed because they have heard that bed rest is important whenever bleeding occurs during pregnancy. Although this need not be discouraged, one should not make patients think it is essential. Bed rest will not prevent the inevitable abortion. The only effect exogenous progesterone therapy may have on the course of abortion is to delay evacuation of the uterus.

Transvaginal ultrasound may be helpful in determining the probable outcome when bleeding occurs during early pregnancy. With an intact, normal-appearing sac that contains a normal embryo or fetus, the prognosis is favorable. If the sac is broken or empty, there is no chance of a normal pregnancy, and the uterus should be emptied promptly.

A combination of serial ultrasonic exams and HCG assays provides the best prognostic information in women who bleed during early pregnancy. A favorable outcome can be anticipated if the embryo continues to grow at the anticipated rate and has normal heart action, and if HCG secretion increases steadily. Conversely, low or falling concentrations of HCG coupled with inadequate embryonic growth are associated with a high probability of abortion.

Because the diagnosis of inevitable abortion implies that irreversible progress toward uterine evacuation already has taken place, treatment should be directed toward reducing blood loss and pain. The administration of oxytocics is unnecessary because these substances do not hasten the process and serve only to increase the discomfort. When the abortion occurs between the tenth and the fourteenth weeks, uterine evacuation usually will be incomplete regardless of whether uterine stimulants are given. When bleeding is profuse it is preferable to empty the uterus surgically.

Placental tissue remaining in the uterus after an incomplete abortion should be removed. It can become infected and, in addition, may be responsible for continued and excessive bleeding. Most clinically recognized abortions occur between the eighth and the twelfth weeks of pregnancy; and, as the passage of the products at this period is likely to be incomplete, a planned program for their management will keep complications at a minimum.

Patients with incomplete abortions require uterine evacuation by suction. The procedure often can be performed in an office or outpatient setting with paracervical anesthesia and some sedation.

Surgical evacuation of the uterus should be considered for most patients with early abortions, even when the material that has been passed appears to represent the entire conceptus. Many who have had "complete" abortions between the eighth and the fourteenth weeks of pregnancy continue to bleed until the remaining placental tissue has been removed surgically.

The uterus should be evacuated promptly when there is evidence of endomyometritis or parametritis. When infection is present, antibiotics should be administered. In these cases close observation for sepsis is necessary.

Missed abortions can be treated expectantly with some products being expelled spontaneously, after which the uterus is curetted. However, it is desirable to hasten the process in most patients.

Before one evacuates the uterus, the diagnosis must be confirmed. Missed abortion can be suspected when the uterus is smaller than it should be for the presumed duration of pregnancy, when the uterus is becoming smaller from week to week, or when fetal heart activity that had been clearly detected can no longer be identified by sonography.

A coagulopathy, initiated by the release of tissue thromboplastin into the maternal bloodstream from the necrotic decidua and placenta, may occur after prolonged retention of a dead fetus (dead fetus syndrome). Clotting defects rarely occur in association with missed abortion during the first half of pregnancy but become progressively more likely if the pregnancy is advanced. The defect develops slowly and often is not seen unless the dead fetus is retained for at least 6 weeks. Fibrinogen, fibrin degradation products, and platelet levels should be checked periodically after fetal death has been diagnosed because the coagulopathy usually develops without any evidence of abnormal bleeding. This condition is becoming rare because of advances in early pregnancy diagnosis.

Recurrent pregnancy loss

The outlook for women who have aborted more than once is considerably less bleak than the 80% rate after three consecutive abortions that was initially suggested. Warburton and Fraser calculated the risk of a repeated abortion to be about 25%. There was no appreciable increase in the risk after subsequent abortions, except for couples who had no living children.

ETIOLOGY. The etiologic factors responsible for repeated abortion include congenital and acquired structural defects in the uterus and cervix, chromosomal abnormalities, chronic infections, hormonal deficiencies, perhaps psychogenic factors, and causes such as immunologic deficiencies that are even less clearly delineated.

A significant etiologic factor or combination of factors responsible for habitual aborters can be identified in *only 50%* of couples. Although the specific mechanism of action can be speculated for

Table 11-1. Causes of recurrent pregnancy loss in a retrospective study of 195 couples

Cause	Rate (%)
Uterine abnormalities	28.2
Corpus (15.4%)	
Cervix (12.8%)	
Infection	14.9
Endocrine dysfunction	5.1
Chromosomal disorders	2.6
Miscellaneous	5.6
Sperm disorders (4.1%)	
Systemic illness (1.0%)	
Smoking (0.5%)	
TOTAL "KNOWN" CAUSES	56.4
TOTAL "UNKNOWN" CAUSES	43.6

Modified from Stray-Pedersen B, Stray-Pedersen S: Etiologic factors and subsequent reproductive performance in 195 couples with a prior history of habitual abortion, *Am J Obstet Gynecol* 148:140, 1984.

the "known" entities, the exact pathogenesis often is unclear. Finally, it must be remembered that a clinical event associated with a single spontaneous abortion is not necessarily the explanation for recurring losses.

DIAGNOSIS. Stray-Pedersen and Stray-Pedersen categorized the causes in 195 couples who had a history of three or more consecutive spontaneous abortions. A summary of their observations can be seen in Table 11-1. Structural abnormalities can include uterine anomalies or the presence of a leiomyoma, usually submucosal. Either condition can reduce the available endometrial surface or provide the endometrial surface with abnormal vascularization, and presumably inhibit normal implantation and placentation. Some uterine fusion defects limit the capacity of the uterus to enlarge as the pregnancy grows. A

cervix that has been injured during a prior pregnancy or surgical procedure or one that is congenitally defective may not be able to remain closed as the pregnancy advances (incompetency of the internal os). Characteristically, the patients have had pregnancies that have terminated in the second trimester in a characteristic manner: the cervix effaces and dilates painlessly, with the membranes rupturing and labor being initiated. On the basis of the work of Danforth, it has been postulated that some patients have an excessive amount of uterine muscle in the cervix and a decrease in the normal concentration of fibrous tissue. This muscle relaxes during pregnancy, as does other smooth muscle in the body, and the cervix dilates prematurely. If the characteristic history is present, the diagnosis becomes more probable if a No. 8 Hegar's cervical dilator can be passed through the canal in the nonpregnant state without meeting resistance.

Although chromosomal abnormalities were identified in only 2.6% of the couples in the Stray-Pedersens' series, most authors report around a 5% incidence of chromosomal problems—usually a balanced translocation. It should be remembered that if the couple has a history of recurrent pregnancy wastage and a fetus with a malformation, the probability of a chromosomal abnormality increases fivefold.

Although hormonal abnormalities have long been considered a major cause of early pregnancy wastage, they probably are responsible for only about 5%. Diabetes mellitus and hypothyroidism receive the most attention. If either of these endocrinopathies is present, it would not necessarily be the only cause. A luteal phase deficiency also has been suggested as a probable cause of early pregnancy wastage. Premenstrual endometrial biopsy with histologic findings that lag more than 2 days behind the menstrual dates is considered the most useful method of making this diagnosis. Serial progesterone levels also have been used. It is important that more than one cycle be studied before a diagnosis is made and therapy instituted. Once pregnancy has occurred, it is difficult to make the diagnosis of a progesterone deficiency based on serum progesterone levels.

Endometrial and cervical infection or, more correctly, colonization of the latter areas probably should receive greater attention. *Ureaplasma urealyticum* has been identified in up to 44% of the women with recurrent pregnancy wastage; *Mycoplasma hominis* is cultured less frequently. Although significant systemic bacterial infections and viral infections have been associated with single pregnancy losses, it appears unlikely that they play a significant role in consecutive abortions.

Some miscellaneous disorders have been postulated as causes for consecutive abortions, including systemic illness (e.g., ulcerative colitis), nutritional deficiency, semen abnormalities, and excessive smoking. Although one should attempt to identify these problems and correct them if possible, again the pathogenesis remains unclear.

Women who have recurrent pregnancy losses may have several problems under the classification of immune disorders. They may share more human leukocyte antigens with their partners, have reduced cell-mediated immune response, lack maternal blocking antibody, and have lower lymphocytotoxic antibody titers.

Lupus anticoagulant, an abnormal immunoglobulin (Ig), probably IgM, has been identified in women having recurrent abortions or unexplained fetal deaths. How this IgM results in the demise of an embryo or fetus is unclear, but it is thought to facilitate thrombus formation through its effect on prostaglandins. Anticardiolipin antibodies also should be measured. They characterize part of the antiphospholipid syndrome.

A summary of the assessment of the couples who have experienced repeated abortions can be seen in Table 11-2.

THERAPY. The effective treatment of habitual abortion must be instituted before concep-

---

Table 11-2. Basic evaluation of recurrent pregnancy loss
HISTORY
Include documentation of pregnancy loss, symptoms of systemic illness
PHYSICAL EXAM
Emphasis on pelvic examination to detect leiomyoma or uterine anomaly
HYSTEROSALPINGOGRAM
Hysteroscopy may be used
KARYOTYPE
Special banding technique required to identify translocations
HORMONAL*
Thyroid-stimulating hormone 2-Hr postprandial blood sugar
PREMENSTRUAL ENDOMETRIAL BIOPSY
At least two cycles assessed; collated with basal body temperature recordings or timed (mid-luteal) serum progesterone
IMMUNE ASSESSMENT
Lupus anticoagulant Anticardiolipin antibody
CERVICAL CULTURES
Ureaplasma and Mycoplasma
*Depending on other clinical evidence.

---

tion. It is not unusual for these couples to achieve pregnancy during the course of the workup; therefore the physician may wish to advise the couple to use some contraceptive measure for a brief period during the course of the evaluation. The physician should approach this assessment in a positive manner. If the cause can be identified, many problems can be treated. If no cause can be found, the couple can be reassured that they have approximately a 75% chance of carrying the next pregnancy to completion. It seems prudent to attempt to correct any nutritional deficiencies and eliminate tobacco smoking, and any alcohol or illicit drug consumption.

SURGERY. Surgical procedures are seldom necessary to treat habitual abortion and should not be considered until the entire assessment has been completed and other potential causes have been corrected. More evidence is being accumulated that the correction of a septate uterus via hysteroscopy is feasible and offers patients satisfactory repair without transabdominal metroplasty. Concomitant laparoscopy may be required to ensure safety of the hysteroscopic approach. In carefully selected patients, removal of a submucous leiomyoma may return the cavity to a normal configuration.

Correction of cervical incompetence usually is performed in the second trimester when the cervix shows evidence of effacement and dilatation. The risk of ruptured membranes and infection increased during the second half of pregnancy. Although cervical cerclage has been recommended by several authors with a variety of suture material, the McDonald type of repair—with a large monofilament nonabsorbable suture—usually is preferred (Fig. 11-3).

HORMONE THERAPY. The most common entity to be treated in this category is luteal phase deficiency. This problem is characterized by a deficiency in progesterone but has several causes, ranging from poor follicular development to a progesterone receptor deficiency in the endometrium. During pregnancy, estrogen and progesterone are secreted by the corpus luteum and later by the trophoblastic cells. It is more likely that progesterone is the most important for the maintenance of an early human pregnancy. Progesterone therapy should be used only in patients who have a documented luteal deficit on the basis of study of at least two cycles. Progesterone vaginal suppositories (25 mg twice a day) or progesterone in oil (12.5 mg intramuscularly daily) have been used. Although there is no scientific evidence that these substances are teratogenic, they are not currently approved for use during pregnancy by the U.S. Food and Drug Administration. Other progestogens such as medroxyprogesterone and the 19-norsteroids, norethindrone, and norgestrel should not be used. Their androgenic activity has been associated with masculinization of the external genitalia of female fetuses.

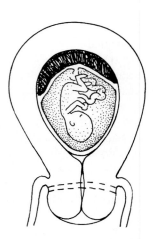

Fig. 11-3. Incompetent internal cervical os. Suture is in place to assist in retention of fetus.

PSYCHOTHERAPY. Some women who undergo pregnancy loss have extremely intense grief reactions. The most significant response is characterized by guilt. It is logical to assume that some compounding of this emotional distress takes place with frequent and consecutive pregnancy wastage. Every woman who has aborted will certainly become anxious and fearful as soon as she realizes that she is pregnant again. A sympathetic approach with a special sensitivity to the problem and patience on the part of the physician are potent factors in achieving an ultimately successful outcome of a pregnancy following repeated abortion, regardless of the cause.

There have been two noteworthy studies of the treatment with psychotherapy of women who were habitual aborters. Mann studied 160 pregnant women who had aborted repeatedly. Of the 145 women who did not have a demonstrable organic cause and were treated with psychotherapy, 81% completed the pregnancy successfully. Tupper and Weil treated a group of habitual aborters with psychotherapy regardless of the cause of the previous abortions, and also reported a similar pregnancy rate.

OTHER THERAPY. In culture-proved infections involving ureaplasma, an appropriate course of tetracycline therapy may result in improved pregnancy outcome. If a male has been identified as carrying a balanced translocation, donor insemination may be discussed as an option. Transfusions of paternal leukocytes for suspected isoimmune etiology should be considered experimental because there may be significant risks.

High daily doses of corticosteroids combined with low doses of aspirin have resulted in increased embryo and fetal salvage in women who have antiphospholipid syndrome or when lupus anticoagulant is present.

Questions

1. If a 23-year-old woman has some spotting and lower abdominal discomfort 6 weeks following her last menstrual period, a positive pregnancy test, and a closed cervix, she most likely has:
   A. An inevitable abortion
   B. A therapeutic abortion
   C. An incomplete abortion

CRITICAL POINTS

- Spontaneous abortions occur in approximately 15% of clinically recognized pregnancies and are associated with chromosomal abnormalities over 50% of the time.
- Slight vaginal spotting with mild lower abdominal discomfort is common in early pregnancy. When heavier, bright red bleeding is present and associated with pelvic cramps and cervical dilatation, the loss is inevitable. Progesterone therapy is futile.
- Most patients undergoing spontaneous abortion will empty their uterus completely. A curettage is not necessary. The patient should be monitored for possible infection.
- A systematic assessment should be conducted on patients who lose two consecutive first trimester pregnancies. A clearly identifiable cause will be found in only 50% of the patients.
- An abortion, whether induced or therapeutic, has significant emotional consequences for the woman. The provider should pay special attention to emotional care while dealing with the medical issues.

D. A threatened abortion
E. A septic abortion
2. The most common cause of a spontaneous abortion in the first trimester is:
    A. Defective placentation
    B. Uterine anomaly
    C. Chromosomal abnormality
    D. Cigarette smoking
    E. An immune disorder
3. When evaluating recurrent pregnancy loss, the following statements are true *except:*
    A. An identifiable cause is found in only 50% of the cases.
    B. A uterine cause is one of the common etiologies.

C. Hypothyroidism is a common cause of recurrent pregnancy loss.
D. Karyotyping the couple is an important consideration.
E. Lupus anticoagulant and antiphospholipid antibodies should be measured in recurrent pregnancy loss.

Answers

1. D
2. C
3. C

12

Medical and surgical conditions in pregnancy

APGO LEARNING OBJECTIVE #12

Jordan H. Perlow

> *Medical and surgical conditions may alter the course of pregnancy, and pregnancy may have an impact on the management of these conditions.*

The student will demonstrate a knowledge of the following conditions in pregnancy:

A. Anemia
B. Diabetes mellitus
C. Urinary tract disorders
D. Infectious diseases, including:
   1. Herpes
   2. Rubella
   3. Group B streptococcus
   4. Hepatitis B
   5. Human immunodeficiency virus and other sexually transmitted diseases
   6. Cytomegalovirus and varicella
E. Thyroid disease
F. Cardiac disease
G. Asthma
H. Alcohol, tobacco, and other drugs of abuse
I. Acute abdominal symptoms

OVERVIEW

The diagnosis and clinical management of pregnancy complicated by medical or surgical conditions is quite challenging and uniformly guided by the understanding that "pregnant women get sick too." That is to say that pregnancy is not a protective state for the mother; in fact it may increase the risks associated with some medical complications. The diagnosis and management of medical and surgical complications during pregnancy require an overall understanding of the normal physiologic changes that occur during pregnancy, the pathophysiology of the disorders and their implications particular to pregnancy, and an understanding of therapeutic options—taking into account the risks and benefits of various pharmacologic and surgical interventions. The student should approach the study of medical and surgical complications of pregnancy asking, "How does the state of pregnancy affect the patient's medical or surgical condition?" and "How does the patient's disease affect the pregnancy?" with respect to perinatal outcome.

ANEMIA

The hematologic system undergoes significant changes in response to pregnancy, beginning as early as 10 weeks' gestation. Plasma volume increases, plateauing at 30 to 34 weeks' gestation. The red blood cell mass also increases; however, because its increase is not proportional, a relatively decreased hematocrit is noted, often termed the "physiologic anemia of pregnancy." The hematocrit may rise slightly during the latter part of the third trimester as increasing red blood cell mass continues to increase until term, long after the plateau in plasma volume. It should also be recognized that multiple gestations demonstrate a greater increase in plasma volume than do singletons.

Women often enter pregnancy with poor or marginal iron stores secondary to menstrual blood loss. Pregnancy presents a significant physiologic demand for iron; if not met, this demand ultimately results in iron deficiency anemia. Women who do not receive iron supplementation during pregnancy will demonstrate lower hemoglobin concentrations, serum iron, and serum ferritin levels by term. It has been estimated that it would take the unsupplemented woman 2 years to replace her iron stores following pregnancy with dietary iron alone. Therefore iron supplementation during pregnancy is appropriate to prevent maternal iron deficiency. Sixty mg of elemental iron, equivalent to 300 mg of ferrous sulfate daily, is an appropriate supplement during pregnancy uncomplicated by anemia.

Once the anemic state is identified a careful history of underlying disease, the use of drugs, or the presence of gastrointestinal or genitourinary bleeding is sought. The next step in patient evaluation is a critical analysis of the components of the complete blood count (CBC). In addition to the erythroid values, the CBC provides red blood cell indices. In pregnancy the mean corpuscular volume (MCV) is 80 to 100 fl, and the mean corpuscular hemoglobin concentration is 31 to 36 g/dl. The morphology of the erythrocytes should be evaluated for sickle cells, spherocytes, schistocytes, and helmet cells. Evaluation of the white blood cell count, platelet count, and reticulocyte count provides additional information. Bone marrow aspiration is rarely indicated.

Iron deficiency anemia

Approximately 75% of anemia in pregnancy is iron deficiency anemia. Serum iron and the percentage saturation of transferrin fall, followed by a rise in total iron binding capacity. Finally, the CBC demonstrates a fall in hematocrit and the release of microcytic, hypochromic red blood cells. Therefore, in addition to the CBC, the evaluation of serum iron, serum ferritin, and/or transferrin saturation may be useful. The diagnosis is confirmed by demonstrating either low serum ferritin, or low serum iron and elevated iron-binding capacity. Treatment consists of patient education and the prescribing of oral ferrous sulfate, 325 mg given 3 times daily.

The effect of iron deficiency anemia on perinatal outcome has been difficult to assess because of confounding variables, such as nutritional and socioeconomic status. Nonetheless, increased risks for preterm delivery and low birth weight have been reported as associated complications.

Megaloblastic anemia

Megaloblastic anemia—characterized by macrocytic, normochromic erythrocyte indices—is the second most common nutritional anemia seen in pregnancy. It occurs as a result of folic acid deficiency and, less commonly, vitamin B_{12} deficiency. The diagnosis is based on the CBC findings and an evaluation of serum vitamin B_{12} and folic acid serum levels. Hypersegmented polymorphonuclear leukocytes also may be noted. Decreased folic acid levels may be seen in women taking oral contraceptives, anticonvulsants, and sulfa-containing antibiotics. Treatment consists of the appropriate vitamin supplementation.

The use of folic acid supplementation before and during pregnancy has gained significant attention recently because studies have shown a decreased risk in fetal neural tube congenital malformations in appropriately supplemented women.

Spherocytosis

Hereditary spherocytosis is the most common inherited hemolytic anemia. The inheritance pattern is autosomal dominant with variable penetrance. Hemolysis appears to occur as a result of increased erythrocyte osmotic fragility caused by a cell membrane defect. Diagnosis is made based on the CBC findings and family history. Folate supplementation has been recommended to maintain normal marrow functions. In the absence of severe untreated anemia, spherocytosis does not appear to affect perinatal outcome negatively.

Thalassemia

The thalassemias are a group of disorders characterized by a decreased rate of normal hemoglobin synthesis. An increased prevalence for this type of anemia is noted in patients of Mediterranean, African, or Asian heritage. The findings of a decreased hemoglobin level (typically 8 to 10 g/dl), microcytosis (a significantly low MCV), a low reticulocyte count, and the exclusion of iron deficiency should prompt consideration of thalassemia. Severity may range considerably from only mild suppression of synthesis of the affected globin chain (as in the heterozygous state) to its complete lack of production (as seen in patients with homozygous disease). Heterozygous patients are usually clinically asymptomatic and detected by CBC evaluation, often prompting a hemoglo-

bin electrophoresis study. The diagnosis is confirmed by an elevated percentage of hemoglobin A_2 (greater than 3.5%). Patients with thalassemia minima are asymptomatic and not at increased risk for abnormal perinatal outcome. Patients with thalassemia intermedia, however, often are symptomatic, with splenomegaly and significant anemia. They frequently are transfusion-dependent during pregnancy and can develop high output cardiac failure. Folic acid supplementation and transfusion when appropriate are the mainstays of therapy. These patients require intensive surveillance during pregnancy, including antepartum fetal testing and serial ultrasound fetal growth evaluations.

The homozygous state is termed thalassemia major, or Cooley's anemia. These patients are transfusion-dependent and rarely survive to reproductive age. Patients found to have thalassemia should have hematologic evaluation of their partner to evaluate the potential for the fetus to be affected. Such patients should receive genetic counseling.

Sickle cell anemia

Sickle cell anemia is a structural hemoglobinopathy. Whereas the structures of globin chains are normal in thalassemia, sickle cell anemia is characterized by a structurally abnormal globin molecule. Amazingly, the simple single substitution of the amino acid valine for glutamic acid at the sixth position of the β-polypeptide chain leads to significant changes in the "behavior" of this hemoglobin (hemoglobin S)—causing unimaginable morbidity, premature mortality, and serious impact on pregnancy outcome.

One in 12 adult African-Americans is heterozygous for hemoglobin S (hemoglobin AS), and thus has sickle cell trait. One in 708 has sickle cell disease, homozygous for hemoglobin S. Patterns of inheritance follow mendelian principles for autosomal recessive patterns of inheritance. The identification of a woman with sickle cell trait or disease should prompt an evaluation of her part-

Table 12-1. Sickle cell anemia: benefits and risks of prophylactic exchange transfusion

Benefits	Risks
Decrease vasoocclusive crisis	Transfusion reactions
Decrease Hb S production	HIV exposure
Decrease % Hb S; increase % Hb A	Hepatitis exposure
Increase O_2 carrying capacity	Alloimmunization

Hb, Hemoglobin; *HIV,* human immunodeficiency virus; O_2, oxygen.

Table 12-2. Hemoglobin percentages in sickle hemoglobinopathies

	S	A	A$_2$	F	C
Hb SS	80-95	0	2-3	3-20	0
Hb AS	20-40	60-75	2-3	2-5	0
Hb SC	40-45	0	2-3	1-3	50-60
Hb S β-thal	55-80	10-35	2-3	3-10	0
Normal	0	95	2-3.5	<2	0

Hb, Hemoglobin; β-*thal,* β-thalassemia.

ner. Genetic counseling and prenatal diagnosis are appropriate components in the prenatal care of these patients.

With the exception of an increased risk for urinary tract infection, patients with sickle cell trait are not at increased risk for complications in pregnancy. Patients with sickle cell disease chronically suffer from hemolysis, vasoocclusion, and an increased risk for infection. The course of sickle cell disease appears to worsen during pregnancy, with increased frequency and severity of complications. Severe anemia, megaloblastic crisis, sequestration and splenic infarcts, painful crisis (sickle cell crisis), preeclampsia, cholecystitis, pyelonephritis, pneumonia, osteomyelitis, and pulmonary embolism may seriously compromise maternal health. Cardiac failure may accompany these morbidities. Fetal complications include intrauterine growth restriction, low birth weight, fetal distress, and intrauterine fetal death. Increased maternal and perinatal mortality have also been reported.

Treatment is largely symptomatic and includes hydration, oxygen, pain management, blood transfusions, and the aggressive diagnosis and treatment of infection. Pneumococcal vaccina-

tion and folic acid supplementation also are recommended. The use of prophylactic red cell transfusion is controversial (Table 12-1). Transfusion-related morbidities such as isoimmunization, infectious disease transmission, and transfusion reaction are worrisome and must be taken into account when using this therapy. The goal of transfusion is to reduce the occurrence of sickle cell crisis and other complications by maintaining the percentage of hemoglobin A at greater than 40% and the hematocrit at less than 35%. Partial exchange transfusions with phlebotomy have been used to increase more effectively the percentage of hemoglobin A and to reduce stress on the cardiovascular system. This technique is typically begun at 24 to 28 weeks' gestation.

Intensive fetal surveillance with fetal movement assessment, antepartum fetal heart rate and biophysical testing, and serial ultrasound examinations to evaluate fetal growth and amniotic fluid volume are important components of third trimester management.

Combined structural hemoglobinopathies

Several inherited combinations of hemoglobinopathies may occur (Table 12-2). Hemoglobin SC disease is the most common, occurs in 1 of 757 adult African-Americans, and is characterized by an individual who is heterozygous for both hemoglobin S and hemoglobin C. Hemoglobin SC disease is similar to sickle cell disease with respect to clinical presentation, associated complications, and maternal-fetal management. Pregnancy has a deleterious effect on this disease and increases maternal and perinatal mortality.

The combined inheritance of hemoglobin S β-thalassemia occurs in 1 of 1672 adult African-Americans. These individuals are characterized hematologically by the presence of increased hemoglobin A and hemoglobin F levels. Hemoglobin S is present and exceeds the percentage of hemoglobin A. Perinatal concerns are similar to those in sickle cell disease, but the clinical course is typically milder.

DIABETES MELLITUS

We undertake the study of diabetes during pregnancy by recognizing the distinction between preexisting diabetes mellitus (pregestational diabetes) and diabetes first occurring or diagnosed during pregnancy (gestational diabetes). Each disorder has special implications for the mother and her developing fetus and is approached individually.

Pregestational diabetes

Before the discovery of insulin by Banting and Best (1922), pregnancy was a rare event in the lives of diabetics, and one fraught with very high rates of maternal and fetal death. Along with the discovery of this important hormone and an increased understanding of the pathophysiology of diabetes came marked improvement in the unacceptably high risks faced by pregnant diabetics. With modern intensive perinatal management of diabetics, fetal and neonatal mortalities have fallen dramatically, from approximately 65% to a corrected rate nearly equivalent to that of nondiabetic patients. Poorly controlled diabetes,

however, considerably increases the incidence of such complications as retinopathy, nephropathy, diabetic ketoacidosis, hypertension, severe preeclampsia, preterm labor and delivery, birth defects, fetal growth aberrations, intrauterine asphyxia and fetal death, and neonatal metabolic derangements.

In pregestational diabetes, where there is an inherent deficiency of endogenous insulin, significant maternal hyperglycemia occurs in the absence of exogenous insulin. As there is a very close correlation between maternal glucose level and fetal glucose uptake, maternal hyperglycemia leads to fetal hyperglycemia. The fetal pancreas responds with beta-cell hyperplasia, which leads to fetal hyperinsulinemia. It is believed that hyperglycemia and hyperinsulinemia contribute to the multiple fetal morbidities and increased mortality noted among fetuses developing within diabetic mothers.

In 1949, Priscilla White published her observations that the duration of time a patient has been diabetic and the presence of vascular complications correlated progressively with perinatal risks. This led to what has been termed "White's Classification," which is illustrated in Table 12-3.

The diabetic is at significantly increased risk for having a baby with major congenital malformations—birth defects that may be fatal, necessitate surgery, or have significant long-term effects. These malformations include caudal regression syndrome, anencephaly, spina bifida and hydrocephalus, cardiac anomalies such as transposition of the great vessels, atrial and ventricular septal defects, and renal anomalies. Approximately 1% of nondiabetic women will have such affected fetuses. Among insulin-dependent diabetics, however, the risk is 7 to 13 times greater!

Aggressive glucose control with insulin is the cornerstone to the management of diabetes during pregnancy and may decrease the risk of malformations noted above. In fact, patients managed in aggressive diabetes treatment programs *before conception* may have major malformation

Table 12-3. Modified White's classification of diabetes in pregnancy

Class	Age of onset (yr)	Duration (yr)	Treatment	Associated disease
A	During pregnancy		Class A1—Diet therapy Class A2—Insulin therapy	None
B	>20	<10	Human insulin	None
C	10-19	and/or 10-19	Human insulin	None
D	10	and/or 20	Human insulin	Benign retinopathy
F	Any	Any	Human insulin	Nephropathy
R	Any	Any	Human insulin	Proliferative retinopathy
H	Any	Any	Human insulin	Cardiac disease
T	Any	Any	Human insulin	Renal transplant

rates similar to those of nondiabetics. Our challenge is to actively promote preconceptional counseling and aggressive periconceptional diabetes management. Diabetic women capable of reproduction should be certain to consume 0.4 mg of folic acid daily before pregnancy to decrease the risk of fetal neural tube defects and should be provided prenatal vitamins when pregnancy is suspected.

Perinatal management components include: (1) patient education and laboratory evaluation for multi-organ disease; (2) appropriate dietary consultation; (3) administration of insulin to achieve euglycemia; (4) home glucose self-monitoring; (5) serial fetal ultrasound evaluations to detect congenital malformations and growth disturbances; (6) fetal surveillance to decrease risks for intrauterine fetal asphyxia and death; and (7) continued specialized care during the intrapartum period.

Insulin requirement is often calculated based on patient weight and trimester, but frequent adjustments and increasing insulin requirements during pregnancy are the rule. To achieve a steadier state of glucose control, regular and neutral protamine Hagedorn (NPH) insulin are provided before breakfast and dinner. Of the total insulin dose, two thirds is given in the morning,

Table 12-4. Diabetes in pregnancy: target plasma glucose levels

Time of glucose check	Target value (mg/dl)
Fasting (prebreakfast)	60-90
Before lunch, dinner	60-105
2 hr postmeals	120
Overnight (2 AM-6 AM)	60-90

with two thirds of that dose consisting of NPH insulin and the remaining one third regular insulin. The predinner dose (one third of the total) has equal quantities of regular and NPH insulin. Patients are then required to perform glucose self-monitoring and to record their results in a log for review at each prenatal visit or by phone on a more frequent basis. Adjustments are made as needed to maintain blood sugar within the ranges noted in Table 12-4.

Delivery management varies based on clinical circumstances. Any worsening of maternal or fetal status may necessitate evaluation for delivery irrespective of gestational age. As term approaches, many clinicians will perform amniocentesis at 37 to 38 weeks' gestation to evaluate for fetal pulmonary maturity by testing amniotic fluid for the lecithin/sphingomyelin ratio and phosphatidyl-glycerol. It is also reasonable to follow patients to term and allow for spontaneous labor as long as maternal and fetal status remain uncompromised. For patients at highest risk—those with a history of prior stillbirth, renal disease, hypertension, noncompliance with medical care, and/or vasculopathy—timing of delivery is often based on the determination of fetal pulmonary maturity, followed by induction of labor or scheduled cesarean section, depending on individual clinical circumstances.

Ultrasound evaluation of the estimated fetal weight is frequently used to help plan delivery management. While controversial and not uniformly accepted, the estimate of a fetal weight at 4000 to 4500 g in the mother affected by diabetes often will prompt consideration of cesarean section to decrease the potential for shoulder dystocia and birth trauma.

During the process of labor and delivery, patients are managed with fetal heart rate monitoring, and often an insulin infusion is administered. It is helpful to have pediatric personnel present at delivery to evaluate for any congenital anomalies, birth injury, or respiratory distress and to provide for appropriate newborn management. The neonate born to the diabetic gravida is at risk for hypoglycemia, hypocalcemia, and hyperbilirubinemia, all of which necessitate prompt recognition and treatment.

Insulin requirements in the early postpartum period decrease dramatically; therefore dosing readjustments are necessary.

Gestational diabetes

Gestational diabetes (GDM) is carbohydrate intolerance with onset or first recognition during pregnancy. Practically speaking, most obstetric practices perform routine screening on all pregnant patients at 24 to 28 weeks' gestation. Other

Table 12-5. Risk factors for gestational diabetes

Maternal age >30 years
Family history of diabetes
Prior delivery of a macrosomic infant
Obesity
Chronic hypertension
History of stillbirth
Prior infant with congenital malformation
Polyhydramnios
Native American population

practitioners screen patients only with traditional risk factors (Table 12-5). A risk factor screening approach, however, has been estimated to miss up to 75% of affected pregnancies. A GDM screening test can be performed in the fasting or fed states and consists of a 1-hour 50-g oral glucose challenge. Patients with a 1-hour test result of greater than 140 mg/dl are considered at increased risk for GDM and should undergo a 3-hour 100-g glucose tolerance test (GTT). For the GTT, the patient must have consumed at least 150 g of carbohydrate for the 3 days before the test; and the GTT must be performed in the fasting state. Patients with two or more abnormal values meet diagnostic criteria for GDM (Table 12-6) or White's class A diabetes.

The fetus of the gestational diabetic is at increased risk for macrosomia, polycythemia, and the metabolic derangements of hypoglycemia, hypocalcemia, and hyperbilirubinemia. Unlike preexisting diabetes, an increased risk for congenital malformations has not been observed. Patients with GDM should begin an American Diabetes Association diet, usually consisting of between 2000 and 2500 kcal per day. Monitoring these patients consists of following fasting and postprandial blood glucose levels at least every 2 weeks. Many practitioners utilize home glucose monitoring for patients with GDM, as practiced for pregestational diabetics. Most patients can

Table 12-6. Diagnosis of gestational diabetes*

100 g oral GTT	Plasma glucose: normal (mg/dl)
Fasting	<105
1 hr	<190
2 hr	<165
3 hr	<145

*Diagnosis of gestational diabetes requires two abnormal values.
GTT, Glucose tolerance test.

be adequately managed with dietary therapy (White's class A1 GDM). Patients who are well controlled with diet therapy alone are not at increased risk for perinatal mortality; therefore antepartum fetal surveillance, other than fetal movement counting, is not routinely recommended. Patients who require the addition of insulin for adequate GDM management should be placed in an antepartum testing protocol similar to that for pregestational diabetics. Serial evaluation of fetal growth using ultrasound may be useful to evaluate for macrosomia, which can complicate up to 50% of GDM-affected pregnancies. As with pregestational diabetes, significant concerns exist for the potential complications of fetal macrosomia, shoulder dystocia, and birth trauma to the fetus and maternal genital tract. Although ultrasound may provide clues to the presence of macrosomia, it is not predictive of complications; and compulsive attention to the course of labor and judicious use of operative vaginal delivery become critical aspects of management.

Approximately 50% of patients with GDM will develop non–insulin-dependent diabetes over the 5 years following their affected pregnancy. Therefore all patients diagnosed with GDM during pregnancy require a 75-g 2-hour GTT at their 6-week postpartum checkup.

THYROID DISEASE

Thyroid disease is not uncommon among reproductive-age women and may complicate 0.2% of pregnancies. Although the exact nature of thyroid effects on pregnancy are incompletely understood, maternal and fetal well-being clearly depend on normal thyroid function. Therefore an understanding of these disorders and implications of treatment is warranted.

Physiology in pregnancy and laboratory assessment

Many normal physiologic changes in thyroid metabolism occur during pregnancy. Understanding these is critical to an understanding of the disease state in pregnancy. Renal clearance of iodine is increased because of increased glomerular filtration rate. With marginal iodine intake, a deficiency may result. The iodine in iodized table salt and prenatal vitamins usually prevents this problem in industrialized countries.

Enlargement of the thyroid in pregnancy (once used as a "pregnancy test" by ancient Egyptians) is thought to represent a compensatory mechanism to maintain gland activity despite decreased iodine levels. Therefore the availability of iodine in the diet can influence the appearance of goiter in the pregnant population.

As in the evaluation of most disease states in pregnancy, one should not interpret thyroid function as for the nonpregnant woman because dramatic changes occur that are related to the hormonal changes of pregnancy (primarily hyperestrogenemia) (Table 12-7). The most dramatic change is an increase in thyroxine-binding globulin (TBG) to levels double nonpregnant levels by only 12 weeks' gestation. Because more than 99% of thyroid hormone is bound to TBG, and given

Table 12-7. Pregnancy and thyroid function tests

Test	Normal pregnancy	Hyperthyroidism
TSH	No change	Decreased
TBG	Increased	No change
Total T_4	Increased	Increased
Free T_4	No change	Increased
Total T_3	Increased	Increased
Free T_3	No change	Increased

TSH, Thyroid-stimulating hormone; *TBG,* thyroxine-binding globulin; *T_4,* thyroxine; *T_3,* triiodothyronine.

that biologic activity is only affected by the unbound free fraction, the total thyroxine (T_4) value will be falsely elevated. Therefore the free fraction is best assayed for, and free T_4 and free triiodothyronine (T_3) are the tests one should use to evaluate hyperthyroid states. These "free" levels do not change significantly in pregnancy; however, they may be slightly increased early in pregnancy with parallel rises in human chorionic gonadotropin. The availability of assays for free T_4 has negated the need for estimations and derivations of thyroid function using the free T_4 index or free T_3 index.

Hyperthyroidism

Thyrotoxicosis is seen in 1 of 2000 pregnant women. The most common cause is Graves' disease, named for the Irish physician Robert James Graves (1796-1853). Other contributing factors are noted in Table 12-7. Graves' disease is an autoimmune process that occurs as a result of stimulatory antibodies leading to increased T_4. This stimulatory immunoglobulin (Ig) G antibody may cross the placenta and has been found in thyrotoxic neonates. These antibodies therefore mimic thyroid-stimulating hormone (TSH), resulting in the clinical manifestations of hyperthyroidism. Exophthalmos is also characteristic of this disorder, resulting from antibody complex deposition within the extraocular muscles. Most women with mild to moderate disease appear to tolerate pregnancy well, and fortunately there is no clear evidence that pregnancy worsens the disease or makes it more difficult to treat.

Hyperthyroidism also may result from thyroid gland destruction or disruption that causes release of thyroid hormone. In these women another antibody, antimicrosomal antibody, may be present. This antibody is frequently seen in patients with Hashimoto's thyroiditis.

The perinatal outcome in women with thyrotoxicosis depends on the ability to achieve metabolic control. Untreated or suboptimally treated patients are at increased risk for preeclampsia, congestive heart failure (CHF), intrauterine growth restriction (IUGR), and stillbirth. Preterm labor and preterm delivery contribute to an overall increase in perinatal mortality and morbidity.

Mild disease may be difficult to diagnose because many of the "hypermetabolic" aspects of pregnancy mimic hyperthyroid symptoms and signs. Resting tachycardia, thyromegaly, exophthalmos, onycholysis, and failure to gain weight despite normal caloric intake are helpful diagnostic signs. An increased free T_4 is confirmatory and typically is seen in conjunction with a suppressed TSH.

Treatment of hyperthyroidism is aimed at providing medication directed at blocking the glandular production of hormone (thiourea compounds) and/or the peripheral manifestations of thyroid hormone (β-blockers). The thiourea compound propylthiouracil (PTU) crosses the placenta and thus has the potential to cause fetal hypothyroidism and goiter. Therefore it is critical to monitor such pregnancies closely, using the least amount of medication to achieve the appropriate effect. Fetal and neonatal thyroid disease also may be caused by transplacental effects of maternal stimulating and blocking antibodies.

When treating hyperthyroidism during pregnancy, PTU is the drug of choice. Long-term follow-up studies on exposed fetuses show no intelligence quotient deficiencies. The usual beginning dose of 300 mg/day is empiric and needs monitoring and potential adjustment. Maintaining the patient on a PTU dose such that the free T_4 level is in the upper range of normal usually is ideal. A change in dose may take 3 to 4 weeks to demonstrate itself in follow-up laboratory tests. The PTU exerts its action by inhibiting thyroglobulin synthesis, iodination of thyroglobulin, and the conversion of T_4 to the more active T_3. Maternal side effects include rash, drug fever, and pruritus (5%). Agranulocytosis may occur in 0.1% of users.

Thyroidectomy may be performed after thyrotoxicosis has been controlled medically. This procedure may be important for noncompliant patients, in those whose medical therapy is suboptimal, or for those who have had thyroid storm.

THYROID STORM. Thyroid storm is a life-threatening condition in which the signs and symptoms of thyrotoxicosis are greatly exaggerated. It is an endocrinologic emergency that may occur in undiagnosed and partially treated hyperthyroid patients. Fortunately it is uncommon in pregnancy, but it may occur in association with labor and delivery, infection, or surgery. More common is the appearance of CHF from the long-standing chronic myocardial effects of T_4. These symptoms may be exacerbated by pregnancy, preeclampsia, anemia, multiple gestation, or combinations of these. Treatment consists of PTU and potassium iodide orally or via a nasogastric tube. Rehydration and thermoregulation are critical components of treatment. Aggressive treatment of infection, hypertension, and anemia are also crucial. Goals of therapy include the control of hormone production and release, reversal of peripheral hormonal effects, identifying and preventing precipitating factors (infection, diabetic ketoacidosis, myocardial infarction, pulmonary embolism), and the treatment of hypotension, hyperthermia, severe tachycardia, CHF, and

dehydration. The intensive care unit is the appropriate setting for the management of this serious condition.

FETAL AND NEONATAL EFFECTS OF TREATMENT. As noted previously, intellectual and physical development and thyroid function in children born to thyrotoxic mothers treated with PTU during pregnancy have not been shown to be adversely affected. The risk of hypothyroidism to the fetus has been estimated at no greater than 2%. Because prolonged administration of iodide significantly increases the risk of hypothyroidism and goiter in the infant, its use is restricted to preoperative treatment before thyroidectomy and in thyroid storm. Taking PTU is not a contraindication to breast-feeding. Infants of mothers with thyrotoxicosis and who have autoantibodies are at risk for hyperthyroidism. Persistent fetal tachycardia may be a hint to the occurrence of this problem in postnatal life. Neonatal thyrotoxicosis has been estimated to occur in about 1% of infants of mothers with Graves' disease. Likewise, the infant exposed to these antibodies and drugs may not manifest symptoms until days to weeks after birth, thus requiring close pediatric follow-up.

Hypothyroidism

Hypothyroidism is manifested by a rise in TSH and a decrease in free T_4 or a failed increase in total T_4. The disease may not be clinically apparent in its milder forms. Severe disease is uncommon because it typically is associated with infertility. Hypothyroidism is usually secondary to Hashimoto's disease, thyroid gland ablation by iodine-131, surgery, or antithyroid medications. Iodine deficiency in the United States is very rare, and secondary hypothyroidism from hypothalamic or pituitary failure also is uncommon.

Hypothyroidism, if not corrected, is clearly associated with adverse perinatal outcome. Risks for preeclampsia, intrauterine fetal death (IUFD), low birth weight, and placental abruption are all increased. Likewise, CHF also may complicate the maternal condition. Treatment consists of thyroid hormone replacement (typically T_4-synthroid). Treatment usually is begun at 0.05 to 0.10 mg/day, with the dose increased as needed to a maximum of 0.20 mg/day. It is important for the physician to recall that replacement requirements typically will increase during the course of the pregnancy. The clinical importance of subclinical hypothyroidism in pregnancy is less clear, although a high incidence of this thyroid condition has been reported in pregnant women with type I diabetes and normal T_4 levels before conception.

FETAL AND NEONATAL EFFECTS. Infants born to hypothyroid women typically are healthy and without evidence of thyroid dysfunction. However, if the mother was rendered hypothyroid by iodine-131 during pregnancy, the fetal thyroid gland also may have been adversely affected, rendering the fetus-neonate hypothyroid. Congenital hypothyroidism may not be apparent at birth; therefore government-mandated screening programs are in effect. The causes include thyroid dysgenesis (1 in 4000 births), inborn errors of thyroid metabolism (1 in 30,000), drug-induced hypothyroidism (1 in 10,000), and endemic iodine deficiency. Most if not all sequelae of congenital hypothyroidism can be prevented with prompt recognition and treatment of these disorders.

Postpartum thyroid dysfunction

Clinical or laboratory evidence of thyroid dysfunction is encountered in 5% to 10% of postpartum women. These disorders include both hypothyroid and hyperthyroid states, may occur 1 to 8 months following delivery, and therefore are not frequently detected. Symptoms of fatigue, palpitations, depression, and memory and concentration impairment well after the routine postpartum visit need to be followed up because they may be significant. Women who are positive for antimicrosomal antibodies tend to have a greater risk of postpartum thyroid dysfunction. Patients with other autoimmune diseases are also at greater risk. Postpartum thyroiditis, not unexpectedly, has a tendency to recur in subsequent postpartum states.

SYSTEMIC LUPUS ERYTHEMATOSUS

Systemic lupus erythematosus (SLE) is an autoimmune disease that occurs most frequently in women of reproductive age—hence its importance to the obstetrician. Although the spontaneous abortion rate is increased, this may be due to the presence of a lupus anticoagulant or to anticardiolipin antibodies often associated with SLE. It is a serious chronic disease whose natural history is often unpredictable in pregnancy.

Preconception counseling is aimed at identifying the status of the patient's disease and a determination of multisystem organ involvement. Such patients (e.g., those with hypertension and renal disease) are at the greatest perinatal risk. Laboratory evaluation consists of antibody tests, frequently positive for antinuclear antibodies and anti–deoxyribonucleic acid (DNA) antibodies. The presence of Anti-Ro is associated with neonatal lupus and congenital heart block, often diagnosed in utero.

Pregnancy has been shown to increase the risk of SLE exacerbations, particularly in early pregnancy and the postpartum period. Although not entirely predictive, the maternal disease status at the initiation of pregnancy seems to correlate best with maternal and fetal outcome. The pregnancy must be observed for the development of SLE exacerbation, preeclampsia (often confused with SLE exacerbation), congenital heart block, and fetal growth restriction. Given the increased risk of fetal mortality, antepartum testing beginning at fetal viability is advised. Induction of labor near term, when fetal lung maturity is documented by amniocentesis, is an option often chosen in delivery management.

Corticosteroids are the most effective treatment and are not contraindicated in pregnancy. High doses of steroids during labor and delivery may decrease the risk for postpartum exacerbation. In severe cases, cytotoxic agents and/or anti-malarial drugs may be required.

DISORDERS OF THE URINARY TRACT

Clinically significant anatomic and physiologic changes to the urinary system are observed during pregnancy. The kidneys enlarge, the ureters become significantly dilated, and urine transport from kidney to bladder is delayed. Renal ultrasound during the third trimester may demonstrate mild hydronephrosis. Increased rates of glomerular filtration, renal plasma flow, and creatinine clearance are also pregnancy-related changes.

A working knowledge of these physiologic changes is essential for the proper interpretation of tests of renal function during pregnancy. Clearance of endogenous creatinine is a very useful test for evaluating renal function during pregnancy. Results of a 24-hour urine creatinine clearance study that may be read as "within normal range" by a reference laboratory may in fact demonstrate a result consistent with significant renal disease with deteriorating function. Similarly, because of the sustained increase in glomerular filtration (by 50% over nonpregnant values), a serum creatinine greater than 0.7 mg/dl should make one suspect renal dysfunction. These pregnancy-related changes also account for increased renal protein excretion. During pregnancy women normally may excrete protein up to 500 mg/24 hr. Glycosuria may be a normal finding during pregnancy, relating to increased glomerular filtration and a reduction in the renal threshold for glucose reabsorption.

Asymptomatic bacteriuria

Asymptomatic bacteriuria (ASB) occurs in 2% to 10% of all pregnant women; although asymp-tomatic, it is a significant urinary tract infection. It is diagnosed when more than 100,000 colonies per ml of a single organism are identified in a catheterized or clean-voided urine specimen. *Escherichia coli* is the most commonly isolated pathogenic organism.

Untreated, approximately 40% of patients with ASB will develop symptomatic urinary tract infection. Appropriate antibiotic therapy of ASB can prevent 70% of symptomatic infections, and most cases of pyelonephritis are prevented. Besides symptomatic urinary tract infection, some have reported increased risks for preterm birth and low birth weight among ASB-affected pregnancies.

Cystitis

Cystitis (symptomatic lower urinary tract infection) occurs in 1% to 2% of pregnant women. The common presenting symptoms include urinary frequency, dysuria, and suprapubic pain and tenderness. Typically, patients are afebrile. Urine analysis demonstrates white blood cells and bacteria, and tests for nitrite and leukocyte esterase frequently are positive. Because of increasing resistance of *E. coli* to ampicillin, many practitioners use antibiotic treatment regimens of sulfonamides, cephalosporins, or nitrofurantoin. Traditionally 7- to 10-day courses of therapy have been used, but cures may be effected with shorter course and single-dose treatment regimens. The pharmacologic treatment of any medical condition during pregnancy necessitates that the practitioner be aware of a given medication's potential undesirable effects on the fetus and/or mother. Tetracyclines are not recommended during pregnancy. Tetracyclines can be deposited in the enamel of fetal teeth, leading to a permanent yellow, mottled discoloration. Nitrofurantoin may cause hemolysis of red blood cells and megaloblastic erythropoiesis in women with glucose-6-phosphate dehydrogenase deficiency. Sulfonamides enter the fetal circulation freely and, if not eliminated, cause dissociation of bilirubin from its binding to albumin, leading to fetal hyperbilirubinemia. As bilirubin transfers across the placenta, concern with the use of sulfonamides is focused on their use near delivery, especially for the prematurely delivered neonate.

Pyelonephritis

Acute pyelonephritis, or acute upper urinary tract infection, is a serious medical complication that occurs in 1% to 2% of pregnant women. Screening and treatment for ASB has been shown to reduce significantly the incidence of acute pyelonephritis. Patients frequently present with symptoms of fever, chills, back pain, malaise, and anorexia. Markedly elevated temperature and exquisite tenderness to palpation of the costovertebral angles frequently are noted. Laboratory findings include leukocytosis with bandemia and urine analysis that demonstrates large numbers of white blood cells (frequently in "clumps") and bacteria. Up to 15% of patients will have positive blood cultures, indicating bacteremia. Patients may present concurrently in preterm labor. They may have symptoms of respiratory distress (caused by pulmonary edema) or adult respiratory distress syndrome resulting from endotoxin-mediated pulmonary injury.

A first generation cephalosporin (e.g., cefazolin) is appropriate initial therapy that can be "fine-tuned" pending urine and blood culture sensitivity reports. Intravenous antibiotics are continued until the patient is afebrile and with diminished symptoms and signs for 24 to 48 hours. Appropriate oral antibiotics are then provided and continued for 7 to 10 days on an outpatient basis. Most patients will respond within 48 hours; however, if clinical improvement is not apparent by 72 hours, the patient should be evaluated for possible urinary tract obstruction.

Patients with recurrent pyelonephritis, high-risk patients (e.g., sickle cell disease), or those with positive follow-up cultures may benefit from prophylactic antibiotic suppression therapy, often consisting of a single dose of nitrofurantoin daily until after delivery.

Nephrolithiasis

Urinary calculi occur infrequently in pregnant women. Ureteral and renal calculi may produce fewer symptoms in pregnancy because of the physiologic decreased muscle tone and dilatation of the urinary tract. Possible hyperparathyroidism should be considered in patients noted to have calcium based stones. Flank pain, hematuria, and coexisting urinary tract infection are the common signs and symptoms. Ultrasound or an abbreviated "one-shot" intravenous pyelogram are helpful imaging techniques. Symptomatic patients are provided with hydration, analgesia, and antimicrobial treatment of any underlying infection. The urine is strained to help in identifying the passage of renal calculi. If these measures are unsuccessful, some patients may require stone removal, usually by a snaring basket via cystoscopy. Limited information on lithotripsy in pregnancy exists; therefore its use is not currently recommended.

Chronic renal disease

Until the 1980s women whose pregnancies were complicated with chronic renal insufficiency often were advised to terminate the pregnancy. More recent information suggests that 90% of these patients may anticipate a "successful" pregnancy. This however implies that 10% will suffer severe health consequences in pregnancy; therefore it becomes critical to identify which patients are the best candidates for successful pregnancy and to provide counseling that will allow each patient with chronic renal insufficiency the information necessary to make this important decision. In general, patients who are normotensive, with only minimal and stable renal dysfunction in the periconceptional period, appear to do well, with no significant effect on perinatal outcome or maternal health. This generalization must be qualified for certain nephropathies that have a propensity to affect pregnancy and maternal renal status adversely during pregnancy. These diseases include lupus nephropathy, membranoproliferative glomerulonephritis, and renal disease associated with scleroderma and periarteritis nodosa. Thus many authorities advise against pregnancy when these clinical situations are present.

Antepartum findings of superimposed preeclampsia, worsening hypertension or renal function, IUGR, or abnormalities of antepartum fetal heart rate or biophysical assessment will determine the advisability of continued pregnancy. Often such findings result in a decision for preterm hospitalization and delivery.

Renal transplantation

Renal transplantation is not necessarily a contraindication to pregnancy when normal renal function exists. A pregnancy success rate of 92% has been reported. Again, the literature supports the concept that the better the renal function and blood pressure before conception, the better the pregnancy prognosis. Outcome also appears to be improved when the transplant comes from a living donor. Diabetics whose renal failure was treated with kidney transplantation appear to do worse in pregnancy than others do.

The patient with a renal transplant who is considering pregnancy should undergo *preconception* counseling. Recommendations have been provided for these patients to wait 1 to 2 years before attempting pregnancy so that health status may be studied over that time. Stable renal function with creatinine preferably less than 1.5 mg/dl, absence of rejection signs, minimal or absent proteinuria, and normal blood pressure or easily controlled hypertension are recommended findings before conception. Maintenance levels of antirejection medications also are advised.

PERINATAL INFECTIOUS DISEASE

Human immunodeficiency virus

In 1993, nearly 17,000 women were newly reported as having acquired immunodeficiency syndrome (AIDS). Human immunodeficiency virus (HIV) is the causative virus in the pathogenesis of this disease for which no cure now exists. The virus has a predilection to infect the CD4 lymphocyte, leading to destruction and lowering of the CD4 cell population, and ultimately to an increased susceptibility to a variety of opportunistic infections and malignancies. Most women acquire the infection through intravenous drug use, but in a large percentage (37%) heterosexual sex is the only risk factor. The minority populations of Hispanic and African-American women represent the majority (nearly 75%) of all AIDS cases. Women constitute the fastest growing population of HIV-infected persons, and HIV infection is the fifth leading cause of death for reproductive-age women in the United States.

No words can adequately describe the tragedy of HIV infection. Unfortunately, the increasing number of infected women provides a less traditional means of acquiring infection—vertical transmission of this incurable virus from mother to child. On average, approximately 20% to 30% (range: 7% to 39%) of exposed neonates become infected in this manner. Women with AIDS are at increased risk for adverse perinatal outcome, including preterm labor, preterm delivery, and IUGR. Cofactors—such as drug abuse, poverty, smoking, and other sexually transmitted diseases (STDs)—may contribute to these outcomes. Untoward obstetric outcomes have not been observed in asymptomatic HIV-infected women. Pregnancy does not alter the course of HIV infection.

Management of HIV-infected pregnant women should involve a multidisciplinary team approach consisting of obstetric care providers and others with experience in the management of HIV infection. Psychosocial support services are an integral part of this team. Counseling is critical to allow for an informed reproductive choice. Since HIV is sexually transmitted, screening and treatment for other STDs is important. A tuberculosis purified protein derivative skin test should be placed. Vaccinations to hepatitis B, pneumococcus, and influenza are indicated for susceptible individuals.

Serial determinations of the CD4 count are made, and counts below 200 per mm warrant prophylaxis against *Pneumocystis carinii* pneumonia. The prenatal course is followed closely for the development of any infection, and treatment is aggressive. Other opportunistic infections—such as toxoplasmosis, cytomegalovirus (CMV) infection, and herpes simplex virus (HSV) infection—also are associated with perinatal complications and are described below. At the present time, there appears to be no advantage to cesarean delivery in decreasing the perinatal transmission rate. Fetal scalp electrodes should be avoided.

Recent research has demonstrated a significantly decreased risk of perinatal HIV transmission with the prophylactic use of AZT (zidovudine) during pregnancy. This emphasizes the importance of offering voluntary HIV screening to all pregnant women. Given the large amounts of blood, amniotic fluid, and other body secretions we are exposed to, all obstetric personnel should be diligent in practicing "universal precautions" to decrease the chance of becoming HIV-infected. Although exceptionally rare, medical personnel have developed HIV infection from patient care exposures. Medical students should become familiar with these precautions before engaging in obstetric patient care.

Cytomegalovirus infection

Cytomegalovirus is another of the double-stranded DNA herpes viruses, and is the most common cause of congenital viral infection. Unfortunately, there are no therapies or perinatal interventions capable of modifying or preventing the neonatal consequences of infections. Although most maternal infections are asymptomatic or associated with nonspecific symptoms, up to 2.2% of all live-born infants develop congenital infections. Unfortunately, a primary infection does not grant complete immunity; however, the fetal implications of recurrent maternal infection are less severe.

The greatest risk to the fetus occurs with primary maternal CMV infection in the first trimester. Seronegative mothers have a 1% risk of infection during pregnancy and will transmit the virus to the fetus in 30% to 40% of cases. Of those infected fetuses, up to 4% will be severely affected at birth, but others may present later with deafness and motor or mental retardation. Structurally damaged neonates often are noted to demonstrate hepatosplenomegaly, chorioretinitis, and microphthalmia. Microcephaly, hydrocephalus, symmetric IUGR, and cerebral calcifications are findings often seen on antenatal ultrasound evaluation. Amniotic fluid can be cultured for CMV and can be sent for polymerase chain reaction studies to identify CMV.

Varicella

Primary maternal varicella infection (chickenpox) is caused by the varicella zoster virus (VZV), which is one of the DNA herpes viruses. Secondary infection, herpes zoster, is caused by the same virus, which may replicate and reactivate following a latent phase where the virus remains in the spinal dorsal root sensory ganglia.

Perinatal concerns about primary VZV infection in pregnancy center on the increased risk of varicella pneumonia occurring during pregnancy, the increased risk of maternal mortality, the increased fetal morbidity and mortality associated with congenital varicella infection, and the use of immune globulin to prevent or modulate infection in the nonimmune exposed gravida. Approximately 95% of all adults are immune to VZV infection based on the presence of protective antibodies resulting from prior infection. Interestingly, even among those who do not recall a primary infection, an immune state exists in 80%. Therefore the occurrence of varicella in pregnancy is quite rare—less than 1 case per 1000 pregnancies.

In the absence of antiviral chemotherapy, varicella pneumonia is associated with a 40% mortality. Therefore pregnant women with varicella deserve close observation and surveillance and should be hospitalized and provided with antiviral chemotherapy in the presence of disseminated infection.

Maternal primary infection can cause severe fetal consequences, including increased risks for spontaneous abortion; IUFD; and congenital malformations consisting of cutaneous scars, limb hypoplasia, malformed digits, muscle atrophy, mental and motor retardation, microcephaly, brain atrophy, cataracts, chorioretinitis, and microphthalmia. This constellation of findings has been termed *varicella embryopathy,* and can occur by transplacental infection in the first half of pregnancy. The reported risk for intrauterine infection or varicella embryopathy ranges from 0% to 24%.

Varicella infection of the newborn occurs in up to 20% of infants delivered to mothers who develop primary VZV infection between 5 days before and 2 days after delivery, with an associated 20% to 30% mortality. Patients should not be electively delivered within 5 days of developing primary VZV infection, and tocolysis can be attempted for those in spontaneous labor. If these measures are unsuccessful in preventing delivery during this critical period, varicella zoster immune globulin (VZIG) should be administered to the neonate; and contact between the newborn and maternal lesions is avoided.

At the first prenatal visit, pregnant women should be asked about a prior history of varicella. If the woman is uncertain of her immune status, a varicella titer is obtained. If she is susceptible, she is counseled to avoid contact with infected individuals. If she is exposed to an individual with chickenpox, she should be counseled appropriately and offered VZIG to prevent maternal infection. If the contact occurs in an individual who does not know her immune status, serologic tests of immunity must be performed and the results made available quickly because VZIG must be administered within 96 hours postexposure to be effective.

Toxoplasmosis

Toxoplasmosis is an infection caused by the protozoan *Toxoplasma gondii.* It complicates 0.1% to 0.5% of all pregnancies. Toxoplasmosis is caused by eating the meat of animals that contain the infective cysts or by inhaling or ingesting oocysts. Oocysts are excreted in the feces of cats; therefore it is inadvisable for pregnant women to have direct contact with cat litter and feces. Routine screening is not currently recommended given the inaccuracy of available tests and the low disease prevalence.

Fetal infection may result in chorioretinitis, hydrocephalus, and microcephaly, and can lead to significant neurologic impairment. An infant who seems normal at birth may demonstrate signs of infection at a later date. Congenital infection is more likely to occur following maternal infection in the third trimester. First trimester infection, although leading to less frequent congenital infection, results in more severe sequelae.

Ultrasound findings of hydrocephaly, microcephaly, symmetric IUGR, and intracranial calcifications should prompt maternal testing for toxoplasmosis.

Serology is the best method for diagnosing toxoplasmosis. The presence of toxoplasma antibodies indicates acute disease or prior infection and immunity. Toxoplasma-specific IgM testing (by a reliable reference laboratory) provides differentiation of acute infection from prior infection and immunity. Should acute infection be confirmed, counseling is essential and prenatal diagnosis of congenital infection may be undertaken. Amniotic fluid and fetal blood provide specimens suitable for evaluating congenital infection. Determination of congenital infection is critical, because pharmacologic therapy with spiramycin, pyrimethamine, and sulfonamides has been shown to reduce the occurrence and severity of congenital toxoplasmosis.

Parvovirus infection

Erythema infectiosum, or fifths disease, is a viral exanthem caused by human parvovirus B19. Maternal infection during pregnancy is frequently the result of viral transmission from infected school-age children. Nonimmune women with other children at home; teachers and school aides; and other women exposed to infected contacts have a 30% to 50% risk of infection. Adult infection often is asymptomatic but may be associated with arthralgia and fever. Fortunately, 50% of pregnant women are immune, having had the infection at some earlier time.

Transplacental intrauterine infection can produce nonimmune hydrops and fetal death. Approximately one third of affected gravidas will transmit the virus to the fetus. Fetal loss is increased when transmission occurs before 20 weeks' gestation; however, fetal infection does not necessarily correlate with adverse fetal outcome. A maximum 10% risk of fetal death has been calculated after maternal infection. No specific B19 Ig is available for maternal prophylaxis.

Management is focused on serologic diagnosis using IgG and IgM titers. With confirmation of diagnosis, serial ultrasound examinations of the fetus are performed to detect hydrops and growth restriction. Fetal hydrops sometimes has been noted to resolve in utero; however, some have used invasive fetal percutaneous umbilical blood sampling to determine the extent of fetal anemia, provide red cell transfusion to the fetus, and direct fetal digitalization to treat myocardial dysfunction and anemia—thus reversing the hydropic process. This technique also allows for fetal serologic studies and polymerase chain reaction identification of virus within the fetal circulation.

Rubella

Rubella, or German measles, is caused by a ribonucleic acid virus and is spread by air-borne droplets or direct contact with infected oronasopharyngeal secretions. The infection—characterized by rash, adenopathy, fever, and arthralgia—confers lifelong immunity. In 1941, an association was made between infection during pregnancy and the findings of congenital heart disease and cataracts in the neonate. Neonatal hearing loss, low birth weight, thrombocytopenia, bone lesions, hepatitis, hepatosplenomegaly, hemolysis, jaundice, encephalitis, and failure to thrive are associated findings with this perinatal infection. Infection during the first 16 weeks of gestation results in a 75% risk of congenital malformations. There is no specific treatment to decrease fetal risks. Definitive confirmation of rubella infection during pregnancy necessitates that the patient be counseled with respect to risks and that the option of pregnancy termination be discussed, depending on the period of gestation.

All women of childbearing age should be tested and vaccinated if not immune. Pregnancy is not recommended for the first 3 months following vaccination, although no significant increased risk for congenital rubella has been documented should pregnancy occur earlier or even with vaccination during pregnancy. Nonimmune gravidas should be advised to avoid contact with those with rubella and ideally should be vaccinated before hospital discharge after delivery.

Genital herpes

Appropriate identification and management of genital herpes is critical because neonatal infection resulting in congenital herpes will result in at least a 25% mortality. Infants with central nervous system or disseminated disease have a 40% mortality. Survivors are at extreme risk for lifelong neurologic disability, including deafness, blindness, seizures, and mental retardation. Unfortunately, despite appropriate management, cases of neonatal congenital herpes infection will occur.

Herpes simplex virus is a double-stranded DNA virus. Type 1 or 2 HSV can result in perinatal infection. Unfortunately, a clinical characteristic of this virus is its ability to become a chronic latent infection and to escape destruction by the immune system. The infection is sexually transmitted and is classified as primary or secondary. Vesicular lesions often are noted on the cervix and mucocutaneous areas of the perineum. The lower back, buttocks, and perirectal region are also areas where lesions may be noted. The symptoms of primary infection are more severe and consist of intense pain, pruritus, and burning at the infected areas; and the patient frequently will have constitutional symptoms of anorexia, malaise, fever, and myalgia. Inguinal adenopathy is often noted. Fortunately, secondary herpes infection is associated with milder symptoms. Approximately 80% of infected patients will have symptomatic recurrences during pregnancy.

The greatest perinatal risk occurs when primary infection occurs during pregnancy. Although some cases of transplacental fetal infection have been reported, these are rare compared with the usual route of ascending or contact infection through fetal exposure to the birth canal. Approximately half of fetuses delivered vaginally during a primary HSV infection will develop neonatal HSV infection.

Patients with positive histories are monitored closely for infection. Should infection occur, a viral culture is taken to confirm the diagnosis. Weekly cultures, once standard prenatal practice, have been shown inadequate in predicting infection at delivery and thus are unnecessary for perinatal management.

Delivery management revolves around the issue of active infection. When labor begins, patients with a history of HSV infection are examined thoroughly. Those without evidence of visible lesions or symptoms of infection are allowed a vaginal delivery. Patients with symptoms or lesions are delivered by cesarean section to decrease the risk of congenital HSV infection. Although acyclovir has been used in the management of primary infection and as a means of decreasing recurrent infections, its use in pregnancy has been limited to disseminated infection or in patients with a compromised immune system.

Human papillomavirus

Human papillomavirus (HPV) appears to be epidemic and may play a significant role in the development of cervical dysplasia, but it seems to have little effect on perinatal outcome. This virus causes condylomata acuminata, or exophytic genital warts, that may increase in size and number during pregnancy and typically affect the urogenital and anorectal areas. In some cases, growth can be markedly accelerated, and vaginal and perineal warts can obstruct vaginal delivery. These warts also increase risks for bleeding from episiotomy or tearing of infected maternal tissues. Laser ablation and cryotherapy have been used in the second and third trimesters to treat these lesions. One of the concerns about the effect of this virus on the fetus is the development of juvenile laryngeal papillomatosis because this is caused by the same virus. Given the high prevalence of HPV among pregnant women and the low incidence of juvenile laryngeal papillomatosis, the risk of transmission is estimated to be extremely low. Cesarean section to prevent fetal exposure to the virus is not currently recommended.

Hepatitis B

Hepatitis B is a viral disease with significant public health and perinatal significance. Over 1 million Americans are chronic carriers of the virus (hepatitis B surface antigen [HBsAg] positive). Acute infection occurs in 1 to 2 cases per 1000 pregnancies, whereas chronic infection is present in 5 to 15 cases per 1000 pregnancies. Risk factors for acquiring hepatitis B infection include illicit drug use, STDs, multiple sexual partners, prior blood transfusion, presence of a tatoo, work in patient-contact health care fields, household contact with an infected person, and residence in a prison.

Approximately 10% to 20% of women positive for HBsAg will transmit the virus to the fetus or neonate in the absence of immunoprophylaxis. Eighty-five percent to 95% of perinatal transmission occurs as a result of intrapartum fetal exposure to infected secretions. For this reason, and because of the high morbidity and mortality associated with chronic infection, routine universal screening for hepatitis B is recommended at an early prenatal visit. Women at high risk for infection without evidence of prior infection should be offered vaccination, whereas those found to be HBsAg-positive are counseled. Liver function tests and tests for sexually transmitted diseases should be obtained. Infants born to these women should have combined passive and active immunization consisting of hepatitis B immune globulin and hepatitis B vaccination before hospital discharge. Recently, it has been recommended that all newborns receive hepatitis B vaccination, regardless of maternal antigen status.

Bacterial vaginosis

Bacterial vaginosis is a vaginitis caused by bacteria that drastically change the vaginal bacterial ecology from one dominated by lactobacilli to include a 100-fold increase in anaerobes (including *Mobiluncus* species), *Mycoplasma hominis,* and *Gardnerella vaginalis.* The clinical presentation is a vaginal discharge with a fishy odor. Diagnosis is aided by a wet-mount examination of vaginal discharge demonstrating "clue cells," epithelial cells with large numbers of adherent bacteria. Addition of potassium hydroxide tends to accentuate the foul odor.

Bacterial vaginosis recently has been shown to increase risks for preterm labor, preterm delivery, intraamniotic infection, and endometritis. Studies evaluating the effect of treating asymptomatic women or screening all women to reduce these risks have yet to be performed. Symptomatic patients are treated with either oral or intravaginal

metronidazole if beyond the first trimester. Clindamycin is an alternative treatment.

Gonorrhea

Gonorrhea complicates between 0.5% and 7% of pregnancies, depending on the population studied, and is caused by the bacterium *Neisseria gonorrhoeae.* As with other STDs, risk of infection is increased by multiple sexual partners, prostitution, drug use, and low socioeconomic status. Nearly half of all women with this infection will be coinfected with *Chlamydia trachomatis.*

Gonorrhea infection is associated with adverse pregnancy outcome. Increased risks exist for septic abortion, preterm labor, preterm delivery, chorioamnionitis, and postpartum maternal infection. If infected, the neonate may develop neonatal gonococcal ophthalmia, arthritis, and sepsis. Because treatment has been shown to decrease these risks, women are screened at the first prenatal visit with a cervical culture. Syphilis, chlamydia, and HIV screening are also performed. Patients found to have gonorrhea are treated with ceftriaxone (125 mg administered intramuscularly). Many recommend treating also for chlamydia, given the high rate of concurrent infection. Follow-up cultures are performed later in gestation to confirm cure.

Chlamydia

Genital infection with the sexually transmitted bacterium *Chlamydia trachomatis* is the most common STD in women. Women at risk are those with multiple sexual partners or other STDs. Unlike the nongravid state, most pregnant women with chlamydia are without symptoms. The effect of chlamydia infection on pregnancy is controversial; however, recent infection may be associated with increased risks for preterm labor and delivery and preterm ruptured membranes. Postpartum, chlamydia infection may cause late-onset endometritis. The neonatal consequences of maternal chlamydia infection include the development of neonatal chlamydia conjunctivitis and pneumonia. Maternal screening and antepartum maternal treatment may be important because up to 20% of chlamydia-exposed neonates will develop conjunctivitis, despite universal standard ophthalmologic preventive treatment in the delivery room. The drug of choice in pregnancy is erythromycin. Amoxicillin is an alternative medication.

Group B β-streptococcus

Group B β-*Streptococcus* (GBS) infection is the leading cause of perinatal infectious morbidity and mortality; and the total number of annual cases exceeds all congenital infections caused by rubella, herpes, toxoplasmosis, and syphilis!

There are two forms of GBS infection in the neonate. Early-onset GBS infection may occur in utero or in the first week of life and constitutes 80% of GBS infection in the newborn. It is acquired by vertical transmission from mothers whose genital tracts are colonized by GBS, with most infection acquired in utero and during labor and delivery. Mothers may be entirely asymptomatic or may have signs and symptoms of chorioamnionitis. The infected neonate suffers from pneumonia, shock, and an overall perinatal mortality of 10% to 20%. Symptoms of GBS typically are apparent within hours of birth. It is a leading cause of neonatal sepsis, with 12,000 to 15,000 cases reported annually. Late-onset disease occurs 1 to 16 weeks after birth and is characterized by meningitis. Less than half of these infections are believed to be due to maternal transmission of infection. Fifty percent of the survivors of late-onset disease will have permanent neurologic sequelae. Chorioamnionitis, endometritis, cystitis, and pyelonephritis are maternal manifestations of GBS infection.

Depending on the methodology and population studied, GBS is cultured from the genital tract or rectum in 15% to 40% of pregnant women and exists without causing maternal symptoms. Pregnancy does not appear to increase the risk of being colonized, and the identification of GBS is not associated with the presence of other sexually transmitted pathogens, suggesting a limited role for sexual transmission. Indeed, the bacteria are found in the lower digestive tract, wherefrom the organisms intermittently colonize the genital tract. Occasionally GBS causes urinary tract infection, which—unlike asymptomatic genital tract colonization—has been associated with increased risks for premature preterm ruptured membranes, preterm delivery, and fetal death. African-American and Hispanic women are more often colonized than are white women; Asian women have the lowest rate of carriage. Vaginal colonization has been noted to be intermittent, with as many as 20% of women with negative cultures at midgestation demonstrating positive vaginal cultures at term. Similarly, in one study, 7.4% of women with negative cultures at midgestation had positive cultures at term. Therefore one can readily see that universal culture and treatment at midgestation will fail to identify a number of patients colonized at term. In fact, two thirds of treated colonized patients at midtrimester will remain colonized at term. Recolonization following treatment from the digestive tract reservoir probably negates the usefulness of midgestation treatment.

Although 70% of infants born to GBS-colonized mothers will become colonized themselves, fortunately, on average, only 1% to 2% of colonized infants will be affected by GBS infection. Although the overall rate of infection is low, several factors identify high-risk groups. These factors include premature delivery, prolonged rupture of the amniotic membranes (more than 12 hours), labor complicated by maternal fever, a previous affected pregnancy, and diabetes. In fact, infants born to GBS-colonized mothers without risk factors have only a 1 in 200 chance of developing GBS infection; but the risk for GBS infection in the presence of risk factors is 1 in 25. Mortality appears highest for the most premature infants, accounting for one third of GBS-related mortality.

Management of this perinatal infection is an area of controversy. This stems from the fairly high colonization rate, and the relatively low infection rate. For this reason, the identification of high risk factors, with their attendant increase in infection rate and mortality, provides practitioners an area to focus antimicrobial infection prophylaxis efforts. This approach has been shown to decrease neonatal GBS morbidity and mortality. Nevertheless, some believe in universal culturing of pregnant women in the third trimester. This is a strategy recommended by the American Academy of Pediatrics (AAP). The American College of Obstetricians and Gynecologists does not make the same recommendation because research supporting such a recommendation is lacking. The arguments against the AAP recommendation include the lack of predictability of an antepartum GBS culture to the maternal colonization state at labor, the estimated $110 million cost associated with universal screening, and antibiotic-associated risks (allergic reaction, development of bacterial resistance).

The development of a rapid test to detect GBS colonization ultimately will prove helpful in determining which patients to treat intrapartum. Presently such a test does not exist, nor is a vaccine close to commercial use. Therefore the management, identification, and prophylaxis of GBS infection remains an area of controversy and research. Current Centers for Disease Control and Prevention (CDC) recommendations promote a strategy to reduce early-onset GBS sepsis using either a risk factor protocol (intrapartum prophylaxis for risk factors only) or prenatal screening cultures at 35 to 37 weeks. Current treatment recommendations advocate intrapartum penicillin G, 5 million U initially followed by 2.5 million U every 4 hours. For penicillin-allergic women, clindamycin or erythromycin may be used.

Syphilis

Syphilis is caused by the spirochete *Treponema pallidum,* which can cross the placenta and cause fetal infection. Increased rates of syphilis in pregnancy have paralleled the rising use of illicit drugs during pregnancy and lack of prenatal care. Without treatment, approximately 50% of newborns born to women with primary or secondary syphilis will develop congenital syphilis, characterized by hepatosplenomegaly, mucocutaneous lesions, and bony and dental abnormalities. Preterm labor and delivery, IUFD, IUGR, and nonimmune hydrops also are findings associated with maternal infection.

Universal syphilis screening during pregnancy is performed, and patients found to have a positive nonspecific screening test (rapid plasmin reagin or Venereal Disease Research Laboratory) should have a specific test for treponemal antibody (e.g., fluorescent treponemal antibody).

Intramuscular penicillin is the drug of choice, with dosage determined by the stage of infection. Penicillin-allergic patients are desensitized and treated because alternative drugs are not effective at preventing congenital syphilis. Patients treated for syphilis in pregnancy are followed up closely for evidence of therapeutic response. This is determined by the observation of a fourfold decline in the nontreponemal antibody titer by 3 to 4 months after treatment for primary or secondary syphilis, and by 6 to 8 months for early latent syphilis. Fortunately, it has been observed that penicillin therapy cures early maternal infection and prevents neonatal syphilis in 98% of cases.

CARDIAC DISEASE

Heart disease affects approximately 1% of pregnant women and is a major contributor to maternal mortality. The proper care of the woman whose pregnancy is complicated by cardiac disease necessitates an understanding of the physiologic cardiovascular changes that occur during pregnancy, integrated with knowledge of the pathophysiology of the cardiac lesion itself.

Physiologic changes

Pregnancy leads to an increase in intravascular volume, consisting of increased plasma volume and red cell mass. This increase is 50% in the third trimester and is appreciably higher with multiple gestations. Furthermore, a 50% increase in cardiac output is observed during labor and delivery. Physiologic changes are well tolerated by the healthy gravida but may lead to morbidity and mortality for women with compromised cardiac function. Women whose heart lesions result in a limited cardiac output have difficulty tolerating the increased load, and this may lead to heart failure or cardiac ischemia. The volume shift caused by the acute loss of blood with delivery and postpartum hemorrhage may be poorly tolerated among women whose cardiac output is dependent on adequate preload (e.g., pulmonary hypertension) or in those with a fixed cardiac output (e.g., mitral stenosis). Decreased systemic vascular resistance in pregnancy also may contribute to the problem of maintaining adequate preload for women whose lesions result in a relatively fixed cardiac output (e.g., idiopathic hypertrophic subaortic stenosis). This change may also affect those with right-to-left shunts, which are increased by the fall in systemic vascular resistance during pregnancy. The hypercoagulable state of pregnancy is a physiologic change important in the consideration of anticoagulation for patients with artificial heart valves and atrial fibrillation.

General considerations

The activity level of the patient with heart disease who is pregnant or contemplating pregnancy is a prognostic indicator. The New York Heart Association (NYHA) classification is widely used. Patients without symptoms or who have symptoms only with greater than normal activity (NYHA classes I and II respectively) typically have a favorable pregnancy prognosis, yet it is clear that functional status may worsen. Women with symptoms of cardiac disease with their usual activity or while at rest (NYHA classes III and IV respectively) typically will have a less than favorable outcome.

With respect to the fetus, IUGR is a common complication when pregnancy is complicated by cardiac disease. Serial ultrasound to evaluate for appropriate fetal growth and the utilization of antepartum fetal heart rate or biophysical monitoring are essential components of pregnancy care. Patients with congenital heart disease should be counseled of a 5% to 10% risk for the fetus being affected by either the same or a different cardiac lesion. Fetal echocardiography is therefore useful in evaluating for this risk. Obstetric patients with cardiac lesions often are provided with antibiotics for endocarditis prophylaxis.

Specific cardiac lesions

- **MITRAL VALVE PROLAPSE.** Mitral valve prolapse is a common congenital occurrence noted in up to 17% of women. Most patients are without symptoms, but some will have bothersome palpitations that may respond to β-blocker therapy.
- **RIGHT HEART VALVULAR DISEASE.** Patients with tricuspid or pulmonic valve disease generally tolerate pregnancy, labor, and delivery. The normal increase in vascular volume increases preload, allowing for maintenance of pulmonary perfusion.
- **MITRAL INSUFFICIENCY.** Because mitral insufficiency usually is related to rheumatic heart disease, typically other heart valves also are involved. Rarely does CHF occur, and thus this lesion usually is well tolerated. Perhaps the most significant risk is the potential for atrial enlargement and atrial fibrillation, which may increase in pregnancy. Therefore patients with severe mitral insufficiency are often recommended digitalis.
- **MITRAL STENOSIS.** Mitral stenosis is the most common rheumatic valvular abnormality noted in pregnancy and has the potential for significant morbidity and mortality. Although patients may tolerate their antepartum course well,

↓ c̄ Mitral Stenosis ↓

the onset of labor and delivery and the postpartum periods are times of greatest risk.

There are two keys to management: (1) the prevention of tachycardia, to allow for adequate ventricular diastolic filling; and (2) the maintenance of preload to allow for adequate filling pressure of the left ventricle. These goals are best achieved by using β-blockers and maintaining the patient in a well-hydrated state, often resulting in high-normal or even elevated capillary wedge pressure. The use of epidural-mediated sympathetic block may result in hypotension and decreased preload. Postpartum blood loss also may contribute to decreased ventricular filling pressure; therefore this also represents a critical time that necessitates continued close management and maintenance of adequate wedge pressure. These patients require intensive cardiac monitoring, preferably in an obstetric intensive care setting.

AORTIC STENOSIS. Aortic stenosis is also most commonly caused by rheumatic heart disease and therefore coexists with other such lesions. It is generally well tolerated in pregnancy owing to the physiologic pregnancy-related increased vascular volume, which results in the maintenance of cardiac output. With severe disease, however, cardiac output may not be adequate to maintain adequate coronary or cerebral perfusion. The consequences include syncope, angina, myocardial infarction, and sudden death. Increased rest throughout gestation often is recommended. During delivery, anything that might result in hypotension and/or decreased preload (decreased venous return) must be avoided to prevent decreased cardiac output. Invasive cardiac monitoring during labor and delivery in the obstetric intensive care setting is indicated.

AORTIC INSUFFICIENCY. A finding of aortic insufficiency may be due to rheumatic heart disease, a congenital bicuspid aortic valve, or collagen vascular disease such as lupus or rheumatoid arthritis. This lesion typically is well tolerated because of the increased heart rate of pregnancy and decreased vascular resistance, which may decrease the extent of regurgitant blood flow. Severe cases, however, may result in left heart failure, with prevention of bradycardia and afterload reduction, cornerstones of management.

ATRIAL SEPTAL DEFECT. Atrial septic defect is the most common congenital heart lesion noted in pregnancy. It is typically well tolerated and asymptomatic during pregnancy. Rarely, however, dysrhythmia, CHF, and death have been reported.

VENTRICULAR SEPTAL DEFECT. Although small ventricular septal defects (VSDs) may be well tolerated, outcome appears to be correlated with VSD size. Patients with larger lesions are at risk for CHF, dysrhythmia, and/or the development of pulmonary hypertension (Eisenmenger's syndrome).

EISENMENGER'S SYNDROME. Eisenmenger's syndrome occurs when pulmonary hypertension develops as a result of a congenital left-to-right shunt (e.g., VSD). With the development of pulmonary hypertension, the shunt then becomes reversed or bidirectional. Pregnancy termination is recommended, given the 30% to 50% maternal mortality. Thromboembolic complications contribute substantially to maternal death. Patients continuing pregnancy are hospitalized and given continuous oxygen, serial ultrasound exams to evaluate fetal growth, and antepartum fetal monitoring. Despite optimal management, fetal distress and death are common occurrences. Intrapartum management consists of preventing hypotension to maintain pulmonary blood flow and serial observations of cardiac function and blood gas parameters by invasive cardiac monitoring.

TETRALOGY OF FALLOT. Tetralogy of Fallot is a congenital complex of disorders that consists of VSD, an overriding aorta, right ventricular hypertrophy, and pulmonary stenosis. With successful pediatric surgical correction, many women born with this disorder are now entering reproductive age. Fortunately for these patients, pregnancy outcome appears good. Women who are symptomatic or who have uncor-

Tet of Fallot = VSD, RVH, overriding aorta, Pul stenosis.

rected tetralogy of Fallot have a particularly poor prognosis.

PRIOR MYOCARDIAL INFARCTION. Ischemic heart disease is rare in the reproductive-age population. Patients who have had a myocardial infarction in the recent past are at high risk of death if they undertake the hemodynamic burden of pregnancy. A 35% risk of maternal mortality has been reported, with greater risk of infarction and death in the third trimester.

PERIPARTUM CARDIOMYOPATHY. Peripartum cardiomyopathy is a dilated cardiomyopathy that develops in the last month of pregnancy or the first 6 months of the postpartum period in a patient without prior history of cardiac disease and after exclusion of other known causes of heart failure. Because of a hypokinetic heart, thrombi may form and embolize. Progressive dilated cardiomyopathy and death occur in up to 50% of cases. The remaining 50% of patients tend to recover and do well. Future pregnancy, however, poses a significant risk of recurrence and is not recommended.

ASTHMA

Asthma is the most common obstructive lung disease seen in pregnancy and affects between 1% and 5% of all pregnancies. Asthma prevalence and mortality is rising significantly in the United States. The disease is characterized by chronic inflammation of the respiratory tract, with intermittent acute episodes of bronchoconstriction resulting from a variety of stimuli, including allergens, environmental irritants, cold air, exercise, and viruses. With proper treatment and control, it is believed that asthmatic women can maintain a normal pregnancy with minimal risk. Nonetheless, retrospective data exist that demonstrate appreciably increased risks for perinatal morbidity when pregnancy is complicated by asthma. It appears that the course of a patient's asthma during pregnancy is related to the severity of disease. In other words, women with mild asthma typically can expect their disease state to remain unchanged or improve, whereas women with severe asthma will in most cases experience a significant worsening of symptoms.

Women with asthma need continued treatment during pregnancy. The medications used during pregnancy to treat asthma are safe and not teratogenic. Therefore women should be encouraged to maintain compliance and should be reassured that their medications will improve perinatal outcome rather than adversely affect the fetus. The concept that the patient is "breathing for two" cannot be overemphasized.

Patients with asthma should be provided with a means of objectively measuring their pulmonary function at home. A spirometer that measures peak expiratory flow is suitable for this purpose. Patients are instructed to report changes from their "personal best" measurement, and additional therapy is then instituted. Patients need to be educated about the various triggers causing asthma exacerbation and provided means of decreasing their exposure.

Pharmacologic therapy consists of medications to prevent exacerbations, as well as to treat the acute asthma attack. Such medications include antiinflammatory drugs such as cromolyn, which stabilizes mast cells, prevents their degranulation, and is useful as prophylaxis for cold- or exercise-induced asthma. Beclomethasone and prednisone are potent steroid antiinflammatory drugs; the inhaled route of administration is preferred. Acute attacks are often managed with bronchodilator therapy consisting of an inhaled β_2-agonist. Theophylline, previously used as first-line therapy, is now recommended for control of patients with nocturnal symptoms. Dosages of these medications and frequency of administration are based on patient symptoms and objective measurement of pulmonary function (Figs. 12-1 and 12-2).

Serious asthma exacerbations are life threatening to the mother and fetus and should be managed in an intensive care setting. Therapy consists of subcutaneous terbutaline or aero-

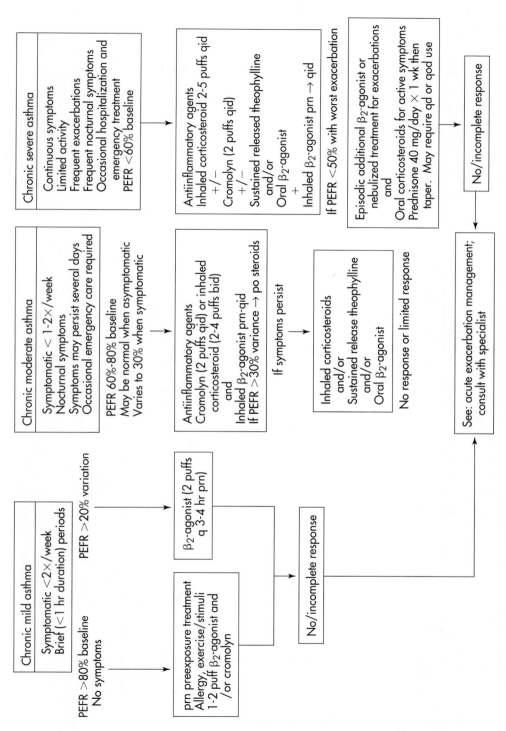

Fig. 12-1. Outpatient management of chronic asthma during pregnancy. *PEFR*, Peak expiratory flow rate; *prn*, as required; *q*, every; *qid*, 4 times daily; *bid*, twice a day; *po*, by mouth; *qd*, every day.

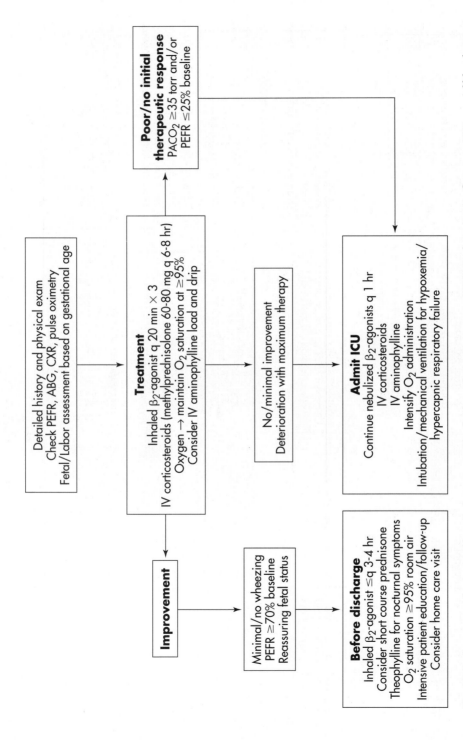

Fig. 12-2. Acute exacerbation and hospital management of asthma during pregnancy. *PEFR,* Peak expiratory flow rate; *ABG,* arterial blood gases; *CXR,* chest x-ray; *q,* every; *IV,* intravenous. *(Adapted from National Institutes of Health: Management of asthma during pregnancy, National Asthma Education Program, NIH Publication No 93-3279A, 1993.)*

solized β_2-agonist therapy. Oxygen administration is critical, and the maternal oxygen saturation must be maintained at 95% to maintain proper fetal oxygenation. These women will also benefit from the prompt administration of systemic corticosteroids.

SUBSTANCE ABUSE DURING PREGNANCY

The use of illicit drugs during pregnancy appears to be widespread and growing. This tragedy crosses all racial and socioeconomic lines. It is not uncommon for practitioners at large medical centers to deal with drug abuse and pregnancy on a daily basis. The motivation for such destructive behavior during pregnancy is complex and multifaceted, and clearly deserves our most intensive efforts to combat its practice. The adverse effects of these habits comprise the whole of adverse perinatal outcome, ranging from preterm labor and delivery to the complications associated with prematurity, abnormal behavioral and neurodevelopment, and congenital malformations. Coexisting risks for STDs and infectious complications associated with drug abuse, including hepatitis and HIV infection, must be recognized and evaluated. The use of alcohol and tobacco and their perinatal effects also must be considered. Clearly the effects go beyond the individual pregnancy; they negatively impact the whole of society, both socially and economically.

Cocaine

Cocaine use during pregnancy has been the focus of intense media attention during the past several years. Placental abruption, fetal limb reduction defects, fetal genitourinary and other malformations, fetal stroke, IUGR, stillbirth, low Apgar scores, preterm birth, and neonatal neurobehavioral disorders have been associated with cocaine use in pregnancy. Users of crack-cocaine have been clearly demonstrated to have infants with head circumference below the tenth percentile for gestational age.

Heroin

Opioid use during pregnancy is related to increased fetal wastage and IUGR. Withdrawal during pregnancy is related to increased fetal death from fetal withdrawal. Neonates are at risk for neonatal abstinence syndrome and long-term neurobehavioral changes. Concurrent complications of heroin abuse include the potential infectious complications associated with intravenous drug abuse, including HIV and hepatitis infections, and contamination of the drug with other teratogenic agents, such as quinine. Methadone is the treatment of choice for heroin addiction in pregnancy, and its use has been shown to improve both maternal and fetal outcome.

Amphetamines

It appears the use of methamphetamines during pregnancy is increasing, particularly the smokable forms "ice" or "crystal meth." Reported perinatal complications include IUGR and preterm birth. Animal data have shown the occurrence of cerebral ischemia and infarction, and human neonates have an increased incidence of intraventricular hemorrhage. We have recently observed an occurrence of in utero intraventricular hemorrhage associated with amphetamine use, and a massive abruption resulting in fetal death and profound disseminated intravascular coagulation. Most available data fail to support an association between amphetamine use in pregnancy and specific structural congenital malformations.

Marijuana

Although marijuana is the most frequently used illicit drug among reproductive-age women, other illicit drugs often are used concurrently. This adds difficulty in determining the impact of prenatal marijuana exposure on pregnancy outcome. Some studies have demonstrated reductions in gestation, birth weight, and neonatal length; but the clinical significance of these findings appears minimal. Similarly, the reported impact on neurobehavioral development has not been consistent. No specific congenital malformations have been associated with prenatal marijuana use.

Alcohol

Literally thousands of scientific publications have addressed the effects of alcohol as a contributing factor in fetal dysmorphogenesis. Fetal alcohol syndrome is a recognized pattern of malformations associated with prenatal alcohol exposure to the fetus. It is characterized by fetal and postnatal growth restriction, central nervous system abnormalities, and craniofacial deformities. Because no minimum amount of "safe drinking" has been identified, and because the fetal alcohol syndrome is the most common cause of recognized mental retardation, it is recommended that pregnant women refrain from all alcoholic beverages.

Smoking

Smoking has deleterious effects on pregnancy. In fact, the Surgeon General has a specific tobacco warning for pregnancy placed on packages of cigarettes and printed with cigarette advertisements. Increased risks for spontaneous abortion, IUGR, low birth weight, oligohydramnios, premature placental aging, premature labor and birth, placental abruption, and placenta previa have all been noted. Given the preponderance of evidence correlating cigarette smoking with adverse perinatal outcome, practitioners should invest time counseling their smoking pregnant patients—increasing their awareness of their general health risks, perinatal risks, and the positive information that decreasing the amount smoked may result in improved pregnancy outcome. Furthermore,

pregnancy offers an opportune time to cease smoking, given the risks above, as well as the risks associated with second-hand smoke for the newborn. Increased occurrences of upper respiratory tract infections, otitis, asthma, and pneumonia have been reported. Ultimately, long-term exposure to second-hand smoke has been linked to increased cancer risks.

ACUTE ABDOMINAL SYMPTOMS

Pregnancy does not protect the patient from appendicitis, pancreatitis, or cholecystitis, and indeed, may make a diagnosis more obscure and difficult. A patient who has signs of an acute condition in the abdomen needs meticulous evaluation, and the tendency to ascribe symptoms to the "general discomforts" of pregnancy should be avoided. A complete history and physical evaluation are crucial; and physical findings, as well as laboratory data, need to be evaluated, taking into account the normal physiologic changes of pregnancy.

Physiologic changes associated with pregnancy can increase the difficulty of early diagnosis. The common occurrence of nausea and vomiting is one of early pregnancy (first trimester), does not begin later, and usually is not associated with abdominal pain. Leukocytosis is present during pregnancy at 6000 to 16,000 per mm^3 in the second and third trimesters. Granulocytosis and bandemia, however, are not physiologic changes. During labor the white blood cell count may rise as high as 20,000 to 30,000 per mm^3. The erythrocyte sedimentation rate is not useful in the diagnosis of inflammatory disorders during pregnancy.

Abdominal pain must be differentiated from benign discomforts caused by the enlarging uterus and the stretching of pelvic ligaments. Urinary tract infection, renal calculus, and a bleeding or torsed corpus luteum also may cause acute abdominal pain. Differentiation is critical because treatments are disease-specific.

Frequently, preterm labor is noted following abdominal surgery during pregnancy, particularly in the presence of infection. Besides antibiotic therapy, tocolytic agents are used when appropriate and with caution. An increased risk for pulmonary edema resulting from pulmonary capillary injury caused by bacteremia has been noted.

Appendicitis

Acute appendicitis occurs with the same frequency in pregnant as in nonpregnant women, but pregnancy often makes the diagnosis more problematic, resulting in delayed diagnosis and increased maternal and fetal complications. It is the most common nonobstetric acute surgical complication in pregnancy. The enlarged uterus may obscure the appendix, which tends to be displaced upward and laterally in the direction of the right iliac crest. Abortion or preterm labor may occur if the infection involves the uterine serosa (visceral peritoneum). Preterm uterine contractions may be quite difficult to control, despite aggressive efforts, in the presence of peritonitis.

Nausea and vomiting, epigastric pain localizing in the right side of the abdomen, and tenderness anywhere from McBurney's point to the right flank are suggestive of appendicitis. Elevated temperature and tachycardia usually are present. An increased white blood cell count may be seen in normal pregnancy; however, a serial rise in the count or the presence of increased band forms suggests the presence of an acute infectious process. Use of ultrasound to aid in the diagnosis of appendicitis in pregnancy has been described.

Appendicitis complicating pregnancy necessitates surgery as soon as the diagnosis can be established. Depending on the trimester, this may include laparoscopy or laparotomy. Because of the extreme morbidity and even mortality associated with delayed or missed diagnosis, it has been stated that a rate of finding a normal appendix in 30% of cases is acceptable. At surgery, should perforation be noted, copious antibiotic irrigation should be used to decrease bacterial contami-

nation. Doses for parenteral antibiotics recommended for serious infection should be used. Postoperatively, close observation and management of preterm labor are critical as noted previously.

Intestinal obstruction

Gravidas presenting with symptoms of an acute condition in the abdomen, abdominal distention, rebound tenderness, nausea and vomiting, constipation, and a history of previous abdominal or pelvic surgery should be considered at risk for intestinal obstruction. If not diagnosed and treated promptly, perforation and peritonitis may occur, causing significant maternal and fetal morbidity and mortality. Surgical exploration is required where findings may include adhesions from prior surgery—causing kinking, constriction, or volvulus of the bowel. Prompt decompression and release of adhesions is necessary, with attention to fluid and electrolyte replacement. At times the uterus must be evacuated in the third trimester because uterine size can impede one's ability to visualize the abdomen and pelvis well enough to identify the obstruction and correct it surgically.

Gallbladder disease

Pregnancy has been associated with an increased predisposition to gallstone formation, but not an increased risk for acute cholecystitis. In early pregnancy, a positive Murphy's sign and jaundice help differentiate cholecystitis from simple gestational nausea and vomiting. In late pregnancy, gallbladder disease must be differentiated from severe preeclampsia and hemolysis, elevated liver enzymes, and low platelet count (HELLP) syndrome. This cannot be overemphasized. Many women have been monitored conservatively and worked up with multiple tests for gallbladder disease while severe preeclampsia with liver involvement went unrecognized. Given the finding of elevated liver enzymes, hyperbilirubin-

CRITICAL POINTS

- When evaluating any medical or surgical complication during pregnancy, one should ask oneself not only how the condition affects maternal and fetal status, but also how the physiologic state of pregnancy may affect the diagnosis and natural history of the condition in question.
- What is commonly referred to as the "physiologic anemia of pregnancy" in fact is not a deficiency in erythrocyte mass, but rather a relative decrease in hematocrit that is due to an increase in plasma volume accompanying normal pregnancy.
- Dysuria in the pregnant woman should be investigated thoroughly and lower urinary tract infection treated aggressively to prevent the development of pyelonephritis, which—in addition to significant maternal morbidity—plays an important role as a cause of premature labor.
- The greatest help the physician may offer in treating diabetes in pregnancy is assisting the patient in achieving euglycemia in the preconceptional period, which has been shown to reduce the risks of major congenital malformations and first trimester pregnancy loss.
- The interpretation of thyroid function tests in pregnancy is assisted by the knowledge that total T_4 increases significantly in normal pregnancy; whereas the free, unbound fraction does not. A TSH evaluation is not affected by pregnancy in terms of laboratory interpretation.
- Women with a history of genital herpes simplex infection do not always require a cesarean section to prevent viral transmission to the neonate. Cesarean section is reserved for the patient with active lesions and/or symptoms at the time of labor and delivery.
- The CDC recommends using one of two strategies to prevent the complications of GBS infection in pregnancy: (1) intrapartum antibiotic prophylaxis is offered to women identified as carriers of GBS through prenatal screening cultures collected at 35 to 37 weeks' gestation and to women who develop premature onset of labor or rupture of membrane at less than 37 weeks' gestation; or (2) intrapartum antibiotic prophylaxis for women who develop one or more risk conditions at the time of labor or membrane rupture including delivery at less than 37 weeks' gestation, duration of ruptured membrane of more than 18 hours, intrapartum fever greater than 100.4° F, GBS bacteria noted at any time in the pregnancy, and/or history of having previously delivered an infant who had GBS sepsis.
- All pregnant women should be offered HIV screening. This is emphasized by important data that demonstrate a reduced risk of neonatal HIV infection when the HIV-positive gravida is treated with AZT during pregnancy.
- Despite the universal recommendation that all newborns begin a vaccination series for hepatitis B, routine screening for hepatitis B in pregnancy remains important to identify chronic carriers of hepatitis B and allow also for the provision of passive immunization (hepatitis B immune globulin) to the newborn of an infected mother.
- Given the potentially serious and potentially lethal complications of cardiac disease during pregnancy, preconceptional counseling is critical for women who have cardiac disease—allowing them to make informed choices with respect to reproduction.
- The pregnant woman with abdominal pain poses a most difficult but critical diagnostic dilemma. An understanding of the physiologic changes in pregnancy; the history and physical examination; knowledge of the gestational age; and appropriate interpretation of selected laboratory tests will assist in the formation of a differential diagnosis and implementation of a treatment plan. An ability to distinguish between obstetric and nonobstetric causes is imperative to enhance perinatal outcome.

emia, epigastric pain, and liver tenderness, one can see that this differentiation may not be clear at all times. Ultrasound evaluation of the gallbladder and ducts is an integral part of patient evaluation.

If possible, medical management is preferred, using withdrawal of food, intravenous hydration, and antibiotics. Patients may benefit from restriction of fat from the diet. Patients with recurrent episodes may require operative intervention. Depending on the trimester, surgical management options include cholecystectomy by either laparotomy or laparoscopy; and, in skilled hands, fiberoptic endoscopic cannulation retrieval of stones may be successful. Dissolution of gallstones with chenodeoxycholic acid or lithotripsy is contraindicated in pregnancy.

Questions

1. The prognosis of which of the following conditions is most influenced by pregnancy?
   A. Varicella pneumonia
   B. Mild asthma
   C. Appendicitis
   D. Mitral valve prolapse
   E. Acute hepatitis B
2. In which medical or surgical condition would termination of pregnancy be considered?
   A. Pyelonephritis
   B. Cholecystitis
   C. Eisenmenger's syndrome
   D. Mitral valve prolapse
   E. Class B diabetes mellitus
3. Fetal outcome may be improved via either maternal or direct fetal therapy for which of the following infectious diseases?
   A. Human immunodeficiency virus
   B. Human parvovirus B19
   C. Varicella
   D. Syphilis
   E. All of the above
4. Which of the following conditions has the most "impact" on perinatal outcome?
   A. Mild asthma
   B. Appendicitis
   C. Class F diabetes mellitus
   D. Varicella
   E. Thalassemia

Answers

1. A
2. C
3. E
4. C

Preeclampsia-eclampsia syndrome

APGO LEARNING OBJECTIVE #13

William H. Clewell

> *Preeclampsia-eclampsia syndrome accounts for significant morbidity and mortality in both mother and newborn.*

The student will demonstrate a knowledge of the following:
A. Definition(s) and classification of hypertension in pregnancy
B. Pathophysiology of preeclampsia-eclampsia syndrome
C. Symptoms, physical findings, and diagnostic methods
D. Approach to management
E. Maternal and fetal complications

Preeclampsia is a condition unique to human pregnancy. No comparable condition occurs in men or in nonpregnant women, and no similar condition occurs in other animals. These facts have made study of this condition difficult. Hypertensive disorders are the most common medical complication of pregnancy, and the most common hypertensive complications of pregnancy are preeclampsia or preeclampsia superimposed on chronic hypertension.

DEFINITION

In addition to the problem of there being no animal or nonpregnant model for this disease, the interpretation of clinical studies is complicated by inconsistent definitions of the condition. The Committee on Terminology of the American College of Obstetricians and Gynecologists and the National Institutes of Health Working Group on Hypertension in Pregnancy (1990) have recommended the following classification:

Chronic hypertension
Preeclampsia-eclampsia
Preeclampsia superimposed on chronic hypertension
Transient hypertension
Unclassified

Chronic hypertension is defined as high blood pressure that was present before pregnancy or diagnosed before 20 weeks of gestation. For this purpose, hypertension is defined as a pressure greater than 140/90 mm Hg.

Preeclampsia-eclampsia is defined as hypertension with edema, proteinuria, or both. Since many women of reproductive age have low baseline blood pressures, ideally one would define hypertension as a rise of 30 mm Hg systolic or 15 mm Hg diastolic over baseline values. In practice, a prepregnant value for comparison or even a first trimester blood pressure often is not available. In these circumstances a blood pressure greater than 140/90 after 20 weeks of gestation should be considered abnormal. Proteinuria greater than 0.3 g/24 hr or 0.1 g/L (2+ on clinical testing) is considered significant. Edema is a common feature of normal pregnancy; but excessive swelling, especially of the face and hands, or rapid weight gain (greater than 2 kg/wk) may indicate preeclampsia.

Mild preeclampsia is distinguished from severe preeclampsia. The characteristics of severe preeclampsia are as follows:

1. Blood pressure of 160 mm Hg systolic or 110 mm Hg diastolic on at least two occasions more than 6 hours apart with the patient at bed rest
2. Proteinuria of 5 g or more per 24 hours
3. Oliguria
4. Cerebral or visual disturbances
5. Epigastric pain
6. Pulmonary edema or cyanosis

Eclampsia is the occurrence of seizures or coma in a patient with preeclampsia when there is no other cause.

Transient hypertension is elevated blood pressure during pregnancy or immediately postpartum with no other signs of preeclampsia.

The term *unclassified hypertension* refers to the condition of those patients who do not fit into other classes.

This classification is far from perfect. As is demonstrated in the section on diagnosis, there is no perfect diagnostic test for preeclampsia; and many cases that appear to fit the preceding criteria are not truly preeclampsia. Some patients with the most severe forms of preeclampsia are not hypertensive and may not have proteinuria or clinically evident edema.

PATHOGENESIS

Since there is no animal model in which to test physiologic hypotheses, our understanding of the pathophysiology of preeclampsia is based on attempts to link the various observations of physiologic changes in human cases into a coherent model. Such models of disease remain incomplete and at this time cannot completely explain all of the features of the disease. One of the first abnormalities noted in women who will become preeclamptic is a relative failure of the second wave of trophoblastic invasion of the spiral arteries of the endometrium. This process normally converts the muscular spiral arteries into passive, widely dilated, noncontractile vessels. Another characteristic of these women is a relative deficiency of blood volume expansion and a less than normal increase in cardiac output. These changes may account for some of the abnormalities in renal, hepatic, placental, and brain function. There also appears to be an imbalance in the proportions of the prostaglandins thromboxane and prostacyclin in these women. This imbalance, with a relative increase in thromboxane, may account for some of the observed endothelial damage, vasospasm, and coagulation abnormalities. How all of these abnormalities are related, and which are primary and which are secondary, remains to be determined.

Arterial pressure results from cardiac output and peripheral vascular resistance. The hypertension in preeclampsia is primarily caused by generalized vasospasm. The cardiac output in most cases of preeclampsia is normal or slightly less than normal for pregnancy. Elevated blood pressure results from increased peripheral vascular resistance. The mechanism of this increased vascular tone is uncertain. Attempts to find a circulating pressor substance in the serum of preeclamptic women have been unsuccessful. It appears that the microcirculation in these patients is unusually sensitive to normal levels of pressor substances. Studies of normal pregnant women have shown that they are relatively resistant to the pressor effect of angiotensin II. Women who will develop preeclampsia have increased sensitivity to the pressor effect of angiotensin II when compared with pregnant women who will not become preeclamptic. The mechanism of the decreased sensitivity in normal pregnant women is unknown, as is the mechanism of the increased sensitivity in preeclamptic women.

In many preeclamptic women there is evidence of activation of the coagulation system. Most commonly this is seen as a consumption of platelets. In severe cases this may progress to severe thrombocytopenia (less than 50,000), but in most cases it is detectable only as a decline in platelet numbers on serial counts. Other evidence of activation of the clotting system, such as a decrease in fibrinogen or elevation in fibrin degradation products, occasionally is seen. Since fibrinogen is normally quite high in pregnancy, serial values may be needed to detect a decline.

SYMPTOMS AND SIGNS

One of the first signs of developing preeclampsia is sudden weight gain caused by the development of pathologic edema. Routine weight measurement at each prenatal visit is intended to detect such a sudden gain. An increase greater than 2 kg in a week is reason for concern. A rise in blood pressure even less than that which defines hypertension should be evaluated carefully. Urine testing for proteinuria is routine in prenatal care as a means of detecting the development of preeclampsia. None of these features alone points to the diagnosis of preeclampsia, and some patients with severe preeclampsia will not show any of these changes until the disease is far advanced or may not manifest them at all. The usual prenatal medical record, in which these parameters are serially charted, is designed to detect the development of preeclampsia before it becomes severe. When it is suspected that preeclampsia may develop, laboratory evaluation should be performed.

LABORATORY-DIAGNOSTIC STUDIES

As with clinical evaluation, no laboratory test is specifically diagnostic of preeclampsia. Abnormalities in renal, hepatic, and hematologic function can support a clinical diagnosis. Serum uric acid concentration is one of the most sensitive indicators. In normal pregnancy the serum urate concentration is less than 4.5 mg/100 ml (0.27 mmol/L). Serum creatinine values greater than 0.8 mg/100 ml should also be considered suspicious. It should be noted that these values for uric acid and creatinine are lower than the upper limit of normal for nonpregnant women. Printed laboratory reports usually do not flag these values as abnormal. Since one of the physiologic features of preeclampsia is failure of plasma volume expansion, a rising hematocrit or hemoglobin concentration is a feature of developing disease. Because many pregnant women are anemic, serial values are most useful. Platelet consumption is a common feature of preeclampsia, especially in severe disease. Serial platelet counts are very useful in diagnosis and in assessing the progression of disease. Some patients develop a microangeopathic hemolysis caused by intravascular coagulation. Elevations of the liver enzymes serum glutamic-oxaloacetic transaminase (SGOT) and serum glutamate pyruvate transaminase (SGPT) are common in severe disease. Occasionally patients will have manifestations of hepatic, hematologic, and renal function abnormalities with little or no hypertension or edema. Only a suspicion based on trends of clinical findings will lead to the laboratory diagnosis of these cases. The combination of hemolysis, elevated liver enzymes, and low platelet count is identified as the HELLP syndrome. Patients with this syndrome often have little or no edema and may not be hypertensive.

MANAGEMENT

There is no known effective prevention for preeclampsia. Certain groups of patients are at particular risk and deserve extra attention. Adolescent and older (over age 35) pregnant women are both at greater risk, as are women with chronic hypertension, diabetes, or renal disease. The risk of preeclampsia increases with fetal number in multiple gestation and reaches nearly 100% in quadruplet gestation by 34 weeks if premature delivery does not end the pregnancy first. Women who have had preeclampsia in one pregnancy are at high risk (30%) of recurrence in subsequent gestations. Several studies have suggested that low doses of aspirin (81 mg/day) may reduce the occurrence in high-risk patients. Calcium supplementation also has been shown to reduce the risk. Both of these therapies appear to be relatively safe for use in high-risk populations.

The only cure for preeclampsia is delivery. When it develops near term, management consists of stabilization of the woman and delivery of the fetus. When preeclampsia develops at immature gestational ages, management becomes much more difficult. In these cases attention must be paid to both maternal and fetal well-being while attempting to achieve optimal fetal maturity before delivery. Management of preeclampsia in these women usually entails hospitalization with bed rest and close surveillance of maternal and fetal status. The administration of glucocorticoids to accelerate fetal lung maturity is important in patients of less than 34 weeks' gestation. This therapy requires 48 hours to achieve optimal benefit. In some cases the maternal condition is so severe or progresses so rapidly that one cannot wait 48 hours after steroid administration for delivery. Maternal condition is rarely a contraindication to giving steroids. The rate of disease progression is unpredictable, and it is likely that giving steroid therapy for less than 24 hours may be of some benefit to the fetus. This is especially true for the extremely premature fetus (less than 30 weeks' gestation).

The preeclamptic patient is at risk for developing renal and hepatic failure, seizures, coma, or cerebral edema. Seizure prevention is usually achieved by administering magnesium sulfate ($MgSO_4$ $7H_2O$). This can be given by intramuscular injection; but more consistent, controllable, and predictable serum concentrations are achieved with intravenous administration. Generally a 4-g loading dose is given over 5 minutes followed by a constant infusion of 1 to 2 g/hr. Occasionally higher or lower infusion rates are needed to achieve therapeutic serum concentrations. Therapeutic levels can be assessed clinically by noting depression of deep tendon reflexes until they are present but not brisk. This generally corresponds to a serum level of 4 to 7 mEq/L. As long as the patellar reflex is present, magnesium toxicity is unlikely. Reflexes should be checked every 30 minutes during magnesium administration. This is generally sufficient to prevent seizures. Clinical assessment usually is sufficient to monitor magnesium therapy, but occasionally it is useful to check serum concentrations. Magnesium is excreted by the kidney, and in patients with preeclampsia there may be rapid changes in renal function.

In addition to preventing seizures, one must control the maternal blood pressure at safe levels. Magnesium sulfate has only a very weak antihypertensive effect. Repeated small intravenous doses of hydralazine or labetalol usually lower the arterial pressure in a controlled fashion to safe levels. Too rapid or extreme lowering of maternal pressure may result in acute fetal decompensation and distress. Generally the diastolic blood pressure should be maintained between 90 and 100 mm Hg.

The development of oliguria may necessitate placement of the patient in an obstetric intensive care unit. Often oliguria can be corrected by expanding maternal blood volume with saline infusions. However, these patients are at risk for developing pulmonary edema, and volume expansion should be done with care. Occasionally, invasive cardiovascular monitoring is needed to manage these patients safely. If pulmonary edema or central nervous system (CNS) complications develop, intubation and ventilation occasionally are needed.

Serial assessments of maternal hematologic, hepatic, renal, and CNS function are needed to determine both the severity and the rate of change of the maternal condition. It is difficult to set absolute limits for any of these parameters. When the disease progresses rapidly, one should set a much lower threshold for ending the pregnancy. The proximity to fetal maturity must also be taken into account in deciding when to deliver the baby. The development of seizures, cerebral edema, or coma is an absolute indication for expeditious delivery of the fetus regardless of gestational age.

The fetus is at jeopardy in preeclampsia for both antepartum and intrapartum distress and for placental abruption. At times fetal growth restriction with or without oligohydramnios is the first manifestation of the disease. This probably results from placental dysfunction. The fetus is also at risk for acute asphyxia. With advancing gestation and progression of preeclampsia the risk of fetal compromise rises. In the relatively stable patient, twice weekly fetal nonstress tests and weekly amniotic fluid volume assessments seem adequate to ensure fetal well-being. In the patient with a rapidly changing condition or during the initiation of blood pressure control, more frequent or even continuous fetal monitoring may be needed.

The route of delivery in these patients can be by induction of labor and vaginal delivery or by cesarean section. The choice is dictated by the urgency of the maternal condition, the favorability of the cervix for induction, and the fetal tolerance for labor. The development of maternal thrombocytopenia or coagulation abnormalities often must be taken into account in this decision. Since induction of labor is often successful in these patients, it should be attempted if maternal and fetal conditions allow it.

MATERNAL AND FETAL OUTCOMES

Maternal mortality generally is uncommon in preeclampsia. With the development of eclampsia or HELLP syndrome the risk increases, but should still be less than 5%. Cerebral hemorrhage, hepatic necrosis, heart failure, and acute renal failure may contribute to maternal mortality. Fetal morbidity and mortality are most commonly related to prematurity. Intrauterine or intrapartum fetal death can occur because of placental insufficiency or abruption. Fetal growth restric-

CRITICAL POINTS

- Preeclampsia is a relatively <u>common</u> complication of pregnancy and a <u>significant</u> cause of maternal and fetal morbidity and mortality.
- Serial assessments of maternal weight, blood pressure, and urine for protein are intended to detect the development of this problem and to allow timely intervention. Some patients may develop severe preeclampsia without developing any of these signs.
- The fetus is at risk during the antepartum and intrapartum period. Fetal growth retardation may be the first clinical manifestation of disease.
- Delivery is the only cure for the condition, but this may not be optimal for the fetus because of prematurity.
- Protecting maternal health and life while also attempting to achieve optimal fetal maturity poses the most difficult management problem in this condition.

tion or intrauterine growth retardation (IUGR) is a frequent complication.

Questions

1. Preeclampsia is characterized by:
   A. Elevated peripheral vascular resistance, expanded maternal blood volume, and normal cardiac output.
   B. Normal peripheral vascular resistance, elevated cardiac output, and normal maternal blood volume.
   C. Elevated peripheral vascular resistance, reduced maternal blood volume, and normal cardiac output.
   D. Reduced placental perfusion, decreased renal perfusion, and increased maternal blood volume
   E. Reduced placental perfusion, reduced cardiac output, and increased renal perfusion
2. Fetal risks in preeclampsia include:
   A. Intrauterine growth retardation, intrapartum asphyxia, prematurity, and abruption
   B. Prematurity, fetal malformation, and intrapartum asphyxia
   C. Antepartum asphyxia, neonatal death, and postmaturity
   D. Abruption, fetal renal failure, and IUGR
   E. Intrapartum fetal distress, IUGR, and fetal malformation
3. Treatment of preeclampsia includes:
   A. Maternal magnesium sulfate, antihypertensive drugs, and fluid restriction
   B. Induction of labor, control of blood pressure, and magnesium sulfate
   C. Glucocorticoids, fluid restriction, and delivery
   D. Magnesium sulfate, expansion of blood volume, and cesarean section
   E. Immediate delivery by cesarean section

Answers

1. C
2. A
3. B

14

D isoimmunization

APGO LEARNING OBJECTIVE #14

William H. Clewell

The problem of fetal hemolysis from maternal D isoimmunization has been greatly lessened in the past few decades. Awareness of the red cell antigen-antibody system is important to help further reduce the morbidity and mortality from isoimmunization.

The student will demonstrate a knowledge of the following:

A. Antigens of the Rh system
B. Use of immunoglobulin prophylaxis during pregnancy
C. Clinical circumstances under which D isoimmunization is likely to occur
D. Methods used to determine maternal isoimmunization and severity of fetal involvement

Red blood cell isoimmunization occurs when a woman is exposed to foreign red cell antigens by blood transfusion or fetal-to-maternal red cell leakage during pregnancy or delivery. If the woman's body mounts an immune response to these antigens, the antibody can cause fetal red cell destruction in a subsequent pregnancy if the fetus carries the sensitizing antigen. The fetal or neonatal consequences of such hemolysis were recognized before 1932, but it wasn't until Landsteiner described the Rh antigen in 1940 that the pathophysiology of the condition began to be understood. Various red cell antigens can be involved in isoimmunization, but the D antigen in the Rh system is the most important in terms of the numbers of patients at risk. Approximately 15% of people in North America are Rh-negative or lack the D antigen. Thus an Rh-negative woman has a high likelihood (85%) of marrying an Rh-positive husband.

PATHOGENESIS

Of the red blood cell antigens, the D antigen is the one most frequently involved in significant isoimmunization and fetal effects. The Rh antigen system includes five antigens, D, C, c, E, and e. They are inherited as six alleles on three loci, D/d, C/c, and E/e. There is no antigen associated with the d gene. A person is considered Rh-positive if the red cells carry the D antigen and Rh-negative if the antigen is absent. To be Rh-negative the person must be homozygous d/d. Homozygous D/D and heterozygous D/d individuals type as Rh-positive and cannot be distinguished from each other. Exposure of persons to red cell antigens that they lack can result in isoimmunization. In the case of the D antigen as little as 0.3 ml of Rh-positive red cells is sufficient to provoke a primary immune response. Other antigen systems may require larger antigen doses to cause sensitization.

Once sensitization has occurred and the immune response is mature and producing immunoglobulin (Ig) G, the fetus is at risk. The class G Ig's cross the placenta from the maternal circulation to the fetus. The Ig's bind to their antigens on the fetal red cells, and these antibody-coated cells are destroyed by the fetal reticuloendothelial system. Hemolysis results in anemia and an erythropoietic response in the fetus. Hemolysis also results in increased bilirubin production in the fetus and an elevated amniotic fluid bilirubin concentration. The serum bilirubin in the fetus never gets high enough to be dangerous because it is cleared by the placenta into the maternal circulation. If the fetal anemia becomes severe enough, extramedullary hematopoiesis occurs and erythroblasts will be found in the fetal circulation. Fetal hepatosplenomegaly occurs because extramedullary hematopoiesis and ultimately fetal hydrops develops owing to high-output heart failure and hypoproteinemia. This can progress to fetal or neonatal death.

After delivery infants with severe sensitization may develop hyperbilirubinemia caused by continuing hemolysis and the inability of the immature liver to conjugate and eliminate the excess bilirubin. The excess unconjugated bilirubin can be deposited in the basal ganglia of the brain, leading to kernicterus.

SIGNS AND SYMPTOMS

Except in rare and extremely severe cases, D isoimmunization causes no symptoms in the woman. When the fetus is hydropic, polyhydramnios may develop—leading to uterine overdistention and perhaps preterm labor. In very rare cases the woman may become preeclamptic in response to a severely affected hydropic infant and placental enlargement. Because of its superficial similarity to hydrops, this has been referred to as the maternal "mirror syndrome." Generally when this occurs the fetus is very near death from hydrops.

DIAGNOSIS AND LABORATORY TESTS

Diagnosis of sensitization

Detection and prevention of isoimmunization rely on laboratory studies. Except in the most severe cases there are no symptoms in the affected woman. Testing of all pregnant women for blood types ABO and Rh must be done at their first prenatal visit. They also need an antibody screen. This is a nonspecific screen for any significant red cell antibodies. If antibodies are found they should be identified as to specificity. Table 14-1 lists the antibodies that are significant for their ability to cause fetal hemolysis. If the antibody identified can cause significant fetal problems, it should be titered. In general there is little risk to the fetus with titers less than 1:16. It is often useful to type the father of the fetus. If the father does not carry the sensitizing antigen, the fetus will not inherit it and is at no risk from the sensitization. This is often the case with non-Rh antigens. Patients are not routinely matched for

Table 14-1. Antibodies causing hemolytic disease*

Blood group system	Antigens related to hemolytic disease	Severity of hemolytic disease
CDE	D	Mild to severe
	C	Mild to moderate
	c	Mild to severe
	E	Mild to severe
	e	Mild to moderate
Lewis	Le^a	Not a proved cause of hemolytic disease of the newborn
	Le^b	Not a proved cause of hemolytic disease of the newborn
Kell	K	Mild to severe with hydrops fetalis
	k	Mild to severe
Duffy	Fy^a	Mild to severe with hydrops fetalis
	Fy^b	Not a cause of hemolytic disease of the newborn
Kidd	Jk^a	Mild to severe
	Jk^b	Mild to severe
MNSs	M	Mild to severe
	N	Mild
	S	Mild to severe
	s	Mild to severe
Lutheran	Lu^a	Mild
	Lu^b	Mild
Diego	Di^a	Mild to severe
	Di^b	Mild to severe
Xg	Xg^a	Mild
P	PP P^a (Tj^a)	Mild to severe

(Modified from Weinstein L: Irregular antibodies causing hemolytic disease of the newborn: a continuing problem, *Clin Obstet Gynecol* 25:321-332, 1982.)

*Note that conditions listed as being "mild" only can be treated like they are ABO incompatible. Patients with all other conditions should be monitored as if they are sensitized to D.

these antigens for blood transfusion, and so are frequently exposed to non-Rh red cell antigens. With the successful prevention of D sensitization by anti-D Ig, transfusion-induced sensitization to other antigens has become relatively more important.

Amniocentesis

As noted above, fetal red cell destruction results in increased bilirubin production in the fetal compartment. This is reflected in elevated amniotic fluid bilirubin concentration. Lilly performed am-

niocentesis in a number of Rh-sensitized women and noted that the amount of bilirubin in the amniotic fluid depended on both the gestational age and the severity of fetal hemolysis. He measured the amount of bilirubin in the amniotic fluid as the "Delta OD 450." A spectrophotometric scan of the amniotic fluid showed a displacement of the curve at 450 nm, which corresponded to bilirubin (Fig. 14-1). Recently Queenan expanded on Lilly's observation and, in a larger series of patients over a wider gestational age range, defined a relationship of Delta OD 450 to gestational age and disease severity. Figure 14-2 is

Table 14-1. Antibodies causing hemolytic disease—cont'd

Blood group system	Antigens related to hemolytic disease	Severity of hemolytic disease
Public	Y1^a	Moderate to severe
	Y1^b	Mild
	Lan	Mild
	En^a	Moderate
	Ge	Mild
	Jp^a	Mild
	Co^a	Severe
	Co^{a-b}	Mild
Private antigens	Batty	Mild
	Becker	Mild
	Berrens	Mild
	Evans	Mild
	Gonzales	Mild
	Good	Severe
	Heibel	Moderate
	Hunt	Mild
	Jobbins	Mild
	Radin	Moderate
	Rm	Mild
	Ven	Mild
	Wright^a	Severe
	Wright^b	Mild
	Zd	Moderate

drawn after the work of Queenan. Often two or more amniocenteses are needed to define a patient's status as to disease severity.

Developing hemolytic anemia is the primary problem faced by the fetus in isoimmunization. In many cases premature delivery of the fetus is needed to avoid severe anemia and death. Following delivery, the infant is at risk from anemia and continuing hemolysis. If the infant's red cells are coated with maternal antibody they will be rapidly destroyed and the hemoglobin metabolized to bilirubin. Because of the relative immaturity of the newborn liver, bilirubin is not rapidly conjugated for excretion. The unconjugated bilirubin can be toxic to the brain if the binding capacity of serum albumin is exceeded. The infant may require phototherapy or in some cases exchange transfusion to prevent bilirubin toxicity.

In some cases the fetus is so severely affected at such an early gestational age that premature delivery is not a reasonable option. In these cases the fetus is at risk of death in utero from anemia and hydrops. Fetal transfusion is the only option to avoid both fetal death and the complications of extreme prematurity. Ultrasound-guided umbilical cord puncture for fetal blood sampling and

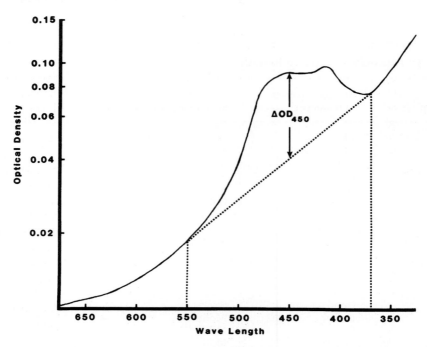

Fig. 14-1. Spectrophotometric scan of amniotic fluid. Peak at 450 nm corresponds to bilirubin. Lilly's method of estimating amniotic fluid bilirubin is demonstrated here.

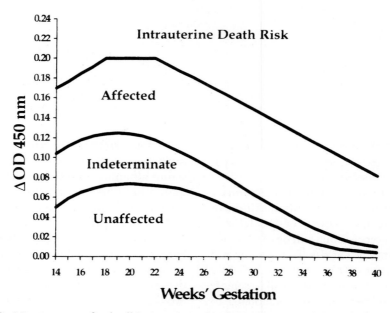

Fig. 14-2. Management of red cell isoimmunization. Queenan expanded on work of Lilly, and using larger patient population and more samples was able to define risk zones shown here.

transfusion is then needed. This procedure carries approximately a 1% risk of procedure-related fetal death for each transfusion performed. In some cases several transfusions may be needed.

MANAGEMENT

Prophylaxis with D immune globulin

It was observed that patients who were ABO incompatible with their infants rarely became Rh-sensitized. Patients with type O blood have anti-A and anti-B antibody in their serum. Likewise, type A patients have anti-B antibody, and type B patients have anti-A antibody. These antibodies are usually of the IgM type and do not cross the placenta. It was presumed that these constitutive antibodies prevented sensitization to the Rh antigen by removing the Rh-positive, type A or B incompatible cells before they could be recognized as foreign by the maternal immune system. Based on this hypothesis it was shown that one could effectively prevent primary immunization with the D antigen by giving a person exogenous anti-D antibody shortly after exposure to D antigen. The prevention of sensitization is more efficient and more specific than can be accounted for by simple removal of the potentially sensitizing red cells. It appears that the treated person's immune system is able to recognize the presence of antibody to the antigen in question (D in the case of Rh isoimmunization) and specifically not respond to it as a primary immunogen.

Since most sensitization occurs through fetal red cell leakage into the maternal circulation at the time of delivery, immunoprophylaxis was first used immediately after delivery. Three hundred micrograms of anti-D Ig given by intramuscular injection within 72 hours of delivery prevented sensitization in most cases. In an untreated population of Rh-negative women delivering Rh-positive babies, 15% of the exposed women became sensitized following each delivery. With postpartum Rh immune globulin treatment,

1.5% of women became sensitized. These sensitizations appear to occur through antepartum fetal-to-maternal red cell transfusions. By giving Rh immune globulin to unsensitized women at 28 weeks' gestation and following delivery, nearly all of these sensitizations can be prevented. Since this material is IgG and capable of crossing the placenta, it could in theory cause some fetal hemolysis. Because of the amount of antibody involved and the dilution in the maternal system, the amount that gets to the fetus is insufficient to cause significant hemolysis.

Any procedure or event that potentially exposes an Rh-negative, unsensitized woman to Rh-positive cells presents an opportunity to prevent sensitization with Rh immune globulin. This includes amniocentesis, uterine bleeding in any trimester, spontaneous or induced abortion after 6 weeks of amenorrhea, ectopic pregnancy, and even mismatched transfusion with Rh-positive blood. The amount of Rh immune globulin administered is adjusted depending on the estimate of the volume of Rh-positive cells that the woman received.

CONCLUSIONS

Red cell isoimmunization can be a devastating problem for the fetus and newborn. Immunoprophylaxis with Rh immune globulin has the potential to eliminate it almost completely. Most sensitizations today occur from excessive fetal-to-maternal transfusion or failure to use this preparation appropriately. Sensitizations to other red cell antigens that can cause fetal problems similar to D sensitization generally occur following blood transfusion. Blood is not routinely matched for these antigens before transfusion, and these antigens make up a larger portion of isoimmunization cases today than in the past. Once sensitization has occurred, management depends on the antigen involved; the titer of the antigen; and, in more severe cases, the amniotic fluid bilirubin content.

CRITICAL POINTS

- Red cell isoimmunization is generally asymptomatic; therefore the diagnosis depends on routine laboratory testing for red cell antigens.
- The main therapy is timely delivery based on direct assessment of the degree of fetal jeopardy by amniocentesis or fetal blood sampling.
- In severe cases direct fetal transfusion can correct the fetal anemia until a time safe for delivery.
- Immunoprophylaxis with Rh immune globulin has greatly reduced the prevalence of this problem.
- Non-Rh isoimmunization remains a problem; because of the reduction in the number of Rh sensitizations it is relatively more common today.

Questions

1. Maternal red cell isoimmunization can occur after:
   A. Uncomplicated delivery of an Rh-positive baby
   B. Spontaneous abortion of an Rh-positive fetus
   C. Third trimester bleeding
   D. All of the above
2. Maternal red cell isoimmunization is diagnosed by finding:
   A. Rh-negative blood type
   B. Antibody to red cell antigens in the mother's serum
   C. An Rh-positive baby

3. In red cell isoimmunization the fetus is at risk for:
   A. Anemia caused by blood loss
   B. Hemolysis and neonatal hyperbilirubinemia
   C. Hypoxia

Answers

1. D
2. B
3. B

15

Multifetal gestation

APGO LEARNING OBJECTIVE #15

John P. Elliott

> *When there is more than one fetus, antepartum, intrapartum, and postpartum management must be modified to minimize adverse outcome for the mother and fetuses.*

The student will demonstrate a knowledge of the following:

A. Etiology of monozygotic, dizygotic, and multizygotic gestation
B. Altered physiologic state with multifetal gestation
C. Symptoms, physical findings, and diagnostic methods
D. Approach to antepartum, intrapartum, and postpartum management

Human reproduction is most efficient when there is one fetus present. Two or more babies accentuate the problems that occur in a singleton gestation and create some that are unique to multifetal gestations. These pregnancies can occur spontaneously or can result from assisted reproductive technology, as shown in Table 15-1. Hellen's rule can be used to estimate the spontaneous rate of multiple gestation. If the rate of twins in a population is known (N), then triplets will occur $1:(N)^2$. In the United States, twins occur 1 in 83 deliveries, so triplets would occur $1:(83)^2$, or 1 in 6889 deliveries; quadruplets would occur $1:(83)^3$, or 1 in 571,787 deliveries; and so on.

PATHOGENESIS

Twin, triplet, or quadruplet pregnancies can result from the splitting of one zygote into two or more embryos; more commonly, more than one egg is ovulated and fertilized. Twins are classified as dizygotic (fraternal) or monozygotic (identical). Monozygotic twinning creates some different circumstances that significantly affect outcome. As illustrated in Fig. 15-1, the time after fertilization when the split occurs determines placental type and fetal complications. If the split occurs in the first 3 days, the embryo retains the

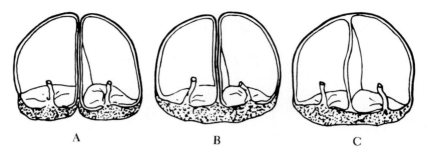

Fig. 15-1. Placenta and membranes in twin pregnancy. **A,** Dizygotic twins with two complete placentas and membranes. **B,** Dizygotic twins with double membranes and fused placenta. **C,** Monozygotic twins with double amniotic cavities enclosed within one chorion.

Table 15-1. Incidence of multifetal gestations

	Spontaneous	Clomid	Pergonal	GIFT*
Twins	1.2 : 100	8%	18%	22%
Monozygotic	40 : 10,000			
Dizygotic	80 : 10,000			
Triplets	1 : 6889	0.5%	3%	4%
Quadruplets	1 : 571,787	0.3%	1.2%	1.2%
≥ Quintuplets	$1 : (47 \times 10^6)$	0.13%		

*Gamete intrafallopian tube transfer procedure.

ability to form a complete chorion, amnion, and fetus—resulting in a dichorionic-diamniotic (Di Di) placenta and two same-sex babies in separate sacs. At 3 days, the embryo loses the ability to make a separate chorion, so splitting between day 3 and day 8 results in a placenta with a single chorion, but separate amnions and babies. The placenta is monochorionic-diamniotic (Mo Di) with same-sex fetuses in separate sacs. If the twinning event occurs between day 8—when the amnion is irreversibly differentiated—and day 14, there will be one chorion and one amnion, but two like-sex fetuses. The placenta is mono-chorionic-monoamniotic (Mo Mo), with both babies in the same sac. Twinning that occurs after day 14, when the fetal cells start to become irreversibly differentiated, results in the rare occurrence of conjoined twins. The placenta is Mo Mo with two like-sex fetuses that are fused and that share some organs in a single sac. Two thirds of twins are Di Di, one third are Mo Di, and 1% are Mo Mo. It should be remembered that when the placenta is Di Di, the fetuses can be either identical or fraternal.

It is important to establish the type of placentation in a multifetal gestation because it will establish the risk for complications and determine optimal management. Real-time ultrasound scanning can help to clarify the placentation. Separate placentas or different-sex fetuses

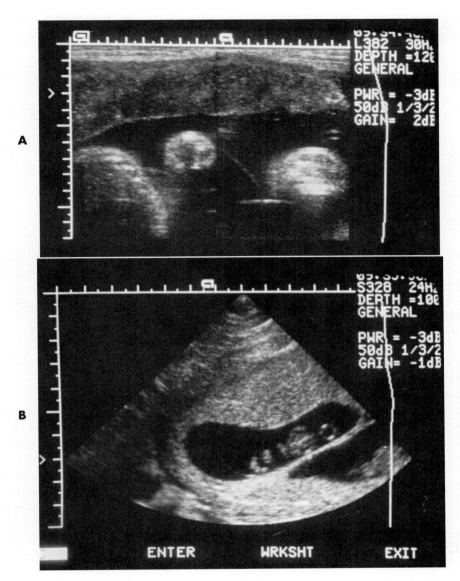

Fig. 15-2. Ultrasound of amniotic membranes. **A** demonstrates thin wispy membrane of monochorionic placenta. **B** demonstrates thicker (more echo-dense) membrane of dichorionic placenta.

will identify Di Di placentas. When the placentas are fused, a thin, wispy membrane suggests monochorionic placentation; a thicker, more echo-dense membrane would indicate dichorionic placentae (Fig. 15-2). Placental tissue extending between the amnions (twin-peak sign) would also indicate two chorions. Monochorionic placentation is associated with a higher rate of fetal loss and places the pregnancy at risk for twin-twin transfusion syndrome.

Table 15-2. Pregnancy complications of multifetal gestation (%)

	Singleton	Twins	Triplets	Quadruplets*
SGA	4.6	17.4	30	10
Antepartum hemorrhage	2.0	2.8	6.7	10
PIH	8.2	23	28	75
Anemia	3.5	23	28	40
Preterm labor	8.4	42.7	84	80
IUFD >20 weeks	1	3.7	6.7	0

*Data from Phoenix Perinatal Associates.
SGA, Small for gestational age; *PIH*, pregnancy-induced hypertension; *IUFD*, intrauterine fetal death.

INCIDENCE

Twins represent about 1.25% of all pregnancies conceived but, because of spontaneous loss, account for only 1 in 83 deliveries. The incidence of identical twins is constant (about 4 in 1000 deliveries) across all populations. Dizygotic or fraternal twins are affected by race (higher incidence in black women than in white women; higher incidence in white women than in Asian women); maternal family history of twins; increasing age; increasing parity; and, most important, ovulation induction. The difference in dizygotic twinning probably relates to differences in gonadotropin production that are related to race, age, and inherited family traits. The father has little influence on twinning.

PHYSIOLOGY

Cardiovascular changes in pregnancy include a 30% to 50% increase in cardiac output, with increase in both stroke volume and heart rate. Twin gestations are associated with an even more profound increase in cardiac output of approximately 70% compared with nonpregnant patients. Systemic vascular resistance is decreased in pregnancy, but presumably not significantly more in twin gestation than singleton. Renal plasma flow in pregnancy is 35% to 40% above nonpregnant levels and probably is increased further in multiple gestation. No information is now available about any further effect of triplets or quadruplets on this physiology.

DIAGNOSIS

Multifetal gestation should be suspected if the uterine size is larger than expected for the presumed gestational age. It is important to make the diagnosis as early in gestation as possible to try to prevent the increased complications observed with these pregnancies. Maternal serum α-fetoprotein (MSAFP) usually is elevated in twin gestation and would prompt ultrasound evaluation. Ultrasound should be used liberally to establish solid gestational age information and should be indicated in high-risk patients, especially when ovulation was stimulated.

CLINICAL COURSE

Pregnancy complications of multifetal gestation are listed in Table 15-2. Complication rates generally increase with each additional baby added to

Table 15-3. Mortality rates of multifetal gestation (%)				
	Number of fetuses			
	1	2	3	4
Fetal	1.1	3.4	3.2	2.9
Neonatal	2.8	11.8	3.5	12.2
Perinatal	3.9	15.2	6.7	15.1

the uterus. Mortality rates (Table 15-3) reflect the same trend. Twins have a higher incidence of congenital malformations (8%) compared with 3% in singleton gestations.

First trimester nausea and vomiting is frequently more severe in multiple gestations and sometimes necessitates parenteral feeding. Diet is important, and ideal weight gain is greater than the 24 lb suggested for a singleton pregnancy. A high-protein, high-calorie diet is suggested, with a target weight gain for twins of 35 to 40 lb, triplets 50 to 65 lb, and quadruplets 75 to 100 lb. Extra iron is suggested, and 2 g/day of supplemental calcium is recommended. Somatic complaints such as heartburn, backache, abdominal distention and discomfort, and difficulty with breathing frequently are observed. The individual growth of the fetuses is generally equivalent to a singleton until about the twenty-seventh week, when a slowing occurs. Growth of the fetuses is supported equally until the total combined weight reaches approximately 7 lb; then subsequent growth of the combined fetal weight is equal. This occurs in twins at about 30 weeks' gestation, 27 weeks' in triplets, and 26 weeks' in quadruplets.

Pregnancy-induced hypertension (PIH) is more frequent in dizygotic twins (27%) than in monozygotic (18%), and it is about 3 to 4 times as common as in singleton gestations (6%). Treatment with supplemental calcium (2 g/day) may reduce the incidence of PIH.

Monochorionic twins are at risk for a special complication of twin pregnancy: twin-twin transfusion syndrome (TTTS). This complication occurs in 6% to 27% of monochorionic pregnancies. Schatz in 1895 described the pathophysiology of TTTS when he described the presence of vascular anastomosis in the placenta. These anastomoses are of three types: arterial-arterial; venous-venous; and arteriovenous. The important type is when an artery from one baby's circulation anastomoses to a low-pressure venous vessel of the twin. These anastomoses go from B to A and from A to B. If the net flow is significantly disproportionate, TTTS can develop (Fig. 15-3). The disproportion of blood volume affects the babies. The recipient fetus develops hypervolemia, which causes ascites, pleural effusion, and pericardial effusion. The fetus attempts to excrete the volume overload, and the polyuria creates polyhydramnios in the amniotic sac of the recipient. The donor twin is hypovolemic, which causes intrauterine growth retardation (IUGR) and oligohydramnios resulting from oliguria.

Severe TTTS occurs in the second trimester and results in what is referred to as the "stuck twin syndrome." The donor twin appears to be stuck to the wall of the uterus because the almost total oligohydramnios wraps the baby in the amnion like a "mummy." The excess amniotic fluid is all in the sac of the recipient. Untreated, TTTS is associated with about 100% mortality as a result of preterm labor or premature rupture of fetal membranes (PROM). Treatment with therapeutic amniocentesis has been associated with 75% survival. The goal of therapeutic amniocentesis is to remove as much fluid as possible from the recipient's sac, attempting to achieve a normal volume. The amniocentesis is repeated as often as necessary to achieve normal fluid volume around both babies. There is also a moderate TTTS, which occurs in the early third trimester and is associated with a better outcome but still a significant risk of premature delivery. The final classification of TTTS is mild, which is characterized by a difference in weight greater than 20% and a difference in hemoglobin concentrations of greater than 5 g. Outcome usually is good in these monochorionic twin pregnancies, which presumably have a more chronic low-grade perfusion differential.

Preterm labor is frequent in multiple gestations, occurring in 40% to 50% of twins, 70% of triplets, and more than 90% of quadruplet pregnancies; PROM also occurs frequently in twins, with an incidence of 12% occurring less than 36 weeks' gestation. The prevention of prematurity is the key to management of multifetal gestations. Important aspects include early diagnosis, frequent ultrasound to detect early TTTS or growth discrepancy, supplemental iron and folic acid, adequate diet, calcium supplementation, frequent cervical exams, bed rest, and contraction assessment. Monitoring uterine activity at home may be helpful in detecting increased uterine activity with cervical change early enough to allow intervention with tocolytic drugs. (See Chapter 19, Preterm Labor.) There does not appear to be a benefit from cerclage or prophylactic tocolytic drugs.

Amniocentesis is frequently indicated in the management of multifetal gestations. Twins are more frequent in older gravidas; and infertility frequently affects older women, placing these gestations at increased risk for chromosomal abnormalities. Sampling the amniotic fluid of each sac necessitates careful, ultrasound-guided technique. It is important to mark the fluid in the sac that is sampled first. This is accomplished by instilling a colored solution such as indigo carmine or Evans blue dye into the amniotic fluid after removal of the first sample. A second amniocentesis is then done into what is presumed to be the other sac. If nonblue fluid is obtained, the physician can be certain that each baby has been sampled. For triplets, dye is inserted into the second sac also, and the third sac is sampled.

Another reason for amniocentesis in multifetal pregnancies is to determine fetal lung maturity before delivery or administration of corticosteroids to enhance pulmonary surfactant production. There is reasonably close agreement of lecithin/sphingomyelin ratios in concordantly growing twins (same size); however, if growth is discordant, both sacs must be sampled. There is no consistent pattern of pulmonary maturity in either the smaller or larger babies.

DELIVERY ISSUES

The timing of delivery in multifetal gestations is an important management decision. Perinatal morbidity and mortality in twin gestation is increased when the gestation extends beyond 38 completed weeks (beyond that is postdates for a twin pregnancy). Elective earlier delivery (35 to 36 weeks with documented pulmonary maturity) should be strongly considered in monochorionic twins because of risk of sudden, acute, severe volume shifts that can occur in seemingly normal-growing monochorionic twins.

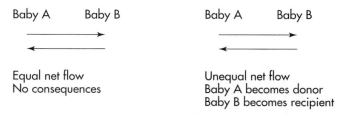

Fig. 15-3. Schematic of blood flow in twin-twin transfusion syndrome (TTTS).

Monoamniotic twins represent a perplexing dilemma because of the risk of cord entanglement. Perinatal mortality is possibly as high as 50% in this situation, most of which occurs prior to 30 weeks. How early should these twins be delivered? Some perinatologists advocate giving corticosteroids and delivering at 32 weeks; others would target 34 weeks to attempt to lower morbidity. This question is controversial, but delivery of monoamniotic twins should be by cesarean section because of increased risk of cord compromise and possibly locked twins (if presentations are breech-vertex).

Delivery of triplets or quadruplets should be by cesarean section. Most of these women are infertility patients and will be delivering premature babies. They do not tolerate labor well and also do not tolerate any delivery trauma well. A vaginal birth after cesarean section can be offered in future pregnancies. Twin delivery offers more options to the obstetrician. Vertex-vertex presentation at any gestational age is a candidate for attempted vaginal delivery. Breech or transverse lie of the first baby should be delivered by cesarean section. Vertex-nonvertex presentations can be delivered by cesarean section or vaginal delivery of the first twin, followed by attempted external cephalic version of the second twin to a vertex with vaginal delivery or breech extraction of the second twin. It is sometimes necessary to perform a cesarean section for the second twin because of failed version, cord prolapse, or placental separation. Labor is usually of normal duration in twin gesta-tions; however, long contractions (greater than 90 seconds) are frequent because of uterine overdistention. Both fetuses should be monitored on an electronic fetal heart rate monitor. Delivery of the first twin is similar to singleton labors. After delivery of twin A, clamp the umbilical cord and check for the position and station of twin B. Ultrasound in the delivery room is helpful in assessing twin B. If the cord is not palpable, oxytocin can be given to reinstitute contractions, which often cease after delivery of twin A. The obstetrician must be prepared for rapid vaginal delivery or cesarean section in the event of cord prolapse or abruption. The best outcomes are achieved when the second twin delivers within 15 to 20 minutes after twin A. Epidural analgesia and anesthesia is preferred in twin labors because it will facilitate interventions for the second baby (breech extraction, external cephalic version, forceps or vacuum-assisted delivery, or prompt emergency cesarean section).

Postpartum hemorrhage is more frequent in twins and high-order multiple gestations because of the overdistention of the uterus. Careful attention must be paid to prevention of this complication if possible. Vigorous manual massage of the uterus is the initial treatment, with concurrent administration of drugs to stimulate contraction of the uterine smooth muscle. Oxytocin (30 to 40 U) diluted in 500 to 1000 ml of intravenous solution should be run wide-open until the uterus firms up. Methylergonovine (0.2 mg) may be given intravenously in the absence of hyperten-

CRITICAL POINTS

- Twins have significantly higher perinatal morbidity and mortality than do singletons.
- Maternal risks include PIH, anemia, gestational diabetes, and postpartum hemorrhage.
- Fetal risks include prematurity, congenital anomalies, TTTS, IUGR, cord prolapse, and entanglement.
- Monochorionic twins are at risk for TTTS.
- Postdates in twin gestations occur after 38 completed weeks of gestation.

sion or, preferably, one ampule of 15 methyl-prostaglandin $F_{2\alpha}$ (250 µg) can be given intramuscularly or, at cesarean section, injected into the uterine muscle. These therapies will be successful most of the time, with operative intervention (hypogastric artery ligation or hysterectomy) reserved for those who do not respond. If blood loss is excessive, transfusion may be necessary.

Questions

1. The most common contributing factor of multifetal pregnancy is:
   A. Black race
   B. Infertility treatment
   C. Twins in mother's family
   D. Multiparity
   E. Increasing maternal age
2. The most common complication of multifetal gestation is:
   A. Twin-twin transfusion syndrome
   B. Discordant twins
   C. Prematurity
   D. Pregnancy-induced hypertension
   E. Anemia
3. Recommended treatment for severe TTTS is:
   A. Observation
   B. Tocolysis with magnesium sulfate
   C. Indomethacin
   D. Therapeutic amniocentesis
   E. Fetal blood transfusion

Answers

1. B
2. C
3. D

16

Fetal death

APGO LEARNING OBJECTIVE #16

Shirley K. Sawai

Early and accurate diagnosis and management will help the patient with emotional adjustments surrounding fetal death and may prevent associated obstetric complications.

The student will demonstrate a knowledge of the following:
A. Differential diagnosis of the causes of fetal death in each trimester
B. Symptoms, physical findings, and diagnostic methods to confirm the diagnosis
C. Management of a patient after fetal death
D. Emotional reactions and their effect on management
E. Maternal complications of fetal death, including disseminated intravascular coagulation

Fetal death has been defined by the World Health Organization as death of the conceptus before the complete expulsion or extraction of the products of conception, regardless of the gestational age. It has been recommended that the term *fetal death* replace the older terms of *abortion* for fetal death after less than 20 weeks' gestation and *stillbirth* for deaths occurring later than 20 weeks or fetuses weighing over 500 g. Fetal deaths are classified as follows:

Group I: Early fetal deaths—less than 20 completed weeks of pregnancy
Group II: Intermediate fetal deaths—20 to 27 completed weeks of pregnancy
Group III: Late fetal deaths—28 or more completed weeks of pregnancy
Group IV: Unclassified

The National Center for Health Statistics in the United States recognizes fetal deaths as those occurring at 20 weeks' gestation or more when reporting vital statistics and calculating fetal mortality. Since most states do not require the reporting of fetal deaths before 20 weeks' gestation, the true fetal death rate cannot be accurately determined. Spontaneous abortion (less than 20 weeks' gestational age) occurs in 10% to 15% of recognized pregnancies. Some studies report that 35%

to 40% of conceptions end in fetal death in the first 4 weeks of pregnancy.

CAUSES

Despite a thorough work-up, the cause of fetal death remains unknown in 25% to 50% of cases. The gestational age at fetal death does, however, make some causes more likely than others. More than 80% of fetal deaths at less than 20 weeks occur in the first trimester, with chromosomal anomalies being the cause of at least half of these early deaths. Genetic causes of fetal death decrease to 36% in the second trimester, and to 5% in the third trimester, compared with a 0.6% occurrence in liveborns. Chromosomal abnormalities are seen more often in fetal deaths with congenital malformations, most commonly trisomy 13, trisomy 18, and monosomy X (Turner's syndrome). Trisomy 21 can also present as a fetal death; however, the physical diagnosis may be more subtle.

Ninety-five percent of chromosomal abnormalities causing fetal death are due to an abnormal number of chromosomes, either in the number of sets of chromosomes or in a change in the number of a single chromosome pair (Table 16-1). Examples of the former are triploidy (three sets of haploid chromosomes) and tetraploidy (four haploid sets). Eighty percent of triploid gestations are due to dispermy (two paternal chromosome sets) and are associated with characteristic cystic changes in the placenta that identify a partial hydatidiform mole. Most of these pregnancies terminate spontaneously at a mean gestational age of 122 days, compared with triploid gestations composed of two maternal chromosome sets, which terminate at a mean gestational age of 74 days. The embryo typically is growth-retarded, even at this early gestational age. Tetraploidy is most often diagnosed clinically as a first trimester loss with an empty gestational sac. Diandry occurs when an egg without a functional set of chromo-somes is fertilized with an X-bearing sperm that then replicates without division, resulting in a diploid complement of chromosomes of paternal origin. This is associated with cystic degeneration of the placenta and lack of embryonic development known as a *complete hydatidiform molar pregnancy*. Digyny refers to a diploid complement of chromosomes of maternal origin that has been reported only in teratomas.

Nondisjunction occurring at the first or second meiotic division results in monosomy or trisomy. Trisomies are the most common genetic abnormality occurring in fetal death, and have been reported for every human chromosome except number 1. Autosomal trisomies are incompatible with survival until term, except for trisomies 13, 18, and 21. Trisomy 16 occurs most often, making up 30% of trisomies in fetal deaths. Increasing maternal age increases the risk for trisomy. It should be noted that spontaneous abortions with normal karyotypes also increase with maternal age.

Monosomy X is the second most common chromosome abnormality in early fetal deaths, with 99.5% spontaneously terminating, usually in the first trimester without a well-formed embryo. Unlike trisomy, monosomy is associated with young maternal age.

Structural abnormalities in individual chromosomes are the result of breakage and rearrangement of chromosome segments, either within the chromosome, as in deletions and inversions, or involving the exchange of material between chromosomes, as in translocations and insertions. Translocations can be *balanced*, with no loss of essential chromosome material (resulting in a normal phenotype) or *unbalanced*, caused by extra or missing chromosome material. Studies have shown that in couples with two or more early pregnancy losses there is a 3% to 5% incidence of a parental balanced translocation. Unbalanced structural rearrangements occurred in only 2.7% of karyotypically abnormal fetuses among 2517 spontaneous abortions in one study, and were

Table 16-1. Causes of fetal death

GENETIC
Abnormal number of sets of chromosomes (triploidy, tetraploidy)
Change in number of a chromosome pair (trisomy, monosomy)
Structural abnormalities (deletions, inversions, translocations)

FETAL ANOMALIES, MALFORMATIONS, AND DEFORMATIONS
Neural tube defects
Cardiac, renal, GI anomalies
Amniotic band syndrome
Potter's oligohydramnios sequence
Twinning abnormalities (conjoined, acardiac)

INFECTION
Bacterial (GBS, *Listeria, Fusobacterium*)
Viral (parvovirus, CMV, rubella, HSV, coxsackie)
Mycotic (*Candida albicans*)
Parasitic (*Toxoplasma,* malaria, *Trypanosoma cruzi*)

MATERNAL MEDICAL CONDITIONS
Diabetes mellitus
Chronic hypertension
Uncontrolled thyroid disease
Cardiac disease
Immunologic
   Alloimmune (recurrent pregnancy wastage)
   Isoimmune (Rh disease, atypical antibodies)
   Autoimmune (antiphospholipid syndrome, SLE, systemic scleroderma, Sjögren's syndrome, mixed connective tissue disease)
Severe anemia (sickle cell disease)
Drug abuse (cocaine, amphetamines)

OBSTETRIC CONDITIONS
Intrauterine growth retardation
Oligohydramnios
Preeclampsia-eclampsia
Postmaturity
Twin-twin transfusion syndrome
Uteroplacental insufficiency
Placental infarcts
Maternal floor infarction

UNPREDICTABLE EVENTS
Cord accidents (knot, prolapse, compression)
Placental abruption
Fetomaternal hemorrhage
Fetal or maternal trauma

GI, Gastrointestinal; *GBS,* group B *Streptococcus*; *CMV,* cytomegalovirus; *HSV,* herpes simplex virus; *SLE,* systemic lupus erythematosus.

fifth in decreasing order of frequency behind trisomy, monosomy X, triploidy, and tetraploidy.

Other nonchromosomal fetal causes of fetal
death are fetal anomalies and malformation syndromes, a partial list of which is presented in
Table 16-1. Potter's oligohydramnios sequence is
a descriptive term for the situation that arises
from any condition that results in a prolonged
period of severely reduced amniotic fluid, usually
beginning before 24 weeks' gestation. This has
been described classically with renal agenesis;
however, obstructive uropathy, dysplastic kidneys, or chronic fluid loss can cause a similar
situation, resulting in the characteristic facial features, pulmonary hypoplasia, and arthrogryposis.
The frequency of some malformation syndromes
leading to fetal death may be determined by the
population being served (e.g., anomalies attributed to diabetes mellitus, fetal alcohol syndrome,
and so on).

Infection is no longer a major cause of fetal
death, although it plays a larger role in neonatal
morbidity, especially in premature infants. Because infection is a treatable cause of fetal death,
the diagnosis should be sought in order to counsel
a patient more accurately about the prognosis for
future pregnancies. Bacteria are believed to cause
fetal death by an ascending route, with subsequent activation of prostaglandin production and
the onset of labor. Neonatal death because of
prematurity is more likely than fetal death. Rarely,
decidual necrosis may occur, leading to abruption
and fetal demise. In the past, syphilis played a
major role as a cause of fetal death; however, in
contemporary medicine it has become rare. Organisms that have been implicated in fetal and
neonatal deaths are group B streptococci, fuso-
bacteria, ureaplasma, mycoplasma, and chlamydia. *Listeria monocytogenes* can cause placental
abscess formation and subsequent fetal septice-
mia, resulting in microabscesses in the fetal lung,
liver, adrenal, and brain. Listeria is an enteric
organism that has been reported in outbreaks
caused by contaminated cheese. *Candida albicans*
can cause a life-threatening fetal infection and has
been reported in association with use of an intrauterine device.

Toxoplasma gondii is a parasitic infection that
can be acquired by ingesting poorly cooked, infected meat or from the dry fecal matter of infected cats. Congenital toxoplasmosis is more
common following *Toxoplasma* infection than is
fetal death or spontaneous abortion. Other parasitic causes of fetal death uncommon in the
United States are malaria and Chagas' disease
caused by *Trypanosoma cruzi* infection. The latter
can cause fetal hydrops as well as death and spontaneous abortion.

Many viral organisms have been associated
with fetal death, but more commonly these cause
a congenital syndrome. Such is the case with
rubella, varicella zoster, cytomegalovirus (CMV),
and herpes simplex virus. Rubella can cause endothelial damage and thromboses in placental and
fetal vessels. Cytomegalic inclusion bodies can be
found in cells in the fetal lung, liver, kidneys, and
other organs, along with local thromboses and
chronic villitis in the placenta. These findings
explain the wide spectrum of clinical sequelae seen
in congenital CMV infection—from intrauterine
growth retardation to microcephaly to chorioretinitis and hepatosplenomegaly. Herpes simplex virus is thought to be a rare cause of fetal
death and can be acquired as an ascending infection transcervically, from maternal viremia resulting from transneural infection through lumbar
spinal ganglia, or possibly from latent endometrial infection. Coxsackie B virus commonly
causes neonatal hepatitis, myocarditis, and encephalitis; however, it also can cause fetal hydrops
and death from myocarditis. Parvovirus B19
can also cause fetal hydrops and death from
hemolysis.

Immunologic causes of fetal death can be categorized into three conditions: (1) *alloimmune:*
maternal immunologic rejection of the conceptus
because of failure of development of normal maternal tolerance mechanisms; (2) *isoimmune:* induction of maternal hemolytic antibodies by fetopaternal red cell antigens that cross the placenta,

causing destruction of fetal erythrocytes; and (3) *autoimmune:* destruction or damage of fetal or uteroplacental tissues caused by maternal autoantibodies directed against maternofetal antigens.

Alloimmune causes of fetal death remain a subject of investigation and include consideration of such topics as trophoblast antigens, cytotoxic antibodies, and parental HLA sharing. The most common cause of isoimmune fetal death is D antigen isoimmunization (Rh isoimmunization), which can result in hydrops fetalis from fetal hemolysis, severe anemia, tissue hypoxia, and eventual cardiac collapse. A hydropic fetus often has ascites, hepatosplenomegaly, cardiomegaly, pleural effusion, skin edema, and placental edema. Hydrops becomes clinically evident with a fetal hemoglobin of 4 g/dl or less. Other fetopaternal red cell antigens also can cause hemolytic disease in the fetus; however, these account for less than 5% of cases, either because they are weaker immunogens or because of fewer numbers of susceptible women. In contrast, the D antigen of the Rh blood group system is a potent immunogen, and 15% of women in the white population are susceptible to isoimmunization.

Several clinical autoimmune diseases have been associated with an increased rate of fetal loss, including systemic lupus erythematosus (SLE), systemic scleroderma, mixed connective tissue disease, and possibly polymyositis-dermatomyositis. Recently certain autoantibodies have been recognized in association with a high pregnancy loss rate even in the absence of clinical autoimmune disease. Antinuclear antibodies (ANA); antibody to soluble tissue ribonucleoprotein (anti-SS-A antibody); and, more strikingly, the antiphospholipid antibodies—lupus anticoagulant (LAC) and the anticardiolipin antibodies (ACA)—have been implicated. In women with LAC the pregnancy loss rate after 13 weeks is reported as 30% to 40%. Of patients with untreated LAC who delivered liveborns, 50% of the pregnancies were complicated by fetal growth retardation, preeclampsia, or both. In addition to a high rate of second trimester intrauterine fetal death (IUFD),

antiphospholipid syndrome also is characterized by a history of thromboembolic phenomena and thrombocytopenia. The treatment to improve pregnancy outcomes is still evolving; however, the currently accepted regimen includes heparin and baby aspirin or heparin and steroids. Anti-SS-A antibody is associated with isolated complete congenital heart block that can be part of a neonatal lupus syndrome comprising a transient lupus dermatitis, hepatosplenomegaly, and hematologic abnormalities. The fetal cardiac conduction system is impaired, resulting in a fetal heart rate of 50 to 60 beats/min and often nonimmune hydrops. Anti-SS-A antibody is associated with maternal SLE and Sjögren's syndrome, although many of the mothers are asymptomatic at the time of delivery and 30% to 60% eventually show signs of autoimmune disease.

Obstetric situations that increase the risk for fetal death often are the result of or cause of uteroplacental insufficiency, such as preeclampsia, intrauterine growth retardation (IUGR), oligohydramnios, and postmaturity. A growth-retarded fetus has a three to eight times greater risk for antepartum asphyxia and perinatal mortality. Other causes of fetal death due to obstetric events are unpredictable, including uncontrollable hemorrhage from placental abruption or previa or umbilical cord accidents that result from cord compression or prolapse. Fetomaternal hemorrhage sufficient to compromise fetal well-being can occur spontaneously or after significant trauma in addition to placental abruption and fetal injury. Maternal medical conditions such as chronic hypertension, diabetes, cardiac disease, collagen vascular diseases, and severe anemia may predispose to uteroplacental insufficiency. Other maternal and obstetric conditions may increase the risk for placental abruption, such as chronic hypertension (11% to 65% risk); preeclampsia-eclampsia; a rapidly distending uterus caused by polyhydramnios or higher order multiple gestations; and drug abuse, especially cocaine and amphetamines. Uncontrolled metabolic disorders such as diabetes and hypo- or hyperthyroidism, although now less common, elevate the risk for untoward outcome, often from congenital malformations in the case of diabetic pregnancies.

DIAGNOSIS

Before the introduction of biochemical assays and radiologic and ultrasonographic techniques, the diagnosis of fetal death was based on the same clinical signs and symptoms that had been taught for centuries. These are essentially the regression or absence of the signs and symptoms associated with a normal pregnancy. The gravida may notice decreased or absent fetal movement, weight loss, or regression of nausea and breast size. Uterine size may not increase on serial examinations, fetal heart sounds are inaudible, and fetal movements are not palpable. The clinical diagnosis based on these signs and symptoms can be made only after the fetus has grown large enough to allow detection of fetal movement or fetal heart tones. Because the disappearance of many of these signs of pregnancy takes an interval of time, there is a delay from the actual time of death until clinical suspicion.

The technologic advances of the twentieth century have increased the sensitivity of diagnostic techniques. Several are now of historic interest only because ultrasonography has become the predominant diagnostic mode, assuming the gestational age of the fetus is greater than the threshold for detection of cardiac activity.

Attempts to diagnose fetal death with several biochemical markers included investigations using urinary estriol (E_3), serum concentrations of the beta subunit of human chorionic gonadotropin (HCG), and maternal serum α-fetoprotein (AFP). The major precursors of E_3, DHAS (dehydroepiandrosterone sulfate) and 16 OH-DS (16 hydroxydehydroepiandrosterone sulfate), originate from the functioning fetal adrenal and liver respectively. A decline in maternal urinary E_3 should, therefore, occur within 24 to 48 hours after fetal demise. The diagnostic accuracy of this test is poor because of many extrinsic factors, including difficulty in obtaining a 24-hour collection, interference by exogenous steroids, and difficulty in performing the assay because of interference by prescription drugs.

Serum concentrations of maternal β-HCG that are lower than should be expected for gestational age should lead one to suspect either inaccurate dating, an abnormally developing intrauterine pregnancy, or an extrauterine pregnancy. This test is more useful in early gestations when the critical threshold for ultrasonographic detection of cardiac activity has not yet been reached. A normally developing early pregnancy is reflected by an approximate doubling in the HCG titer by 48 hours. A decline in serial titers 48 hours apart is suspicious for either a fetal death, impending death, ectopic pregnancy, or a blighted ovum. Because of continued support of placental metabolism by the maternal circulation, the HCG levels may remain positive for up to 1 month after an IUFD.

The AFP is a fetal metabolite that may be elevated in the maternal serum when there is disruption of the integrity of the fetal integument. It may be elevated before or after fetal death but is not specific for fetal death.

Before the use of ultrasound as a means of diagnosing IUFD, four presumptive signs of fetal death were sought on a radiograph of the maternal abdomen. These were gas formation within the fetus as a decomposition by-product, the "halo" sign caused by fluid accumulation beneath the subcutaneous layer of the scalp, overlapping of the cranial sutures, and abnormal angulation of the fetal spine. Gas formation can be seen within 6 hours and 10 days after fetal death; however, it may be difficult to detect because of its transient nature, overlying maternal bowel gas, and its presence only in third trimester fetal deaths. The halo sign, which appears within 48 hours of fetal death, can be mimicked by fetal hydrops. Normal molding of the fetal head in oligohydramnios or during labor can be mistaken for the overlapping suture sign.

Ultrasound is now the most sensitive and specific method of diagnosing fetal death. In addition, other advantages over previous diagnostic methods include its ready availability, ease of application, immediate results, and low cost with an in-office machine. The lack of cardiac motion after 8 weeks' gestation is irrefutable evidence of fetal death if the pregnancy has been dated accurately. Absence of cardiac activity is harder to diagnose than its presence; therefore in ideal circumstances the observation should be confirmed by two independent examiners.

Before 8 weeks' gestation, ultrasonographic evidence of cardiac activity may be inconsistent. The presence of an empty 7- to 8-week size gestational sac is the most specific sign of an early nonviable pregnancy and is considered a "blighted ovum" if there is no evidence of embryonic tissue. Studies have reported that an empty gestational sac greater than 20 or 25 mm mean diameter is 100% predictive of a nonviable pregnancy. Other less sensitive indicators of an IUFD are an irregular contour to the gestational sac, an incomplete or thin decidual ring, or poor daily growth of the gestational sac. The rate of gestational sac growth should be approximately 0.12 cm/day. If the gestational age is uncertain and an empty gestational sac or a fetal pole measuring less than 8 weeks is present, a repeat ultrasound examination in 7 to 14 days should be performed to allow sufficient time for measurable growth and the appearance of cardiac activity.

A less sensitive ultrasonographic indicator of fetal death is lack of fetal movement after 8 to 9 menstrual weeks of gestation. Care must be taken, however, to distinguish the dead fetus from a fetus during the normal physiologic periods of sleep or imposed condition of sedation caused by maternal medications or other pathology. Passive movement transmitted by maternal movement or vascular pulsations must not be mistaken for fetal movement.

Other sonographic signs reflecting fetal maceration after death are similar to the radiographic signs and should be considered secondary diagnostic criteria for fetal death. Overlapping of cranial sutures, scalp edema, fluid collections in the peritoneal and pleural cavities, and intrafetal gas accumulation also may be seen on ultrasound examination. With prolonged in utero retention of a dead fetus, further maceration occurs, and the fetal outline may become unrecognizable.

In addition to making the diagnosis of fetal death, ultrasonographic evaluation also may detect potential causes of death in findings of fetal anomalies; fetal hydrops; evidence of placental abruption; and placentomegaly, which can be seen in triploidy, congenital infections such as syphilis and toxoplasmosis, and anemia.

MANAGEMENT

Because ultrasound now quickly and reliably confirms the diagnosis of fetal death, many women are unwilling to await the onset of spontaneous labor, which usually occurs within 2 weeks in 80% to 90% of patients. Effective new cervical ripening and labor induction methods have provided a safe alternative to expectant management with its psychologic stress and risk of coagulation defects. It is believed that thromboplastin generated from the dead fetus can stimulate a consumptive coagulopathy in the maternal system, primarily of factors V, VII, fibrinogen, prothrombin, and platelets. Fibrinogen is the most useful clinical index of coagulopathy. The probability of developing hypofibrinogenemia correlates with the length of retention of a dead fetus within the uterus. Pritchard reported no instances of a fibrinogen level less than 150 mg/dl in women who retained a dead fetus less than 5 weeks. Approximately 4 weeks after fetal death, the fibrinogen level declines at a rate of 20 to 85 mg/dl/wk in approximately 25% of patients. Potentially dangerous complications can occur at levels of 100 mg/dl or less. One to two percent of those who develop coagulopathy will experience a hemorrhagic event. In patients with an intact circulation, heparin infusion can be used to block the coagulation process when administered over a few days. After correction of the coagulopathy, delivery can be effected, and fibrinogen levels usually will return to normal within 48 hours of delivery.

Because fetal death usually occurs before the natural ripening of the cervix, such cervical ripening techniques as application of 0.5 mg prostaglandin E_2 (PGE$_2$) gel intracervically or 3 to 5 mg intravaginally, or placement of mechanical intracervical dilators such as *Laminaria* or *Dilapan* or placement of an intracervical Foley catheter with extraamniotic infusion of saline, may be done before induction of labor. Labor induction can be accomplished subsequently with either intravaginal placement of 20 mg PGE$_2$ suppositories at intervals of between 2 and 6 hours for gestational ages of less than 28 weeks, or with Pitocin infusion using the same protocol as for term inductions if gestational age is more than 28 weeks. Recent studies have led to several newer methods of labor induction for early pregnancy termination, including the use of intravaginal prostaglandin E_1 (PGE$_1$) tablets (PGE$_1$; misoprostol) every 12 hours and a high-dose Pitocin protocol. The use of PGE$_2$ suppositories necessitates prophylactic medications for nausea and vomiting, diarrhea, and pyrexia, which are some of the side effects experienced with high doses of PGE$_2$. The PGE$_1$ tablets have the advantage of fewer side effects and no need for premedication.

Other, less widely used methods of labor induction for abortion or IUFD are intravenous PGE$_2$, intraamniotic PGF$_{2\alpha}$, and intramuscular 15-ethyl PGF$_{2\alpha}$. Dilatation and evacuation can also be performed by those with experience to do the procedure safely.

The management of the death of a fetus in a multiple gestation must take into consideration the type of placentation and the gestational age of the remaining fetus or fetuses. A monochorionic surviving twin is at risk for bilateral renal cortical necrosis and multicystic encephalomalacia. Vascular shunts in the placenta allowing fetofetal exchange of thromboplastic material or sudden hemodynamic changes are speculated causes of these complications. If the pregnancy is remote from term, expectant management with monitoring of fetal well-being and maternal coagulation parameters is recommended. If heparin therapy is necessary, it is unlikely to reverse any coagulopathy in the surviving fetus since it does not cross the placenta because of its greater molecular weight. In a gestation close to term, or term with a fetus with documented lung maturity, delivery is appropriate. A surviving twin of a dichorionic gestation may still be at risk from exposure to whatever extrinsic factors may have contributed to the first twin's death, such as infection or maternal disease.

After the delivery of the fetus, a thorough work-up for the cause of fetal death would include (Fig. 16-1) an autopsy, placental histopathology looking for supportive evidence for infection or vascular disease, aerobic cultures for group B *Streptococcus, Listeria,* anaerobic cultures for *Fusobacterium,* maternal Kleihauer-Betke smear and lupus anticoagulant, tissue biopsies for genetic studies, and radiographs and photographs. Tissue for genetic studies should be transported to the cytogenetics lab as soon as possible in a clean, closed container with no added liquid, which could promote the growth of contaminating organisms. A follow-up counseling session with the parents to discuss the results of any studies is an essential step in the grief resolution process. During this session any evidence for the cause of fetal death, the recurrence risk, and any alterations in the management of future pregnancies should be discussed. Limited resources often necessitate that the following factors also be considered before making any decision to perform a test: financial cost, the risk or harm of the test, the ease with which one can obtain the study, the effect of missing a positive result, the diagnostic discrimination of a particular test (sensitivity, specificity, predictive value, and so on), the treatability of the condition determined by the test, and legal aspects.

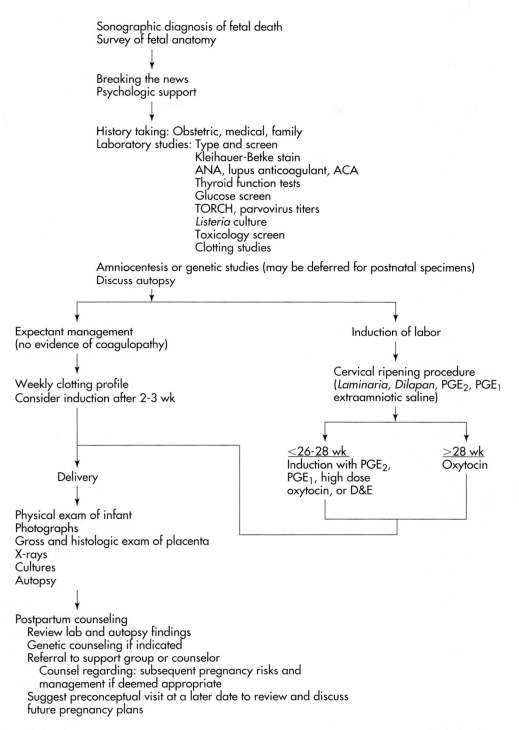

Fig. 16-1. Management of fetal death. *ANA*, Antinuclear antibodies; *ACA*, anticardiolipin antibodies; *TORCH*, toxoplasmosis, other, rubella, cytomegalovirus, and herpes simplex virus; *PGE₂*, prostaglandin E₂; *D&E*, dilatation and evacuation.

EMOTIONAL ASPECTS

In the past, the attachment parents felt toward their unborn fetus was not recognized; therefore their involvement in decision-making and in discussions of the event was minimized. The intent was to spare them the agony of grieving and attachment. For this reason, holding and viewing the child was discouraged, and the mother often was sedated to reduce her memory of the experience. Both actions are now known to complicate the normal grieving process. Recent investigations into grieving responses to fetal loss acknowledge the early bonding of parents with their unborn child and that a fetal loss is mourned with the same intensity as that of an older relative. Normal progression through recognized stages of grieving is encouraged as a healthy response to avoid pathologic emotional responses.

Grieving is an intense and complex but consistent process necessary to detach strong emotional ties to the deceased and allow resumption of normal life. Although stages of grief are often discussed, the process is not linear and the stages may overlap and recur. The stages of perinatal grieving have been identified as shock, searching, disorientation, and reorganization. Normal characteristics of each of these stages are outlined in Table 16-2. The initial response to fetal death is usually shock and numbness, which is a protective adaptive mechanism to allow for emotional adjustment and partial acceptance. The searching stage is characterized by emotional extremes and fluctuations, with severe psychologic pain manifested as crying and despair, preoccupation with thoughts and images of the infant, self-blame and guilt, blame of others and hostility, and anger and protest. Eventually, the intensity of the grief response becomes less pronounced as increasing acceptance occurs and an attempt to return to normal activities is made. During this stage of disorientation, symptoms of depression are apparent, causing a disruption of normal function. This stage may last for 6 months to a year or longer, and peer support groups and counseling

---

Table 16-2. Normal characteristics of stages of grief

SHOCK
Disbelief
Denial
Somatic distress
Anger
Change in social behavior
Sense of loneliness
Sense of emotional and physical detachment
Inability to concentrate
Selective integration of information

SEARCHING
Guilt
Hostility (toward staff, religion, other gravida)
Anger (unfairness)
Emptiness
Rationalizing
Severe psychologic pain (crying, despair)
Flashbacks, preoccupation with image of deceased

DISORIENTATION
Increasing acceptance of death
Depression (lowered self-esteem, listlessness, feelings of aimlessness and futility)
Difficulty returning to normal pattern of life

REORGANIZATION
Gradual adjustment to acceptance of loss
Increased energy and activity
Return to normal activities of daily living
Stabilization of old relationships
Formation of new relationships
Ability to plan for the future

---

may be especially helpful at this time. Finally, in the stage of reorganization there is a gradual adjustment and acceptance of the loss, a return to normal activities and relationships, and renewed ability to plan for the future.

The importance of allowing and encouraging the progression through the normal stages of grieving cannot be overemphasized. Normal grieving is a healthy response to loss and helps to avoid pathologic responses of inhibited, delayed, or chronic grieving with prolonged and distorted

Table 16-3. Areas that determine adjustment to death

CIRCUMSTANCES OF DEATH

Unanticipated versus high risk for perinatal
death

Professional reactions (anxious, avoiding, minimizing behavior versus compassionate, informative)

Long-term follow-up

**RELATIONSHIP WITH
THE DECEASED**

Attitudes toward pregnancy

Gestational age (affects duration of acute grieving but not intensity)

Duration of life of deceased

Birth defects

Loss of a multiple gestation

**CHARACTERISTICS
OF THE MOURNER**

Cultural influences

Incongruent grieving

Sense of guilt

Sense of failure (as a mother, wife, woman)

SOCIAL SUPPORT

Family

Friends

Support groups

Counselors

From Parks CM: Bereavement, *Br J Psychiatr* 146:11-17,
1985.

The goal of grief management is to facilitate the normal grieving process in a compassionate, supportive manner—not to attempt to isolate or protect the patient and family from unavoidable profound feelings of loss. Open communication and exchange of information are essential, as is permission to express feelings and the reassurance that these feelings are normal. The patient should be encouraged to participate in decision-making and to remain alert, although as comfortable as possible, through the delivery process to experience the reality of the birth and death of a loved one and to initiate the steps toward acceptance. An important way to affirm and recognize the child's existence as well as to dispel any exaggerated anxieties about fetal abnormalities is to have the patient and family see and hold the infant. The parents should be prepared for what they will see and should be presented with an infant wrapped in a blanket with the same sensitivity as if it were a liveborn child. Many mothers who do not see their infant have regrets and difficulties during the searching phase of grieving. Because the relationship with the infant cannot be based on experiences and memories, naming the infant and collecting mementos helps to establish a more lasting memory that will acknowledge the baby's reality and importance by giving an identity. Baptism and funeral or memorial services often facilitate the grieving process by affirming the importance of the baby as a family member and by allowing family and friends an opportunity to grieve with the parents and offer their support.

Before discharge from the hospital, a discussion focused on "anticipatory guidance" is helpful in preparing the parents for the intense and sometimes frightening or confusing feelings they will experience during the grieving process. Preoccupation with thoughts of the infant, severe depression, somatic symptoms, and inability to function in daily life may lead some patients to question their sanity. The parents should be reassured that these are normal responses to loss of a loved one. The routine use of tranquilizers and

symptoms. Signs of pathologic grief include overactivity without a sense of loss; exacerbation of psychosomatic symptoms; alterations in relationships; focused furious hostility; psychotic behavior; agitated depression; prolonged loss of patterns of social activity; and activities detrimental to personal, social, and economic existence. Adjustment to perinatal death has been found to be influenced by four important areas: the circumstances of death; the relationship with the deceased; particular characteristics of the mourner; and social conditions and support (Table 16-3).

antidepressants should be avoided because they only prolong the grieving process. A common response to fetal death is to attempt to replace the lost child with another pregnancy to alleviate painful feelings of loss. Parents should be counseled that neither future pregnancies nor existing children at home can replace the need to complete the grieving process. They should also be forewarned that well-meaning individuals may make statements that reveal their lack of understanding of perinatal grieving such as, "You're young and can have another baby." The names and numbers of support groups should be made available because the compassionate support of other parents with similar experiences can be invaluable. Couples also should be counseled that parents often resolve their grief at different rates

in different ways with different feelings; therefore maintaining communication with each other is essential.

A follow-up or series of subsequent appointments is important in reviewing information obtained from tests and autopsy results and in discussing the parents' progression through the grieving process and any difficulties encountered, including social and marital problems that may have arisen. Future pregnancy risks and plans should be discussed. Parents should be cautioned to wait at least 6 months to 1 year in order to avoid placing both them and their future child at psychologic risk. Strong feelings of anxiety, ambivalence, pessimism, and extreme vulnerability can mark a subsequent pregnancy if grief over the loss of a previous pregnancy has not been com-

CRITICAL POINTS

- Fetal deaths are classified as early (less than 20 completed weeks), intermediate (20 to 27 weeks), late (28 weeks or greater), or unclassified.
- The cause of fetal death remains unknown in 25% to 50% of cases.
- Genetic abnormalities as a cause of fetal death decrease from at least half of first trimester deaths, to 36% in the second trimester, to 5% in the third trimester, and 0.6% in liveborns.
- Other causes of fetal death include fetal anomalies and malformations, infections, maternal medical conditions, obstetrically related conditions, and unpredictable obstetric events.
- Ultrasound is the most sensitive diagnostic test for detecting fetal death after 8 weeks' gestation. Before 8 weeks, serial quantitative β-HCG levels can be compared for an appropriate rise.
- The spontaneous onset of labor usually occurs within 2 weeks after fetal death in 80% to 90% of patients.
- A coagulopathy may develop in 25% of patients approximately 4 weeks after the fetal death.
- The management of labor induction can be performed with preinduction cervical ripening techniques and induction with PGE_2 vaginal suppositories, PGE_1 vaginal tablets, or intravenous Pitocin.
- A thorough evaluation for the cause of fetal death includes: an autopsy; placental histopathology; cultures; genetic studies; radiographs; photographs; maternal Kleihauer-Betke smear; and lupus anticoagulant.
- Stages of perinatal grieving are shock, searching, disorientation, and reorganization. Progression through the stages is essential for resumption of normal life and can be facilitated by compassionate, open communication and information.

pleted. Most important, families appreciate a patient, compassionate listener who is comfortable with his or her own ability to deal with the intense emotions associated with grieving.

Questions

1. Which of the following may be a cause of fetal death?
   A. Genetic abnormalities
   B. Intrauterine growth retardation
   C. Motor vehicle accident
   D. Cardiomyopathy
   E. All of the above
2. Which of the following is the most sensitive diagnostic finding of fetal demise?
   A. Absence of fetal movement
   B. Slowly rising β-HCG
   C. Lack of fetal movement on ultrasound exam
   D. Lack of cardiac activity on ultrasound exam after 8 weeks' gestation
   E. Halo sign on flat plate of the abdomen

3. Grief counseling and management should incorporate:
   A. Avoiding discussion of the deceased fetus
   B. Allowing the patient and family to see and hold the infant after delivery
   C. Sedating the patient during the emotionally and physically painful process of labor and delivery
   D. Encouraging the parents to forget the painful experience and get back to normal life as soon as possible
   E. Prescribing tranquilizers and antidepressants to help the patient endure the psychologic strain of the postpartum period

Answers

1. E
2. D
3. B

17

Abnormal labor

APGO LEARNING OBJECTIVE #17

Marlin D. Mills

Labor is expected to progress in an orderly and predictable manner. Careful observation of the mother and fetus during labor will allow early detection of abnormalities so that management can be directed toward reducing the frequency of adverse outcome.

The student will demonstrate a knowledge of the following:

A. Various abnormal labor patterns
B. Methods of evaluating fetopelvic disproportion
C. Fetal and maternal complications resulting from abnormal labor
D. Indications and contraindications for oxytocin administration
E. Management of abnormal fetal presentations
F. Vaginal birth after cesarean delivery

DEFINITIONS

The goal of modern obstetrics continues to be a safe and healthy delivery for both mother and child. *Labor* is defined as the progressive efface-ment and dilatation of the uterine cervix that occurs with contractions of the uterine muscula-ture and results in the complete expulsion from the uterus of the products of conception. Aberra-tions of this process are many and varied.

Premature and *postdates* labor are complications of pregnancies with labor occurring before 37 weeks and after 42 weeks respectively. Contrac-tions without cervical change (Braxton-Hicks con-tractions or false labor) can be uncomfortable and can confuse the determination of the onset of true labor.

Normal labor has been divided into three stages (first, second, and third), with the first stage further subdivided into phases (latent and active). By using the amount of cervical change over time, parameters for the progression of labor have been established for these various stages and phases.

Table 17-1. Abnormal labor patterns

Type of abnormal labor	Definition
Prolonged latent phase	No progress from latent to active phase of labor For nulligravidas: in more than 20 hr For multiparas: in more than 14 hr
Protraction disorders	Prolonged active phase of labor such that the following occur: Cervical dilatation proceeds at less than 1.2 cm/hr for nulligravidas or 1.5 cm/hr for multiparas Descent of the presenting part proceeds at less than 1 cm/hr for nulligravidas or 1.5 cm/hr for multiparas
Arrest disorders	Secondary arrest of dilatation; No more progress in the active phase of labor No cervical dilatation for more than 2 hr for nulligravidas or multiparas No progress in the second stage of labor (*arrested descent*): No descent of the presenting part in more than 1 hr

---

Abnormal duration of these stages and phases is what is most commonly meant when discussing abnormal labor.

Precipitate labor progresses through the stages of normal labor more rapidly than expected. This can occur with normal uterine contractions, particularly in multiparous patients. More commonly it is associated with excessive uterine contractions that occur as a result of stimulation of the uterus by chorioamnionitis, placental abruption, or oxytocin.

Dystocia (difficult labor or childbirth) is the general term applied to abnormal labor that progresses more slowly than expected. There are no established standards for the classification, diagnosis, and treatment of abnormal labor. By using the parameters that have been established for the various stages and phases of labor, the patterns of abnormal labor can be classified as shown in Table 17-1.

A *protraction disorder* results in labor that progresses slower than normal. An *arrest disorder* results in a complete cessation of the progress of labor. *Failure to progress* is another term used to describe the lack of progression of labor resulting from an unspecified or unknown cause.

It is important to recognize lack of progress in labor promptly and to manage it appropriately. Various adverse outcomes significantly increase maternal and fetal morbidity and mortality. Rates for both operative vaginal and cesarean deliveries increase, as do maternal and fetal infection rates. Specific organ exhaustion results in less effective pushing effort, poorer maternal recovery, and an increased risk of uterine atony with resultant postpartum hemorrhage. Only after careful assessment of the factors potentially responsible for the labor abnormal ity can one most effectively manage labor to achieve the desired outcome—a healthy mother and child.

PATHOGENESIS

Dystocia can be the result of anatomic or functional abnormalities of the fetus *(the passenger)*, the maternal tissues that comprise the birth canal *(the passage)*, the uterus *(the power)*, or combinations of these three factors that interfere with the normal mechanics of labor and delivery.

Fetal abnormalities causing abnormal labor include *malpresentation,* where some fetal part other than the vertex is presenting (e.g., breech, transverse lie, face, brow, compound presentation), *malposition* of the fetal vertex (e.g., occiput posterior, asynclitism), and *macrosomia.* The latter is one of the causes of *fetopelvic disproportion,* which is a discrepancy between fetal size and the size and shape of the maternal pelvis so great that vaginal delivery is prevented.

Abnormal fetal anatomy and development also may cause any of the above conditions. Fetal hydrocephalus creating cephalopelvic disproportion; fetal goiter producing face or brow presentation; and fetuses with myotonic dystrophy resulting in malpresentation are just a few examples. Prenatal ultrasound often diagnoses these conditions before labor. *Intrapartum ultrasound* can be used to confirm fetal presentation and position or evaluate fetal anatomy if labor is abnormal and no previous ultrasound has been performed.

If fetal macrosomia (defined as an estimated fetal weight greater than 4500 g in the nondiabetic patient) or fetal abnormalities are present to the extent that a successful vaginal delivery is unlikely, a cesarean delivery may be indicated. Care must be taken in interpreting maternal and fetal risks when assessing for method of delivery. Ultrasound estimates of fetal weight may be useful, but can be inaccurate by as much as ± 10% of actual fetal weight.

Fetal malposition of the vertex can convert to a more favorable position, such as a vertex or face in the case of a brow presentation. Face or occipitoposterior positions may rotate to a mentum anterior or occipitoanterior position respectively, which allows an easier delivery. Face presentation with persistent mentum posterior cannot be delivered vaginally. Persistent occipitoposterior position prolongs descent and may even necessitate forceps rotation to accomplish vaginal delivery. If the abnormal position cannot be corrected by manual or forceps rotations to a more favorable

position for vaginal delivery, delivery by cesarean section may be necessary.

The structures that comprise the birth canal or passage include the maternal bony pelvis and the soft tissues of the cervix, vagina, and perineum. Soft tissue structures that can interfere with labor include uterine fibroids, ovarian cysts, adnexal masses, and distended bladder or colon. The condition of the cervix also is important. If the cervix is long and firm, it may not be ready for labor and may necessitate prostaglandin cervical ripening if induction of labor is necessary. With previous surgery, such as a cervical conization, there may be cervical stenosis and scarring, which also may prolong labor. Conditions of the bony pelvis that cause dystocia include traumatic injury, skeletal dysplasia, severe scoliosis, and musculoskeletal disorders that prevent normal pelvic bone development.

Epidural anesthesia has been shown to delay labor progress in certain patients by relaxing the pelvic floor musculature that provides the support to accomplish internal rotation of the vertex into the more favorable occipitoanterior position.

For the fetus to be pushed through the birth canal, there must be sufficient power created by the uterus and by accessory muscles used during the second stage of labor. Uterine contractions develop fundally and progress toward the pelvis, with the effect of creating descent of the fetus through the pelvis and also producing cervical dilatation. This occurs by pushing the fetus past the cervix, but also by pulling the cervix up, as evidenced by progressive cervical dilatation with a fetus in a transverse presentation that prevents fetal descent. Uterine contractions that are discordant or of insufficient strength or frequency may cause ineffective labor. Conditions that affect maternal expulsive efforts include exhaustion, excessive anesthesia, and neuromuscular disorders. Maternal medical conditions such as previous stroke, cardiac disease, and diabetic retinopathy may preclude a vaginal delivery because of the risk of exacerbating the condition.

The pathogenesis for the specific patterns of abnormal labor may be distinguished. A prolonged latent phase can result from abnormal fetal position, an unripe cervix, excessive anesthesia, fetopelvic disproportion, or dysfunctional or ineffective uterine contractions; it may also simply be false labor. A prolonged active phase may result from fetal malposition, fetopelvic disproportion, excessive use of sedation, inadequate contractions, and premature rupture of membranes before the onset of active labor. Secondary arrest of labor may result from fetal macrosomia, malpresentation or malposition, a contracted pelvis, fetal cephalopelvic disproportion, or ineffective uterine contractions.

SYMPTOMS, SIGNS, AND LABORATORY-DIAGNOSTIC STUDIES

The assessment of labor begins with the information obtained during the antenatal period. Any of the conditions described previously should be evaluated for their potential effect on labor. The initial examination should assess any of the above factors. In addition, the vaginal exam on the first (as well as subsequent) evaluations should obtain the following information: cervical dilatation in centimeters, percent effacement of the cervix, station of the presenting part, position of the presenting part, and presence of caput or molding. This information should be logged graphically on a *partogram* to facilitate assessing the progress of labor. The type of labor abnormality can then be more readily identified (Fig. 17-1). In the event of a labor abnormality, the patient is evaluated to determine the cause and therapy most likely to be effective in treating the abnormality or to establish that a vaginal delivery is not achievable safely so that a timely cesarean delivery can be performed.

Fetal heart rate can be assessed either by auscultation using American College of Obstetricians and Gynecologists guidelines or with continuous electronic fetal monitoring to assess fetal tolerance to the effects of uterine contractions.

Uterine contractions can be assessed to determine strength and frequency by palpation, with an external tocodynamometer or with the use of an intrauterine pressure catheter. Manual palpation is a subjective measure based on indentation of the uterus by the examiner, who must interpret whether the contraction is mild, moderate, or strong. Timing of uterine contractions also can be established by a tocodynamometer, but the actual pressure generated and the assessment of the coordination of the uterine contractions can only be done with an intrauterine pressure catheter. The optimal strength is 50 to 60 mm Hg, with a frequency of three uterine contractions to each 10-minute period. During early labor the uterus may not supply uterine contractions of sufficient strength to affect cervical change; therefore these cannot be assessed until the *active* phase of labor has been achieved. This usually occurs at 3 to 4 cm, but is better defined by a change in the rate at which cervical dilatation occurs with an established uterine contraction pattern of sufficient strength and frequency.

Evaluation of the risk of cephalopelvic disproportion by measuring the maternal pelvis with radiographic or computed tomographic pelvimetry has been shown to be of marginal benefit except in the antepartum or early labor assessment of the patient undergoing evaluation for vaginal delivery of a fetus presenting in the breech presentation.

Leopold's maneuvers can be used to assess fetal presentation. If a vaginal exam and Leopold's maneuvers cannot adequately determine fetal presentation, ultrasonographic examination is indicated to assess basic fetal anatomy—as well as presentation, position of the presenting part, and amniotic fluid volume. Low amniotic fluid volume may be an indication for *amnioinfusion,* a technique in which intraamniotic fluid volume is reestablished during labor to help protect the umbilical cord from compression by uterine contractions.

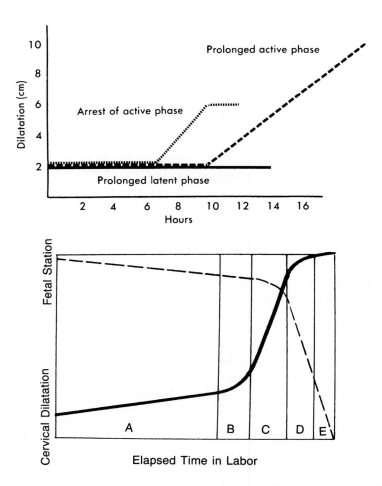

Fig. 17-1. *Top,* Abnormal labor curves. *Bottom,* Characteristic graphic patterns of cervical dilatation *(heavy line)* and fetal descent *(broken line)* against time in labor. *A,* Latent phase; *B,* acceleration phase; *C,* phase of maximum slope; *D,* deceleration phase; *E,* second stage. *B* through *D* represent the active phase of the first stage. (Bottom *from Friedman EA, Acker DB, Sachs BP:* Obstetrical decision making, *ed 2, St Louis, 1987, Mosby–Year Book.)*

MANAGEMENT

Prolonged latent phase

A prolonged latent phase in and of itself does not pose a threat to mother or infant; therefore the following steps provide the most effective management. Prolong the observation period, preferably not in the hospital, to distinguish between latent phase and false labor. Do not use narcotic analgesics and sedatives routinely. Encourage the patient to remain physically active and to continue normal nutrition. Discuss with the patient that long latent phases are not unusual and reassure her about her well-being and that of the fetus. Avoid the early use of oxytocin and amniotomy unless induction or augmentation is otherwise indicated. With a long latent phase that results in maternal exhaustion, consider a therapeutic rest with sedation or analgesia.

Regardless of the type of management interventions, the effect of emotional support to laboring women cannot be underestimated. *The laboring woman should never be left alone.* Supportive interaction includes activities that reduce maternal anxiety such as frequent physical contact; massage; quiet conversation; response to all questions in a quiet, reassuring manner; and attending to the patient's many physical needs during the course of labor.

A laboring woman should be allowed to change position frequently to provide for the most efficient labor. In early labor, she should be encouraged to ambulate with intermittent monitoring until she chooses to lie down. The lateral recumbent position then provides for the greatest intensity and efficiency of contractions. The supine position, in addition to being less labor-efficient, creates the risk of supine hypotension with subsequent fall in maternal blood pressure and interruption of uteroplacental perfusion because of the compressive effect of the uterus on the abdominal aorta and inferior vena cava. If positioning measures are ineffective, stimulation of uterine activity with oxytocin is indicated.

Oxytocin

If causes of prolonged labor other than the possibility of inadequate uterine forces have been ruled out, stimulation of uterine activity is indicated. Oxytocin is currently the drug most commonly used for the treatment of prolonged labor resulting from inadequate uterine tone. Although dosing schedules have varied, the advantage of using this medication is its short half-life. It necessitates administration by continuous intravenous infusion; however, the effects abate quickly, which is an important management and safety feature.

Secondary arrest of labor, which often results from fetal malposition or asynclitism, often responds well to oxytocin stimulation of labor. Women with primary dysfunctional labor may not have as good a response to oxytocin, resulting in a higher rate of cesarean delivery. Alternative measures including ambulation and emotional support may have a greater benefit in this group of patients.

Secondary arrest of labor and induction of labor are the most common indications for the use of oxytocin. Additionally, it can be used to augment a protracted latent phase when other methods have been unsuccessful or are inappropriate. Oxytocin is also used postpartum as a uterotonic to decrease the risk of postpartum hemorrhage.

The treatment modality of *active management* of labor, which is a specific process for the management of labor in nulliparous patients, relies on a labor partogram and action line with early and aggressive use of oxytocin to reestablish labor progress and reduce the number of cesarean deliveries required in this patient population.

All of the studies that demonstrate the benefits of oxytocin also add the qualifier for its "judicious use." That phrase underscores the potential risks associated with oxytocin use. Uterine hyperstimulation is the complication seen most often. This creates the risk of fetal distress and uterine rupture, particularly in multiparous patients and in patients undergoing a trial of labor after a previous cesarean section. Additional risks include water intoxication at high doses, subsequent postpartum uterine atony, acute hypotension with rapid intravenous infusion, and increased use of analgesics.

Many clinical circumstances have been described as contraindications to oxytocin use. They are best characterized by the statement by Cibils, as follows: "the only contraindications to the proper use of oxytocin are those contraindications to spontaneous labor."

The administration of oxytocin necessitates continuous intravenous infusion because of its rapid breakdown. Initial doses of 0.5 to 1.0 mU/min should be used. The doses increase at intervals of 20 to 40 minutes to achieve adequate contraction frequency and strength. Increasing the dose at shorter intervals is associated with an increased risk of fetal distress; longer intervals have slightly greater length of labor and increased cesarean section rates. If fetal distress occurs during oxytocin infusion, the medication is discontinued until the fetus recovers, then restarted at a slightly lower rate if continuing labor is appropriate. An acute tocolytic such as terbutaline can be given to decrease uterine contractions if a more immediate response and in utero resuscitation are desired.

There are special circumstances that of themselves do not cause abnormal labor; however, the labor must be conducted with adjustments to the clinical condition. Among these are malpresentation and vaginal birth after cesarean section (VBAC).

CRITICAL POINTS

- Labor is defined as the progressive effacement and dilatation of the uterine cervix.
- Dystocia (difficult labor or childbirth) is the general term applied to abnormal labor that progresses more slowly than expected.
- Only after careful assessment of the factors potentially responsible for the labor abnormality can one most effectively manage labor to achieve the desired outcome—a healthy mother and child.
- Intrapartum ultrasound can be used to confirm fetal presentation and position or to evaluate fetal anatomy if labor is abnormal.
- If the abnormal position cannot be corrected by manual or forceps rotations to a more favorable position for vaginal delivery, then delivery by cesarean section may be necessary.
- The vaginal exam on the first, as well as subsequent, evaluations should obtain the following information: cervical dilatation in centimeters, percent effacement of the cervix, station of the presenting part, position of the presenting part, and presence of caput or molding.
- The actual pressure generated and the assessment of the coordination of the uterine contractions can be done only with an intrauterine pressure catheter.
- Regardless of the type of management interventions, the effect of emotional support for laboring women cannot be underestimated. The laboring woman should never be left alone.
- Oxytocin is currently the drug most commonly used for the treatment of prolonged labor resulting from inadequate uterine tone.
- All of the studies that demonstrate the benefits of oxytocin also add the qualifier for its "judicious use." That phrase underscores the potential risks associated with oxytocin use.
- If fetal distress occurs while the woman is being given oxytocin, the medication is discontinued until the fetus recovers, then restarted at a slightly lower rate if continuing labor is appropriate.
- Signs of uterine rupture include fetal bradycardia, loss of intrauterine pressure, pain, bleeding, and movement of the presenting fetal part out of the pelvis.
- If oxytocin is used for augmentation of arrested labor in a VBAC patient, there should be a favorable response with labor progression within the first 2 hours.

Malpresentation

With the exception of the fetus presenting as a frank breech presentation, the method of delivery that provides the least risk for mother and infant in all other types of malpresentation (e.g., a transverse, compound, footling breech) is a cesarean delivery. Vaginal delivery of the infant presenting as a frank breech can be accomplished safely in the patient who, by careful assessment using preestablished guidelines, has been shown to be an acceptable candidate for trial of vaginal delivery.

Vaginal birth after cesarean section

The dictum "once a C-section, always a C-section" has been clearly shown not to apply to most circumstances under which women now deliver babies. Patients with a previous cesarean section in which the uterine incision was made transversely through the lower uterine segment are candidates for a trial of labor and vaginal delivery. The success rate varies from 60% to 85%, even if the previous cesarean section was for circumstances thought likely to recur. *Scar dehiscence,* a condition in which the previous scar separates, creating an open window in the uterine wall, occurs approximately 2% of the time and is not associated with significant clinical complications. A *uterine rupture* with complete extrusion of the contents of the uterus is more clinically significant and increases the risk of fetal loss or injury. The likelihood of this complication is low, however, occurring only 0.2% to 0.8% of the time. Signs of uterine rupture include fetal bradycardia, loss of intrauterine pressure, pain, bleeding, and movement of the presenting fetal part out of the pelvis. Management techniques used in normal labor are safe with VBAC, including artificial rupture of membranes, epidural anesthesia, prostaglandin gel cervical ripening, and oxytocin. If oxytocin is used for augmentation of arrested labor in a VBAC patient, there should be a favorable response with labor progression within the first 2 hours. Internal pressure catheter monitoring of uterine contractions should be considered; to reduce the risk of uterine rupture, the contraction pattern should not exceed five to seven contractions in a 15-minute period.

Patients with previous vertical or T-shaped uterine incisions involving the more muscular body of the uterus are not candidates for vaginal delivery. The risk of uterine rupture in this group is 4.5% to 8.5%. Other situations in which labor is contraindicated include previous uterine rupture or dehiscence, a leiomyomectomy that involved the full uterine wall thickness, tubal reimplantation, uterine perforation, or metroplasty.

Questions

1. The most common indications for administering oxytocin during labor include:
   A. Malpresentation
   B. Prolonged latent phase
   C. Secondary arrest of labor
   D. Cephalopelvic disproportion
2. Symptoms of uterine rupture include:
   A. Vaginal bleeding or hematuria
   B. Fetal bradycardia
   C. Loss of intrauterine pressure
   D. All of the above
3. The most common complication of oxytocin use is:
   A. Water intoxication
   B. Uterine hyperstimulation
   C. Hypotension
   D. Anaphylaxis

Answers

1. C
2. D
3. B

18

Third trimester bleeding

APGO LEARNING OBJECTIVE #18

Thomas H. Strong, Jr.

> *Bleeding in the third trimester necessitates immediate patient evaluation. Thoughtful and prompt evaluation and management are necessary to reduce the threat to the lives of the mother and fetus.*

The student will demonstrate a knowledge of the following:

A. Approach to the patient who has third trimester bleeding

B. Symptoms, physical findings, and diagnostic methods that differentiate patients with placenta previa and abruptio placentae from those with other causes of third trimester bleeding

C. Complications of placenta previa and abruptio placentae

D. Immediate management of shock secondary to third trimester bleeding

E. Components of the various blood products and indications for their use

Third trimester bleeding remains a major cause of maternal morbidity and mortality. Indeed, hemorrhage during this period of pregnancy still accounts for a considerable portion of bleeding events that threaten maternal and fetal well-being. Third trimester bleeding occurs in roughly 20% of pregnant women and has a wide range of causes (Table 18-1). While many causes of third trimester bleeding are nonthreatening, some can be rapidly fatal. Approximately 15% of maternal cardiac output (1 L/min) passes through the maternal uterus at term; therefore until the proper diagnosis is secured, it is prudent to assume that all third trimester vaginal bleeding may be life-threatening.

PLACENTAL ABRUPTION

Normally the placenta does not detach from its implantation site until after delivery of the fetus. When placental separation occurs prematurely, placental abruption, or *abruptio placentae,* is present. Abruption develops in up to 2.5% of all pregnancies and accounts for roughly 30% of third trimester bleeding. In subsequent pregnancies, its rate of recurrence is approximately 10%.

Because of its central role in fetal nutrition and gas exchange, the placenta is vital to the development and well-being of the fetus. During placental abruption, fetal intravascular homeostasis and a variety of fetal metabolic processes are disturbed. As the placental implantation site is disrupted, blood can rapidly pass from the vagina or collect unseen inside the reproductive tract as a *concealed* or *occult abruption*. In the latter situation, relatively high-pressure blood in the maternal vessels forcefully separates the layers of myometrium, dissects into the amniotic fluid, or collects as a hematoma retroplacentally or in the maternal broad ligament. In the setting of concealed abruption, which occurs in up to 20% of abruptions, little or no vaginal bleeding may be noted. In this circumstance, the degree of maternal cardiovascular instability frequently can be out of proportion with the observed volume of vaginal bleeding. Frequently, retroplacental bleeding will dissect a path to the edge of the placenta, thereby permitting some blood eventually to pass from the vagina. In contrast to the bright red, clotting blood associated with placenta previa, blood passed during an abruption is usually dark and nonclotting, a characteristic of old, sequestered hemorrhage (Table 18-2).

Risk factors

Acute or chronic maternal hypertension is a considerable risk factor for placental abruption. Occurring in roughly 50% of women with placental abruption, maternal hypertension may be associated with chronic hypertension and preeclampsia, or it may be induced acutely by such illicit substances as cocaine. Additionally, women who have undergone placental abruption in previous gestations also are at increased risk. Maternal trauma, especially to the abdomen or uterus, is another very common antecedent to abruption.

Table 18-1. Causes of third trimester bleeding

Abruptio placentae
Bloody show
Cervical or vaginal neoplasm
Cervicitis
Circumvallate placenta
Genital tract trauma
Placenta previa
Vasa previa

Table 18-2. Differentiating abruptio placentae from placenta previa

	Abruptio placentae	Placenta previa
Risks	Hypertension, trauma, prior abruption, smoking, AMA, fibroids	High parity, prior cesarean delivery
Diagnosis	Clinical	Sonographic
Pain	Yes	No
Bleeding	Dark, nonclotting*	Bright red, clots
Sequelae	DIC, postpartum hemorrhage	Placenta accreta, postpartum hemorrhage

AMA, Advanced maternal age; *DIC,* disseminated intravascular coagulation.
*Bleeding may be scarce or absent in the setting of a concealed abruption.

Diagnosis

Despite the many diagnostic and therapeutic advances in obstetrics, the diagnosis of abruption remains a clinical one, based largely on the patient's history and physical examination. While real-time ultrasonographic assessment of the patient with a suspected abruption is frequently done, the reality is that ultrasound aids in the diagnosis of placental abruption in only a minority of cases. As noted earlier, the gravida with placental abruption will often have a history of hypertension, substance abuse, or trauma. In addition to vaginal bleeding, the patient frequently will complain of intense, very painful uterine contractions. In this circumstance, rapid increase of uterine fundal height suggests an expanding hematoma. At the time of fetal membrane rupture, port wine–colored amniotic fluid will suggest dissection of a retroplacental hematoma into the amniotic space. Examination will reveal the uterus to be hyperactive or tetanically contracted. Uterine rupture occasionally can occur. Excessive uterine activity may precede the abruptive event and frequently may contribute to the genesis of placental separation. Detachment of the placenta from its implantation site diminishes its effectiveness as a respiratory organ. The vigorous uterine contraction pattern observed during an ongoing abruption can contribute to further fetal compromise by reducing uterine blood flow. Typically, fetal death will occur when more than 50% of the placental surface has detached. It can be presumed that a maternal blood loss of 2000 ml (whether seen or unseen) has occurred in a placental abruption sufficiently severe to cause fetal death. Therefore the gravida with a placental abruption associated with fetal demise should be monitored closely for signs and symptoms of hypovolemic shock. If delivery occurs shortly after an abruption, inspection of the placenta will reveal adherent clot at the site of disruption.

Owing to the intensity of uterine contractions, placental tissue fragments can be forced into the maternal circulation. Rich in placental thromboplastin, these fragments can trigger the coagulation cascade, thereby evoking disseminated intravascular coagulation (DIC). Indeed, roughly 20% of all severe abruptions are associated with some degree of coagulopathy. If a cesarean delivery is performed in association with an abruption, the uterine serosa frequently will demonstrate a marbled, petechial pattern known as *Couvelaire uterus*. Couvelaire uterus results from high-pressure, hemorrhagic dissection of myometrial tissue planes during the abruptive event. Uterine atony with secondary hemorrhage should be anticipated following a significant placental abruption.

Management

Should fetal distress or any contraindication to ongoing labor develop during placental abruption, cesarean delivery is warranted. However, there are several disadvantages of cesarean delivery in abruption, including the following:
1. Increased physical insult-risk inherent in a major surgical procedure for a gravida whose cardiovascular status may not be stable
2. Increased potential for significant intraoperative hemorrhage in a patient with a high risk for, or in the throes of, coagulopathy

On the other hand, the advantages of cesarean delivery include the following:
1. Rapid delivery of the fetus from a hostile intrauterine environment
2. Direct access to the uterus and its vascular supply in the event that postpartum hemorrhage develops

Vaginal delivery is the preferred route in the gravida with a stable cardiovascular status and a dead fetus. Fortunately, labor and delivery usually progress relatively rapidly in most active abruptions secondary to uterine hyperactivity.

Management of abruptio placentae includes regular monitoring of hemoglobin-hematocrit, clotting status (prothrombin time–partial thromboplastin time, platelets, fibrinogen and fibrin degradation products), hourly urine output, and vital signs. In the oliguric or unstable gravida, Swan-Ganz monitoring may be indicated. However, the risks and benefits of this invasive modality must be considered within the context of a pathophysiologic process not infrequently associated with significant coagulopathy. Continuous electronic fetal heart rate monitoring is vital to ensure fetal well-being. During an acute abruption with a viable fetus, 2 to 4 units of packed red blood cells should be cross-matched. Four to 6 units should be prepared if the fetus is dead. Severe DIC may be suggested by persistent bleeding from sites of minor trauma such as intravenous sites or minor cuts. Blood, collected in a nonheparinized glass tube, that does not clot within 6 to 8 minutes suggests a clinically significant consumptive coagulopathy with fibrinogen levels frequently below 100 mg/dl. Replacement of clotting factors destroyed by disseminated intravascular coagulation can be achieved by transfusion of cryoprecipitate or fresh frozen plasma.

CHRONIC ABRUPTION

Partial-chronic abruption, or "marginal sinus separation," occurs at least as frequently as the severe variety of placental abruption and may initially display signs and symptoms as acutely threatening as its more life-threatening counterpart. However, the abruptive process fails to progress and the clinical picture stabilizes, thereby permitting a more conservative management approach. Not infrequently, placental abruption of this type is diagnosed as preterm labor. Although the use of tocolytics with any type of abruption is controversial, there are those who advocate tocolytic therapy in women with stable, nonacute abruption. In this circumstance, it appears that tocolysis does no harm. However,

Table 18-3. Indications for terminating expectant management of chronic abruption (or placenta previa)

MATERNAL INDICATIONS
Labor that fails tocolysis
Excessive bleeding
Other obstetric indications (preeclampsia, and so on)
FETAL INDICATIONS
Anomalies incompatible with life
Distress
Death
Lung maturity

expectant management of the patient with a non-acute abruption should be tempered with the knowledge that the abruptive process may progress suddenly at any time. Regular assessment of hematologic status should be performed in the patient with chronic abruption. Rapid access to blood products should always be available. In addition, twice weekly assessment of fetal well-being is warranted. Contraction stress testing is contraindicated because of the potential risk for provoking further abruption. Sonographic assessment of fetal growth should be done at regular intervals until delivery. The indications for terminating expectant management of chronic abruption are listed in Table 18-3.

PLACENTA PREVIA

The fertilized ovum may implant anywhere in the uterine cavity. Most commonly, the implantation site is in the upper segment of the uterus. When implantation occurs in the lower uterine segment such that the body of the placenta extends below the presenting part of the fetus, a placenta previa is

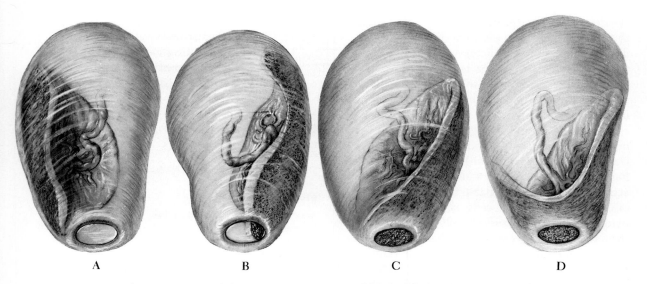

Fig. 18-1. Types of placenta previa. **A,** Marginal. **B,** Partial. **C** and **D,** complete.

present. As the cervix effaces and dilates during late gestation and parturition, the implantation site of a placenta previa can be disrupted, with vaginal bleeding being a worrisome consequence. Among all causes of third trimester bleeding, roughly 20% are attributable to placenta previa. Fortunately, 90% of placentas that implant in the lower uterine segment will be in the upper aspect of the uterus by the late third trimester. This phenomenon is *placental migration.* On occasion, the placenta may be noted to have migrated up to 10 cm from the cervix. Although the exact mechanism of placental migration is not well understood, it most probably does not represent true migration of the placenta. Rather, the phenomenon probably relates to the progressive lengthening ("development") of the lower uterine segment that occurs late in the third trimester of gestation. Therefore it is not the placenta that migrates from the cervical os but the cervix itself that migrates away from the placenta. There are three varieties of placenta previa (Fig. 18-1): (1) marginal, in which the edge of the placenta comes up to but does not overlie the internal cervical os; (2) partial, in which the internal os is partially covered

by the placenta; and (3) complete, in which the internal os of the cervix is totally covered by the body of the placenta.

Risk factors

Any pathophysiologic process that interferes with placental migration will increase the risk for placenta previa. Because the multiparous uterus generally experiences less lower uterine segment development than does a nulliparous one, the risk for placenta previa increases with parity. Indeed, placenta previa occurs infrequently in the nulliparous gravida. Advancing maternal age is also a risk factor for placenta previa but may simply be another reflection of increased parity. Surgical scarring of the lower uterine segment also appears to increase the risk for placenta previa. This particular type of uterine scarring may impede the development of the lower uterine segment and prevent sufficient placental migration. Disruption of the myometrial and decidual architecture at the old uterine incision site may alter the normal process of placentation in a fashion that also inhibits migration.

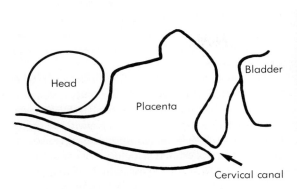 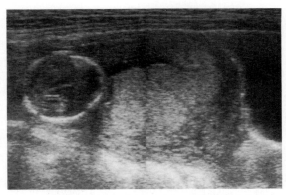

Fig. 18-2. Sonogram of complete placenta previa, longitudinal view.

Diagnosis

The presence of a placenta previa should be considered in the setting of painless, bright-red vaginal bleeding and the passage of clots. Most commonly, the onset of bleeding is quite sudden, without apparent provocation. Nevertheless, uterine contractions may be demonstrated in 25% of patients. The first episode of hemorrhage usually occurs in the early third trimester of pregnancy, with a peak incidence between 30 and 34 weeks' gestation. The initial bleeding event is generally not life-threatening unless provoked by a vigorous digital examination of the internal cervical os. Commonly, the gravida will undergo multiple, small bleeding events before a catastrophic episode occurs. Pelvic examination, intercourse, or douching sometimes will provoke bleeding of an unsuspected placenta previa. Because placenta previa occupies the lower uterine segment, fetal malpresentation is often noted. Therefore the obstetrician should consider the possibility of placenta previa whenever a malpresenting fetus is noted late in gestation.

As opposed to the situation in placental abruption, real-time ultrasonography has become an extremely accurate modality for diagnosing placenta previa (Fig. 18-2). It currently is the diagnostic tool of choice for this complica-

tion of pregnancy. In experienced hands, the accuracy of this technique exceeds 90%. Transvaginal or perineal scanning may provide a greater degree of accuracy, but their utility must be balanced against the theoretic potential to provoke vaginal bleeding.

Management

An attempt at vaginal delivery in the setting of placenta previa is potentially life-threatening and is unwarranted. The combination of intense uterine contractions, cervical dilatation, and frequent digital examinations may provoke considerable, catastrophic hemorrhage. Therefore cesarean delivery remains the standard approach for this pregnancy complication. Because it is sometimes difficult to differentiate a low-lying placenta from a marginal placenta previa, a "double set-up" examination sometimes is warranted if a trial of labor is contemplated. A double set-up examination is merely a digital examination of the cervical os performed in the delivery suite with full readiness for cesarean delivery. Should significant vaginal bleeding be provoked or if a placenta previa is confirmed, a cesarean delivery can be performed rapidly. Should the placenta be determined to be clear of the cervical os, an attempt at vaginal delivery may be pursued.

In modern obstetrics, the goal is to optimize outcome for both mother and fetus. Therefore to the extent that a cesarean delivery is the necessary mode of delivery, timing of delivery will be the key to successful management. It is presently desirable to delay delivery until fetal pulmonary maturity if this can be accomplished without unduly increasing risk to the mother. Cautious, expectant management of placenta previa is generally associated with improved maternal and fetal outcome. The mother benefits from cesarean delivery of a baby that she cannot safely deliver vaginally, and the fetus benefits from prolongation of pregnancy until pulmonary maturity is achieved. Moreover, delayed delivery may permit placental migration to occur, thereby affording some patients a vaginal delivery.

Expectant management should be terminated at the point where the risks outweigh the benefits of delaying delivery (Table 18-3). Clearly, there is no benefit in prolonging pregnancy beyond the development of fetal pulmonary maturity. Additionally, it is not prudent to prolong gestation when the well-being of the mother or fetus is at risk, irrespective of fetal pulmonary status. Expectant management of the gravida with a placenta previa is considered a reasonable option based on the premise that (1) catastrophic, life-threatening bleeding rarely occurs from unprovoked vaginal bleeding; and (2) the major cause of perinatal death is prematurity. Additionally, in selecting a conservative course of management, the following assumptions apply: (1) cesarean delivery can be performed immediately at any hour of the day should it become necessary; (2) the fetus has a reassuring heart rate tracing; (3) vaginal bleeding has stopped or is minimal; and (4) the mother's cardiovascular status is stable.

Upon sonographic confirmation of placenta previa, strict pelvic and bed rest are important. Although it is unclear whether bed rest is useful in preventing preterm uterine contractions, it does appear to be associated with greater fetal growth, thereby benefiting the fetus should preterm delivery be required. Pelvic rest (abstinence from digital examination, intercourse, douching, tampons, and so on) is necessary to avoid traumatic exacerbation of bleeding or stimulation of uterine contractions.

In placenta previa it is only a matter of time until vaginal bleeding recurs. With sufficient blood loss, the mother will eventually become anemic and unstable. Keeping in mind the infectious potential of blood components, it is reasonable to use a maternal hemoglobin of roughly 8 to 9 g/dl as the limit below which transfusions should be considered during the antenatal period. Maintenance of maternal hemoglobin in this range should allow adequate fetal oxygenation and maternal cardiovascular stability in the patient at bed rest. Throughout this period, properly typed and screened blood should be readily accessible. In the patient who requires serial transfusions because of ongoing vaginal bleeding, the obstetrician must determine whether ongoing expectant management is warranted.

Because placental migration may occur as gestation advances, sonographic reassessment of the placenta is recommended every 2 to 3 weeks. Moreover, because intrauterine growth retardation and fetal anomalies occur more frequently in placenta previa, it is also advisable to assess fetal growth and anatomy. When clinically indicated, nonstress testing or fetal biophysical assessment is recommended to ensure fetal well-being. As with placental abruption, contraction stress testing in the setting of a placenta previa is contraindicated.

Tocolytic therapy is recommended should preterm uterine contractions develop. However, selection of an appropriate tocolytic agent is somewhat controversial. β-Agonist tocolytics may worsen cardiovascular instability in the hypovolemic patient. Additionally, nonsteroidal antiinflammatory drugs may increase the risk of bleeding by interfering with platelet aggregation. Therefore in placenta previa an acceptable first-line tocolytic agent is magnesium sulfate. Among those patients at greatest risk for preterm delivery, use of betamethasone to accelerate fetal lung maturation is recommended.

Cesarean delivery should be performed when fetal pulmonary maturity is documented (i.e., a lecithin/sphingomyelin ratio of 2.0 or greater, and/or the presence of phosphatidyl glycerol in the amniotic fluid). Approximately one half of all fetuses at 34 weeks' gestation will have mature lungs. Therefore amniocentesis beyond 34, and no later than 36, weeks should be performed. If the fetal lungs are not mature, amniocentesis should be repeated in 7 to 14 days.

A growing body of data suggests that outpatient management may be successful in selected patients. However, widespread contemporary clinical experience with this modality is not sufficient to justify its widespread use. The use of cervical cerclage to improve pregnancy outcome in the setting of placenta previa is popular in some countries but has thus far received only limited study in the United States.

Complications

Although cesarean delivery is the recommended treatment for placenta previa, it may be complicated by a variety of problems. First, a considerable portion of the placenta may be under the site where the uterine incision is to be placed. Although the incision can be modified, placental laceration frequently occurs and may be associated with considerable maternal and fetal blood loss. When the placenta is transected, the umbilical cord should be quickly clamped and the placenta quickly extracted through the uterine incision to minimize hemorrhage. Second, because the lower uterine segment is less muscular than the upper segment, it contracts less effectively. Because tonic myometrial contraction is the primary hemostatic mechanism following delivery (see Chapter 22, Postpartum Hemorrhage), placental implantation in the lower uterine segment sometimes is associated with increased postpar-

tum bleeding. Finally, placenta accreta, the abnormal adherence of placenta to the underlying myometrium, is associated with placenta previa. Usually, only part of the placenta is unduly adherent. Placenta accreta occurs secondary to the absence of Nitabuch's layer and decidua basalis at the implantation site. Consequently, the placenta's anchoring villi attach directly and irreversibly to the uterine wall. As with placenta previa, placenta accreta also tends to occur at the site of old uterine incisions. If attempts to remove the adherent placenta manually fail, blood loss can be torrential and life-threatening. The standard treatment for placenta accreta remains hysterectomy, although data are accumulating that expectant management coupled with the use of chemotherapeutic agents such as methotrexate may have use.

TRANSFUSION OF BLOOD COMPONENTS AND DERIVATIVES

From time to time, third trimester bleeding will cause sufficient instability in the hemodynamic or hematologic status of the patient to warrant transfusion of blood components or derivatives.

Although whole blood has long been the mainstay of transfusion therapy, in recent years the use of blood components has become the preferred modality. Blood products may be subdivided into cellular and plasma components. The most commonly used cellular components include red blood cells (RBCs) and platelet concentrates. The most commonly utilized plasma components are fresh frozen plasma and cryoprecipitate.

Cellular components

TRANSFUSION OF RED BLOOD CELLS. Transfusion of whole blood usually is indicated only for rapid replacement of both blood volume and oxygen-carrying capacity, an extremely uncommon occurrence. Blood component therapy allows the physician to treat the specific derangement in a patient's blood system. Thus most patients requiring replacement of RBCs should receive packed RBCs. Transfusion of one unit of packed RBCs into a 70-kg woman usually will increase her hemoglobin level by 1 g/dl (Table 18-4). Because one unit of packed RBCs contains less fluid than one unit of whole blood, there is a reduced risk of fluid overload. Pregnant women with anemia who exhibit cardiovascular instability, a hemoglobin below 8 to 9 g/dl, or evidence of fetal compromise should be considered as candidates for RBC transfusion. Autologous blood donation-transfusion is being used with increasing frequency in placenta previa. It appears to have use in properly selected patients.

PLATELET CONCENTRATES. Platelets are separated from whole blood and suspended in small volumes of plasma. They may be collected from single or multiple donors. Platelet transfusion is indicated for the treatment of clinically significant thrombocytopenia or platelet dysfunction. Although thrombocytopenia is considered to be present when the platelet count falls below 100,000 per mm^3, bleeding following trauma or major surgery rarely occurs until the platelet count falls below 50,000 per mm^3. One unit of platelets is generally equivalent to the number of platelets typically found in one unit of whole blood. When one unit of platelets is transfused into a 70-kg woman, her platelet count should be expected to rise by 7500 platelets per mm^3 (Table 18-4). Because platelet concentrates contain considerable numbers of serum-bound RBCs, the possibility of Rh sensitization may occur in the Rh-negative recipient. Therefore when the Rh-negative woman receives platelet transfusions, Rh immune globulin prophylaxis is prudent.

Plasma components

FRESH FROZEN PLASMA. Fresh-frozen plasma (FFP) is extracted from whole blood and typically contains 700 mg of fibrinogen per unit. Generally, FFP is used to correct deficiencies of multiple clotting factors as may occur in disseminated intravascular coagulation, liver disease, or vitamin K deficiency. It also may be used to correct deficiencies of factors II, V, VII, IX, X, or XI, and may be used for rapid reversal of warfarin.

One unit of FFP usually will increase the maternal fibrinogen level by 10 to 15 mg/dl. When considering FFP therapy, a reasonable starting dose is 15 ml/kg. It must be remembered that roughly 30 minutes are required to thaw FFP in the blood bank. Additionally, consideration must

[handwritten margin note: FFP treats DIC]

Table 18-4. Blood components

Component	Indications	Approx. volume	Expected effect
Packed RBCs	Increase red cell mass	300 ml	Increases Hct 3%/U Increases Hgb 1 g/U
Platelet count	Platelet count below 50,000 per mm^3	50 ml	Increase total platelet 7500/U
Fresh-frozen fibrinogen plasma	Treatment of coagulation disorders	250 ml	Increase total fibrinogen 10-15 mg/U
Cryoprecipitate fibrinogen	Hemophilia A; von Willebrand's disease; fibrinogen deficiency	40 ml	Increase total 10-15 mg/U

RBCs, Red blood cells; *Hct,* hematocrit; *Hgb,* hemoglobin.

be given to the fact that one unit of FFP contains approximately 250 ml of fluid. Should large volumes of FFP be required, the patient may be at risk for fluid overload.

CRYOPRECIPITATE. Cryoprecipitate is the cold-insoluble fraction of FFP that precipitates when frozen, whole blood is allowed to thaw. Cryoprecipitate is rich in factor VIII, XIII, fibrinogen, and von Willebrand's factor. Because one unit of cryoprecipitate contains roughly 40 ml of fluid, it will raise the fibrinogen level more efficiently without posing the risk for fluid overload that FFP does.

Risks of blood product transfusion

The risks from blood product transfusion increase in proportion to the number of units transfused. The risks posed by transfusion therapy may be subdivided into infectious and immunologic processes.

Among the infectious risks from blood products, the hepatitis C virus had been the most common pathogen. With the development of hepatitis C screening, it is anticipated that the incidence of hepatitis C among transfusion recipients will decline to the same level as hepatitis B (approximately 1 per 300 units transfused). The risk of acquiring the human immunodeficiency virus (HIV) ranges from 1 in 40,000 to 1 in 1,000,000 units of transfused blood products. Although a screening test is available for the presence of HIV antibody, this antibody screen can take 6 months or more to convert following infection. Therefore blood donated by an HIV-infected person during this time period would give a false-negative antibody screen and accounts for the majority of transfusion-associated HIV infections. Other pathogens that may be transmitted through administration of blood products include cytomegalovirus, bacterial and endotoxin associated disease, malaria, parvovirus, Epstein-Barr virus, babesia, and T-cell viruses.

Most commonly, transfusion reactions are initiated by antigens located on the surface of red and white blood cells. The hemolytic type of transfusion reaction occurs once per 6000 units of transfusion and is fatal in 1 per 100,000 units of transfused blood. The nonhemolytic transfusion reaction usually is characterized by febrile or urti-

CRITICAL POINTS

- Intravenous access with at least one and preferably two large-bore intravenous catheters is important.
- Continuous electronic fetal heart rate monitoring is prudent until the condition of the mother and fetus is established.
- Left lateral displacement of the uterus can optimize maternal cardiac output and uteroplacental perfusion. In third trimester bleeding, this maneuver is always prudent.
- As a result of normal physiologic changes, a pregnant woman may not demonstrate significant changes in vital signs until 25% to 30% of her intravascular volume has been lost. In many instances, the fetus will demonstrate fetal heart rate abnormalities before the mother evidences clinical signs of intravascular depletion.
- Until placenta previa has been ruled out, direct digital examination of the cervical os is absolutely contraindicated.
- Women with placenta previa or abruptio placentae are at increased risk for recurring bleeding and postpartum hemorrhage.

carial reactions and occurs much more frequently (1 per 100 units of blood) than the more worrisome hemolytic reaction. Additionally, alloimmunization can produce platelet antibodies that diminish the therapeutic response to platelet transfusions. In the immunocompromised individual, graft-versus-host disease occasionally can occur following transfusion of certain blood products.

Questions

1. Abruptio placentae should be considered in the setting of:
   A. Painless, bright red bleeding
   B. Tetanic uterine contractions and passage of nonclotting blood
   C. Fever and passage of blood clots
   D. Severe maternal anemia
   E. Late fetal heart rate decelerations

2. The primary modality for diagnosing placenta previa is:
   A. Clinical presentation
   B. Ultrasound
   C. Cervical examination
   D. Maternal laboratory analysis
   E. Kleihauer-Betke screening

3. The risk of acquiring HIV following transfusion of one unit of packed RBCs:
   A. Is increasing
   B. Is higher than that for hepatitis B
   C. May be as high as 1 in 40,000
   D. Is influenced by gestational age
   E. Is unknown

Answers

1. B
2. B
3. C

19

Preterm labor

APGO LEARNING OBJECTIVE #19

John P. Elliott

Prematurity is the most common cause of neonatal mortality and morbidity. The reduction of preterm birth remains an important goal in obstetric care. Understanding the causes and recognizing the symptoms of preterm labor provide the basis for management decisions.

The student will demonstrate a knowledge of the following:

A. Factors predisposing to preterm labor
B. Signs and symptoms of premature uterine contractions
C. Causes of preterm labor
D. Principles of tocolysis

Prematurity is the leading cause of newborn mortality and morbidity. Approximately 6% to 8% of all births in the United States are considered premature (delivery less than 37 completed weeks of gestation). The current perinatal mortality rate in the United States is 10.4 per 1000 live births. Morbidity occurs in 10% of survivors with severe handicaps and in about 30% with mild to moderate handicaps. In addition, premature babies have a 5 to 20 times increased risk of dying in the first year of life compared with term deliveries. Preterm babies also have an increased risk of hospital admission for complications during the first year of life. A breakdown of gestational age at delivery would show about 1% deliver at less than 28 weeks' gestational age, 1% at 28 to 32 weeks, and 5% at 32 to 36 weeks.

Efforts to prevent prematurity have been largely unsuccessful. Figure 19-1 shows the birth weight of babies in the United States from 1979 to 1985 and illustrates the flat trend in deliveries at each birth rate. This trend continues into the 1990s without change. Table 19-1 illustrates the improvement in both morbidity and mortality with advancing gestation at delivery; and Table

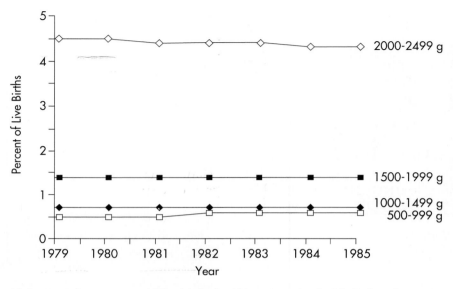

Fig. 19-1. Annual percentages of live births by 500-g categories for births less than 2500 g in United States from 1979 to 1985.

Table 19-1. Mean birth weight, estimated neonatal survival, and expected improvement in rate of survival per week and per day at various gestational ages

Gest. age (wk)	Approx. mean birth weight (g)	Survival (%)	Improvement in survival	
			Per wk (%)	Per day (%)
22	500	0	4	0.6
23	575	4	13	1.9
24	650	17	13	1.9
25	775	30	21	3.0
26	900	51	13	1.9
27	1025	64	11	1.6
28	1150	75	6	0.9
29	1250	81	6	0.9
30	1400	87	6	0.9
31	1550	93	2	0.3
32	1750	95	2	0.3
33	2000	97	1	0.1
34	2200	98	1	0.1
35	2400	99	1	0.1
36	2600	99+	<1	<0.1

19-2 shows the improvement in survival without major handicap on a weekly and daily basis. These tables illustrate that each day gained before delivery is extremely important at gestational age less than 28 weeks and not as significant at 35 to 36 weeks.

Premature delivery can be grouped into three main categories based on the reason for delivery: preterm labor (PTL), 25%; preterm premature rupture of the membranes (PPROM), 30%; and medical complications, 45%. Preterm premature rupture of the membranes tends to be more frequent in lower socioeconomic status populations, and PTL as a cause of preterm delivery occurs more frequently in predominantly middle class populations. Preterm labor is responsible for about 25% of the prematurity rate.

PATHOGENESIS

Preterm labor is defined as regular uterine contractions occurring four in 20 minutes or eight in 60 minutes with evidence of cervical change (either greater than or equal to 2 cm dilatation or 80% effacement), occurring between 20 and 37 weeks' gestation.

Preterm labor represents a final common pathway that may have a number of different causes. Faulty placentation may be associated with abruptio placentae; infection (either clinical or subclinical) of the decidual tissue (chorioamnionitis); immunologic causes; cervical incompetence; uterine factors (uterine anomalies, leiomyoma uteri); maternal systemic infection; trauma; fetal anomalies; overdistention of the uterus (polyhydramnios,

Table 19-2. Mean birth weight, estimated survival without major handicap, and expected improvement in rate of survival without major handicap per week and per day at various gestational ages

Gest. age (wk)	Approx. mean birth weight (g)	Estimated survival without major handicap (%)	Improvement in survival without major handicap	
			Per wk (%)	Per day (%)
22	500	0	2	0.3
23	575	2	7	1.0
24	650	9	9	1.3
25	775	18	23	3.3
26	900	41	13	1.9
27	1025	54	13	1.9
28	1150	67	7	1.0
29	1250	74	7	1.0
30	1400	81	6	0.9
31	1550	87	3	0.4
32	1750	90	3	0.4
33	2000	93	2	0.3
34	2200	95	2	0.3
35	2400	97	1	0.1

multifetal gestations); drugs (cocaine, methamphetamine); and idiopathic causes. The most common conditions associated with PTL are infection and abnormal placentation (abruptio placentae). Frequently there will be two or more possible identifiable causes for PTL. It is important to try to determine the cause of PTL so that it can be addressed, if possible, to make treatment more effective.

SIGNS AND SYMPTOMS for PTL

Every pregnant patient is at risk for PTL and should be aware of the signs and symptoms of PTL, including uterine contractions (71%), pelvic pressure (50%), backache (47%), increased vaginal discharge (47%), and menstrual-like cramps (43%). Other symptoms that can be present are intestinal cramping or diarrhea, spotting or bleeding, and a general feeling that "things are not right." These signs and symptoms are common in normal pregnancy, which often delays the early diagnosis of PTL. There are certain risk factors for PTL that should be recognized, and patients who have these should be managed more intensively (Table 19-3).

The prevention of PTL involves a high degree of suspicion and some preventive tactics. All patients should be counseled about the signs and symptoms of PTL and an inquiry should be made at each prenatal visit. Cervical exam should be done at the start of the third trimester (24 weeks) and again at 30 weeks, seeking unsuspected cervical change. The life-style of patients identified as at increased risk for PTL should be examined, with modifications made to reduce stress. A strenuous, stressful work environment or several small children in the house frequently contribute to a poor outcome.

Obstetric care providers must also prioritize prematurity prevention as the most important goal of prenatal care. The providers should respond to maternal calls with complaints of symptoms of PTL with direct evaluation of the symptoms, not telephone advice such as "Get off your feet," "It can't be labor," or "You're not due yet!"

MANAGEMENT

Treatment of preterm contractions or PTL involves a graduated response. The patient arrives for evaluation and is placed on a fetal monitor. She is positioned on her left side. If contractions are

Table 19-3. Preterm labor risks and incidence of preterm delivery

	Incidence of PTD (%)
History of PTL and PTD × 1	40
History of PTL and PTD ≥2	70
History of PROM	30
Incompetent cervix—cerclage placed <18 wk	16
Uterine anomaly (including fibroids)	20
Second trimester abortion >1	30-40
Black indigent patient (nulliparous)	16
Twins	55
Triplets	90
Quadruplets	100
Cocaine use during current pregnancy	10-20
RISKS IN CURRENT PREGNANCY	
PTL	70
Acute incompetent cervix—cerclage placed >19 wk	91
Second trimester vaginal bleeding	40
Polyhydramnios	20
False labor	34

PTL, Preterm labor; *PTD,* preterm delivery; *PROM,* premature rupture of the membranes.

documented, the next step in management is to perform an evaluation of the cervix. If the cervix does not show evidence of significant change, then intravenous (IV) hydration may improve intravascular volume and increase oxygen delivery to the uterus, which may stop the contractions. If there is cervical change present (dilatation 2 cm or greater; effacement 80% or greater) tocolysis should be initiated immediately. Terbutaline should be given 0.25 mg subcutaneously initially while IV drugs are being prepared.

Tocolytic drugs will reduce contractions of the uterine smooth muscle. Drugs that have been used successfully as tocolytics include magnesium sulfate; β-sympathomimetic agents (ritodrine or terbutaline); prostaglandin synthetase inhibitors (indomethacin, ibuprofen); calcium channel blockers (nifedipine); and the antihypertensive drug diazoxide. These drugs vary in efficacy, side effects, route of administration, cost, and complications.

There are questions about the efficacy of tocolytic drugs. Why? There is lack of consensus on the definition of success with a tocolytic drug. Is it prevention of delivery for 24 hours, 48 hours, 1 week, to term? The indications for use are not clear. Ten percent of patients will develop PTL, and another 10% will have "false" labor. Who should be treated and how aggressively? Tocolytic drugs also are frequently given in inadequate dosage and for too short a time. All of these reasons contribute to very poor documentation of efficacy. Tocolysis is also a treatment of relative desperation and has a high rate of failure. It is a general response to a final common pathway (labor) that does not address the underlying disorders.

SELECTION OF TOCOLYTIC DRUGS

Preterm labor is an identifiable event of indeterminate duration (several hours to several days). Effective tocolysis must be maintained for the duration of the risk period. The most popular tocolytic agents are the β-sympathomimetic drugs (ritodrine, terbutaline). These drugs are effective tocolytics when given IV. The recommended duration of IV therapy is 12 hours; then a switch is made to oral therapy. This short duration of IV treatment limits the success of these drugs when PTL lasts more than 12 hours. Prolonged IV therapy increases complications, including pulmonary edema, arrhythmias, and cardiac ischemia. The β$_2$-cardiovascular side effects of these drugs include tachycardia, increased cardiac output, and decreased peripheral vascular resistance; and these effects limit the use of the drugs in patients with hypertension, cardiac disease, diabetes, or active vaginal bleeding from abruptio placentae or placenta previa.

Magnesium sulfate should be the IV tocolytic drug in all circumstances. The only absolute contraindication to magnesium sulfate is myasthenia gravis, but caution should be observed in patients with severe renal disease. An initial bolus dose of 6 g of magnesium sulfate is given over 20 minutes; then maintenance therapy is initiated at 3 g/hr. This dosage is adjusted up or down, depending on response of the contractions and maternal side effects. Therapeutic serum levels of magnesium range from 5.5 to 7.5 mg/dl. Magnesium sulfate is the preferred drug for IV tocolysis because it has fewer side effects, fewer contraindications, lower cost, and is equally efficacious as the β-mimetics. In addition, obstetricians are more familiar with the drug; there is an antidote for overdosage (calcium); and, most important, it can be used for prolonged periods—up to months, if necessary.

Prostaglandin synthetase inhibitors are effective tocolytics. These drugs inhibit cyclooxygenase, which converts arachidonic acid into PGG$_2$. Indomethacin is administered either rectally or orally (50 mg initially, then 25 mg every 6 hours). There are some side effects that must be considered, including maternal gastrointestinal problems (peptic ulceration, bleeding) and thrombocytopenia. Fetal problems include oli-

Table 19-4. Results of magnesium sulfate tocolysis: singleton pregnancy with intact membranes (274 patients)

Dilatation in centimeters	Number of patients	Number of patients (%) for time gained after initiation of tocolysis						Number of patients (%) with			
		24 Hours	48 Hours	72 Hours	>7 Days	Term gestation	Abruptio placentae	Clinical infections	Pathologic infections	Fetal distress	
Closed	91	78 (86)	76 (84)	73 (80)	62 (68)	45 (50)	18 (20)	3 (3)	1 (1)	8 (9)	
1	33	32 (97)	32 (97)	32 (97)	26 (79)	24 (73)	5 (15)	1 (3)	1 (3)	0 (0)	
2	49	43 (88)	42 (86)	36 (73)	23 (47)	21 (43)	7 (14)	1 (2)	3 (6)	4 (8)	
3	48	33 (69)	32 (67)	28 (58)	17 (35)	9 (19)	11 (23)	3 (6)	3 (6)	1 (2)	
4	24	15 (63)	14 (58)	12 (50)	8 (33)	6 (25)	6 (25)	1 (4)	1 (4)	0 (0)	
5	13	7 (54)	7 (54)	6 (46)	3 (23)	1 (8)	1 (8)	1 (8)	0 (0)	0 (0)	
6	11	5 (46)	4 (36)	4 (36)	1 (9)	0 (0)	0 (0)	1 (9)	1 (9)	0 (0)	
7	4	1 (25)	1 (25)	0 (0)	0 (0)	0 (0)	1 (25)	2 (50)	0 (0)	0 (0)	
8	1	0 (0)	0 (0)	0 (0)	0 (0)	0 (0)	0 (0)	0 (0)	0 (0)	0 (0)	
Total	274	214 (78)	208 (76)	191 (70)	140 (51)	106 (39)	49 (18)	13 (5)	10 (4)	13 (5)	

gohydramnios (from decreased fetal renal blood flow) and possibly some constriction of the ductus arteriosus, which usually is transient and reversible. Administration of indomethacin at term (after 36 weeks) may cause primary pulmonary hypertension and tricuspid insufficiency in the neonate. PSIs should not be used for prolonged periods and should be discontinued by 32 to 34 weeks' gestation.

Calcium channel blockers such as nifedipine can be used for oral tocolysis. These drugs have not been studied as thoroughly as the other drugs and represent second line drug therapy. Diazoxide can cause profound hypotension and is not useful for tocolysis.

What is "success" with a tocolytic agent? It is suggested that if the cervix is dilated less than 2 cm, success should be defined by a delay of delivery for at least 1 week and probably to term; however, if the cervix has dilated 3 cm or more, success should be measured by reaching 48 hours without delivery. This would allow steroids to be administered and achieve their maximum effect in the fetus. Table 19-4 shows the success of tocolysis with magnesium sulfate based on cervical dilatation. Tocolytics can be used in patients with advanced cervical dilatation if expectations are 48 hours' delay before delivery, not achievement of term gestation.

If tocolysis is successful, management of the patient is based on several factors. What is the gestational age? What factors contributed to the onset of PTL, and are these factors still present (e.g., twins or polyhydramnios)? What is the current cervical examination? What social and economic factors are important? Should the patient be managed in the hospital, or is home management appropriate? If the patient can be removed from IV tocolysis, will oral tocolytic drugs be used (there is no scientific documentation of efficacy for oral tocolysis)? All of these questions must be considered before attempting long-term management in patients successfully treated for PTL. It must be remembered (Table 19-3) that PTL in the current pregnancy that is successfully treated still has a 70% chance of delivery at less than 37 weeks' gestation. The patient requires careful monitoring and follow-up, whether in the hospital or at home. If the patient experiences PTL and preterm delivery, she is at an increased risk (40%) of having the same problem in a subsequent pregnancy, and the risk rises to 70% if PTL happened in two previous pregnancies. Please note also that false labor is a risk factor for preterm delivery. If a patient is evaluated for PTL and cervical change is not documented, and contractions cease with hydration and left-side recumbent position, she still must be followed carefully.

CRITICAL POINTS

- The diagnosis of PTL is difficult, and the clinician must have a high index of suspicion.
- Preterm labor has many associated clinical findings that should be evaluated to assist in developing an effective treatment plan.
- Tocolysis is a treatment of desperation and has a high rate of failure.
- Preterm labor may last for several days; effective tocolysis often must be maintained for an extended time.
- Inadequate dosing of tocolytic drugs often is associated with failure.
- More than one tocolytic drug may be needed (combination therapy).
- Tocolysis is an *art,* not a science.

Questions

1. Which of the following risk factors is associated with the greatest risk of PTL?
   A. Preterm labor in the current pregnancy
   B. History of PTL and delivery in one previous pregnancy
   C. Quadruplets
   D. False labor in the current pregnancy
   E. Polyhydramnios
2. All of the following are signs or symptoms of PTL *except:*
   A. Backache
   B. Intestinal cramping
   C. Increased vaginal discharge
   D. General feeling that things aren't right
   E. Severe heartburn
3. The most important aspect of treatment of PTL is:

A. Transport of the patient to a tertiary perinatal center
B. Prophylactic tocolytic drugs
C. Early identification and diagnosis of PTL
D. Tocolytic drugs
E. Bed rest
4. What is the definition of successful tocolysis?
   A. 24-hour delay before delivery
   B. 48-hour delay before delivery
   C. 1-week delay before delivery
   D. Delay until term before delivery
   E. Depends on cervical dilatation

Answers

1. C
2. E
3. C
4. E

20 Premature rupture of membranes

APGO LEARNING OBJECTIVE #20

Daniel F. O'Keeffe, Jr.

> *Rupture of the membranes before labor is a complication in both term and preterm pregnancies. Careful evaluation of this condition may affect fetal and maternal outcome.*

The student will demonstrate a knowledge of the following:

A. History, physical findings, and diagnostic methods to confirm rupture of the membranes
B. Conditions favoring expectant management versus timely delivery with premature rupture of the membranes
C. Methods to monitor maternal and fetal status in expectant management

Premature rupture of the membranes (PROM), or amniorrhexis, is one of the most confusing and controversial dilemmas in obstetrics today. Premature rupture of the membranes is probably the single most common precipitating factor in preterm delivery. In addition, maternal and fetal-neonatal infection, fetal distress, adverse influences on fetal development, and increased cesarean rates with concomitant increased morbidity and mortality are significant complications of PROM.

DEFINITION

One confusion associated with the problem of PROM is the lack of uniformity in defining it. Most studies define it as rupture of the fetal membranes any time before onset of labor. Strictly speaking, the definition does not include a gestational age requirement. From a management standpoint, however, it is useful to distinguish between preterm premature rupture of the membranes (PPROM) and PROM. It is particularly important not to confuse PROM with prolonged rupture of the membranes, which usually means rupture of membranes for more than 24 hours. The incidence of PROM, using the definition as described, is approximately 8% to 10% of all pregnancies.

ETIOLOGY

Much attention has been paid to discovering the cause of PROM, but little definitive knowledge is yet available. Attempts to correlate clinical variables with the incidence of PROM generally have been disappointing. Studies usually have failed to demonstrate any relationship between PROM and maternal age, parity, maternal weight, trauma, or meconium. Correlations have been shown between a higher incidence of PROM and antepartum bleeding, cervical operations and lacerations, multiple gestations, smoking, and polyhydramnios. A large body of evidence has accumulated that infection may cause a significant number of preterm deliveries with PROM.

COMPLICATIONS

The main complications of PROM are labor and infection. Premature labor can be expected within 24 hours following PROM in 80% to 90% of the patients. The precise figure varies, however, with gestational age at the time of membrane rupture. Generally the earlier in the pregnancy membrane rupture occurs, the longer the latent period that can be expected. An important clinical question in managing patients with PPROM is the likelihood of labor in the woman who presents with PROM but is not in labor at the time of her admission. Studies show that by 4 days after PROM most preterm patients are in labor. These figures indicate that the likelihood of achieving a substantial additional amount of time in utero for infants of preterm women with PROM is low.

The incidence of chorioamnionitis varies with gestational age and the population studied, and, at least at term, with the duration of ruptured membranes. Of all pregnancies, the incidence is 0.5% to 1%. In prolonged (more than 24 hours) PROM, the incidences have been reported at 3% to 25%. In PPROM, chorioamnionitis occurs in 6% to 22% of patients. Maternal consequences of chorioamnionitis include sepsis and all its possible complications, endometritis, abscesses, fistulas, and infertility. These infections remain potentially lethal to the mother. It appears that, with aggressive intervention including delivery and antibiotics, the risks one must take to buy time for fetal maturity may not be as great as previously thought.

Neonatal consequences of chorioamnionitis vary significantly with gestational age. At term, the consequences of chorioamnionitis to the fetus/neonate are slight. Neonatal mortality at term and the presence of amniotic infection, especially due to infectious causes, are considerably less frequent—probably on the order of 1% to 2%, which nonetheless is a 50% to 100% increase in death rate over uninfected low-risk patients.

The preterm infant fares far worse than its term counterpart. Looking specifically at the prenatal consequences of preterm chorioamnionitis, it has been found that perinatal mortality increases from 3% to 11%; the rate of serious newborn infections increases 2.5 times; and the rate of respiratory distress syndrome doubles.

It has been recognized for many years that the incidence of umbilical cord prolapse has increased in the setting of PROM to about 1.5%, compared with 0.5% in all deliveries. This is particularly so when PROM and malpresentation coexist. Even in the absence of frank cord prolapse, the incidence of fetal distress from umbilical cord compression is substantially greater. The only other significant complications of consequence in PROM are the effects on fetal development subsequent to amniotic fluid loss, particularly when PROM occurs in the first half of the second trimester. Included in these effects are pulmonary hypoplasia, abnormal facies, and associated anomalies of the hands, feet, and ears. While the risks of infection are not trivial, it is generally believed that the consequences of prematurity are 2 to 3 times more likely than infections to cause death in preterm neonates. Therefore one can generalize that complications of prematurity, especially hyaline membrane disease, are the major causes of perinatal mortality in PPROM. Although efforts aimed at prolonging pregnancy may well result in improved outcomes, it appears that these efforts must also include earlier identification of infection and fetal hypoxia so that babies are not lost or damaged from these causes during attempts to gain maturity.

EVALUATION OF THE PATIENT

Management of PROM depends first on establishing the correct diagnosis. Making the correct diagnosis depends on the combination of history, physical examination, findings, and laboratory information.

A typical history of amniorrhexis generally includes a large gush of fluid from the vagina, followed by continuous leakage. Fluid is generally clear but is often blood-tinged and occasionally frankly bloody. Explanations for incorrect diagnosis based on patient history include urinary leakage, excessive vaginal and/or cervical mucus secretion, cervicitis and/or vaginitis, and bloody discharge.

The examination should be conducted with a sterile speculum. Often the perineum is moist; as the sterile speculum is inserted, pooled fluid in the posterior vagina can be seen. Occasionally Valsalva's maneuver is necessary to determine whether any fluid comes from the cervix.

While the sterile speculum is in place, a nitrazine test should be performed. During pregnancy, the pH of the vagina usually is between 4.5 and 6. The pH of the amniotic fluid ranges from 7 to 7.5. The nitrazine paper will change color from yellow-green to a dark blue with a pH above 6 to 6.5. False-positive rates for the nitrazine test range from 1% to 17%, and false-negative rates range from 0 to 10%.

The most commonly used and reliable test probably is the fern test. A swab or an aspiration tube should be used to obtain fluid from the posterior fornix and the fluid placed on a dry, clean slide. After 5 to 7 minutes for drying, an easily recognized arborization of crystals can be seen under the microscope when amniotic fluid is present. Many substances may interfere with or prevent ferning. Blood, meconium, heavy discharge, and lubricants may give false-negative results. Prolonged membrane rupture also may give false-negative results. Occasionally (about 5% to 30% of cases), cervical mucus ferns in pregnancy and can be confused with amniotic fluid; care must be taken to avoid the cervix in taking the sample. Many other tests have been developed to look for PROM but have not become clinically popular.

In some cases where it is difficult to determine whether PROM has occurred, the use of obstetric ultrasound, either alone or in conjunction with amniocentesis, and an injection of indigo carmine dye may be of great help.

In making the diagnosis of PROM it is crucial that one not increase the likelihood of infection in the process. It has been documented that even a single digital examination increases the risk of maternal and fetal infection. Digital examinations should not be performed in the evaluation of PROM. A sterile speculum examination is the preferable method, and all necessary tests and inspections of the cervix can be done without digital examinations.

At the time of sterile speculum examination, cervical culture should be taken—especially for group B *Streptococcus* (GBS).

Fluid can also be obtained to assess fetal lung maturity by doing a phosphatidylglycerol test on the cervical fluid.

Once the diagnosis of PROM has been made, the next step is to review the dates to assess gestational age. Menstrual history, the results of early examinations, early pregnancy testing, and the findings of early ultrasound, when available, must all be reviewed. An ultrasound examination at the time of initial assessment of the patient with PROM helps to confirm dates, as well as the diagnosis of PROM; assesses fetal presentation and lie; and occasionally reveals unexpected information, such as the presence of congenital malformation, twins, or fundic presentation. Once gestational age has been assessed, it may be desirable to assess fetal lung maturity. Indications for assessing fetal lung maturity are not fixed. Generally, if fluid can be obtained from the vaginal vault during sterile speculum examination, it would be wise to do so. The use of transabdominal amniocentesis to determine fetal lung maturity, advocated a number of years ago, generally is not done today unless one also is assessing whether any concomitant amniotic infection is present.

RULING OUT INFECTION

Once gestational age and, when appropriate, fetal maturity have been established, the next question is whether intraamniotic infection is present. Many of the signs and symptoms of infection are sensitive, but not specific, to this kind of infection. Leukocytosis to a moderate degree (more than $15,000/ml^3$), fetal tachycardia (more than 160 beats/min), maternal tachycardia (more than 100 beats/min), uterine tenderness, and foul-smelling fluid are all helpful but not specific. One cannot be absolutely sure of the diagnosis of chorioamnionitis in the absence of fever (more than 100° F), positive Gram stain, or culture. Chorioamnionitis must be looked for carefully. If the patient is infected, delivery and antibiotics are the treatment.

Patients are generally monitored for fetal heart rate from 12 to 24 hours for the following reasons: (1) To evaluate the patient for labor. Since it is desirable to avoid digital examination, there is a need to know whether the patient is contracting and, if so, if the cervix is changing. The monitor gives us an idea of the contractions, and a sterile speculum can examine the cervix for any changes. (2) Fetal distress is more common in PROM and probably is a significant contributor to fetal morbidity and mortality.

The use of corticosteroids in PPROM is controversial and often will depend on the beliefs of physicians in a regional area. Use of tocolytic agents in PPROM also is controversial. The efficacy of tocolytic agents in PPROM is open to serious question. If used, they should be employed only to prolong pregnancy for 48 hours to allow physicians who wish to administer steroids to give them. Otherwise, there does not appear to be any great evidence that tocolytic agents will prolong the pregnancy significantly. It is generally believed that a culture should be done for GBS on all patients with PPROM. A broad spectrum antibiotic to cover GBS should be started until the culture results are known. At that time, further use of antibiotics can be individualized.

The management of PROM, beside the generalizations that have been made, should be individualized based on the gestational age at the time of delivery.

PREMATURE RUPTURE OF MEMBRANES AT LESS THAN 24 WEEKS

Compared with later gestational ages, the special situation of PROM at a previable gestational age creates a completely different set of variables that determine management. First, the fetuses that are delivered immediately have virtually no chance of survival; indeed, 50% of women will deliver within 1 week. Second, maternal risks are greater than at later gestational ages. There is nearly double the rate of chorioamnionitis and a subsequent risk of hemorrhage from retained placenta, often necessitating blood transfusions. Thus the mother is taking a sizable risk if she elects to wait for delivery and buy time for her fetus to mature. Unfortunately, the likelihood of a successful outcome is not great. A composite of studies looking at outcome with expectant management suggests an overall survival rate of

40%, of which about 30% will have major neurologic handicaps. The mother is then left with two choices: whether to deliver the fetus or opt for the risk of expectant management. If she chooses expectant management after the appropriate tests have been done and infection has been ruled out, she can go home and remain housebound, where pelvic rest is prescribed along with taking her temperature every 4 hours. She is instructed to come in or call immediately if labor or fever develops. When she reaches 25 weeks she is then generally admitted to the hospital and managed differently.

PREMATURE RUPTURE OF MEMBRANES AT 25 TO 32 WEEKS

At this early gestational age, prematurity is the overwhelming concern, and efforts to deal with its sequelae are primary. If chorioamnionitis is discovered, delivery should take place immediately, along with the administration of antibiotics. Cesarean section should be reserved for the usual obstetric indications. Patients should have fetal testing (i.e., nonstress testing, biophysical profile) to make sure that there is no fetal distress. These tests should be done on a regular basis anywhere from twice a week to daily. Delivery should be considered if fetal lung maturity has been achieved or 36 weeks of pregnancy reached. In labor, amnioinfusion may be used prophylactically or therapeutically for those who exhibit variable decelerations before 8 to 9 cm of dilatation.

PREMATURE RUPTURE OF MEMBRANES AT 33 TO 36 WEEKS

In very early gestational ages (24 to 30 weeks) prematurity is the overwhelming concern. Later, when neonatal survival rates increase substantially, the concerns about prematurity may become secondary; and efforts to identify the specific risks of prematurity for a given patient may allow selective management to prevent complications from infection. At this gestational age it is important to determine fetal lung maturity. If the lungs are mature, infection becomes the overriding concern, and delivery would be indicated. When fetal lungs are immature they should be tested every 4 to 7 days for maturity. Delivery is indicated at any time for labor, fetal distress, or chorioamnionitis. Patients should have fetal testing (i.e., biophysical profile, nonstress test) to make sure that no fetal distress is occurring. These tests should be done on a regular basis anywhere from twice a week to daily. Delivery should be considered for any pregnancy that reaches 36 weeks or longer. Amnioinfusion may be used prophylactically in all patients or therapeutically in those exhibiting variable decelerations before 8 to 9 cm.

PREMATURE RUPTURE OF MEMBRANES AT MORE THAN 37 WEEKS

For patients who are not in labor, not infected, and show no signs of fetal distress, two reasonable options exist. In all cases the patient should remain in the hospital until she delivers. A reasonable amount of time (12 to 24 hours) should be allowed for the patient to go into labor. After that time, if labor has not started spontaneously, oxytocin induction should begin. The duration of latent phase allowed before resorting to cesarean section should be at least 12 hours (up to 18 hours) after beginning oxytocin and establishing a reasonable labor pattern. Digital examination of the cervix should be avoided completely until the patient appears to be in active labor. The alternative to this form of management involves the use of prostaglandins. A protocol is available for the placement of prostaglandin E_2 to ripen the cervix. One can use from one to three applications, and then start the patient on oxytocin. Patients who have not delivered by 18 hours following PROM should have an antibiotic given for GBS prophylaxis unless they are known to be GBS-negative by prenatal cultures.

Premature rupture of the membranes continues to be a controversial area in obstetrics. One hopes that continued research and new technologies will help improve outcomes in this very difficult diagnostic area.

CRITICAL POINTS

- Incidence: 8% to 10% of all pregnancies.
- Etiology: Largely unknown, but infection may cause a significant number of preterm deliveries with PROM.
- Complications: Labor; infection; consequences of prematurity in the neonate.
- Evaluations: Do not do a digital examination; it markedly increases the risk of infection.
- Management should be based on the gestational age at the time of PROM.

Questions

1. Incidence of PROM:
   A. 2% to 4%
   B. 5% to 7%
   C. 8% to 10%
   D. 11% to 13%
2. All have shown a correlation with PROM *except:*
   A. Smoking
   B. Antepartum bleeding
   C. Parity
   D. Infection
   E. Multiple gestations
3. All are part of a work-up of PROM *except:*
   A. Fern
   B. Speculum exam
   C. Nitrazine
   D. Digital examination
   E. Ultrasound
4. All are appropriate methods to monitor the fetus with PROM *except:*
   A. Biophysical profile
   B. Doppler studies
   C. Nonstress tests
   D. Fetal movement counts

Answers

1. C
2. C
3. D
4. B

21

Intrapartum fetal distress

APGO LEARNING OBJECTIVE #21

Daniel F. O'Keeffe, Jr.

Intrapartum fetal evaluation allows detection of changes during labor that may jeopardize the fetus.

The student will demonstrate a knowledge of the following:

A. Techniques of intrapartum fetal surveillance, including auscultation, electronic fetal monitoring, and fetal scalp sampling
B. Reassuring fetal heart rate patterns
C. Recognition and management of nonreassuring fetal heart rate patterns

There is no generally agreed upon definition of fetal distress because the term has various meanings for different people. Although not interchangeable, the terms *fetal distress, fetal asphyxia,* and *asphyxia trauma* often are freely substituted and erroneously equated. The term fetal distress probably should not be used in obstetrics; in its place one should determine whether there is a reassuring or nonreassuring fetal heart rate pattern and describe what the patterns are. The correlation between fetal heart rate diagnosis and ultimate outcome is far from perfect. The term

birth asphyxia should be applied only in a clinical condition defined by the following:

1. Profound umbilical artery, metabolic, or mix acidemia (pH less than 7, base deficit greater than 20)
2. 5-minute Apgar score of 0 to 3
3. Neonatal neurologic sequelae such as seizures, coma, and hypotonia
4. Multiorgan system dysfunction such as that involving cardiovascular, gastrointestinal, hematologic, renal, and/or pulmonary systems

Techniques for intrapartum fetal surveillance include the following:

1. Auscultation
2. Electronic fetal monitoring
3. Fetal scalp sampling
4. Scalp stimulation test (vibroacoustic stimulation test)

Fetal heart rate patterns can be divided into *reassuring* heart rate patterns and *nonreassuring* heart rate patterns. Reassuring heart rate patterns include those with accelerations, normal baseline, and good variability. Early decelerations and mild variable decelerations are associated with normal fetal blood gases, scalp pH, and Apgar scores and perinatal outcome. Nonreassuring heart rate patterns include the more severe forms of variable decelerations, any degree of late decelerations, and various atypical or preterminal patterns including prolonged decelerations. Baseline fetal heart rate changes of tachycardia and loss of variability should be interpreted in light of the clinical situation and associated periodic changes present on the fetal monitor strip. Nonreassuring heart rate patterns can occur in the presence of a correctable maternal disease. Included in these diseases are severe anemia, respiratory failure, diabetic ketoacidosis, and so on. These are potentially correctable problems, and the abnormal fetal heart rate tracing can be reversed if therapy is initiated. A complete understanding of the entire clinical picture is necessary to correctly interpret and manage fetal heart rate changes in a compromised patient.

Variable decelerations are the most frequent periodic change observed in patients in labor. They usually result from umbilical cord compression. The pattern is characterized by an abrupt fall in fetal heart rate to as low as 50 beats/min. The pattern varies from one moment to the next and may be influenced by such things as maternal position changes. The vast majority of variable decelerations are generally considered a reassuring pattern unless the cord compression is frequent, prolonged, and severe. The problem with variable decelerations is that they may suddenly get more severe. There is much less predictability from one moment to the next with variable decelerations than with late decelerations, which tend to follow a slowly deteriorating course. Thus this type of deceleration is difficult to manage, especially in a hospital lacking the capability to move rapidly to an operative delivery. Variable decelerations are considered to be nonreassuring when the following are true:

1. The decelerations last more than 45 to 60 seconds on a repetitive basis.
2. There is a rising fetal heart rate baseline.
3. There is a loss of fetal heart rate variability.
4. There is a delay in return to baseline at the end of the variable deceleration.

It is common to see variable decelerations lasting more than a minute at 2- to 3-minute intervals during the second stage of labor when the mother is pushing. The medical management of nonreassuring variable decelerations includes the following steps:

1. Change the mother's position to where the fetal heart rate pattern is most improved (patient's left side, right side, or Trendelenburg).
2. Discontinue oxytocin if being used.
3. Check for cord prolapse or imminent delivery by vaginal examination.
4. Administer oxygen.
5. If variable decelerations are persistent, but reassuring, consider therapeutic amnioinfusion. Scalp pH is of little value with variable decelerations.

Late decelerations are found in association with uteroplacental insufficiency. It also suggests some degree of fetal hypoxia. The appearance of late decelerations is the earliest marker that we now have for fetal hypoxia. The pattern characteristically is described as uniform, appearing consistently from one contraction to the next, starting about midcontraction and ending after the contraction. Generally, the depth of the deceleration is not greater than the magnitude of the contraction. When the fetus is severely compromised, the depth of the deceleration can be quite small. Medical management includes the following steps:

1. Place the mother in the lateral position.
2. Hydrate the mother.
3. Discontinue oxytocin if being used.
4. Administer oxygen.

Again, as with variable decelerations and late decelerations, one must look carefully at the clinical picture to make sure that there is no maternal disease or any iatrogenic state, such as oxytocin infusion or conduction anesthesia, that may have caused the late decelerations. With persistent decelerations one can try the above medical management up to 15 to 30 minutes to correct them. If they are not corrected at that time, one might either consider the use of fetal scalp sampling or proceed directly to delivery. The discussion thus far has concerned the management of late decelerations in association with good variability. A fetal heart rate pattern of persistent late decelerations with complete absence of variability or tachycardia is much more ominous, and almost always is associated with fetal acidosis. When this is encountered, expedient delivery by cesarean section is recommended.

Prolonged decelerations are seen when the fetal heart rate tracing goes below 100 for more than 90 seconds. Prolonged decelerations occur more or less as isolated events and can be observed in association either with or without identifiable causes. If there is no known cause, prolonged decelerations are more ominous because they may present severe umbilical cord compression or a catastrophic event such as a sudden abruption or ruptured uterus. The following known causes of prolonged deceleration may be identified and managed during the intrapartum period:

1. Tetanic contraction (spontaneous or oxytocin-induced)
2. Vaginal examination
3. Application of internal or fetal scalp electrode
4. Prolapsed umbilical cord
5. Paracervical block
6. Epidural block
7. Supine hypotension
8. Prolonged umbilical cord compression often associated with rapid descent of the fetus during expulsion

In all cases where there is an identifiable cause, the cause should be treated first and the patient should not be rushed to cesarean section. Treatment of prolonged decelerations should consist of looking for an identifiable cause, changing the position of the patient, and administering oxygen.

TOCOLYTIC THERAPY FOR ABNORMAL FETAL HEART RATE PATTERNS

β-Sympathomimetic agonists (terbutaline, ritodrine) or magnesium sulfate to help relax the uterus in the presence of an abnormal fetal heart rate pattern have been used successfully. When there are persistent late decelerations that cannot be improved by medical management, when there are severe variable decelerations that cannot be managed medically, and when there is prolonged deceleration from overstimulation of the uterus, then a tocolytic agent may allow one time to proceed to an expedient cesarean delivery. Tocolytics can also be used for hyperstimulation and tetanic contractions resulting from overstimulation by oxytocin.

FETAL SCALP SAMPLING

Agreement on indications for fetal scalp sampling does not exist. In most community hospitals, capability to do scalp sampling is limited or nonexistent. The skill to do a fetal blood scalp sample following residency training has decreased because there is seldom need to do it. It would be much wiser to understand fetal heart rate patterns well and to use either fetal scalp and/or acoustic stimulation as a substitute for pH sampling.

SCALP STIMULATION OR ACOUSTIC STIMULATION TEST

Accelerations in response to fetal movement or manual, visual, or auditory stimuli provide assurance of normal fetal metabolic state. Fifteen seconds of gentle digital scalp pressure followed by a 15-second application of an atraumatic Allis clamp to the scalp (or the use of vibroacoustic stimulation) following the same method used in the antepartum period is an excellent method to use in place of scalp sampling. Studies have shown that if an acceleration was present, no fetus had a scalp pH below 7.19. This appears to be a more reasonable approach in view of the nonavailability of scalp sampling in most community obstetric centers.

The goal of intrapartum fetal monitoring is the prevention of any permanent sequelae from fetal hypoxia during that period.

CRITICAL POINTS

- The term *fetal distress* should not be used. Use *reassuring* or *nonreassuring* pattern and describe what it is.
- The term *birth asphyxia* should be used only if the clinical situation meets the correct definition.
- Know the nonreassuring patterns and how to treat them.
- Fetal scalp sampling generally is not feasible in a community hospital. Use scalp vibroacoustic stimulation.
- The goal of intrapartum monitoring is to prevent any permanent sequelae from hypoxia during the intrapartum period.

Questions

1. The techniques for intrapartum fetal surveillance are as follows *except:*
   A. Auscultation
   B. Ultrasound
   C. Electronic fetal monitoring
   D. Scalp and vibroacoustic stimulation
2. Nonreassuring heart rate patterns include all of the following *except:*
   A. Late decelerations
   B. Prolonged decelerations
   C. Early decelerations
   D. Severe variables
   E. Tachycardia
3. Management of late decelerations includes all of the following *except:*
   A. Hydration
   B. Oxygen
   C. Left lateral position
   D. Walking
   E. Discontinuing oxytocin

Answers

1. B
2. C
3. D

Postpartum hemorrhage

APGO LEARNING OBJECTIVE #22

Thomas H. Strong, Jr.

Postpartum hemorrhage continues to be a major, although often preventable, cause of maternal morbidity and mortality.

The student will demonstrate a knowledge of the following:
A. Risks associated with postpartum hemorrhage
B. Immediate management of the patient with postpartum hemorrhage, including inspection for laceration and use of contractile agents

Parturition is invariably associated with blood loss, especially during the third stage of labor while the placenta detaches from its implantation site in the uterus (Fig. 22-1). Not surprisingly, the most common problem encountered in the postpartum period is hemorrhage, occurring in roughly 5% to 10% of all deliveries. Indeed, the relative frequency of heavy bleeding following childbirth sometimes can delay recognition of this potentially life-threatening process until a considerable volume of blood has been lost. Traditionally, postpartum hemorrhage has been considered to be present when more than 500 ml of blood is lost following a vaginal birth or when more than 1000 ml is lost during a cesarean delivery.

Not all instances of postpartum hemorrhage are sudden or torrential. Steady flow, if neglected, also can place the mother in jeopardy. Because even experienced obstetricians frequently underestimate maternal blood loss at delivery and because a parturient will tolerate relatively large blood losses before demonstrating cardiovascular instability, postpartum hemorrhage will not infrequently be unrecognized until a significant volume of blood has been lost. Experience has taught that a definition of postpartum hemorrhage that relies solely on estimated blood loss will have little practical application. Rather, a definition that incorporates the clinical situation (i.e., vital signs, physical findings, volume and duration of bleeding, and so on) will be of greater clinical use and increase the likelihood that appropriate care is rendered.

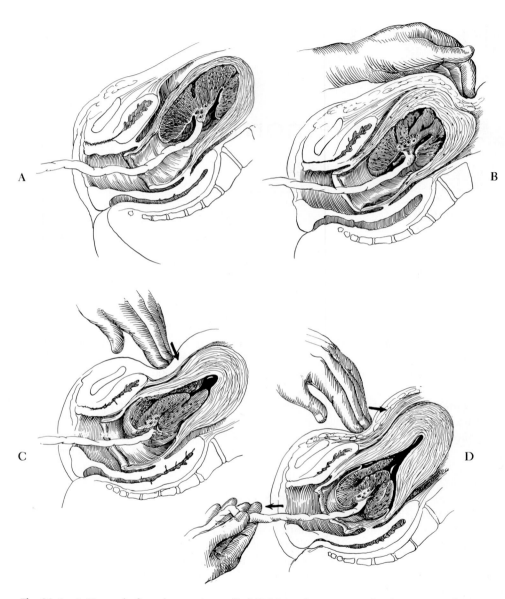

Fig. 22-1. A, Uterus before placenta is expelled. **B,** Manual pressure on fundus as uterus begins to contract aids expulsion of placenta into lower segment **(C)**, from where it can be expressed by upward pressure on contracted fundus and tension on cord **(D).**

MATERNAL SAFEGUARDS

The gravida undergoes a variety of physiologic changes during gestation that may minimize blood loss at delivery. In an uncomplicated singleton gestation, maternal intravascular volume increases by 30% to 50%, and the mother's blood becomes relatively hypercoagulable. Indeed, the maternal serum concentrations of fibrinogen and factors VII, VIII, IX, and X are increased. While the clotting time is typically unchanged, the prothrombin time and partial thromboplastin time values may be shortened somewhat. At the time of delivery, tonic uterine contractions can force 300 to 500 ml of blood from the uterine vasculature into the central maternal circulation, thereby providing an autotransfusion for the parturient. The end-result is a woman less likely to bleed than her nongravid counterpart; at the same time, she is better able to tolerate considerable losses of intravascular volume. In fact, because of the physiologic adaptations of pregnancy, the gravida may not show significant changes in her vital signs until 25% to 30% of her intravascular volume has been lost. Therefore, a patient evidencing unstable vital signs in association with a postpartum hemorrhage has likely lost a profound volume of blood.

ETIOLOGY

Following expulsion of the placenta, blood loss from the vascular implantation site in the uterus is minimized through tonic myometrial contraction. Any pathophysiologic process that alters the normal uterine anatomy or physiology may predispose the patient to hemorrhage from this area by interfering with efficient uterine contraction. A well-contracted uterus will not bleed significantly in most circumstances. The female genital tract may be segregated into contractile and noncontractile components (Table 22-1). Ongoing, heavy vaginal bleeding in the presence of a firm, globular uterus should arouse suspicion of bleeding from minimally contractile or noncontractile

---

Table 22-1. Postpartum bleeding sites

CONTRACTILE TISSUE
Upper uterine segment

MINIMALLY CONTRACTILE OR NONCONTRACTILE TISSUE
Uterine septum
Broad ligament
Round ligament
Lower uterine segment or cervix
Vagina or vaginal septum
Perineum
Lower urinary tract

---

tissue, such as the lower uterine segment, cervix, or vagina. However, it is worth noting that identification of bleeding at one site in the genital tract does not preclude the possibility of bleeding from other sites. It is best to start the search for hemorrhage in the more superior aspects of the genital tract, since heavy downflow of blood makes visualization of the more inferior landmarks less easy. Real-time ultrasound frequently is useful for identifying large placental fragments high in the uterine cavity. Failing this, manual exploration of the endometrial cavity must suffice. Manual placental extraction and/or curettage is indicated when retained placental tissue is identified. A variety of identifiable risk factors may predispose a patient to postpartum hemorrhage (Table 22-2). In many instances, those who experience severe postpartum bleeding have multiple antecedent risk factors.

UTERINE ATONY

The most common cause of severe postpartum hemorrhage (bleeding in excess of 1000 ml following vaginal delivery) is uterine hypotonia or atony. Bleeding secondary to uterine atony usually occurs shortly after delivery, often while the patient is still in the delivery room. Typically, vaginal

Table 22-2. Causes of postpartum hemorrhage

ALTERED MYOMETRIAL ACTIVITY (ATONY)
Amnionitis or endometritis
Grand multiparity
Magnesium sulfate
Myasthenia gravis
Precipitate or prolonged labor
Uterine overdistention (multiple fetuses, poly-
hydramnios, and so on)

ALTERED ANATOMY
Traumatic
Dührssen's incisions
IUPC or FSE injury
Genital tract laceration
Uterine scar disruption
Nontraumatic
Congenital uterine anomalies
Fibroids
Retained placenta or placental fragments
Uterine inversion

OTHER
Coagulopathy
History
    Prior postpartum hemorrhage
    Placenta previa or abruptio placentae

IUPC, Intrauterine pressure catheter; *FSE,* fetal scalp electrode.

vascular lower uterine segment can be brisk and at times torrential. Recognition of lower uterine segment atony frequently will be delayed because the uterine fundus will be firm to palpation. Successful management of this worrisome problem includes prolonged manual compression of the lower uterine segment until adequate hemostasis can occur at the placental implantation site. Occasionally, laparotomy will be necessary to ligate the vascular supply of the placental implantation site (see Surgical Treatment section of this chapter).

The anticipation and early recognition of uterine atony should allow a timely, considered response to this vexing postpartum complication. When the parturient's history includes factors associated with increased risk for postpartum uterine atony (Table 22-2), proper preparations should be made for the possibility of significant postpartum hemorrhage. Early in the course of labor, blood should be typed and cross-matched and a large-bore intravenous catheter should be inserted. Obstetric nursing and anesthesia staff should be alerted to the patient's increased risk for hemorrhage. Uterine stimulants (oxytocin, ergots, and prostaglandins) and full preparation for potential operative intervention should be immediately available.

RETAINED PLACENTAL FRAGMENTS

Retained placenta or placental fragments contribute to uterine atony by interfering with efficient uterine contraction at the placental implantation site. Normally, expulsion of the placenta occurs within 30 minutes of childbirth, with the implantation site contracting to a fraction of its former area (Fig. 22-2). Following expulsion of the placenta, its fetal surface should be carefully examined to make certain that no fragments are missing. Retained placental fragments can be a source of either acute or delayed postpartum hemorrhage. Late postpartum hemorrhage generally is

bleeding is accompanied by a soft, boggy uterus. Risk factors for uterine atony include amnionitis or endometritis, high parity, magnesium sulfate, myasthenia gravis, precipitate or prolonged labor, and uterine overdistention (Table 22-2).

Less muscular than the uterine fundus, the lower uterine segment is generally less contractile. Because tonic myometrial contraction is the primary hemostatic mechanism following expulsion of the placenta, bleeding from the less contractile lower uterine segment can be particularly difficult to control. This condition develops most frequently after expulsion of a low-implanted placenta or placenta previa. Bleeding from the very

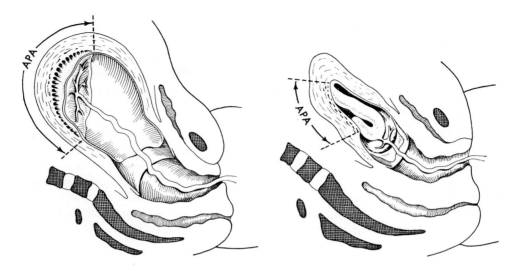

Fig. 22-2. Reduction in size of area of placental attachment *(APA)* as upper segment contracts, separates placenta, and expels it into lower uterine segment.

defined as hemorrhage that occurs more than 24 hours after delivery.

TRAUMA

Traumatic injury of the genital tract is the third major cause of acute postpartum hemorrhage. While hemorrhages caused by genital tract lacerations generally are less profuse than those from the placental implantation site, delayed identification of this not uncommon pregnancy complication can result in significant maternal morbidity. Although traumatic injury can occur at a variety of sites in the genital tract (Table 22-1), most lacerations can be localized to the birth canal, cervix, and uterus.

Birth canal

Lacerations of the perineum and vaginal sidewalls often are iatrogenic (episiotomy, forceps-assisted delivery, and so on) or secondary to difficult vaginal delivery (e.g., compound presentation, shoulder dystocia). Most such injuries are minor and relatively easy to repair, but some lacerations may extend high into the vaginal canal or fornices. Hematomas containing up to 1 L of blood and clot may develop as a result of extension or dissection of birth canal lacerations.

Cervical lacerations

Cervical lacerations can occur after either vaginal or cesarean delivery. If unrecognized, they can contribute to considerable blood loss. If not properly repaired, they may contribute to cervical incompetence in future pregnancies. Therefore, inspection of the cervix is of vital importance following delivery, especially if an instrumented (forceps or vacuum delivery) or precipitate delivery has occurred.

Uterine rupture

Spontaneous rupture of an unscarred uterus is rare. Among women with prior cesarean deliveries, the incidence of uterine scar disruption is also quite low, occurring in less than 1% of vaginal deliveries. Following a vaginal birth after cesarean delivery, many recommend manual inspection of the lower uterine segment to determine the status of the uterine scar. Uterine scar disruption should be suspected in the setting of profuse bleeding from the cervical os of a firmly contracted uterus.

MISCELLANEOUS CAUSES

Placenta accreta

A placenta accreta is present when the placental villi invade and attach directly to the myometrium. As a result, normal placental separation is prevented and normal postpartum tonic uterine contraction is prevented. Potentially life-threatening hemorrhage can result. Because placenta accreta commonly is associated with placenta previa, it is discussed in Chapter 18, Third Trimester Bleeding.

Coagulopathy

In the postpartum period, a tonically contracted uterus will minimize bleeding, even in the presence of a systemic coagulopathy. Most commonly associated with amniotic fluid embolism, placental abruption, or severe preeclampsia, disseminated intravascular coagulation may occasionally contribute to excessive postpartum blood loss. Other causes of systemic coagulopathy include factor deficiency, anticoagulant medications (platelet binding inhibitors, heparin, or warfarin), and abnormalities of platelet function or number.

Abnormal uterine anatomy

Any process that alters the normal anatomy of the uterus will adversely affect efficient myometrial contraction, thereby predisposing the patient to postpartum bleeding (Table 22-1). Uterine fibroids (particularly large ones) may interfere with effective tonic myometrial contractions following delivery, thereby contributing to excess blood loss.

Uterine or vaginal septa, if lacerated, also may be a source of significant postpartum bleeding. Perhaps the anatomic abnormality with the greatest risk of significant maternal morbidity and mortality is uterine inversion. Complete inversion of the uterus following childbirth is typically the result of excessive traction on an umbilical cord attached to a placenta implanted in the uterine fundus (i.e., iatrogenic). Fundal placentation, primiparity, and uterine hypotonia appear to increase the risk for uterine inversion. Prompt reestablishment of the uterus into its normal anatomic configuration appears to be the key to managing this potentially life-threatening problem.

MANAGEMENT

As mentioned earlier, anticipation and early recognition of postpartum hemorrhage should evoke a timely, considered response to this common pregnancy complication. An orderly, stepwise protocol for managing postpartum hemorrhage is of vital importance and should be well understood and rehearsed by all obstetric care providers. Women at increased risk for postpartum hemorrhage should have their blood typed and crossed at the onset of labor. Identification of acute postpartum bleeding should provoke an immediate and systematic search for the source of hemorrhage. A second large-bore intravenous catheter should be placed to ensure adequate vascular access. Although oxytocin is always indicated in the setting of postpartum hemorrhage, concentrations of more than 30 to 40 U/L of intravenous fluid do not increase myometrial contraction and may increase the risk of fluid overload secondary to the antidiuretic characteristics that this hormone possesses.

Firm but gentle uterine massage frequently will reverse uterine atony. However, care must be taken to avoid uterine massage so vigorous that the large blood vessels in the broad ligament are injured. Uterine exploration, manual placental extraction (Fig. 22-3), and sharp uterine curettage

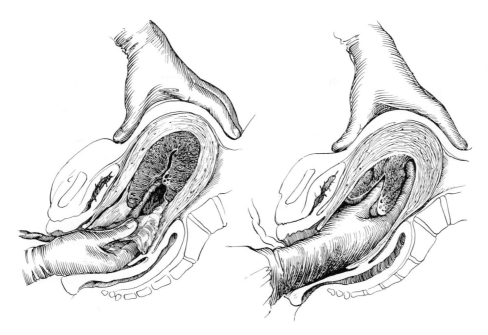

Fig. 22-3. Technique of manual removal of retained placenta.

may be necessary. Should massage of the uterine fundus in concert with intravenous administration of oxytocin fail to alleviate uterine atony, ergot preparations such as ergonovine and methylergonovine (0.2 mg intramuscularly) are warranted. Administration of these potent vasoconstrictors are contraindicated in the presence of hypertensive disease, including preeclampsia. Prostaglandin $F_{2\alpha}$ is a potent stimulator of myometrial contraction. Should oxytocin and ergot administration fail to reverse uterine atony, prostaglandin $F_{2\alpha}$ may be given vaginally, rectally, intramuscularly, or intravascularly. Because this preparation can evoke a considerable degree of bronchoconstriction, prostaglandin $F_{2\alpha}$ should not be used in patients with asthma. This preparation also can cause significant pulmonary vasoconstriction and is contraindicated among women with pulmonary hypertension. If necessary, oxytocin or prostaglandin can be injected into the myometrium transabdominally. However, extreme caution must be taken to avoid puncture or laceration of intestinal, urinary, or

vascular tissue. Intravascular injection of undiluted oxytocin can result in profound hypotension and/or cardiac arrest. Therefore only dilute solutions of oxytocin should be administered intravascularly.

Excessive bleeding from the lower uterine segment is a worrisome situation because it is less responsive to uterotonic medications and difficult to suture from the vagina. At times laparotomy is necessary. For similar reasons, repair of upper vaginal or cervical lacerations can be extremely difficult. When placing sutures in this area, it is important to have adequate exposure and visualization of the laceration. Care must be taken to avoid perforating the maternal bladder or bowel during suture placement. Likewise, inadvertent injury or occlusion of the urethra must be avoided. Insertion of a straight rubber catheter frequently will reduce the risk of inadvertent urethral ligation. When placing sutures in this area it is advisable to use absorbable suture to prevent maternal discomfort. When placing sutures in the cervical or upper vaginal area, it is also important to avoid excessive or prolonged packing of the vaginal canal. When packs are used, it is always prudent to leave a "tail" protruding from the vagina to remind the operator of the indwelling packing. It is important to remember that packing may provide the operator with a false sense of security by preventing the escape of active bleeding. Additionally, packing sometimes can obscure a laceration that necessitates repair.

Surgical treatment

When acute postpartum hemorrhage does not respond to standard medical treatment, surgical therapy is indicated. Despite the wide range of surgical options available for treating this common postpartum problem, the most effective surgical procedure for controlling severe postpartum hemorrhage remains hysterectomy. Because of its detrimental impact on a woman's fertility, most obstetricians prefer to use hysterectomy only as a last resort. At the same time, it must be remembered that none of the alternative surgical techniques have the same efficacy as hysterectomy. Therefore, in torrential bleeding or hemodynamic instability, delay of definitive therapy (hysterectomy) is not advised. Other surgical procedures used for treating severe, refractory postpartum bleeding include the following: (1) uterine artery ligation; (2) uteroovarian arterial anastomosis ligation; (3) placental implantation site oversewing; and (4) bilateral internal iliac (hypogastric) artery ligation. In certain situations, various combinations of the above techniques will be more effective than any one surgical modality alone. However, owing to its greater technical difficulty, bilateral hypogastric artery ligation generally is reserved until ligation of the other vascular sites has been deemed unsuccessful. At times, transabdominal compression of the aortic bifurcation may be used as a temporizing measure. Compression of the bifurcation against the maternal vertebrae can be a life-saving technique.

Military antishock trousers (MAST) were perfected during the Vietnam War. The MAST suit may be indicated in the gravida with persistent bleeding or the patient for whom surgical reexploration is best avoided. The MAST suit appears to force peripheral blood centrally by way of a direct pressure effect. Additionally, when the abdominal portion of a MAST suit is sufficiently inflated, the increase in intraperitoneal pressure may reduce the escape of blood from intraabdominal bleeding sites. During MAST suit use, the circulatory status of the lower extremities must be monitored vigilantly. Pressure injury to the peroneal nerve from prolonged or overag-

CRITICAL POINTS

- The primary mechanism for controlling postpartum uterine bleeding is tonic myometrial contraction.
- Because of physiologic adaptations imposed by pregnancy, a parturient may not demonstrate significant changes in her vital signs until 25% to 30% of her intravascular volume has been lost.
- The three most common causes of postpartum hemorrhage are uterine atony, retained placental fragments, and lacerations of the genital tract.
- When acute postpartum hemorrhage does not respond to standard medical treatment, surgical therapy is indicated. The most effective surgical procedure for controlling severe postpartum bleeding remains hysterectomy.

gressive MAST suit inflation can result in maternal footdrop.

Other techniques

Although less studied and in less widespread use, a variety of alternative techniques are available for controlling postpartum hemorrhage. These modalities include uterine lavage, uterine packing, and arterial embolization. In certain circumstances, these approaches may be life-saving, even though they are not considered to be standard parts of routine postpartum hemorrhage management protocols.

Questions

1. Following expulsion of the placenta, blood loss from the placental implantation site is minimized by:
   A. Tonic myometrial contraction
   B. Hypercoagulable maternal blood
   C. Reduced blood flow to the uterus
   D. Oxytocin
   E. Ergot alkaloids
2. The initial step in the management of uterine atony includes:
   A. Antibiotics
   B. Uterine massage
   C. Exploratory laparotomy
   D. Manual extraction of the placenta
   E. Repair of lacerations
3. The definitive surgical treatment of torrential, unremitting postpartum hemorrhage is:
   A. Bilateral hypogastric artery ligation
   B. Uterine artery ligation
   C. Unilateral hypogastric artery ligation
   D. Hysterectomy
   E. Placental implantation site oversewing

Answers

1. A
2. B
3. D

Postpartum infection

APGO LEARNING OBJECTIVE #23

Jordan H. Perlow

> *Early recognition and treatment of postpartum infection will decrease maternal morbidity and mortality.*

The student will demonstrate a knowledge of the following:

A. Risk factors for postpartum infection
B. Evaluation and management of the patient with postpartum infection
C. Pathogenic infectious organisms capable of contributing to this obstetric complication
D. Rationale and use of prophylactic antibiotics

Infectious complications of pregnancy remain an important cause of maternal death. Studies in the early 1970s indicated that infection was responsible for up to 50% of direct obstetric-related maternal deaths. Although more recent studies clearly show a decline, infection remains a major contributor to maternal mortality. Recently published work from data collected in the 1980s indicates that obstetric infection contributes to 10% to 15% of direct maternal deaths in the United States. An understanding of the pathogenesis and treatment of this complication should provide the student with the tools necessary to recognize patients at high risk for postpartum infectious complications; to diagnose such patients; to treat them appropriately; and thus to contribute to reduced maternal morbidity and mortality.

Postpartum or puerperal infection generally is considered to be any infection of the genital tract following delivery. The most commonly used definition of postpartum infection relates to the finding of maternal fever—defined as a body temperature determined orally of at least 100.4° F (38° C) and occurring in any 2 of the first 10 days postpartum, exclusive of the first 24 hours. Although this definition of the United States Joint Committee on Maternal Welfare is quite useful, it has certain limitations. It is important to recognize that elevated temperature in the first 24 hours may be clinically significant; and, although postpartum fever most commonly relates to pelvic infection, other causes (pyelonephritis, pneumonia, thrombophlebitis, mastitis) should be considered.

The first 24 hours postpartum traditionally have been excluded from this definition because it has been found that up to 8% of women delivered vaginally will have an elevation in body temperature that will resolve spontaneously in 80% of patients. It remains unclear what mechanisms are responsible for these transient temperature elevations, although proposed theories include necrotic decidua obstructing the cervical os, atelectasis, breast engorgement, and subclinical intraamnionic infections resulting in transient uterine bacterial infection. It must also be recognized that, with shorter hospital stays following both vaginal and cesarean deliveries, many patients will be diagnosed and treated for postpartum infection as outpatients; and others will be diagnosed before meeting strict definitions of febrile morbidity. Therefore the findings of fever, uterine tenderness, odoriferous lochia, and malaise postpartum most commonly suggest endometritis. Several histopathologic terms have been applied to the clinical findings consistent with postpartum infection of the uterus, the most common being *endometritis*. The terminology may be confusing because postpartum uterine infection has been shown to involve a variety of pelvic tissues, including the decidua, myometrium, and parametrial tissues, leading to use of such other terms as *metritis, endomyometritis,* and *endomyoparametritis.*

ENDOMETRITIS

Before moving toward an understanding of its diagnosis and treatment, it is imperative to review the many factors that place the gravida at increased risk for endometritis.

Risk factors and epidemiology

Cesarean section is the single greatest risk factor for the development of endometritis. This gives added significance to the recent overall increase in cesarean section rates. Studies have shown that the overall risk of endometritis in vaginal delivery is no more than 3%, but 50% or more of women who undergo cesarean delivery may develop this infection. Overall, cesarean section patients are at 5 to 30 times the risk for endometritis when compared with women delivered vaginally. Women who develop endometritis following cesarean section also are at greater risk for additional infectious complications, including pelvic abscess, septic pelvic thrombophlebitis, and life-threatening sepsis. Efforts to reduce the number of cesarean sections will, if successful, undoubtedly lead to a significant decrease in maternal morbidity and mortality.

While the overall increased risk for infection among women delivered by cesarean section is clear, some within this group are at greater or lesser risk. Women not in labor and with intact amniotic membranes who have scheduled cesarean sections demonstrate significantly fewer infectious complications when compared with patients operated on while in labor after prolonged membrane rupture or with frank chorioamnionitis (intraamniotic infection). Adolescents undergoing cesarean section also appear to be at greater risk than adults. Prophylactic perioperative antibiotics (discussed later in this chapter) have been shown to decrease the occurrence of postoperative endometritis by 50% to 60%.

Patients of lower socioeconomic class appear to be at greater risk of cesarean-related pelvic and wound infections. The increased presence of sexually transmitted disease, anemia, poor nutritional status, and inadequate hygiene have all been noted as contributory. Endometritis has been reported to occur in as many as 45% to 85% of these women. Patients who are diabetic, obese, or being treated with systemic steroids for a variety of disorders also may be at increased risk for postcesarean endometritis and/or wound infections and dehiscence. Although obese patients are at significant risk for a variety of cesarean section–related morbidity and mortality, the risk for endometritis is approximately 8 times that for nonobese women.

Women delivered following premature labor or premature preterm ruptured membranes also are at increased risk for postpartum endometritis, perhaps because up to 60% of such patients are found to have bacterial contamination of the amniotic fluid before delivery.

Controversy exists as to whether frequent cervical examinations and the presence of internal fetal-uterine monitoring devices contribute to postpartum endometritis. Patients subjected to these variables often are those with protracted labor and prolonged rupture of membranes, thus making it difficult to sort out which factors are truly predictive. Recent information using sophisticated statistical techniques suggests that these variables may facilitate postpartum endometritis—while cesarean section, the presence of highly virulent bacteria, *Mycoplasma hominis,* and bacterial vaginosis organisms predict endometritis.

PATHOGENESIS AND MICROBIOLOGY

Typically, postpartum endometritis is an infection of polymicrobial etiology, involving both aerobes and anaerobes. These bacteria are believed to represent cervicovaginal flora that ascend into the uterus where, under appropriate conditions, infection develops. The vast majority of women (70% to 80%) delivered vaginally can be demonstrated to have significant bacterial growth from endometrial cavity isolates. It is interesting to postulate why so few (1% to 4%) develop clinical endometritis, especially given the environment of necrotic decidua and an open cervix, allowing for the ascent of cervicovaginal flora. Theories on this matter include the types and combinations of bacteria present, the extent of genital tract trauma, and the presence of retained placental tissue.

Cesarean section results in the iatrogenic disruption of the uterus, devitalization of tissue, and placement of foreign bodies (suture materials). Colonizing bacteria during labor and surgery may later invade and thrive in the periincisional hematomas and necrotic uterine tissues. With progression, the infection may invade the myometrium and parametrial tissues. This is believed to be accomplished by direct extension and/or lymphatic spread. Ultimately, the broad ligament (parametritis), peritoneal surfaces (peritonitis), and pelvic veins (septic pelvic thrombophlebitis) may become involved. Bacteremia may occur in 10% to 25% of patients, and rarely septic shock may ensue.

The most common organisms isolated in patients with endometritis are gram-positive aerobes such as groups B and D *(Enterococcus) Streptococcus,* gram-negative aerobes (e.g., *Escherichia coli, Gardnerella vaginalis*), gram-positive anaerobes (including *Peptostreptococcus, Peptococcus,* and *Bacteroides* species), and the genital mycoplasmas (*M. hominis, Ureaplasma urealyticum*). *Chlamydia trachomatis* has been associated with late-onset endometritis; in addition, *G. vaginalis,* a bacterium frequently encountered in patients with bacterial vaginosis, is isolated most often among adolescents who develop postcesarean endometritis. Although an average of two to three organisms are recovered from the infected uterus, the isolation of these organisms is not required to formulate a diagnosis and begin treatment.

SYMPTOMS AND SIGNS

Fever is the cardinal sign of postpartum endometritis. Other signs and symptoms elicited by history and physical examination may include uterine and/or pelvic tenderness, lochia with an atypical or foul odor, abdominal or pelvic pain, and rigors associated with temperature "spikes." The presence or absence of these findings will vary with the severity of infection. Persistent postpartum fever must lead the clinician to suspect endometritis.

DIAGNOSIS AND LABORATORY TESTS

In the evaluation of a postpartum patient with fever, the clinician can rely primarily on a thorough review of the patient's labor and delivery course, assessing her risk factors for developing postpartum endometritis. Therefore this is a disease that can be anticipated for selected high-risk patients, and treatment can begin expeditiously. In clinical practice it is not always necessary to await the patient's exact fulfillment of the definition of febrile morbidity before making the diagnosis and initiating treatment. For example, the patient who undergoes a cesarean section after a protracted 36-hour labor with prolonged rupture of membranes and who demonstrates a temperature of 39° C on the first postoperative day should not have evaluation and treatment of endometritis delayed until the fever persists for a second day (see standard definition of puerperal morbidity above). Therefore clinical judgment is extremely important. It is as important to search for signs and symptoms of endometritis as it is to rule out this infection. Thus the physical examination should not be directed only toward detecting the signs of endometritis but also should evaluate for other possible causes of postpartum infection, including pyelonephritis, pneumonia, atelectasis, and wound infection.

Careful palpation of the uterine fundus often can provide useful information to the experienced clinician in differentiating the tenderness inherent to the postsurgical state from that of uterine infection. Bimanual pelvic examination may be useful to evaluate for parametrial tenderness and retained placental tissue, which frequently can be palpated at the opening of the cervix. Elicitation of costovertebral angle tenderness may suggest pyelonephritis; pulmonary auscultation may demonstrate findings consistent with pneumonia or atelectasis. Breast examination may demonstrate marked engorgement, cellulitis, or abscess. For patients delivered by cesarean section, careful inspection and palpation of the surgical wound are essential components of the physical evaluation. Wound infection, hematoma, and cellulitis all may be associated with postpartum fever and must be considered in the differential diagnosis. The diagnosis of endometritis often can be made without sophisticated and expensive laboratory tests. The clinical value of a complete blood count is limited because of the physiologic leukocytosis that exists postpartum, with white blood cell counts as high as 20,000 per mm^3 being normal. Obtaining endometrial cultures is fraught with the risk of contamination from lower genital tract flora, and therefore these are not used routinely on many clinical services. They may be considered when therapy does not bring clinical improvement. Blood cultures will be positive in up to 20% of women with postcesarean endometritis. Routinely obtaining blood cultures probably is unnecessary. It has been suggested that such cultures be reserved for patients who appear quite ill or who have very high temperatures (greater than 39° C). Urinalysis and culture are useful in the evaluation of pyelonephritis or cystitis. Radiologic imaging techniques using ultrasound, computed tomography (CT), and magnetic resonance imaging (MRI) may be useful in very select cases of therapeutic failure where complications of postpartum infection are suspected (discussed later in this chapter).

MANAGEMENT

The treatment of postpartum endometritis is based on our understanding of its polymicrobial nature, and therefore antibiotics should be chosen for their ability to cover those pathogens most frequently encountered—while posing the least risk to the patient. Fortunately, a number of safe antibiotics exist. When these are used by themselves or in various combinations, they offer a high degree of therapeutic efficacy.

Patients with mild endometritis after vaginal delivery respond well to a variety of antibiotics. Although a broad spectrum oral antibiotic may be appropriate in the mildest cases, the vast majority of these patients—and those with postcesarean endometritis—require intravenously administered broad spectrum antibiotics. Because of the increased glomerular filtration rate associated with normal pregnancy, increased clearance of antibiotics excreted by the kidney can be expected; therefore using doses of these medications (penicillins, cephalosporins, and aminoglycosides) at the upper end of "normal" is appropriate.

Effective broad spectrum single agent antibiotics include the extended spectrum cephalosporins (e.g., cefoxitin, cefotetan, cefotaxime), combination penicillin and β-lactamase inhibitors (e.g., ampicillin-sulbactam, ticarcillin-clavulanate), and extended spectrum penicillins (e.g., mezlocillin, piperacillin). These drugs have become popular because of their demonstrated efficacy as well as their cost-effectiveness when compared with combinations of antibiotics.

Since the late 1970s the combination of clindamycin and gentamicin has been considered the "gold standard" by which other therapies are judged. This is based on early studies demonstrating a cure rate of approximately 95% with this antibiotic regimen. It is, however, not without its risks; and recent studies have shown less optimistic therapeutic results, especially with infections complicated by the presence of enterococci. Also, clindamycin has been associated with the development of pseudomembranous colitis, a rare but serious disorder caused by selective colonic overgrowth of *Clostridium difficile*. Treatment consists of vancomycin or metronidazole and supportive measures, including replacement of fluids and electrolytes lost as a result of profuse diarrhea. While rare at therapeutic levels, nephrotoxicity and ototoxicity are reported complications with aminoglycosides.

In patients treated with gentamicin, it is controversial whether peak and trough levels are mandatory in all patients. They certainly add to the costs associated with treatment; and, since most patients exhibit a prompt response to therapy, their routine use is questionable. Doses of 1.5 mg/kg after a loading dose of 2 mg/kg have been recommended. Peak and trough levels are perhaps best used when therapeutic response is not as expected or when renal compromise is known or suspected. In the latter case, other less nephrotoxic antibiotics may be preferable.

To avoid concerns associated with the gentamicin-clindamycin combination therapeutic regimen, several alternatives to treatment are available. Aztreonam is a monobactam providing the aerobic gram-negative coverage of gentamicin but without the need for blood level assessment and without nephrotoxic risks. Dosage does need to be adjusted, however, in patients with renal compromise. Comparison studies have shown equal efficacy between clindamycin-gentamicin and clindamycin-aztreonam regimens. Given the increased costs of aztreonam, it may best be used when significant concerns for aminoglycoside toxicity exist.

Single-agent broad spectrum antibiotics offer the advantage of increased safety and lower costs. The commonly used cephalosporins are such examples. Cefoxitin provides excellent coverage for most pathogens encountered in patients with endometritis. Cure rates of 90% or more have been reported, and side effects are rare. Other cephalosporins (e.g., cefotetan) provide for a longer dosing interval than does cefoxitin; however, there are concerns about side effects associated with elevation in hepatic transaminases and platelet dysfunction.

Such extended spectrum penicillins as mezlocillin, ticarcillin, and piperacillin offer broad spectrum coverage for postpartum infection. They appear to offer cure rates comparable with such multiple drug combinations as gentamicin-clindamycin therapy. Efficacy has been reported at 75% to 91%.

Ampicillin-sulbactam and ticarcillin-clavulanate are penicillins combined with a β-lactamase inhibitor. This combination offers these penicillins an extended spectrum of activity to include β-lactamase–producing bacteria such as *E. coli, Haemophilus influenzae, Bacteroides* species, and *Staphylococcus aureus.* β-Lactamase inhibitor–containing antibiotics have been demonstrated to be comparable to combination therapy with gentamicin-clindamycin.

Patients responsive to antibiotic therapy have decreased signs on physical examination, typically demonstrated as a decrease in uterine tenderness. Patients often appear more energetic and experience defervescence. Once these findings are noted, the antibiotic regimen should be continued for 24 to 48 hours after the patient becomes afebrile and is without other signs and symptoms. Until recently, patients have been discharged home with instructions to complete a course of oral antibiotics. Recent research has shown that this practice is without basis, and patients will do well without continued outpatient antibiotic therapy. It is also uncertain whether patients with positive blood cultures require continued outpatient antibiotic therapy after a successful course of intravenous antibiotics. It has been recommended, however, that patients bacteremic with *S. aureus* complete an outpatient oral antibiotic regimen.

Prophylactic antibiotics

The success in decreasing infectious complications following vaginal hysterectomy by administering antibiotics preoperatively prompted studies to determine whether similar benefits could be had with cesarean section–related endometritis risk. Indeed, a great many studies have documented the efficacy of prophylactic antibiotics given at the time of umbilical cord clamping in decreasing the risk of postcesarean endometritis and wound infection by up to 50%.

Single-dose prophylaxis has been shown as effective as multiple doses for several types of antibiotics. Therefore, to avoid additional risks, expense, and the potential for selecting resistant and more virulent pathogens, single dose prophylaxis is recommended for those patients at significant risk for postoperative infections. Patients in labor with prolonged membrane rupture and/or intrapartum fever would be among the candidates suitable for this intervention. Comparative studies have shown virtually no difference in efficacy with respect to which antibiotics are used or the number of doses administered. A first-generation cephalosporin (e.g., cefazolin) has been shown as effective as more costly second- or third-generation cephalosporins. The "drug of choice" for cesarean section prophylaxis should be a drug with documented efficacy, safety, and cost-effectiveness. Suitable drugs meeting these requirements include ampicillin and a first-generation cephalosporin. Broader spectrum and more potent antibiotics are more expensive and have not been shown to improve outcome; therefore they should be reserved for the specific treatment of endometritis. It is of interest that irrigation of the uterus and pelvis with antibiotic-containing saline solution may be as effective as administering the antibiotic intravenously.

Treatment failure

Patients with clinical endometritis who have not responded to therapy within 48 to 72 hours need a detailed reevaluation, and consideration must be given to other causes or possibly to incomplete antibiotic coverage. Every attempt should be made to identify other sources for infection and to begin appropriate treatment promptly. It is often at this time that patients being treated with a single antibiotic will be changed to "triples" consisting of ampicillin, gentamicin, and clindamycin. Patients receiving the combination therapy of gentamicin-clindamycin may benefit from the addition of ampicillin to cover for *Enterococcus.* Patients developing endometritis should not be treated with the same antibiotic they received for prophylaxis.

If the patient's infection persists despite appropriate antibiotic selection, physical examination may reveal a wound infection. Wound infection has been reported to be the most common cause of antibiotic treatment failure among patients treated for endometritis. Approximately 3% to 7% of patients having cesarean section will develop wound infection. It is significantly more common among patients with endometritis and typically appears on the fourth postoperative day. Thus patients may present after hospital discharge with wound drainage, erythema, and pain. Frequently patients will respond favorably to antibiotics and opening of the wound to allow drainage of the abscess. Probing the wound is an important aspect of the evaluation to determine whether the fascia is intact.

Pelvic examination may demonstrate a mass consistent with pelvic abscess or retained placental fragments or membranes. Radiologic techniques including ultrasound, CT scan, and MRI may be useful. Uterine curettage to remove these products is indicated. A pelvic abscess has the potential for rupture and the subsequent development of life-threatening peritonitis. Pelvic abscess may be drained either percutaneously with radiographic guidance or via colpotomy, where access to the abscess is via the posterior cul-de-sac, depending on abscess location. Occasionally laparotomy may be required. Antibiotic therapy should be continued for a prolonged period, and it has been recommended that metronidazole may be preferable to clindamycin in this clinical situation.

SEPTIC PELVIC THROMBOPHLEBITIS

Occasionally, despite continued antibiotics, a patient persists with spiking fevers yet no longer appears acutely ill. Patients with septic pelvic thrombophlebitis often demonstrate these findings and typically have minimal to no pelvic pain. This infection occurs when organisms associated with endometritis (typically anaerobes) gain access to the pelvic veins, resulting in thrombosis and inflammation. Potential serious complications include septic pulmonary emboli, bacteremia, and the formation of metastatic abscesses.

Diagnosis may be made using CT scan or MRI, or, alternatively, by observing a rapid return to normal temperature in response to heparin therapy. This is, however, controversial because some studies have shown that in documented septic pelvic thrombophlebitis resolution occurs with continued antibiotic therapy in the absence of heparin. Nevertheless, standard heparin anticoagulation is an accepted therapy in conjunction with continued antibiotics for this clinical entity. Therapy typically is recommended for 5 to 10 days. Longer therapy consisting of prolonged oral warfarin is required if pulmonary embolism has occurred.

OTHER POSTPARTUM INFECTIONS

Episiotomy infection

One would expect that, given the bacterial contamination of the perineum at delivery, episiotomy and perineal laceration infections would be frequent. Fortunately this is not the case, and these infections are reported in only 0.35% of vaginally delivered patients. Dehiscence of the episiotomy is reported to occur in approximately 0.5% of patients. When this complication occurs, the vast majority (80%) are associated with infection of the episiotomy site. Patients typically present with perineal pain and discharge and may have urinary retention. In the past, definitive repair was delayed several months to allow for antibiotic therapy, resolution of infection and edema, and neovascularization of the tissues. Recent studies, however, have demonstrated excellent outcomes with a more expeditious approach to repair. An uncommon but often life-threatening complication of perineal infection is necrotizing fasciitis. This is also a polymicrobic infection involving anaerobes, *E. coli*, *Klebsiella* species, *Proteus* species, and *S. aureus*. Treatment must be prompt and includes intensive antibiotic therapy, radical surgical debridement, and intensive medical supportive care.

Mastitis

Puerperal mastitis is an infection of the breast that typically occurs in nursing women 1 to 3 weeks after delivery. It is most often unilateral. *S. aureus* is the most commonly isolated causative bacteria. Other commonly cultured pathogens include streptococci and *H. influenzae*. The infection is transmitted from the colonized oronasopharynx of the nursing infant and may enter the milk ducts via small fissures in the nipple area. Neonates frequently are colonized by the organism while in the hospital nursery. Breast engorgement and milk stagnation also may contribute to

CRITICAL POINTS

- Even today, postpartum infectious complications remain an important cause of maternal mortality.
- Postpartum infection is commonly defined as fever (oral temperature greater than 100.4° F) occurring in any 2 of the first 10 days postpartum, exclusive of the first 24 hours. Practically, however, elevated maternal temperature in the first 24 hours necessitates close evaluation and is often treated in the appropriate clinical circumstances.
- The triad of postpartum fever, uterine tenderness, and odoriferous lochia suggests endometritis.
- Cesarean section is the single greatest risk factor for the development of endometritis. Other risk factors include preterm delivery, prolonged labor and ruptured membranes, frequent cervical exams and internal fetal-uterine monitoring, adolescent age group, low socioeconomic class, diabetes, and obesity.
- The gram-positive aerobes (groups B and D *Streptococcus*), gram-negative aerobes (*Peptostreptococcus, Peptococcus,* and *Bacteroides* species), and the genital mycoplasmas are the most common organisms isolated in patients with endometritis, though typically the infection is polymicrobial.
- Prophylactic antibiotics have been shown to decrease the occurrence of postoperative endometritis by 50% to 60%.
- A single dose of ampicillin or cefazolin is as effective for endometritis prophylaxis at cesarean section as more costly antibiotics and is appropriate for use as prophylaxis at the time of cord clamping. Alternatively, irrigation of the pelvis with antibiotic-containing saline may be as effective.
- Anticipate and observe carefully for the development of endometritis in high-risk patients because women developing endometritis are also at greater risk for pelvic abscess, septic pelvic thrombophlebitis, and life-threatening sepsis.
- Treatment of endometritis is based on our understanding of its polymicrobial nature, and therefore broad spectrum antibiotic therapy is used. Extended spectrum cephalosporins, combination penicillin and β-lactamase inhibitors, and extended spectrum penicillins offer excellent therapeutic and cost efficacy.
- Wound infection, pelvic or abdominal abscess, urinary tract infection, and septic pelvic thrombophlebitis should be considered in the differential diagnosis of the patient with presumed endometritis unresponsive to appropriately selected antibiotics.
- Women with mastitis may typically be allowed to continue nursing their infants while treated with penicillinase-resistant synthetic penicillins or cephalosporins.

the pathogenesis. The infection frequently is characterized by patient complaints of high fever and shaking chills accompanied by breast engorgement, pain, and erythema. Diagnosis is based on the clinical presentation and confirmatory physical findings. Culture of expressed breast milk often is performed.

Therapy should begin promptly to prevent the more serious complication of breast abscess. Treatment consists of appropriate antibiotics to cover the most likely organisms, supportive measures including analgesics, and such local measures as breast support and ice application to the affected breast. Appropriate antimicrobial choices include the penicillinase-resistant synthetic penicillins (e.g., dicloxacillin, oxacillin, nafcillin) and the cephalosporins. Erythromycin may be used in penicillin-allergic patients. If culture and sensitivity testing indicate a methicillin-resistant staphylococcal infection, vancomycin may be required. Outpatient therapy has been shown effective for most patients.

Patients typically will respond to therapy within 24 to 48 hours and are not discouraged from nursing. In the absence of breast abscess, no ill-effects are noted in the newborn from continued breast milk ingestion. Breast-feeding is only discouraged in breast abscess or when discomfort prohibits it. In these cases, gently using a breast pump is helpful to maintain drainage of the breast and may inhibit abscess formation.

Fortunately, with timely administration of antibiotics the complication of breast abscess is uncommon. Nevertheless, physical examination should search for the signs of breast abscess (fluctuance and exquisite tenderness) because surgical drainage is an essential addition to antibiotic therapy.

Questions

1. Which of the following scenarios is least likely to suggest a patient with postpartum endometritis?
   A. A 16-year-old who is without prenatal care, 16 hours after vaginal delivery that was complicated by prolonged ruptured membranes and chorioamnionitis, now has a temperature of 101.3° F, a pulse of 118, and foul vaginal discharge.
   B. A 32-year-old obstetrician's secretary, who is now 24 hours post–elective repeat cesarean section and tubal ligation, is noted by the nurse to have a temperature of 100.8° F and found to have marked tenderness of the uterine fundus on abdominal examination.
   C. A 20-year-old college student who develops low grade fever and uterine tenderness 10 days following cesarean section for breech. Her prenatal history includes the finding of a positive *Chlamydia* culture.
   D. A 300-lb patient who had a scheduled repeat cesarean section and tubal ligation. Her medical history is significant for asthma. She now complains of shortness of breath and cough and was noted to have a temperature of 101.4° F.
   E. A 15-year-old who was discharged from the hospital 8 hours following vaginal delivery. She presented in active labor stating her "water bag broke" several days prior. She now presents to the prenatal clinic with a foul-smelling discharge, uterine tenderness and rebound, and a temperature of 103.5° F.

2. Which of the following organisms are most likely encountered in culture from patients with endometritis?
   A. *E. coli, C. difficile, Klebsiella* species
   B. Group B streptococci, *Bacteroides fragilis,* gonnococci
   C. ***Bacteroides bivius, G. vaginalis,*** peptostreptococci
   D. *C. trachomatis,* group B streptococci, *Proteus mirabilis*
   E. *Pseudomonas* species, *Clostridium perfringens, S. aureus*

3. Complete the following statement with the correct choice. Prophylactic antibiotic ad-

ministration during cesarean section at the time of cord clamping:

A. Is best dosed for 48 hours if the patient's membranes have been ruptured at least 8 hours before surgery
B. Can prevent at least 75% of postcesarean endometritis cases
C. Has the best chance of being successful when both gentamicin and clindamycin are given
D. Should be used for all cases of cesarean section
E. Should consist of a single dose of a first-generation cephalosporin in high-risk cases only

4. The treatment of endometritis consists of:
A. An understanding of the polymicrobial nature of the infection
B. Broad spectrum monotherapy or drug combinations covering both gram-positive and gram-negative aerobes and anaerobes
C. Thorough patient history and physical examination to rule out extrauterine sources of infection
D. Continuation of therapy until the patient is without signs and symptoms of infection for 48 hours
E. All of the above

Answers

1. D
2. C
3. E
4. E

24

Psychologic and psychiatric issues

APGO LEARNING OBJECTIVE #24

Dorothy Kammerer-Doak
Laura Weiss Roberts
Melissa Schiff
Teresita A. McCarty
Lisa M. Fromm

Pregnancy is a significant life event and may be accompanied by anxiety and depression. Recognition of psychologic disturbance is essential for early intervention.

The student will demonstrate a knowledge of the following:

A. Normal emotional responses to pregnancy changes
B. Signs and symptoms of postpartum depression and psychosis
C. Management of patients with psychiatric illnesses

A woman's life is marked by many transitions, some of which may be related to reproduction. One such significant life event is becoming a mother. Each pregnancy is a unique experience for a woman and her family. Although physiologic changes take place in a progressive and orderly fashion, the same is not true of the complex psychologic changes—and, at times, psychiatric illnesses—accompanying pregnancy and childbirth. In this section, first the psychologic issues arising in pregnancy are discussed, including the acceptance of pregnancy; development of the maternal role; relationship with the partner and changes in body image; concerns and fears; relationship with the fetus; and grief after miscarriage. Second, a common experience of mild, transient depression related to childbirth (the "baby blues") and three distinct psychiatric illnesses unique to pregnancy and the postpartum period—postpartum depression, anxiety, and psychosis—are discussed.

ACCEPTANCE OF PREGNANCY

When she learns she is pregnant, a woman immediately experiences a reaction to the physical and emotional reality of pregnancy. Not all women are happy. In fact, approximately 50% of women are ambivalent about a pregnancy or reject it regardless of whether pregnancy was planned. A first pregnancy is the most highly accepted. The acceptance of subsequent pregnancies varies; however, subsequent pregnancies are more readily accepted when there is a longer space between children and fewer children. Age, financial status, relationship with the partner, anticipated life-style changes, and interference with career goals also influence acceptance of pregnancy. Sharing the knowledge of the pregnancy with others assists in confirming and accepting the pregnancy.

During the second trimester, fetal movements and body changes cause an increased awareness of a new life, making the pregnancy more real to the mother. This sense of reality and attachment is enhanced when the fetal image in utero is visualized ultrasonographically. By the third trimester, the overwhelming majority of women come to accept their pregnancies. The physical and psychologic changes that occur during the course of pregnancy facilitate this acceptance. It is not unusual, however, for some ambivalence to persist throughout pregnancy, during labor and delivery, and into the postpartum period.

DEVELOPMENT OF THE MATERNAL ROLE

As pregnancy progresses, a woman prepares herself for her new role as a mother. This process of maternal identity formation changes a woman's self-understanding significantly and occurs whether the woman is pregnant with her first child or already is a mother. Frequently, a pregnant woman recalls her childhood experience and wonders about her own mother's pregnancy, labor and delivery, family traits, and child-rearing practices. Additionally, she draws from society for the ideal images of qualities, traits, attitudes, and achievements that form the maternal identity. The baby's health, developmental capabilities, and the "goodness of fit" between the temperaments of mother and infant also have been related to the mother's comfort and acceptance of the maternal role.

Pregnant women must adjust to less freedom and more responsibility. This is particularly true for a woman who works away from home. Many difficult decisions must be made when addressing conflicts between a work role and a new or expanded maternal role: the length of maternity leave, whether to return to work at all, how to arrange for day care, and how to balance other family responsibilities. Seldom are these issues resolved before the postpartum period.

RELATIONSHIP WITH THE PARTNER AND CHANGING BODY IMAGE

Couples experience a change in their relationship during pregnancy. The majority experience a deeper sense of closeness and commitment. Others may experience more conflict and strain. For those who had unresolved marital difficulties before the pregnancy, the probability of conflict is greater. Women who feel emotionally alone and burdened by the physical and emotional changes of pregnancy may feel resentment toward the partner. Sexual activity within a relationship can be greatly influenced by the changes in pregnancy. See Chapter 53, Sexuality, for more detail.

A woman's body image undergoes changes throughout pregnancy, and these changes also may influence the relationship with her partner. Women who have a positive body image before pregnancy often continue to have a positive body image during pregnancy. If the individual is happy and accepts the pregnancy, the physical changes may be even desired and welcomed. With increasing abdominal size, some women report a more negative feeling about their body—as it begins to seem more alien and different, and as the pregnant body shape increasingly differs from society's ideal body image, that of a thin woman. The partner's attitude about the pregnancy and the changes it brings to the woman's body also may greatly affect their sense of intimacy and comfort together.

Communication and empathy within the relationship are especially important at this time in a woman's life. As the couple learns to communicate and nurture each other during both the happy and difficult times of pregnancy, they prepare themselves for their new role as parents.

CONCERNS AND FEARS

Many women experience some fear and anxiety during pregnancy. Common concerns relate to the health and well-being of the unborn child; the changing marital relationship; the new role as mother; and, if the mother works away from home, how her work role may be affected by motherhood. Open discussions in which the patient's worries are elicited and addressed, information is provided, and reassurance is generously offered may greatly assuage the woman's distress.

During the third trimester, specific fears about labor and delivery increase. Because the physical changes and the process of labor and delivery are inevitable and outside the pregnant woman's control, she may experience a general feeling of powerlessness. Labor and delivery education classes may help alleviate some of these feelings.

RELATIONSHIP WITH THE FETUS

During pregnancy a unique relationship develops between the mother and her unborn child. During the first trimester, the pregnant woman begins to incorporate the idea of being pregnant and her anticipated new role as a mother into her concept of herself. Fetal movement helps to confirm the reality of the pregnancy and initiates the process of differentiation: that is, establishing that another being is within her body. The second trimester is characterized by a turning inward or "binding in" with the unborn child. Many women have vivid dreams and fantasies as they develop a very personal relationship with their unborn baby. As the third trimester progresses and delivery approaches, the process of separation begins. The parents choose names for the baby and acquire clothes and furniture in anticipation of the baby's arrival. Although many women are anxious to have the pregnancy over and finally to see their baby, they also experience sadness over the separation.

PSYCHOLOGIC ISSUES ACCOMPANYING MISCARRIAGE AND ABORTION

The loss of a pregnancy is a complicated, distressing event. It is accompanied by grief for most women, even those who decide to end an unwanted, unexpected, or unhealthy pregnancy. Women whose pregnancies end prematurely experience many emotions: sadness and despair, self-blame and failure, fear about future pregnancies, hopelessness, social stigma, and isolation. Should miscarriage or elective abortion occur once fetal movement has been felt, or after ultrasound has shown the clear presence of a developing baby, a woman's grief reaction is more intense. In addition, women who have undergone miscarriage or abortion may be vulnerable to disquieting mood swings, fatigue, and irritability; and they are at risk for the more serious psychiatric syndromes accompanying the postpartum period described below.

PSYCHOLOGIC AND PSYCHIATRIC ISSUES IN THE POSTPARTUM PERIOD

The postpartum period can be both happy and stressful. The birth of a baby brings enormous physical, social, and emotional changes, and, for some women, brings psychiatric difficulties as well (Table 24-1). Although pregnancy itself does not appear to be associated with an increased

---

Table 24-1. Overview of postpartum syndromes and disorders

Psychosis	Postpartum blues	Postpartum depression and anxiety*	Postpartum psychosis
Onset	3-10 days	3 days-1 yr Depression: insidious Anxiety: often sudden	3-30 days; often very sudden
Incidence	26%-85%	10%-20%	0.1%-0.3%
Dangers	Evolution to depression	Infant: abuse, neglect, risk of infanticide Mother: risk of suicide	Infant: abuse, neglect, risk of infanticide Mother: risk of suicide
Interventions	Usually self-limited; give support	Psychiatric evaluation; psychotropic medications	Emergency psychiatric evaluation

*Postpartum anxiety presents with predominant symptoms of fear and worry rather than sadness.

---

incidence of psychiatric illness, the physical and physiologic changes accompanying pregnancy and concerns about the developing fetus greatly influence the management of patients who experience psychiatric symptoms. It is essential to recognize preexisting psychiatric syndromes; the development of postpartum blues ("baby blues") associated with childbirth; and the emergence of new, serious psychiatric illnesses, such as postpartum depression, anxiety, and psychosis.

Women with preexisting psychiatric illnesses often become mothers or are mothers already. Pregnancy may worsen or, in some instances, may offer relief from psychiatric symptoms. These symptoms include sadness, lack of pleasure in life, hopelessness, poor self-esteem, irritability, worry, poor self-care, stress-related physical complaints, poor concentration, impulsivity, hallucinations, delusions, and disorganized thinking and behavior. Not only must serious consideration be given to the care of patients with these symptoms, but also to the therapeutic interventions, which may harm the developing fetus. Benzodiazepines (e.g., Valium, Ativan), antidepressants (e.g., Elavil, Prozac), neuroleptics (e.g., Haldol, Mellaril), anticonvulsants (e.g., Tegretol, valproic acid), and lithium are drugs that have been associated with

teratogenic effects. For these reasons, collaboration with a psychiatrist for treatment is crucial to the well-being of the patient, her family, and the unborn child. Psychiatrists may be helpful in providing the patient with additional structure and support; recognizing serious and/or endangering symptoms; administering necessary medications; and, rarely, in providing treatments (e.g., psychiatric hospitalization, electroconvulsive therapy) to address potentially life-threatening difficulties experienced by the pregnant woman.

Postpartum blues, in contrast to preexisting psychiatric illnesses, are so common (up to 85% of all mothers) that they are understood to be a "normal," predictable event of the pregnancy and birth process (Table 24-1). Symptoms generally begin 3 to 10 days after delivery and include worry, depression, irritability, insomnia, tearfulness, fatigue, and labile mood. This disorder has only a minimal effect on the woman's ability to function in her role as a mother, does not necessitate psychiatric referral, and generally resolves spontaneously within a few weeks with support and reassurance.

Serious psychiatric syndromes can occur in the postpartum period. Several related factors seem to place some women at risk for more such serious

Table 24-2. Symptoms of postpartum psychiatric illnesses

PHYSICAL SYMPTOMS

Loss of appetite

Multiple physical complaints without clear basis

Severe insomnia and fatigue (unrelated to infant care)

Episodes of palpitations, trembling, fear, sweating, and so on

Unexplained pain

EMOTIONAL SYMPTOMS

Frequent crying without clear basis

Excessive concern about well-being of the infant

Avoidance of the baby

Uncharacteristic silence, reclusiveness, talkativeness

Extreme feelings of sadness, inadequacy, fear, emptiness

Extreme feelings of exuberance, energy, grandiosity

COGNITIVE SYMPTOMS

Bizarre thoughts or beliefs

Poor concentration

Memory lapses

Disorientation, confusion

Disorganized thoughts

Odd behavior

Hallucinations

Obsessive ideas or images

---

poorly understood relationship with the woman's own mother.

Three especially important psychiatric syndromes that can arise during the postpartum period include postpartum depression, postpartum anxiety, and postpartum psychosis. Recognition of the physical, emotional, and cognitive symptoms that may occur is essential to the diagnosis of these disorders (Table 24-2).

Depression

Postpartum depression, which can occur at any time in the first 6 months after delivery, affects 10% to 20% of mothers. The symptoms of postpartum depression are similar to those of postpartum blues but are more severe and interfere with the mother's ability to function. The bond between mother and baby may be disrupted. Postpartum depression has been associated with twin and preterm delivery. History of depression or postpartum depression is associated with an increased risk. The recurrence rate in subsequent pregnancies is 20% to 30%. Consultation with a psychiatrist usually is necessary for a patient with postpartum depression. Its treatment, like that of nonpuerperal depression, includes psychotherapy and antidepressant medication. Recovery within 1 year occurs in about two thirds of patients.

Anxiety disorders

Postpartum anxiety disorders have recently become recognized as important psychiatric illnesses associated with pregnancy, although their prevalence has not yet been well documented. With postpartum panic disorder women experience episodes of extreme distress without more prominent depressive symptoms. The episodes resemble panic attacks in other patients and involve palpitations, sweating, breathlessness, choking sensations, trembling, dizziness, and fear of losing control, dying, or "going crazy." Psychiatric consultation and psychotropic medications are indicated if the panic episodes recur and cause the

psychiatric syndromes. Included among these risk factors are the following elements: (1) biologic factors, such as preexisting psychiatric illnesses, complications during pregnancy and delivery, history of difficulty becoming pregnant, or family history of psychiatric illness; (2) psychologic factors, such as ambivalence or negative attitude toward motherhood, history of difficulty coping with life transitions, stresses related to caring for a premature or ill baby, or past experiences of abuse; and (3) interpersonal factors, such as poor marital relationship, poor temperamental fit between mother and child, social isolation, and difficult or patient significant distress. If untreated, the symptoms may worsen dramatically, leading to a more severe anxiety disorder, perhaps complicated by a depressive disorder and increased risk of suicide. Another anxiety disorder, obsessive-compulsive disorder, may arise or worsen during the postpartum period. Obsessions (e.g., about contamination) and compulsive behaviors (e.g., handwashing, repetitive checking behaviors) are understandably provoked by caring for a newborn. The incidence and duration of postpartum obsessive-compulsive disorder is unknown, but the symptoms can become exhausting and may interfere with the new mother's ability to function effectively. Embarrassment and confusion about these difficulties may prevent the mother from seeking help for her thoughts and behaviors. Psychiatric treatments can, however, be extremely effective in reducing symptoms and restoring function.

Psychosis

Postpartum psychosis is the least common and the most severe of the postpartum mental disorders, affecting less than 1% of new mothers. The delivery of a child is a known precipitating factor for psychosis, with the incidence of psychosis increased 20 times in the postpartum period. Risk factors related to this disorder include personal or family history of psychosis, absence of partner involvement, cesarean section, and perinatal death. History of bipolar disorder is a significant risk factor, with up to 25% of these women developing postpartum psychosis.

Symptoms of psychosis—such as hallucinations, paranoia, delusions, compromised reality-testing, and disorganization of thoughts and behavior—typically develop 2 days to 3 weeks after delivery. In general, postpartum psychosis does not appear to be different from other psychoses in terms of symptoms, treatment principles, outcome, or genetic predisposition. The recurrence rate in subsequent pregnancies is approximately 14%.

Women with postpartum psychosis require immediate psychiatric referral. Hospitalization usu-ally is necessary because injury to the newborn—usually through neglect, confusion, or delusional acts—is a serious concern. Most patients require antipsychotic medications for several months and long-term follow-up therapy.

PRINCIPLES OF PREVENTION AND TREATMENT

Prevention of pregnancy-related psychiatric illnesses begins well before delivery. First, taking a careful history to identify biologic and psychologic risk factors is extremely important. Second, just as the obstetrician prepares a woman for each stage of pregnancy, anticipatory guidance about the realities of the immediate postpartum period may ease the stresses of that transition. Third, dispelling myths about mothers as unlimited sources of love, as instinctively knowledgeable about babies, and as finding ultimate fulfillment through the experience of childbearing may prevent unrealistic expectations and subsequent disappointment. Fourth, helping the pregnant mother to develop a set of practical plans (e.g., encouraging friends and family to help with meals, housework and laundry, choosing a pediatrician) and emotional supports (e.g., answering questions, providing an opportunity to express fears) before the birth of the baby is especially important. Finally, although the emphasis is often on the immediate postpartum period, becoming a mother has long-term implications for every woman. By beginning a discussion of the changes that motherhood brings in a woman's self-understanding and life experience, an obstetrician will start a dialogue of great value within the doctor-patient relationship.

Effective treatment strategies must take into consideration how complex biologic, psychologic, and social factors may contribute to the symptoms experienced by a woman with postpartum psychiatric syndromes. Consultation with a psychiatrist can facilitate this comprehensive approach. Adequate evaluation of physical symptoms (Table 24-2) and of reversible medical causes of psychiatric symptoms (e.g., hypothyroidism or hyperthyroidism, electrolyte abnormalities, severe pain) is essential in addressing the biologic issues. Use of appropriate medication regimens and careful clinical follow-up for mother and baby are crucial as well. Treatment of psychologic factors may involve identification of emotional and cognitive symptoms (Table 24-2); clarification of stressors; and provision of supportive interventions for the mother (e.g., reassurance, encouragement of the mother's effort to take care of herself as well as the baby, psychotherapy), the infant (e.g., evaluation of infant's health; establishment of appropriate sleeping, eating, and comfort routines), and the father (e.g., identifying new role, reassurance). Through these efforts, the physical and emotional well-being of the mother and her infant can be better assured.

CRITICAL POINTS

- Pregnancy is a normal developmental stage in the lives of many women. It is an event of great magnitude, however, and many psychologic adjustments are necessary.
- Pregnancy adaptation issues include the following:
    Acceptance or rejection of the pregnancy
    Emotions generated by miscarriage or abortion
    Changes in body image
    Fears related to the baby and to the mother's new sense of self
    Different relationship with partner and other family members
    Effects on other roles (e.g., job)
    Realistic expectations concerning the maternal role
- Anticipation and preparation for the realities of having a baby help to prevent some psychiatric sequelae.
- So many women experience postpartum blues shortly after giving birth that it is considered by many to be a normal process, not usually necessitating psychiatric intervention.
- Psychiatric illnesses that occur postpartum tend to be serious for both mother and baby; they include postpartum depression, postpartum anxiety, and postpartum psychosis.
- Postpartum psychosis is a medical emergency and necessitates immediate psychiatric evaluation.

Questions

1. All of the following present an increased risk for the development of postpartum psychosis *except:*
   A. Bipolar disorder
   B. History of psychosis
   C. Family history of psychosis
   D. Perinatal death
   E. Vaginal delivery

2. Which of the following is an accurate statement about postpartum "baby blues"?
   A. It is relatively rare.
   B. It inevitably progresses to postpartum depression.

C. It typically develops 3 to 7 days after delivery.

D. It interferes significantly with a woman's ability to function in her role as mother.

E. It represents a psychiatric emergency.

3. The acceptance of pregnancy is influenced by:

A. Financial status

B. Emotional support from spouse

C. Career goals

D. Age

E. All of the above

4. Maternal identity formation occurs only during the first pregnancy.

A. True

B. False

5. Sexual activity during pregnancy may be influenced by:

A. Stage of pregnancy

B. The woman's body image

C. Unnecessary fears of harming the fetus

D. Physical discomfort

E. All of the above

6. All of the following are stages experienced by the mother in her relationship with the unborn child *except:*

A. Assimilation

B. Incorporation

C. Separation

D. Differentiation

7. Common fears and concerns experienced during pregnancy include:

A. Finances

B. Health of unborn child

C. Maternal role changes

D. Effect on marital relationship

E. All of the above

8. Fatigue, irritability, odd behavior, and hallucinations may accompany which of the following?

A. Postpartum anxiety

B. Postpartum depression

C. Postpartum psychosis

D. "Baby blues"

E. All of the above

9. Women who undergo miscarriage or elective abortion are vulnerable to the same psychiatric syndromes that accompany the postpartum period in women who have full-term pregnancies.

A. True

B. False

10. Appropriate treatment of preexisting and postpartum psychiatric syndromes involves:

A. Providing guidance about the realities of the postpartum period

B. Discussing openly the emotional changes accompanying motherhood

C. Identifying physical, emotional, and/or cognitive psychiatric symptoms

D. Addressing reversible medical causes of psychiatric symptoms (e.g., hypothyroidism)

E. All of the above

Answers

1. E
2. C
3. E
4. B
5. E
6. A
7. E
8. C
9. A
10. E

25 Perinatal and maternal mortality

APGO LEARNING OBJECTIVE #25

Michael F. Koszalka, Jr.

Maternal and perinatal mortality are infrequent but catastrophic events for women of reproductive age. Comprehension of terminology is critical to appreciate the frequency of these events in clinical practice. Awareness of predisposing factors allows better insight to diagnosis required for therapy to reduce these adverse outcomes.

The student will be able to do the following:
A. Classify relationships of maternal, fetal, and infant deaths with reference to the time from the last menstrual period to the end of pregnancy
B. Identify how maternal and perinatal mortality is reported, and recognize trends for each over the past 1 to 2 decades
C. Discuss factors associated with increased maternal or perinatal mortality
D. Present conceptual guidelines for women's health care management directed toward reducing maternal and perinatal mortality

Maternal and perinatal mortality represent the worst of all potential outcomes that could occur with a healthy mother and a normal infant. Understanding the terminology used to report these unfortunate events and knowing how to examine associated factors are necessary to gain insight into this group of grave clinical problems.

MATERNAL MORTALITY

Maternal mortality is the number of maternal deaths occurring during pregnancy or within

42 days of its termination, irrespective of the duration or site of pregnancy, from any cause related to or aggravated by the pregnancy or its management but not from accidental or incidental causes (World Health Organization [WHO] revision, 1993).

The maternal mortality rate indicates the likelihood of a pregnant woman dying of maternal causes. Rates are computed on the basis of the number of live births. The maternal mortality rate is reported as the number of maternal deaths from direct causes per 100,000 live births. In 1990 the maternal death rate was 8.2 per 100,000 live births from deliveries, complications of pregnancy, childbirth, and puerperium. Analysis of maternal mortality by race for 1990 notes a persisting discrepancy between white and black women. Deaths for white mothers were 5.4 per 100,000 live births; for black mothers and mothers of other races, deaths were 19.1 per 100,000 live births. Trends in maternal death from 1985 through 1989 were 7.8, 7.2, 6.6, 8.4, and 7.9 per 100,000 live births, respectively. In 1930, maternal mortality was 600 per 100,000 live births. Although the most dramatic declines occurred after 1930, later declines were noted, with perinatal mortality dropping nearly 50% each year from 1961 through 1981, with rates of 36.9 in 1961, 21 in 1970, and 8.5 in 1981.

Causes of death associated with pregnancy vary by outcome in the pregnancy. As pointed out in 1994 by Grimes, the leading causes of maternal death today are pregnancy-induced hypertension, hemorrhage, and pulmonary embolism. Grimes also noted that ectopic pregnancy was substantially more dangerous (38 deaths per 100,000 events) than either childbirth (9 deaths per 100,000 events) or legal abortion (less than 1 death per 100,000). Among the deaths in ectopic pregnancy, 90% were caused by hemorrhage.

In 1987, of the 272 maternal deaths reported in the United States, puerperal complications were associated with 75, or 27.5%. The second, third, and fourth most frequent causes were toxemia, ectopic pregnancy, and hemorrhage, occurring at frequencies of 14.7%, 13.2%, and 9.9% respectively. Major causes of maternal deaths from nonabortive pregnancies (excluding ectopic pregnancies) were, in order, as follows: (1) pulmonary embolism; (2) hypertensive disorders of pregnancy; (3) uterine hemorrhage; and (4) sepsis. Unfortunately, owing to reporting mechanisms, overlap of contributing factors often is not recognizable because the primary cause of death may be the only one listed on the death certificate. In addition, indirect and nonobstetric deaths may be listed under such specific causes as heart disease, which may not appear as deaths of pregnant or recently delivered women.

Internationally, maternal mortality remained high until the early part of the twentieth century. A decline occurred starting in the mid-1930s, and mortality rates since then have been halved approximately every 10 years until 1980. Interestingly, varied approaches were used internationally to reduce mortality rates. In the United States, obstetrician and hospital-based delivery systems were developed. In the Netherlands, combinations of highly trained midwives with home deliveries were used; and in New Zealand, trained midwives with deliveries at hospitals were adopted. Britain settled for a compromise of specialist obstetricians who consulted with better-trained midwives and general practitioners. These variations and approaches had little differential effect on the decline in mortality rates. Although the initial downturn in mortality was attributed to antibiotics such as sulfonamides and penicillin, the benefits have not been universal. On a global basis, wherever overall mortality is highest, deaths from hemorrhage and infection still account for a large percentage of excess maternal mortality. The largest reductions in more developed countries have been due to the decreased frequency of maternal mortality from hemorrhage, abortion complications, pulmonary embolism, and hypertensive disease. Many of these conditions improved because of better recognition of risk and appropriate aggressive medical management.

RISK FACTORS FOR MATERNAL MORTALITY

Maternal mortality, when analyzed retrospectively from 1979 through 1986, shows increased rates of mortality in older women. Historically, women in their 40s were 8.6 times more likely to die in pregnancy than women aged 20 to 24, when pregnancy risk was lowest. Additional risk factors include marital status and lack of education and prenatal care. Unmarried women have a 3 times higher mortality than married women. Educational attainment is inversely related to the risk of death. This discrepancy widens with age, so that at 35 there is a threefold increase in maternal mortality risk in women with less than a high school education.

Maternal mortality for blacks has been 3 to 4 times higher than that of whites for the past 20 years and remains so. In 1990, mortality for black mothers was 22.4, compared with a mortality rate of 5.4 for whites per 100,000 live births. Black women were twice as likely as white women to have received either late or no prenatal care. Lack of prenatal care increases the risk of maternal death sixfold. Delays in establishing prenatal care and lack of availability of prenatal care frequently have been cited as causes of the maternal mortality differential between the races. Recently, however, individual level variables (i.e., biology and behavior) have been noted as equally, if not more, significant concerns.

Hypertensive disease is associated with a significantly increased risk for maternal mortality. When preeclampsia progresses to eclampsia, then coma, vascular accidents, and death may occur. Eclampsia-related deaths have fallen from the 7% to 17% range in the 1970s to 0.4% reported in 1984. In developed countries, hypertensive disorders have risen as a relative cause of mortality, whereas hemorrhage and infection have declined—bringing hypertensive disorders to the forefront in many regions of the world. Although the standard of care for preeclamptic therapy in the United States uses magnesium sulfate, alternative agents are undergoing study in South America, Africa, and Asia. Several trials of preeclamptic prevention have suggested the potential of baby aspirin to reduce the frequency of preeclampsia; however, the effectiveness and safety of these agents remains controversial in low-risk populations. General anesthesia also is noted to increase maternal risk, especially when intubation was impossible, or where there was anatomic airway distortion. Aspiration of gastric contents caused by the delay in gastric emptying time of the pregnant patient further increases the risk of the general anesthesia procedure.

TERMINOLOGY OF PREGNANCY LOSS

The duration of gestation is the critical element in defining the type of reproductive loss. The terminology is categorized by the number of weeks of gestation achieved (Fig. 25-1). The period of gestation is defined as the number of completed weeks elapsed between the first day of the last normal menstrual period (LNMP) and the date of delivery. The first day of the LNMP is used as the initial date because it can be determined more accurately than the date of conception, which usually occurs 2 weeks after LNMP.

FETAL DEATH

Fetal death was defined in 1950 by the WHO as the death of a product of conception before the complete expulsion or extraction from its mother, irrespective of the duration of pregnancy. Death is indicated by the fact that after such separation, the fetus does not breathe and shows no other evidence of life, such as a beating heart, pulsation of the umbilical cord, or other definite movement of voluntary muscles.

The WHO has recommended the term *fetal death* to replace such older terms as "stillbirth" or "abortion." Deaths are classified as *early death* when they occur at less than 20 completed weeks

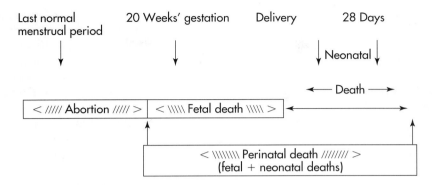

Fig. 25-1. Terminology categorization of pregnancy loss.

of pregnancy, *intermediate death* when they occur at 20 to 27 completed weeks of pregnancy, and *late death* when they occur 28 weeks or later during pregnancy. Statistics from 1987 show that the fetal mortality rate was 7.7 per 1000 live births. The actual number of fetal deaths, however, cannot be accurately determined because most states do not require reporting deaths from pregnancies of less than 20 weeks' duration. Many states require fetal death certification when gestation is 20 weeks or greater.

The most common causes of fetal death are anoxia, congenital anomaly, and infection. Anoxic causes may be attributable to abruption, placenta previa, prolapsed cord, hypertension, and abnormal labor. In nearly half of fetal deaths, no cause can be determined.

LIVE BIRTH

A liveborn infant is one born with signs of life, including any of the following: breathing, cord pulsation, heart beat, and voluntary muscle movement detectable after complete expulsion from the vagina.

NEONATAL DEATH

A neonatal death is the death of any liveborn within the first 28 days of life. Neonatal deaths are reported as the number of deaths per 1000 births of liveborn infants. The neonatal mortality rate for 1987 was 6.5 per 1000 live births. Earlier neonatal mortality statistics showed a gradual decline from 39.2 in the 1920s, to 20 in 1951, and 10.5 in 1976.

PERINATAL MORTALITY

Perinatal mortality is defined as the sum of fetal deaths and neonatal deaths. Because most perinatal deaths occur in low-birth-weight infants, prematurity is attributable to the cause of death in nearly 50%. The most obvious way to reduce neonatal mortality, therefore, is to reduce the premature delivery rate. Since many neonatal deaths occur in high-risk pregnancies, it is essential that women with conditions associated with increased perinatal mortality be given special attention antepartum and intrapartum.

PREVENTION OF NEONATAL MORTALITY

Reduction in preterm delivery is the mainstay of reduction in neonatal mortality. Identification of pregnancies with high-risk conditions allows use of high-risk perinatal services and centers to optimize patient management. Pregnancies in unmarried women and pregnancies at the extremes of the reproductive years also are accompanied by an increased risk of prematurity and higher fetal and neonatal death rates. It is essential, therefore, that sexually active teens and, especially, older women who desire no future pregnancies be provided with highly reliable contraceptive means. Perinatal mortality from all causes is higher in poor women than in middle class and upper class women. The general health of those who are more affluent is better; they are often better nourished and have greater awareness of the availability of medical resources, and they use these resources. Adequacy of prenatal care alone is important in influencing the outcome of a high-risk pregnancy; however, it is only an incomplete solution to reproductive problems associated with poverty. Epidemiologic analysis of persisting suboptimal pregnancy outcomes as associated with race and ethnicity have suggested we are dealing with biopsychosocial problems that have proved refractory to the traditional mortalities of prenatal care. In a review by James, new conceptual models are proposed that acknowledge the strong connection between structural factors (cultural and economic) and individual variables (*behavioral:* unprotected teenage sex, smoking, alcohol and illicit drugs, late or nonuse of prenatal care, physical exertion at work; and *biologic:* poor nutrition, poor weight gain, anemia or abnormal hemoglobin, urinary tract infections, hypertension [preeclampsia or toxemia]) in determining risk for poor pregnancy outcomes.

Examination of the differential and neonatal mortality rates between nonHispanic whites and blacks finds death rates of 5.2 for nonHispanic whites, and 10.9 deaths per 1000 live births for blacks. Hispanic-Americans of Mexican descent have a neonatal death rate of 5.2 per 1000 live births. What factors protect the Mexican-American against the increased frequency of neonatal death among the economically disadvantaged and those with lower use of prenatal medical care service? Analysis by public health experts cites the degree of adherence to traditional cultural orientation. For Mexican-American women with predominantly Mexican cultural orientation, the frequency of low-birth-weight and neonatal death was significantly lower than that of the Mexican-American women with predominantly U.S. cultural orientation. This protective association was independent of age, parity, education, household income, and cigarette smoking status. Low educational status was associated with an increasing probability of having a low-birth-weight child only for women with a predominantly U.S. cultural orientation. Findings of this study raised the possibility that the traditional culture protects Mexican-American women, especially those most economically disadvantaged, against having suboptimal pregnancy outcomes.

Prenatal services and the types of provider have been evaluated for their effect on changing suboptimal outcomes in pregnancy. Prenatal programs directed toward identifying and addressing psychosocial needs of the expectant mother, in addition to monitoring the usual physiologic parameters, appear essential. Counseling—including nutritional discussions, other aspects of personal health care, and aggressive follow-up for missed appointments—was associated with significant improvements. These comprehensive programs appear to provide low-income women an extended, highly knowledgeable social support system capable of meeting the demands of the contemporary urban environment, in much the same way that older, more knowledgeable women traditionally guided and supported young, inexperienced expectant mothers. When prenatal programs can be established that provide the equivalent environment for guidance and support, the success of programs to improve perinatal outcomes will be improved.

An additional factor in changing perinatal death rates has been the improved prognosis for extremely low-birth-weight infants. Introduction of surfactant therapy has significantly improved the survival rate of neonates weighing between 600 and 1500 g. Since most neonatal deaths occur in low-birth-weight infants, an appreciation of the recent change in trends of survival is important. A 1987 report from the Office of Technology Assessment of the U.S. Congress made the following assessment of neonatal intensive care for low-birth-weight infants: In 1960, 722 neonatal deaths occurred per 1000 unborn infants delivered at level III hospitals where birth weights were 1500 g or less. From 1971 to 1975, the neonatal death rate fell to 542. Following initiation of neonatal intensive care units for the low-birth-weight infant, neonatal death rates have fallen to 272. In extremely low-birth-weight infants (less than 1000 g), in 1960 919 neonatal deaths were reported. From 1971 to 1975, 805 neonatal deaths were reported; from 1980 to 1985, neonatal death rates fell to 476 per 1000 unborn infants. This dramatic trend has continued to improve. Many sick infants who previously would have died are now surviving, and the overwhelming majority of survivors are normal.

CRITICAL POINTS

- Maternal mortality, the number of maternal deaths occurring during pregnancy or within 42 days of termination of the pregnancy, indicates the likelihood of a pregnant woman dying of maternal causes.
- Ectopic pregnancy mortality is substantially (38 times) greater than mortality from abortion, and 4 times greater than mortality from childbirth. Childbirth has a mortality 9 times greater than does abortion.
- Internationally, maternal mortality has declined by 50% every 10 years from 1930 until 1980. Rates in the United States have varied slightly in the past 10 years, varying from 7 to 8 deaths per 100,000 live births.
- Historical factors associated with maternal mortality have been maternal age greater than 40, hypertensive disease, lack of prenatal care and/or education, and unwed status. Mortality for blacks has been 3 to 4 times higher than that of whites for 20 years and remains higher to date.
- Perinatal mortality is the sum of fetal deaths and neonatal deaths.
- Neonatal mortality is affected by behavioral (teen sex, drugs, nonuse of prenatal care) and biologic (hypertension, urinary tract infections, poor nutrition, and so on) maternal factors. Comprehensive care including psychosocial evaluation, support, and guidance demonstrates enhanced effectiveness as compared with the usual prenatal care that is focused solely on physiologic parameters.
- The perinatal death rate has improved dramatically by surfactant therapy and neonatal intensive care unit development. Many sick infants that previously would have died are now surviving, and the overwhelming majority of survivors are normal.

Questions

1. Maternal mortality rates are computed on the basis of:
   A. Maternal deaths from direct causes per 1000 deliveries
   B. Maternal deaths from direct and indirect causes per 1000 deliveries
   C. Maternal deaths from direct causes per 10,000 live births
   D. Maternal deaths from direct causes per 100,000 live births
2. Neonatal death is the death of a newborn:
   A. Within 24 hours of birth
   B. Within 7 days of birth
   C. Within 28 days of birth
   D. Within 1 year of birth
3. Perinatal mortality represents the sum of:
   A. Abortion deaths and neonatal deaths
   B. Fetal deaths and abortion deaths
   C. Fetal deaths and neonatal deaths
   D. Neonatal deaths and infant deaths

Answers

1. D
2. C
3. C

26

Postterm pregnancy

APGO LEARNING OBJECTIVE #26

Shirley K. Sawai

Perinatal mortality and morbidity may be increased significantly in a prolonged pregnancy. Prevention of complications associated with postterm pregnancy is one of the goals of antepartum and intrapartum management.

The student will demonstrate a knowledge of the following:

A. Normal period of gestation
B. Risks of postmaturity
C. Antepartum fetal surveillance
D. Management of prolonged gestation

The length of a normal-term gestation is from 37 to 42 weeks. A postterm pregnancy exceeds 294 days or 42 weeks from the first day of the last menstrual period (LMP). The incidence of postterm pregnancy ranges from 7% to 12%, with approximately 4% extending beyond 43 weeks. Increasing parity is associated with a decreased incidence of postterm pregnancies. There is a tendency to repeat postterm births: 27.4% risk if

the first pregnancy was postterm as opposed to 12.2% risk if the first one was not. With two previous postterm deliveries the risk of a subsequent one increases to 39.1%; whereas if the first two births are not postterm, the risk for the third decreases to 10.7%.

The term *postdates pregnancy* is synonymous with postterm pregnancy and must be differentiated from a *postmature pregnancy,* which is a postterm pregnancy in which the fetus is compromised by growth retardation, intrauterine malnutrition, and oligohydramnios. The diagnosis of postmaturity or dysmaturity syndrome is made in the neonate, but it is in the postmature pregnancy that increased risk for complications occurs. Many attempts have been made at antepartum detection of postmature pregnancy.

PATHOGENESIS

Since the mechanism by which normal labor begins in a term gestation is unknown, it is difficult to know the etiology of preterm and postterm gestations. Explanations proposed in the past have included the following: (1) a relative estrogen deficiency, which may produce a deficiency in the usual release of arachidonic acid—a precursor for prostaglandins; (2) a subnormal increase in progesterone-binding protein; and (3) a lack of estrogen-induced progesterone-binding protein, which may prevent the removal of a "progesterone block" that suppresses uterine excitability by blocking prostaglandin $F_{2\alpha}$. These theories may explain why some estrogen-deficient conditions—such as anencephaly, fetal adrenal hypoplasia, and placental sulfatase deficiency—are associated with postterm pregnancy.

Cortisol promotes the hydroxylation of progesterone, thereby decreasing progesterone and increasing estrogen precursors. Deficient adrenocortical states in sheep result in prolongation of pregnancy. Anencephalic fetuses have a markedly decreased fetal adrenal mass, and postmature infants have been reported to have lower plasma cortisol levels than term infants. Both of these observations implicate a role for corticosteroids in the etiology of postterm pregnancy.

Another common cause of postterm pregnancy may be the overestimation of gestational age either because of variations in the timing of ovulation or uncertain dates with late prenatal care. It is difficult to determine the true incidence of post-

---

Table 26-1. Clinical parameters in estimation of gestational age*

Priority for estimating gestational age	"Estimated" range for 95% of cases
1. In vitro fertilization	±1 day
2. Ovulation induction	±3-4 days
3. Recorded basal body temperature	±4-5 days
4. Ultrasound crown-rump length	±5-7 days
5. First trimester physical examination (normal uterus)	±2 wk
6. Ultrasound BPD before 20 wk	±5-7 days
7. Ultrasound gestational sac volume	±1-1.5 wk
8. Ultrasound BPD from 20 to 26 wk	±1.6 wk
9. First trimester physical exam	±2 wk
10. LNMP from recorded dates (good history)	±2-3 wk
11. Ultrasound BPD 26 to 30 wk	±2-3 wk
12. LNMP from memory (good history)	±3-4 wk
13. Ultrasound BPD after 30 wk	±3-4 wk
14. Fundal height measurement—before 28 wk	±4 wk
15. Fundal height measurement—after 28 wk	±4-6 wk
16. LNMP from memory (not good history)	±4-6 wk
17. Fetal heart tones first heard	±4-6 wk
18. Quickening	±4-6 wk

From Callen PW: *Ultrasonography in obstetrics and gynecology,* Philadelphia, 1983, WB Saunders.
BPD, Biparietal diameter; *LNMP,* last normal menstrual period.
*The rule is to always use a more reliable indicator in preference to a less reliable one.
A "good" history requires knowledge of both LNMP and the previous period with regular periods and no use of birth control pills for at least 6 months before the LNMP.

term gestations, since up to 22% of pregnancies cannot be assigned a reliable expected date of confinement (EDC) based on the first day of the LMP. The caregiver is then faced with the task of establishing an EDC as early in pregnancy as possible based on the most reliable dating criteria still available. As Table 26-1 demonstrates, there is a sizable range of error in most methods of pregnancy dating except for in vitro fertilization. Although many pregnancies may not truly be biologically prolonged beyond 42 completed weeks, there is no accurate way to identify these pregnancies; and the obstetrician is compelled to manage all pregnancies so-labeled as if they are

abnormally prolonged. Thus early establishment of an EDC cannot be overemphasized as a means to avoid possible unnecessary intervention in pseudo-postterm pregnancies, as well as to avoid unmonitored complications in an underdated pregnancy.

SYMPTOMS AND SIGNS OF COMPLICATIONS

Early reports (1963) by McClure-Brown noted a perinatal mortality rate of 11 per 1000 live births at 40 to 41 weeks, with a doubling of this figure by 43 weeks and tripling by 44 weeks. More recent studies (1987) by Eden reflect an overall perinatal mortality rate for postterm pregnancies that is not statistically different from controls at term, probably at least partially because of antepartum fetal monitoring (Table 26-2 and Fig. 26-1). The postterm group had a lower parity, higher birthweight, higher maternal blood pressure, higher cesarean section rate, lower Apgar scores, and greater meconium staining and aspiration.

In 1987 Arias reported on the increasing incidence of macrosomia (defined as greater than 4000 g in his study) with more prolonged gestation. There was a 10% incidence of macrosomia at 38 to 40 weeks, 20% at 40 to 41 weeks, 34% at 42 to 43 weeks, and 43% at 43 to 44 weeks. Macrosomia (usually defined as greater than 4500 g) increases the risk of dysfunctional labor, cephalopelvic disproportion, forceps delivery, cesarean section, and shoulder dystocia. Arias also reported a rising incidence of complications with increasing length of gestation: 5.6% at 38 to 40 weeks, 20% at 40 to 41 weeks, and 28.5% at 42 to 43 weeks. In one third to one half of these pregnancies the complications were related to hypoxia. Fetal distress risk is increased, especially in the postmature, growth-retarded postterm fetus with oligohydramnios.

Hypoxic complications of postterm pregnancies can be easily understood on examination of

---

Table 26-2. Perinatal outcome of uncomplicated postdates pregnancy

Meconium staining	26.5%
Breech presentation	2.1%
Cord prolapse	0.2%
Delivery	
Forceps	17.0%
Cesarean	17.6%
Shoulder dystocia	1.3%
Macrosomia (>4500 g)	2.8%
Growth retardation (<2500 g)	0.2%
Apgar scores	
1-minute <7	10.2%
5-minute <7	1.7%
Meconium aspiration	1.6%
Congenital anomalies	1.6%
Perinatal mortality (per 1000 births)	
Total mortality	4.9
Antepartum	2.3
Intrapartum	0
Neonatal	2.6
Corrected mortality	4.2
Antepartum	2.1
Intrapartum	0
Neonatal	2.1

From Eden RD et al: Perinatal characteristics of uncomplicated postdate pregnancies, *Obstet Gynecol* 69: 296, 1987.

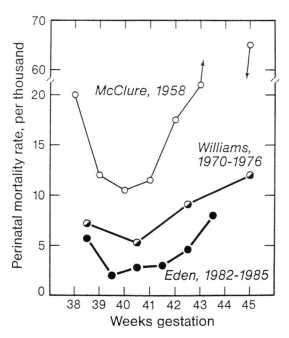

Fig. 26-1. Perinatal mortality in prolonged pregnancy. *(From Dyson DC: J Reprod Med 33:263, 1988.)*

<table>
<tr><td colspan="1">

Table 26-3. Morphologic features of the postterm placenta

Increased syncytial degeneration and fibrotic villi.

Ischemic villous necrosis with hemorrhagic infarcts.

Increased placental calcium and fibrin deposition.

Fibrinoid degeneration of decidual vessels and intervillous space.

Thickened vasculosyncytial membrane.

Thrombosis and hyaline degeneration of villous stem vessels.

Villous changes occur in 40% of postdates pregnancies and often accompany postmaturity.
</td></tr>
</table>

the postterm placenta's morphologic features (Table 26-3). The degenerative changes of aging cause the reserve capacity of the placenta to be exhausted, so that placental insufficiency develops—resulting in impaired placental respiratory, nutritional, and endocrine functions. When the umbilical vein oxygen saturation declines to half of its normal value, meconium passage occurs. Aspiration of meconium can occur in utero or at delivery and can lead to severe respiratory distress from mechanical obstruction of the airways, a chemical pneumonitis, and pulmonary hypertension with persistent fetal circulation (meconium aspiration syndrome).

Amniotic fluid volume decreases as the placenta ages, while the fetus may continue to increase in size, thereby setting the stage for cord compression accidents (Fig. 26-2). The amniotic fluid volume declines from 1100 ml at 38 weeks

to 350 ml at 42 weeks to a few milliliters after 43 weeks.

The postmature infant (Fig. 26-3) develops as a result of these aging processes during gestation. In 1954 Clifford described stages that correlate with gestational length (Table 26-4). The neonatal course of a postmature infant is complicated by dehydration, hypocalcemia, hypoglycemia, glycosuria, albuminuria, and hyperbilirubinemia. Not unexpectedly, Rayburn found that postmature infants had higher incidences of abnormal fetal heart rate tracings before delivery (50% versus 3% in controls); Apgar scores less than 6 (22% versus 3%); and neonatal intensive care unit admissions (19% versus 1%).

LABORATORY-DIAGNOSTIC TESTS

Multiple biochemical markers have been studied in attempts to detect the postterm pregnancy at risk for postmaturity-related complications. Various measurements of estriol—including 24-hour urinary levels, unconjugated plasma levels, and evaluation of single void urine for estriol : creatinine ratio—have yielded low levels of sensitivity. Since human placental lactogen pro-

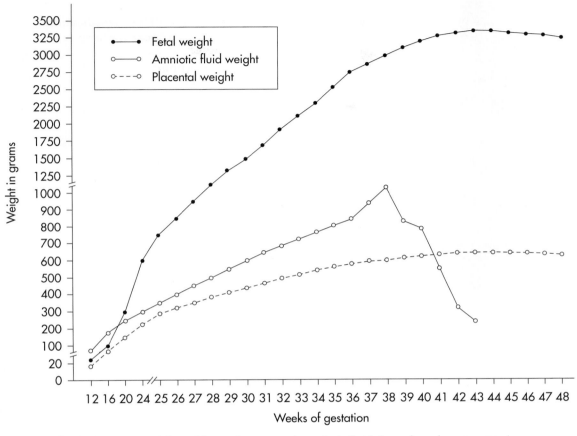

Fig. 26-2. Average weights of fetus, placenta, and amniotic fluid throughout human gestation. Fetal and placental weights are similar during first trimester of gestation. From 16 weeks on, fetus grows more rapidly than placenta; and respective weight curves dissociate. Amniotic fluid correlates to placental weight until 36 weeks' gestation; thereafter amniotic fluid volume declines rapidly. After first half of gestation, fetoplacental weight ratio is 2 to 3:1, increasing to a ratio of about 6:1 at term and remaining so during prolonged pregnancy. Standard deviation for fetal weight during last trimester of gestation is 500 to 600 g; for placental weight and amniotic fluid volume large variations (300 to 600 g) of single values are observed. Volume of amniotic fluid becomes greatly reduced postterm, and only a few milliliters may be found after 43 weeks of gestation. *(From Vorherr H: Placental insufficiency in relation to post-term pregnancy and fetal postmaturity,* Am J Obstet Gynecol *123:67, 1975.)*

duction was believed to decrease with decreasing placental function, several studies examined it as a marker for placental insufficiency; however, it was prone to a significant degree of false-negative and false-positive results.

Physical evaluation for the presence of meconium was studied through amnioscopy and amniocentesis. There was no difference in outcome if induction of labor was based on the presence of meconium on serial amniocentesis or on a

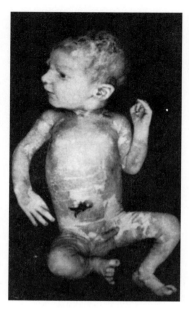

Fig. 26-3. Placental dysfunction syndrome, stage 3. Note long, thin infant with loose, peeling, parchment-like skin; alert expression; and staining of skin and nails. *(From Clifford SH: Postmaturity. In Levine SZ, editor: Advances in pediatrics, vol 9, Chicago, 1957, Mosby-Year Book.)*

Table 26-4. Clifford classification of postmaturity

STAGE 1 (APPROX. 7 DAYS POSTTERM)
Absent vernix caseosa
Thin, dry, cracked, peeling, loose, wrinkled skin
Long nails
Absent lanugo and abundant scalp hair
Alert and apprehensive facies
Depletion of subcutaneous tissue
Relatively long and thin body

STAGE 2 (APPROX. 14 DAYS POSTTERM)
All features of stage 1
Meconium staining (greenish) of skin, umbilical cord, and fetal membranes
Fetal distress or anoxia; birth asphyxia in some cases

STAGE 3
All features of stages 1 and 2
Meconium staining (yellow) of umbilical cord and nails
Perinatal mortality

---

positive contraction stress test (CST), although there was a greater incidence of intervention in the former group.

In the 1980s ultrasonography became more readily available, and studies were undertaken to find sonographic markers of impending postmaturity syndrome. Placental grading proved to be inaccurate, with 21% of patients with a grade 3 placenta delivering postmature infants while 79% delivered normal term–appearing infants. Amniotic fluid volume appeared to be more predictive of postterm-related complications. Decreased volume was associated with an increased incidence of meconium staining, fetal acidosis, cesarean section for fetal distress, low Apgar scores, increased perinatal mortality, and fetal heart rate (FHR) decelerations during nonstress tests (NSTs) and

labor. Many of these complications are related to cord compression caused by a lack of amniotic fluid to provide a protective cushion around the cord. Marks reported on the results of a semiweekly amniotic fluid index (AFI = the sum of the vertical depth of the largest pocket in each quadrant of the uterus in centimeters) in postterm pregnancies. He found that although there was a large range, AFI showed an average decrease of approximately 25% per week in postterm pregnancies and an incidence of oligohydramnios (AFI less than 5 cm) of 11.5%.

The search for predictive biochemical and physical markers yielded to the increased sensitivity of electronic FHR monitoring. Although a nonreactive NST has a high false-positive rate of 80%, in four studies involving 1598 postterm pregnancies the perinatal mortality rate* was reported as 5 per 1000 without variables (tests performed weekly) and 15 per 1000 with variable decelerations. Twice weekly testing is now recommended for antepartum NST. These findings contrast with the perinatal mortality rate of 2.5 per 1000 with a weekly CST in four studies involving 1180 postterm patients. The CST is a reliable indicator of fetal well-being in postterm pregnancies; but it is invasive, work-intensive, and cumbersome. The NST is easier to perform; but when a reactive NST is accompanied by decelerations, there is an increased risk for cesarean section in response to fetal distress, presence of meconium, and Apgar score less than 7 at 5 minutes. A modified biophysical profile (BPP) consisting of an NST and AFI twice weekly measures both acute and chronic parameters of hypoxia. In three studies using 493 postterm patients before AFI (a 1-cm pocket was considered normal) a perinatal mortality rate of 6 per 1000 was reported. Twice weekly BPP has also been shown to identify fetuses at higher risk while reducing interventions for normal fetuses.

Doppler velocimetry has been investigated as a means of antepartum testing in postterm pregnancies. In several studies no significant differences were reported in the uterine or umbilical artery flow velocities in pregnancies with and without complications associated with postdatism.

MANAGEMENT

The management of the postterm pregnancy has historically fluctuated from routine induction at 42 weeks' gestation, to expectant man-

agement, to a middle ground of selective expectant management with induction for any signs of potential fetal compromise. Routine induction of labor regardless of the favorability of the cervix incurs the risks of prolonged labor with an increased risk for infection, failed induction and the surgical morbidity of cesarean section, and fetal distress. Conversely, awaiting spontaneous labor, despite the use of antepartum testing, increases the risk for macrosomia with subsequent shoulder dystocia and birth trauma, oligohydramnios, umbilical cord compression, meconium passage and aspiration, postmaturity syndrome, and fetal distress.

Because gestational age is not always known precisely, so the fetus may be less mature than believed, and because of the increased risk for failed induction with a less favorable cervix, antepartum fetal testing beginning at the best estimate of 41 to 42 weeks has been advocated more recently. Labor is selectively induced when the cervix is favorable (Bishop score greater than 6) or when there is evidence of a failing fetoplacental unit on antepartum tests (nonreassuring NST, CST, or BPP or oligohydramnios with AFI less than 5 cm). The introduction of cervical ripening techniques (prostaglandin E_2 gel, suppository, or pessary; extraamniotic saline infusion; or cervical hydrophilic dilators such as laminaria or Dilapan) has decreased the risk of failed induction for patients in whom induction of labor is indicated before cervical favorability. Although there are several antepartum testing protocols and management schemes for postterm pregnancy, all agree that any prolongation of pregnancy past 42 weeks should undergo some form of fetal surveillance and that the gestation should not exceed 44 completed weeks, although most protocols set a lower limit. A management algorithm using selective induction of labor is depicted in Fig. 26-4.

Intrapartum management includes artificial rupture of membranes as soon as possible to detect the presence of meconium. Continuous FHR monitoring is advisable to detect uteropla-

*In the pregnant population not exclusively postterm, the perinatal mortality rate for antepartum tests are as follows: NST—2.8 per 1000 if performed weekly and 1.2 per 1000 if done twice weekly; CST—0.4 per 1000; BPP—0.6 per 1000; modified BPP twice weekly—0.1 per 1000.

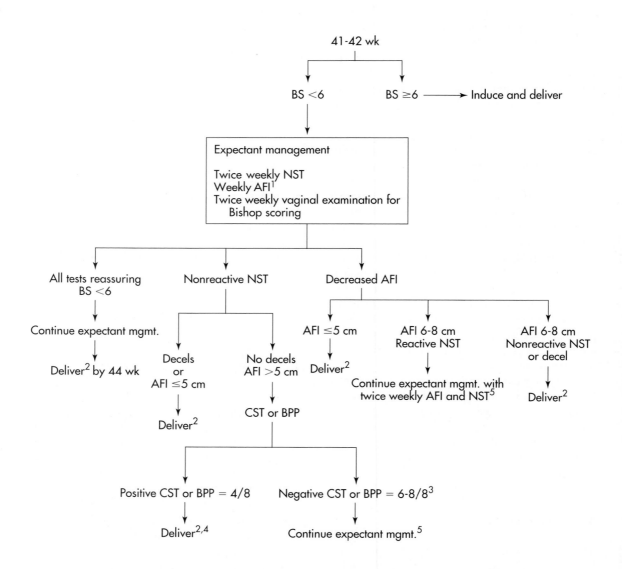

[1]Twice weekly AFI if NST is reactive with variables or previous AFI = 6-8 cm.
[2]If Bishop score (BS) <6, cervical ripening with prostaglandin E_2 before induction of labor.
[3]If BPP = 6/8, repeat testing within 24 hr.
[4]CST has 50% false-positive rate; therefore allow trial of labor (Lagrew, 1986).
[5]Deliver by 44 wk.

Fig. 26-4. Proposed selective induction for postterm pregnancies.

cental insufficiency or fetal compromise, which may be evident only with the stress of contractions. A fetal scalp electrode and intrauterine pressure catheter should be placed if the FHR tracing is questionable or nonreassuring. If meconium is present or no fluid is seen on rupture of membranes, an amnioinfusion of normal saline solution through the intrauterine pressure catheter can be instilled to dilute the concentration of the meconium in the amniotic fluid and hopefully prevent FHR decelerations from lack of fluid and cord compression. If meconium is present, the infant's oropharynx and nasopharynx should be suctioned before delivery of the shoulders, and a pediatric team should be available at delivery to transiently intubate and visualize the airway and to suction out any meconium below the vocal cords, ideally before the first neonatal inspiration. This maneuver decreases the risk of meconium aspiration syndrome, although it does not eliminate it. If vigorous suctioning of meconium is necessary, the 1-minute Apgar score may be depressed and not truly reflective of the intrauterine environment. Therefore cord arterial blood gas measurement is a better parameter to assess oxygenation status in utero. In a fetus showing a macrosomic trend on sonographic estimated fetal weight, preparations should be made in anticipation of shoulder dystocia, traumatic delivery, dysfunctional labor, or cephalopelvic disproportion. Strong consideration should be given to delivering by cesarean section without a trial of labor if the estimated fetal weight is greater than 5000 g.

CRITICAL POINTS

- A postterm pregnancy exceeds 294 days, or 42 weeks.
- A postmature or dysmature pregnancy is a postterm pregnancy in which the fetus is compromised by growth retardation, intrauterine malnutrition, and oligohydramnios.
- Other potential complications of a postterm pregnancy are macrosomia with subsequent shoulder dystocia and birth trauma, meconium staining and aspiration, dysfunctional labor, cephalopelvic disproportion, cesarean section, fetal distress, umbilical cord compression, fetal death, neonatal metabolic imbalances, and Apgar scores less than 6.
- Antepartum fetal surveillance attempts to detect evidence of uteroplacental insufficiency through acute changes in FHR on NST or CST, changes in fetal behavior on BPP, or more chronic changes in amniotic fluid volume on AFI or BPP.
- A postterm pregnancy can be managed "aggressively" with induction of labor at 42 weeks, regardless of cervical favorability; "expectantly" until spontaneous labor occurs, with the use of some form of fetal surveillance; or by selective induction of labor when the cervix is favorable or antepartum testing is nonreassuring.

Questions

1. A postterm pregnancy can be complicted by all of the following *except:*
   A. Oligohydramnios
   B. Neonatal metabolic disturbances
   C. Fetal distress
   D. Hyaline membrane disease
   E. Macrosomia
2. Methods of fetal surveillance for postterm pregnancies not in current use are:
   A. Nonstress test
   B. Serum estriol levels
   C. Contraction stress test
   D. Biophysical profile
   E. Amniotic fluid index

3. Management of a postterm pregnancy may include all of the following *except:*
   A. Amnioinfusion
   B. Cervical ripening
   C. Induction of labor
   D. Antepartum fetal testing
   E. Amnioscopy

Answers

1. D
2. B
3. E

27

Fetal growth abnormalities

APGO LEARNING OBJECTIVE #27

Robert L. Johnson

> *Abnormalities of fetal growth carry increased risks for morbidity and mortality. Monitoring fetal growth is an important aspect of prenatal care and is performed on a regular basis throughout the antepartum period.*

The student will demonstrate a knowledge of the following:

A. Definitions of macrosomia and fetal growth retardation
B. Causes of abnormal growth
C. Methods to detect fetal growth abnormalities
D. Associated morbidity and mortality

Fetal growth abnormalities encompass both extremes of intrauterine development. Intrauterine growth retardation and macrosomia represent these extremes, and each poses a unique risk to mother and fetus. Recognition of normal fetal growth and accretion of fetal tissue is an important component of good obstetric outcome. The normal variation in this growth has contributed to the confusion associated with the diagnosis of growth abnormalities. Expected normal fetal growth, abnormal fetal growth, and methods for detection are discussed.

GESTATIONAL DATING

Although independent observations exist to determine fetal growth asymmetry, no discussion would be complete without gestational dating as a component. Human gestation measured from the first day of the last menstrual period (LMP) to delivery is 280 days ± 14 days. It is prudent to remember that gestational weeks, conceptual weeks, and lunar (months) dating are all different. These unrelated issues frequently lead to confusion in discussions with patients about a delivery date. The discussion should revolve around the

Table 27-1. Estimators for clinical dating of gestation*
1. Last menstrual period
2. Uterine size (early gestation and umbilicus)
3. Audible fetal heart tones
4. Fundal height (late gestation)
5. Quickening (first perception of fetal movement)
6. Positive pregnancy test
*Decreasing predictability from 1 through 6.

Table 27-2. Clinical use of obstetric ultrasound
Gestational dating
Viability
Anomaly detection
Fetal growth
Fetal surgery
Fetal repositioning (external cephalic version)
Amniotic fluid assessment
Fetal motion
Test of fetal well-being (biophysical profile)
Maternal complications of pregnancy

concept of weeks of gestation and the trimester concept of gestational age. Only 5% of pregnancies are delivered on the expected date of confinement (EDC), with 60% being delivered ± 14 days.

The determination of gestational dating may become extremely important when the viability and survival of the fetus are to be discussed with patients. Additionally, other clinical decisions based on gestational age are important in obstetrics. Tools for gestational dating are outlined in Table 27-1.

The LMP remains the most reliable estimator of gestational age. Näegele's rule of EDC is calculated by subtracting 3 from the month of LMP and adding 7 days to the first day of LMP. Multiple variables exist concerning menstrual history. Detailed documentation is required. The first estimate of uterine size and subsequent documentation of uterine growth are important for both gestational dating and subsequent fetal growth. The fundus approaches the umbilicus at 20 weeks and may guide the clinician to early growth or dating problems. Subsequent fundal growth should be recorded with each visit, and a discrepancy of greater than 4 cm from gestational dating using distance from pubic symphysis to fundus should warrant investigation of possible growth abnormalities or dating discrepancy.

Fetal heart tones noted with Doppler ultrasound or fetoscope, quickening (perception of first fetal movement), and early documented hormonal pregnancy testing all can enhance clinical dating. Best dating estimates are 90% ± 3 weeks of EDC.

Ultrasound

Since the 1950s, ultrasound has become a primary tool for assessment of fetal growth, gestational dating, anomaly detection, and fetal well-being. Its biophysics and the imaging principles involved are briefly outlined here.

Ultrasound energy is produced by a transducer, which acts as a generator of sound impulses and a receiver of sound impulses, which are converted to electrical impulses. These impulses are at a high frequency (2-10 MHz). The transducer receives the returning impulse and, depending on the density of the tissue and depth to which it has been transmitted, will convert it to a two-dimensional image using electronic conversion. Therefore bright images (echo-dense) represent tissues of increased density (i.e., bone) and images devoid of echo (echo-lucent) represent areas of less density (i.e., muscle, fat, amniotic fluid, and urine). Total exposure to ultrasound energy during a 15-minute exam may be only 1 second.

Safety of ultrasound was extensively evaluated in 1988 by both the American College of Obstetricians and Gynecologists and the American Institute of Ultrasound in Medicine Bioeffects Committee. Their extensive review stated that no confirmed biologic effects on patients or operators had been found. Therefore the prudent use of ultrasound would indicate a favorable risk/benefit ratio.

The use of ultrasound in pregnancy has unique problems and advantages during each trimester. Errigman and colleagues published a study in 1993 concerning use of ultrasound in low-risk patients (routine antenatal diagnostic imaging with ultrasound [RADIUS] study). It revealed little advantage over routine obstetric care.

The uses of ultrasound in obstetrics are listed in Table 27-2. This discussion is confined to the use of ultrasound to determine abnormalities of fetal growth.

MACROSOMIA

Pathogenesis

Most abnormalities of fetal growth are confined to the last half of pregnancy, particularly the third trimester. Macrosomia is defined as fetal growth above the 90th percentile using population-specific growth curves or estimated fetal weight greater than 4000 g at term. The etiology of macrosomia generally is believed to be multifactorial. Current theories include fetal hyperinsulinemia secondary to increased exposure to transplacental nutrients from the mother. How this mechanism affects fetal growth is not clear. Fetal insulin may alter the metabolic utilization of substrates by enhancing lipogenesis, glycogen synthesis, and protein syntheses. Insulin-like growth factors may be stimulated by the hyperinsulinemia to enhance fetal growth. Further ongoing research is necessary to delineate this complex process.

Perinatal mortality and morbidity in macrosomia may be increased by as much as 2 to 4 times above the average-sized fetus, largely because of birth trauma, asphyxia, stillbirth, and neurologic damage. Therefore the effort to predict macrosomia and establish interventional processes has generated great interest.

Laboratory-diagnostic tests

The diagnosis of macrosomia continues to be both controversial and largely inaccurate. It is readily apparent that diabetic mothers have historically and metabolically been the focus of studies to predict macrosomia reliably. Control of hyperglycemia does not correlate with complete prevention of macrosomia because up to 25% of such patients will still deliver a large-for-gestational-age (LGA) fetus. Therefore, strictly controlled mean maternal glucose does not directly correlate with the risk of macrosomia. Seventeen percent to 25% of well-controlled diabetic mothers still deliver LGA infants. The incidence in the general population is estimated to be 6% to 7%.

Various ultrasonographic and clinical parameters have been used. Previous history of an LGA fetus (greater than 4000 g); previous history of birth trauma (e.g., shoulder dystocia); previous history of cesarean section for perceived LGA fetus for failure to progress; previous history of gestational diabetes; maternal obesity; or such less specific findings as polyhydramnios and stillbirth should alert the care provider to follow the progression of fetal growth closely in a subsequent pregnancy.

Again, well-documented gestational dating and clinical evaluation of fetal size with fundal height and Leopold's maneuvers may signal the need for further investigation.

Various ultrasonographic measurements have been used with less than optimal results. Table 27-3 displays commonly used ultrasonographic measurements to attempt prediction of macrosomia.

Table 27-3. Ultrasonographic measurements

BPD	Biparietal diameter
HC	Head circumference
AC	Abdominal circumference
HC/AC	Head circumference/abdominal circumference ratio
HC/TC	Head circumference/thoracic circumference ratio
EFW	Estimated fetal weight
FL	Femur length

Table 27-4. Risk factors for shoulder dystocia

Diabetes
Postterm pregnancy
Maternal obesity
Previous shoulder dystocia
Abnormal labor
Arrest of labor
Midpelvic delivery
Macrosomia
Oxytocin

Management

Antepartum recognition of macrosomia trending would necessitate screening for gestational diabetes. Other causes such as endocrine or constitutional abnormalities should be investigated.

Intrapartum management of suspected macrosomia relies heavily on the clinical observation of the "conduct of labor." Friedman and colleagues described the conduct of labor in both nulliparas and multiparas. Macrosomia fetuses may not proceed along a normal labor curve such as 1 to 1.5 cm/hr in dilatation and descent of the presenting part. Frequently with complete dilatation and pushing in the second stage, descent of the presenting part is accomplished only with

expulsive effort but returns to the original station after the contraction. A common clinical trap occurs when the temptation to perform operative vaginal delivery overcomes good judgment. Shoulder dystocia and its attendant complications then ensue.

Shoulder dystocia occurs more frequently in fetuses 4000 g or larger in pregnancies complicated by gestational diabetes and in fetuses larger than 4500 g in nondiabetic mothers. Risk factors are listed in Table 27-4. Cesarean delivery may be prudent in these situations, and each patient care plan must be individualized.

GROWTH RESTRICTION OR INTRAUTERINE GROWTH RETARDATION

Pathogenesis

The three strongest predictors of infant birth weight, after length of gestation, are gestational weight gain, pregravid weight, and previous history of growth restrictions. Pathologic decrease in fetal growth less than the 10th percentile is defined as growth restriction (GR), or intrauterine growth retardation. Approximately 5% of pregnancies are affected, and a marked increase in morbidity and mortality has been documented repeatedly. Clinically, serial decline in fundal growth should alert the clinician to investigate further if no other risk factors are present. Risk factors may be maternal, fetal, or uteroplacental. Table 27-5 lists the most common causes. It is important to note that 50% of cases have no cause identified.

Laboratory-diagnostic tests

Ultrasound remains an important technique to evaluate abnormal fetal growth. No reliable in utero method has been described to estimate the ponderal index; therefore other measurements as previously described are used.

Table 27-5. Causes of fetal growth retardation

Maternal	Fetal	Uteroplacental
Drugs	Infections (e.g., viral, protozoan)	Placental abruptions
Smoking	Genetic and chromosomal disorders	Placenta previa
Malnutrition	Congenital anomalies	Multiple gestation
Alcohol		Müllerian anomalies
Diabetes mellitus		Marginal cord insertion
Connective tissue disease		
Prepregnancy weight <50 kg		
Hypertension (chronic)		
Chronic maternal diseases (e.g., cyanotic heart disease)		

$$\text{Ponderal index (PI)} = \frac{\text{Birthweight} \times 100}{\text{Crown} - \text{Heel length}}$$

Biparietal diameter (BPD) either singularly or serially is a poor predictor of GR. Transverse cerebellar diameters have been a valuable tool when correlated with other findings, including femur length to abdominal circumference ratio, FL/AC. The best single indicator of GR is abdominal circumference (AC). It also has the largest intraobserver variation. The decrease in AC may correlate with poor intrahepatic glycogen storage. Varying methods using AC have been evaluated, including BPD/AC, FL/AC, and head circumference (HC)/AC. The ratio of FL/AC is age-independent and may be helpful if gestational age is unknown. Since after 21 weeks' gestation a constant value of 22% ± 2% is normal, increased values (greater than 23.5%) indicate likely GR and should be considered abnormal.

Amniotic fluid volume (AFV) is an important observation because a marked decrease in AFV has a positive predictive value of approximately 90%. This is important because perinatal morbidity and mortality increase as AFV decreases.

Ultrasonography has enabled classifications of GR. Two major categories, symmetric and asymmetric GR, have been described based on certain characteristics.

SYMMETRIC GROWTH RESTRICTION. Symmetric GR usually begins early in gestation, and generally the entire fetus is small for gestational age. This represents approximately 20% to 30% of GR fetuses. This abnormality carries a guarded prognosis since major fetal and neonatal complications have been associated (e.g., viral infections, chromosomal and genetic disorders). Chromosomal aneuploidy may be as high as 25%. Generally, when symmetric GR is suspected the patient and her family should be counseled concerning the need for chorionic villus sampling, amniocentesis, or percutaneous umbilical blood sampling to evaluate fetal karyotype and viral studies. Additional consultation may be necessary for studies to evaluate skeletal dysplasia (dwarfism).

ASYMMETRIC GROWTH RESTRICTION. Asymmetric GR usually is associated with decreased placental function, termed *uteroplacental insufficiency*. This form represents 70% to 80% of GR and is characterized by late gestational onset (greater than 28 weeks), greater BPD/AC ratio, and low AFV. Decreased AFV is associated with redistribution of renal fetal blood flow and decreased fetal urine output. Chronic maternal diseases such as hypertension, renal disease, and collagen vascular disease commonlyare present. Perinatal mortality is increased 5 to 10 times in this clinical setting.

Management

Once fetal GR has been diagnosed, the possibility of intrauterine hypoxia and fetal death must be considered. It is prudent to begin to formulate a care plan that includes therapies to correct fetal growth (e.g., chronic oxygen, reduced-dose aspirin, and immersion therapy). Serial sonography should be done for measurement of interval growth and AFVs. Antenatal fetal monitor testing including nonstress testing and biophysical profiles usually are done.

If slow or almost absent growth and documented fetal lung maturity have been established, delivery should be strongly considered. If the amniotic fluid becomes abnormal, delivery is also indicated.

Intrapartum precautions for possible fetal intolerance to labor should be anticipated. Electronic fetal monitoring, amnioinfusion, preparation for cesarean section, and oxygen therapy are routinely used.

CRITICAL POINTS

- Careful determination of gestational age is important in fetal growth analysis.
- *Macrosomia* is a defined fetal perinatal morbidity; mortality increases 2 to 4 times above the average-size fetus in macrosomia.
- The triad of an LGA fetus, second stage arrest of descent of fetus, and operative vaginal delivery mark an increase in the risk of shoulder dystocia.
- *Growth restriction* is defined as fetal growth less than the 10th percentile.
- Symmetric and asymmetric GR represent separate, unique problems for clinical management.
- Asymmetric GR increases perinatal mortality 5 to 10 times above normal.
- Symmetric GR has been associated with chromosomal abnormalities.

Questions

1. The most reliable estimator of gestational age is:
   A. Uterine size
   B. Crown-rump fetal length
   C. Last menstrual period
   D. Quickening
2. Fetal growth hormone is:
   A. Human chorionic gonadotropin
   B. Human placental lactogen
   C. Insulin
   D. Thyroxine
3. The most reliable indicator of fetal GR is:
   A. Biparietal diameter
   B. Fetal length/abdominal circumference ratio
   C. Abdominal circumference
   D. Biparietal diameter/abdominal circumference ratio
4. Symmetric GR is associated with all of the following *except:*
   A. Genetic disorders
   B. Viral infections
   C. Dwarfism
   D. Uteroplacental insufficiency

5. Possible maternal therapy that has improved
   fetal growth includes:
   A. Oxygen
   B. Low-dose aspirin
   C. Immersion therapy
   D. Restricted activity
   E. All of the above

Answers

1. C
2. C
3. C
4. D
5. E

Obstetric procedures

28

APGO LEARNING OBJECTIVE #28

Thomas H. Strong, Jr.

Knowledge of obstetric procedures is basic to management and counseling of the pregnant patient.

The student will demonstrate a knowledge of the following procedures:

A. Ultrasound
B. Amniocentesis and cordocentesis
C. Chorionic villus sampling
D. Antepartum fetal assessment
E. Induction and augmentation of labor
F. Fetal monitoring
G. Spontaneous vaginal delivery
H. Episiotomy
I. Forceps delivery
J. Vacuum-assisted delivery
K. Breech delivery
L. Cesarean delivery
M. Vaginal birth after cesarean delivery
N. Newborn circumcision

Knowledge of certain obstetric procedures is fundamental to successful management and counseling of the pregnant patient. An overview of this broad subject is presented in this chapter.

ULTRASOUND

The safety of diagnostic ultrasound has long been a major theoretic concern for obstetricians. However, available data suggest that all teratogenic effects attributable to ultrasound occur at energy levels far beyond those used for routine diagnostic imaging. No adverse fetal effects have been reported with diagnostic ultrasound in humans.

First trimester pregnancy detection is one of the most common indications for obstetric ultrasound. Early ultrasonographic assessment is of vital importance when differentiating between intrauterine and ectopic gestations. By transabdominal ultrasound a gestational sac should be visible 6 weeks after the last normal menstrual period. Generally, transvaginal ultrasound will detect pregnancy landmarks 1 week earlier than will the transabdominal modality. A properly performed fetal crown-rump measurement provides the single most accurate sonographic estimation of gestational age, having a margin of error of less than 5 days. Although fetal anatomic imaging is quite limited early in pregnancy, certain severe fetal anomalies (anencephaly, cystic hygroma, omphalocele, and gastroschisis) occasionally may be detected. Early pregnancy ultrasound is also useful for identifying maternal uterine abnormalities. Additionally, cervical length may be measured and lost intrauterine devices located with this modality.

Fetal anatomic assessment is an integral part of second and third trimester ultrasonography and includes evaluation of the fetal head, spine, chest, heart, abdomen, and extremities. Additionally, amniotic fluid volume quantitation, intrauterine growth assessment, placental location, and identification of multiple gestations may be accomplished. Later in pregnancy, accurate prediction of fetal weight can assist clinical management. Moreover, ultrasound may be used as an adjunct for various other surveillance modalities (amniocentesis, chorionic villus sampling, percutaneous umbilical blood sampling, biophysical profile assessment, and so on).

AMNIOCENTESIS, CHORIONIC VILLUS SAMPLING, AND CORDOCENTESIS

For genetic analysis, amniocentesis generally is performed around 15 weeks' gestation. It involves sonographic guidance of a needle into the amniotic space and withdrawal of amniotic fluid for karyotypic, enzymatic, or deoxyribonucleic acid (DNA) analysis. Additionally, amniotic fluid may be evaluated for α-fetoprotein or acetylcholinesterase when evaluating the fetus for possible neural tube defects. With sonographic guidance, the risk of spontaneous abortion from this procedure is generally less than 1%. Amniocentesis performed late in the third trimester of pregnancy can be used to determine fetal lung maturity status, to diagnose intrauterine infection, or to administer medications directly into the amniotic fluid.

Chorionic villus sampling (CVS) generally is performed between 8 and 11 weeks' gestation. It involves transcervical passage of a flexible catheter into the placental bed under sonographic guidance. Using gentle suction, 10 to 25 mg of chorionic villi are aspirated for karyotypic, enzymatic, or DNA analysis. Chorionic villus sampling is not useful for diagnosing neural tube defects. The major advantage of CVS over amniocentesis relates to the earlier point in gestation when the test may be performed, and the concomitant earlier availability of results. Chorionic villus sampling may be associated with increased risk for fetal loss and distal limb reduction abnormalities.

Percutaneous umbilical blood sampling  (PUBS) involves sonographically guided phlebotomy of the umbilical blood vessels. Using this modality, the results of karyotypic analysis generally are available within 3 to 4 days. Likewise, PUBS may be used to evaluate fetal metabolic processes, acid-base status, hematocrit, and platelet count. Additionally, blood products and a wide range of medications may be administered directly to the fetus. It appears that PUBS is associated with a 2% to 3% risk of significant hemorrhage and a lesser risk from fetal trauma or infection.

ANTEPARTUM FETAL ASSESSMENT

Most fetal compromise and death occurs before the onset of labor. Therefore the goal of antepartum fetal surveillance is to prevent stillbirths in high-risk pregnancies. Antepartum fetal heart rate (FHR) testing was derived from experience gained with intrapartum FHR monitoring. The prototypical antepartum FHR test, the oxytocin challenge test, used the notion of intermittent, controlled stress to evaluate placental reserve. Insufficient reserve frequently presents as "late" FHR decelerations in response to spontaneous or evoked uterine contractions. (See the section Fetal Monitoring later in this chapter.) With at least three uterine contractions (each of at least 40 seconds' duration) within a given 10-minute period, a contraction stress test (CST) has been achieved. A CST is interpreted as negative (reassuring) when there are no late decelerations during the entire test. A positive CST is noted when there are persistent late decelerations with uterine contractions. The CST is considered equivocal when there are nonpersistent late decelerations. The CST can be falsely positive in the setting of uterine hyperstimulation (more than five contractions in a given 10-minute period or with individual contractions lasting longer than 90 seconds). An unsatisfactory CST occurs when the frequency of uterine contractions is lower than three per 10-minute window. A negative CST is very reassuring and is associated with an extremely low incidence of fetal death during the ensuing 7 days. Therefore the CST is repeated weekly until delivery in high-risk pregnancies. A positive CST strongly suggests that the fetus is at risk for compromise or death. Contraindications to CST include placenta previa, preterm premature rupture of the membranes, multiple gestations, incompetent cervix, polyhydramnios, prior classic cesarean section, or preterm labor.

Nonstress testing

The occurrence of FHR accelerations in response to fetal movement is predictive of fetal well-being and provides the basis for nonstress testing. The nonstress test (NST) has become the most commonly used antepartum FHR test. In contrast to the CST, uterine contractions are not necessary for NST. At many institutions, the NST is the primary surveillance technique, with CST or biophysical profiling reserved as back-up tests. A reactive (reassuring) NST is defined as the presence of two FHR accelerations of 15 beats/min or greater above the baseline that last at least 15 seconds during a 20-minute observation period. If the above criteria are not satisfied during two successive 20-minute windows, the NST is considered nonreactive and a back-up test is indicated.

The NST is repeated every 3 to 4 days in high-risk pregnancies.

Biophysical profile   *"Test the Baby, MAN"*

Most antepartum fetal assessment tools evaluate a single biophysical parameter (i.e., FHR). With ultrasonography, however, assessment of multiple fetal biophysical features such as fetal breathing and body movement is possible. The biophysical profile (BPP) is essentially a fetal physical examination. The BPP has five components: fetal breathing activity, gross fetal body movement, fetal tone, FHR reactivity, and amniotic fluid volume (AFV). With the exception of AFV, the components of the BPP are considered to be markers of acute acidemia and hypoxemia. The AFV is a marker for chronic hypoxia. Because multiple markers of fetal well-being are evaluated during the BPP, it is considered a more reliable test than the NST or CST alone. As FHR reactivity is the most sensitive biophysical component of fetal assessment, it has been combined with AFV assessment (i.e., a marker for chronic hypoxia) at some institutions as a "modified" biophysical profile (MBPP). This test appears to be comparable to the CST and full BPP for predicting fetal well-being and has the advantage of being more easily and rapidly administered than either modality. Like the NST, the BPP (or MBPP) is repeated every 3 to 4 days in high-risk pregnancies.

Doppler velocimetry

Doppler velocimetric analysis evaluates the adequacy of organ perfusion in the fetus. Using this technique, umbilical, fetal aortic, cerebral, and renal arterial blood flow analyses have been accomplished. Despite the controversy surrounding the usefulness of this technique, there appears to be agreement regarding the poor prognosis associated with absent or reversed umbilical blood flow during fetal diastole. Absent or reversed end-diastolic flow is an infrequent but worrisome finding associated with perinatal mortality rates approaching 90% in some reports. Nevertheless, Doppler velocimetry is not presently considered a primary fetal surveillance tool.

INDUCTION AND AUGMENTATION OF LABOR

Labor induction is the initiation of regular uterine contractions before the onset of spontaneous labor. It may be accomplished by various medical or minor surgical techniques. Labor induction is indicated when the benefits of delivery outweigh the risks of ongoing pregnancy. Obstetric indications for labor induction include chorioamnionitis, chronic hypertension, gestational diabetes, isoimmunization, preeclampsia-eclampsia, premature rupture of the membranes, or fetal death. In general, any contraindication to vaginal delivery is a contraindication to labor induction. This includes any uterine incision other than a low-segment incision, severe maternal pelvic abnormalities, certain fetal anomalies (e.g., massive hydrocephaly), placenta previa, or active herpetic infection of the genital tract. One may predict the ease of induction by evaluating the cervix before induction. With increasing effacement and dilatation of the cervix, the likelihood for a successful induction increases. Similarly, as the consistency of the cervix softens and the station of the presenting part becomes progressively lower, the odds for successful induction increase. Application of synthetic prostaglandin derivatives to the cervix before labor induction frequently softens the cervical stroma, thereby improving the prospects that induced uterine contractions will successfully produce progressive cervical dilatation. Because these compounds occasionally are associated with uterine hyperactivity, they should be used under strict protocols and with appropriate medical supervision.

Oxytocin stimulates myometrial contraction. When this hormone is used in conjunction with amniotomy, regular uterine contractions may be produced. The most reliable and predictable results from labor induction occur when a dilute solution of oxytocin is delivered via continuous intravenous infusion. The infusion rate is gradually increased until uterine contractions lasting 60 to 90 seconds occur every 2 to 3 minutes. Because oxytocin infusion may be associated with uterine hyperstimulation, fetal distress, placental abruption, or uterine rupture, monitoring of uterine activity and FHR is mandatory throughout labor induction.

Labor augmentation involves all of the above-mentioned techniques. However, as the name implies, these techniques are used to modify ongoing uterine contractions. Generally, labor augmentation is performed when uterine contractions are of insufficient frequency to produce cervical dilatation.

FETAL MONITORING

Although the use of continuous intrapartum electronic FHR monitoring has become a standard of care, evidence is accumulating that this modality may be no more efficacious than intermittent FHR auscultation for preventing permanent fetal compromise. Nevertheless, familiarity with this modality is necessary for all obstetricians because of its widespread use.

Three features of the intrapartum FHR tracing are important for assessing fetal well-being: baseline FHR, variability-reactivity of the baseline FHR, and periodic FHR changes. The normal baseline FHR is between 120 and 160 beats/min. Reassuring FHR variability or reactivity suggests an intact, coordinated neural pathway between and including the central nervous system and heart. Reassuring beat-to-beat FHR variability (greater than 5 beats/min) and/or reactivity (repetitive FHR accelerations of 15 beats/min or greater for at least 15 seconds) signifies that the fetal nervous system is functioning normally. Recurring or sustained hypoxic insults will eventually produce asphyxia and the variability-reactivity will decrease or disappear. Periodic changes in the baseline FHR relate to any alteration in the baseline FHR that occurs in concert with uterine contraction. Worrisome periodic changes include late and variable FHR decelerations. The late deceleration is so named because its onset follows the onset of myometrial contraction. This type of deceleration has a gradual onset and resolution and has a uniformly smooth contour; it represents fetal hypoxemia secondary to insufficient gas exchange within the uteroplacental unit. On the other hand, a variable FHR deceleration is of variable shape and timing. Variable decelerations are the result of umbilical cord compression.

Fetal distress is a process that can manifest itself with a wide range of subtlety. In many cases, even ominous intrapartum FHR tracings will be associated with good intrapartum outcomes. This is so because electronic FHR monitoring is much less effective at predicting fetal compromise than fetal well-being. Early recognition and treatment of fetal distress patterns is the aim of the obstetrician. He or she must be able to differentiate reassuring from ominous FHR patterns and implement the proper timing and method of delivery to ensure optimal maternal and fetal outcome.

SPONTANEOUS VAGINAL DELIVERY

No other time during pregnancy carries greater morbidity and mortality than the peripartum period. It is also a time of considerable emotional and physical stress. For successful delivery, the cervix must become compliant and ultimately must dilate sufficiently to allow fetal passage. Physiologic preparation for this process generally begins early in the third trimester. The gravida will detect occasional uterine contractions during this period. Several weeks before the onset of labor, the mother may note that the fetus has settled into the pelvis. This phenomenon is particularly common among nulligravid patients. One to 2 weeks before the onset of labor, the mother may demonstrate

"bloody show," the passage of blood-stained cervical mucus. The release of the mucus plug usually indicates that the cervix has begun gradually to dilate and efface.

The vast majority of gravidas spontaneously initiate labor between 38 and 42 weeks' gestation. Frequently, however, the mother will experience episodes of nonprogressive or "false" labor. Distinguishing between true and false labor can be frustrating for both patient and obstetrician. The contractions associated with false labor usually are irregular and not painful. In many cases the patient experiences discomfort in her lower back with false labor. The uterine contractions associated with false labor are less frequent and of shorter duration than those noted with true labor.

When a patient presents with painful, regular uterine contractions lasting more than 45 seconds and cervical dilatation in excess of 3 cm, it may be presumed that she is in labor. The patient should be assessed with regard to fetal membrane status, fetal presentation, frequency of contractions, cervical dilatation and effacement, station of the presenting fetal part, estimated fetal weight, maternal vital signs, and FHR tracing (if electronic fetal monitoring is being used).

Labor is divided into three distinct stages. The first stage begins with the first true labor pain and ends with complete dilatation of the cervix. Because identification of the actual onset of true labor is unreliable, determination of the exact length of the first stage frequently amounts to an estimation. The second stage of labor begins with complete dilatation of the cervix and ends with delivery of the fetus. The third stage of labor begins with delivery of the fetus and ends with delivery of the placenta. The third stage of labor is fraught with many risks, postpartum hemorrhage being the most common. (See Chapter 22, Postpartum Hemorrhage.) The first two stages of labor comprise what have traditionally been known as the six cardinal movements of labor:

1. *Engagement.* Entry of the fetal head into the maternal pelvis. Engagement is considered

to have occurred when the lowermost aspect of the fetal head passes the maternal ischial spines. This point defines a "zero station" during digital examination of the birth canal.

2. *Descent.* Further passage of the fetus into and through the pelvis.
3. *Flexion.* Flexion of the fetal neck as it negotiates the maternal pelvis.
4. *Internal rotation.* Rotation of the fetal head into a transverse position so that its occipitofrontal diameter occupies the widest diameter of the maternal pelvis.
5. *Extension.* Extension of the fetal neck so that the fetal head successfully passes underneath and around the maternal pubic bone.
6. *External rotation.* Rotation of the fetal head into the position it occupied before entering the maternal pelvis. This is frequently referred to as "restitution."

Once a patient has reached 4 cm of cervical dilatation, she is in active labor. Thereafter the rate of dilatation should follow a relatively predictable course. Similarly, the presenting fetal part should progress downward through the birth canal at a predictable rate. Failure to maintain a minimal rate of labor progression warrants a search for underlying causes. In this circumstance the risk of dystocia is increased considerably.

As the fetal head comes to occupy the vaginal vault, the tissue of the maternal perineum attenuates. Dilatation and eversion of the rectum may be noted. At this point the mother frequently feels the urge to defecate. As the occiput of the fetal head protrudes from the maternal perineum, the fetus is said to be "crowning." Once crowning has occurred, delivery is imminent. If necessary, an episiotomy should be performed at this point. Thereafter the fetal head is eased over the perineum, and delivery is effected in concert with maternal pushing efforts. It is important to prevent the fetal head from bursting out of the perineum. By gradually assisting passage of the fetal head over the perineal body, sudden decompression of the head is averted, thereby minimizing the risk of intracranial hemorrhage.

On delivery of the fetal head, the nose and mouth of the infant are rapidly but gently suctioned. Application of steady, downward traction to the fetal head and neck allows the anterior fetal shoulder to clear the maternal pubic bone. Traction is then applied in an upward direction to facilitate delivery of the posterior shoulder. Once the shoulders have cleared the perineum, the rest of the fetus is delivered quite quickly. Care must be taken to avoid dropping the slippery neonate once the shoulders have delivered.

After delivery the neonatal head is held slightly lower than the trunk to allow drainage of fluids from the pharynx and upper airways. The cord is doubly clamped, then severed. The child is handed to the neonatal attendant for assessment and clothing. Alternatively, the neonate may be temporarily placed on the mother's abdomen if the child appears to be breathing well and has good color. During the third stage of labor, up to 30 minutes may pass before delivery of the placenta. Care must be taken to avoid placing undue traction on the umbilical cord as it protrudes from the parturient's vagina. Excessive tugging on the cord may result in avulsion from the placenta. Unwarranted pulling before placental separation from the uterus has occurred may result in potentially fatal eversion of the uterus.

Complete detachment of the placenta from its uterine implantation site is heralded by a gush of blood from the vagina, sudden lengthening of the protruding umbilical cord, and detection of a globular uterine configuration as it is palpated through the maternal abdomen. The placenta is frequently detected in the vaginal vault at this point. On delivery of the placenta, gentle uterine massage in concert with a dilute intravenous infusion of oxytocin (10 to 20 U/L) promotes sufficient contraction of the uterus to minimize further blood loss. After ensuring adequate maternal hemostasis, the placenta should be carefully inspected to ensure that no cotyledons or membranes have been retained in the uterus or birth canal. The placenta also should be inspected for anatomic abnormalities. Finally, the cervix, vagina, and perineum should be carefully examined for lacerations. The episiotomy and all clinically significant lacerations should be repaired. Only absorbable sutures should be placed. Before suture placement, adequate maternal anesthesia should be administered.

EPISIOTOMY

Episiotomy, incision of the perineum, is the most frequently performed operative procedure in obstetrics. When performing an episiotomy, the intent is to reduce the risk of severe perineal laceration during vaginal delivery. Generally, it is thought to be easier to repair a surgical incision of the perineum than to repair a large, sometimes jagged laceration. The procedure is generally performed under anesthesia (local, pudendal, or regional block).

An episiotomy is performed just before delivery of the fetal head. Premature episiotomy sometimes can result in excessive perineal bleeding. A midline episiotomy is the preferred incision. The procedure is performed with straight-blade scissors. The vaginal mucosa and perineum are cut to a point just anterior to the rectal sphincter. This type of episiotomy is easy to repair and is associated with less postoperative pain than are other varieties.

After delivery, the episiotomy is repaired with absorbable sutures. The incision is closed in layers. To avoid the risk of fistula formation, care must be taken that the sutures do not enter the rectal mucosa. Postoperatively, ice packs and oral analgesia are indicated. By the first postpartum day, sitz baths also may be used. If the rectal sphincter or mucosa were entered, stool softeners are warranted. Hematomas occasionally may develop in the perineal body if hemostasis was incomplete at the time of episiotomy repair. Wound infection and breakdown are infrequent. Secondary repair usually is quite difficult in this circumstance.

FORCEPS AND VACUUM-ASSISTED DELIVERIES

Obstetric forceps

For various reasons forceps delivery has become uncommon. However, elective forceps deliveries are still used to shorten the second stage of labor. Forceps delivery frequently is indicated with maternal cardiac disease or other circumstances where prolonged maternal pushing efforts are not advisable. Appropriate use of forceps necessitates an appreciation of the patient's pelvic architecture as well as fetal size, station, and head position. Additionally, adequate maternal anesthesia must be in effect before forceps application.

The three general types of forceps procedures are outlet forceps, low-forceps, and midforceps deliveries. When the fetal head is at the perineum and the scalp is visible at the introitus between uterine contractions, forceps application is of the outlet variety. It does not appear that proper outlet forceps application and execution increase fetal morbidity. Low-forceps delivery occurs when forceps are placed with the fetal vertex at a + 2 station. Midforceps application occurs when the fetal head is above a + 2 station. Frequently some degree of fetal head rotation (i.e., restitution) is necessary during midforceps delivery. Although fewer midforceps deliveries are being done in contemporary obstetric practices, their use may be appropriate if there is sudden fetal distress or maternal compromise and a cesarean delivery cannot be performed immediately.

A number of complications can arise from forceps deliveries, including vaginal, cervical, or perineal lacerations. Improperly used forceps also may cause various fetal head, face, or neck injuries.

Vacuum extraction

Application of a soft, plastic suction device to the fetal vertex frequently facilitates vaginal delivery by allowing the obstetrician to apply traction to the fetal head in concert with maternal expulsive efforts. Because a significant negative pressure is created by the suction device, a relatively large area of localized swelling may be created on the fetal occiput. Intracranial bleeding, retinal hemorrhage, cephalohematoma, and soft tissue laceration have occurred with vacuum extraction. Nevertheless, most consider vacuum extraction to be less risky than forceps delivery in the term gestation. Moreover, proficiency at vacuum extraction is gained much more readily than is proficiency with forceps, thereby making the technique accessible to a wider range of care givers.

BREECH DELIVERY

Breech presentation occurs in approximately 3% of term pregnancies. Owing to an increased incidence of perinatal complications, vaginal delivery of a breech-presenting fetus is permitted infrequently by contemporary obstetricians. Some degree of molding of the fetal head is necessary to permit its passage through the birth canal. However, the head of a breech-presenting fetus enters the maternal pelvis in a way that may not allow sufficient molding to occur. Additionally, delivery of a breech-presenting fetus results in the delivery of fetal parts that are sequentially less compressible (i.e., the fetal trunk precedes the fetal head), especially among preterm fetuses secondary to the significant discrepancy between the size of the fetal head and abdomen. In this setting, the body may easily deliver through the maternal pelvis and cervix only to have the relatively larger fetal head become entrapped. As a result, delivery may be unduly delayed and result in fetal hypoxia and acidosis. Additionally, the potential for fetal birth trauma may be increased. The risk for umbilical cord prolapse is also increased in breech presentation.

There are three varieties of breech presentation: frank, complete, and footling. A *frank* breech presentation occurs when the fetal legs are flexed onto the fetal chest and abdomen. This type of breech presentation is associated with the best prognosis for vaginal delivery. A *complete* breech presentation is present when the fetal legs are crossed in front of the fetus. A *footling* breech presentation occurs when one or both of the fetal legs are extended in such a fashion that they precede the fetal body through the cervical os. This type of breech presentation is associated with a particularly increased risk of umbilical cord prolapse.

Attempted vaginal delivery of a breech-presenting fetus may be attempted if certain strict criteria are rigidly followed. These include adequate maternal pelvimetry, fetal gestational age of 35 weeks or greater, fetal weight less than 8 lb, delivery staff experienced and skilled at breech delivery, access to appropriate anesthesia, and informed consent of the gravida. Even when all criteria are fulfilled, evidence suggests that the outcome for breech-presenting fetuses is not always as satisfactory as that of breech-presenting fetuses delivered by cesarean section.

CESAREAN DELIVERY

The cesarean delivery rate in the United States has increased considerably over the last 20 years. Fetal and maternal indications for this procedure have increased accordingly. At present, the cesarean delivery rate is between 20% and 25%. The most common indications for cesarean delivery include dystocia, fetal distress, and malpresentation. Despite a growing body of data that suggests that vaginal birth after cesarean section (VBAC) is a safe and reasonable option, many repeat cesarean deliveries continue to be performed.

The appropriate use of anesthesia during a cesarean delivery is a function of the indication for operative delivery as well as the maternal and fetal condition. Although increasingly less common, general anesthesia allows the physician to rapidly induce surgical levels of anesthesia for rapid cesarean delivery (e.g., with fetal distress, torrential obstetric hemorrhage). Fetal depression can occur with general anesthesia, especially when the interval between skin incision to delivery is unduly long. General anesthesia also is associated with an increased risk of maternal aspiration. Moreover, abrupt increases in blood pressure can occur during intubation, something to be considered when using this type of anesthesia on hypertensive gravidas.

There are two types of regional anesthesia: spinal (subarachnoid) and epidural blocks. With spinal anesthesia the subarachnoid space is entered and a local anesthetic is injected. Complications of spinal anesthesia include hypotension, total spinal block, and postanesthesia headache. The risk of hypotension can be reduced by pre-induction intravenous hydration. Should hypotension develop, intravenous administration of ephedrine may return maternal blood pressure into a normal range. Epidural anesthesia has become the most commonly used anesthetic modality for cesarean delivery. Epidural anesthesia has a lower frequency of complications than spinal anesthesia and has the extra advantage that the mother does not lose motor function in the anesthetized area. Moreover, a catheter may be left in the epidural space for continuous, precise delivery of anesthesia.

Most cesarean procedures use an incision placed transversely in the lower aspect of the uterus. This type of incision generally is associated with excellent healing and minimal blood loss. A gravida who has this uterine incision is generally considered a good candidate for a subsequent attempt at vaginal birth. The "classic" uterine incision is a midline incision running from the inferior aspect of the uterus into the fundus. It involves the thickest, most vascular part of the myometrium and is associated with poor wound healing and heavy bleeding. The woman who undergoes a classic cesarean delivery will require repeat cesarean delivery for all subsequent pregnancies.

Complications

The most common complication during cesarean delivery is excessive uterine hemorrhage.

Moreover, the proximity of the urinary and gastrointestinal tracts places them at relatively high risk for intraoperative injury, with the bladder being the most frequently involved site. The risk of intraoperative injury increases in gravidas who have had multiple laparotomies.

Because it is performed in an area of the body that is potentially contaminated, cesarean delivery is associated with a high rate of infection. In the absence of antibiotic prophylaxis, the incidence of postoperative endometritis may approach 85% at some institutions. Postoperative wound infection is another relatively common complication of surgery. Prophylactic antibiotics at the time of cesarean delivery may reduce the risk of endometritis and wound infection. Generally, one to three doses are given following clamping of the umbilical cord at delivery. As with any patient undergoing abdominal surgery, women recovering from cesarean delivery are at increased risk for atelectasis, pneumonia, postoperative ileus, urinary tract infection, bowel obstruction, and thromboembolic phenomena.

VAGINAL BIRTH AFTER CESAREAN DELIVERY

Owing to the anatomic alterations and scar tissue formation that occur after cesarean delivery, repeat cesarean delivery is fraught with risk. An increasing body of data suggests that VBAC is associated with a very low risk for uterine scar disruption. As a result, the indications for VBAC have become progressively broader. Most studies of VBAC note an overall success rate of 70% to 80%. With growing experience, the use of oxytocin, epidural anesthesia, and cervical ripening with prostaglandin preparations do not appear to be unwarranted in the mother who has had a prior cesarean delivery. The one requirement that has remained constant when considering a patient for VBAC is that the patient's previous uterine incisions be of the transverse, lower uterine segment variety. As mentioned previously, this type of uterine incision appears to provide the greatest resistance to uterine scar disruption during labor. See Chapter 17, Abnormal Labor, for a more complete discussion.

NEWBORN CIRCUMCISION

Once performed on a widespread, routine basis, there is no longer any absolute indication for newborn circumcision. Commonly claimed benefits for newborn circumcision include the reduction of phimosis, balanitis, and penile cancer. If circumcision is planned, it is best performed 1 to 2 days following birth after the health and stability of the neonate have been demonstrated. Contraindications include neonatal coagulopathy, illness, prematurity, or congenital abnormalities of the penis. Some note that among males who do not undergo neonatal circumcision, 5% to 10% will eventually develop medical indications for the procedure.

⌐ CRITICAL POINTS ⌐

- First trimester crown-rump measurement provides the single most accurate sonographic estimation of gestational age.
- Generally, CVS is performed between 8 and 11 weeks of gestation.
- Most cases of fetal compromise and death occur before the onset of labor.
- Oxytocin induction-augmentation seeks to produce uterine contractions lasting 60 to 90 seconds that occur every 2 to 3 minutes.
- Reassuring FHR reactivity-variability suggests an intact, coordinated neural pathway between and including the fetal central nervous system and heart.
- The active phase of labor begins at roughly 4 cm of cervical dilatation.
- A midline episiotomy is the preferred type.
- The most common indications for cesarean delivery are dystocia, fetal distress, and malpresentation.
- Candidates for VBAC ideally should have had previous uterine incisions of the transverse, lower uterine segment variety.
- There is no longer any absolute indication for newborn circumcision.

Questions

1. Nonstress testing is:
   A. An effective intrapartum test of fetal well-being
   B. Dependent on uterine contractions
   C. No longer in widespread use
   D. The primary antepartum fetal surveillance modality at most institutions
   E. Contraindicated in the setting of ruptured fetal membranes

2. Epidural anesthesia during labor:
   A. Is associated with neonatal depression
   B. May provoke hypertensive crisis in preeclamptic patients
   C. Is the preferred form of intrapartum anesthesia
   D. Results in temporary loss of maternal motor function
   E. Is more risky than general anesthesia

3. Vaginal birth after cesarean section is:
   A. Overused in some parts of the country

B. Associated with an overall success rate of 70% to 80%
C. Somewhat riskier to the mother than is repeat cesarean delivery
D. Contraindicated with preterm labor and delivery
E. Not appropriate if the parturient has amnionitis

4. The second stage of labor:
A. Begins with delivery of the fetus and ends with delivery of the placenta
B. Begins with complete dilatation of the cervix and ends with the delivery of the fetus
C. Begins with complete dilatation of the cervix and ends with delivery of the placenta
D. Begins with delivery of the placenta and ends with ovulation

Answers

1. D
2. C
3. B
4. B

Gynecology

29

Contraception

APGO LEARNING OBJECTIVE #29

John H. Mattox

Primary care physicians are frequently called upon to provide counseling regarding methods of contraception. An understanding of the medical, as well as the personal, issues involved in a couple's decisions concerning contraceptive methods is necessary to adequately advise these patients.

The student will demonstrate a knowledge of the following:
A. Physiologic or pharmacologic basis of action of the basic methods of contraception
B. Effectiveness
C. Benefits and risks
D. Financial considerations

Increasing social and economic demands make it essential that each individual reach a decision as to when pregnancy is appropriate and the number of children for which they can assume responsibility. Providers, family-planning clinics, and government social agencies share the responsibility for making effective and appropriate contraceptive methods available to those who want them.

Physicians should introduce the subject of contraception during any office encounter with every patient in the reproductive age range. Unless the subject is introduced by the physician, some patients may remain undecided, or an unintended pregnancy could occur. Physicians who choose not to provide contraception for their patients should refer them to another provider or to an agency for this essential service.

CONTRACEPTION IN TEENAGERS

Pregnancy in teenagers is a major problem, and one that has not decreased, despite the availability of effective contraceptive techniques. About half of unmarried women between the ages of 15 and 19 have had intercourse, and many—even among those who are regularly sexually active—do not use any contraceptive method. Each year 1 out of 10 women between the ages of 15 and 19 (about 837,000) conceive. An additional 23,000 pregnancies occur in girls younger than age 15. Elective abortion is chosen as a solution by 14,000 of those under age 15, and between 15 and 17 years the number increases (about 162,000). The emotional trauma and the cost of many of these pregnancies could be avoided if accurate information and contraception were made available to young women approaching menarche and to teenagers. The usual courses in "sex education" given in schools are often inadequate.

It is difficult to ignore one's personal biases when dealing with teenage sexuality. However, one cannot logically handle the issue with a curt refusal even to consider it. Some young girls may be confused by the pressures being put on them by their peers who are already sexually active. They may be asking for help in understanding and resisting the pressures rather than for contraceptive counseling. Others who already are having intercourse need a reliable contraceptive method. A refusal from the provider, particularly when accompanied by a lecture with moral overtones, can be so embarrassing that many young women will not risk exposing themselves to similar experiences by consulting another provider. The inevitable results are pregnancies that could have been prevented.

Although a 1983 Supreme Court ruling stated that minors do not need parental consent to obtain contraceptive counseling through federally funded services, there are times when it is appropriate to include parents in the decision. Ideally, the parents of young teenagers who seek contraceptive advice should be involved. Before approaching the parents, however, one must learn all one can about the girl and her need for contraception and ultimately be ready to support her in her decision. The federal dollars targeted for family planning, Title X money, are continuously being scrutinized by proponents and antagonists of contraceptive programs. Mandatory parental consent is a frequent, polarizing topic of debate.

There is no ready answer to the problem of unplanned or unwanted teenage pregnancy. The solution will require societal recognition and a multifaceted approach involving patients, parents, institutions, and appropriate funding.

CONTRACEPTIVE METHODS

The many contraceptive methods range from relatively simple forms to operative procedures that interrupt the continuity of the fallopian tubes or the ductus deferens. No single method is uniformly satisfactory, and the physician must be familiar with many options and several types so that a patient can select the one best suited to her life-style and medical circumstances.

Theoretic effectiveness refers to the protection offered by a technique when it is used perfectly. *Use effectiveness* refers to the protection offered to large groups of couples, many of whom may use the method carelessly or irregularly. An excellent method that is too difficult for an individual to use or one that is unacceptable for one reason or another will have low use effectiveness.

The use effectiveness for any contraceptive method can be calculated by determining the number of pregnancies per 100 woman-years by using *Pearl's formula,* which permits comparison of methods. *Lifetable analysis* calculates failures for each month of use and is a more effective measure of effectiveness (Table 29-1).

In general, contraceptive methods can be divided into (1) physiologic, (2) chemical, (3) barrier, (4) intrauterine, (5) hormonal, and (6) surgical. Surgical sterilization is covered in Chapter 30, Sterilization. Birth control pills, tubal sterilization, and condoms are the most common forms of contraception.

Table 29-1. Contraceptive failures (first year)

Method	Percent pregnancies	
	Lowest %	Typical %
No method	85	85
Combination pill	0.1	3
Progestin only	0.5	3
IUDs		3
Progesterone IUD	2	>2
Copper T 380-A	0.8	>1
Norplant	0.2	0.2
Female sterilization	0.2	0.4
Male sterilization	0.1	0.15
Depo-Provera	0.3	0.3
Spermicides	3	21
Periodic abstinence ("rhythm")		20
Ovulation method	3	
Symptothermal	2	
Cervical cap	6	18
Sponge (multiparous)	6	18
Diaphragm with spermicides	6	18
Condom	2	12

IUD, Intrauterine device.

Physiologic contraception

In physiologic contraception, no chemical or mechanical device is used. The two methods are coitus interruptus and avoiding coitus during the period of greatest fertility.

COITUS INTERRUPTUS (WITHDRAWAL). Coitus interruptus is the oldest—and, besides breast-feeding, may be the most frequently used—contraceptive method throughout the world.

The penis is withdrawn from the vagina just before ejaculation occurs. This method does not afford maximum protection because fertilization can occur if live sperm are present in the sticky, clear seminal fluid that leaks from the urethra before and during coitus and if the withdrawal is delayed so that part of the semen is discharged within the vagina.

NATURAL FAMILY PLANNING (RHYTHM). Couples who use natural family planning prevent conception by confining coitus to the phases of the menstrual cycle during which conception is unlikely to occur.

It is thought that the human ovum can be fertilized no later than 24 to 48 hours after it is extruded from the ovary. Although motile spermatozoa have been recovered from the uterus and the oviducts as long as 60 hours after coitus, their ability to fertilize the ovum probably lasts no longer than 24 to 48 hours. Pregnancy is unlikely to occur if a couple refrains from intercourse for 4 days before, and for 3 or 4 days after, ovulation *(fertile period).* Unprotected intercourse on the other days of the cycle *(safe period)* should not result in pregnancy. The principal problems with natural family planning are that the exact time of ovulation cannot be predicted accurately in each cycle and that couples may find it difficult to exercise restraint for several days before and after ovulation. A high-quality over-the-counter urinary luteinizing hormone (LH) detection kit helps this method to be more reliable.

Ovulation usually occurs about 14 days (12 to 16) before the onset of menstruation. The fertile period can be anticipated by calculating the time at which ovulation is likely to occur by the length of the menstrual cycles *(calendar method),* by recording the rise in basal body temperature caused by the thermogenic effect of progesterone *(temperature method),* by recognizing the changes in cervical mucus at different phases of the cycle *(cervical mucus method),* or by combinations of all three (Fig. 29-1).

Observations are made on secretions collected by checking the vaginal introitus daily. Ovulation occurs soon after the peak estrogen production, when the mucus at the introitus is abundant, clear, thin, and watery. Women should not engage in coitus after tacky mucus is first recognized and until the watery discharge character-

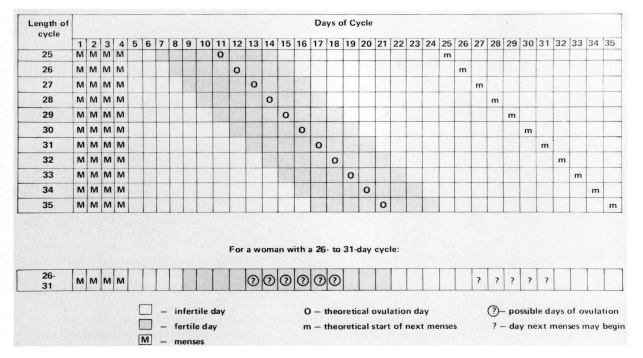

Fig. 29-1. Day of ovulation and fertile period during cycles of varying length. *(From Ross C, Piotrow PT: Birth control without contraceptives. In Population reports: periodic abstinence, Series 1, No 1, Washington, DC, June 1974, Population Information Program, The Johns Hopkins University.)*

istic of ovulation disappears. Coitus can be undertaken toward the end of menses, but many couples find this practice uncomfortable for aesthetic reasons.

Chemical contraception

The chemical methods of contraception involve the deposition of a spermicidal substance, usually *nonoxynl 9,* in the vagina before coitus. This material coats the vaginal wall and the cervix and collects in the fornices, thus exposing the spermatozoa to its destructive action. The chemical is supplied as foam, suppositories, or jelly. In general, chemical contraception affords better protection than the rhythm method and is also used with another form of contraception, that is, condoms or a diaphragm.

Barrier contraception

Before oral contraceptives were developed, the most frequently prescribed method was the combination of a *vaginal diaphragm* with a *spermicidal jelly.* A diaphragm is a dome-shaped cup with a flexible rim. It fits in the vagina with its anterior edge behind the pubic bone, its lateral edges against the vaginal walls, and its posterior edge against the posterior vaginal fornix. The cervix is covered by the diaphragm, and the external os rests in a pool of spermicidal jelly, which immobilizes any spermatozoa that get past the barrier (Fig. 29-2).

It is necessary that a trained health care provider fit the diaphragm, thoroughly instruct the patient in proper use, and make certain, by having the patient insert the diaphragm in the office, that

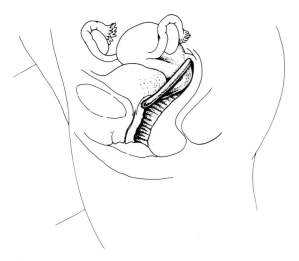

Fig. 29-2. Occlusive contraceptive diaphragm in place.

she can insert it properly. For many women the insertion of a diaphragm is either distasteful or too much trouble, but for those who use one regularly and properly, a diaphragm offers good protection. The diaphragm must be inserted before intercourse and left in place at least 6 hours after ejaculation; additional insertion of contraceptive jelly before subsequent coital episodes enhances protection. The principal reasons for failure are inconsistent use, improper insertion, improper size, and displacement during coitus caused by expansion of the upper vagina associated with penile thrusting.

Possible side effects in diaphragm users are irritation from the spermicidal cream or jelly and an increased incidence of urinary tract infections.

The *condom coated with spermicide* is a common form of barrier contraception that offers good protection but has disadvantages. It may break or slip off the penis. Only *latex condoms* should be used; commercial lubricants can cause other materials to fragment. The reasons for failure are inconsistent use, leakage of semen if the condom is put on late in coitus or as the deflated penis is withdrawn, and breakage.

The regular use of condoms can reduce the chance of contracting gonorrhea, chlamydia, or human immunodeficiency virus infections. To accomplish this it is essential that the condom be used throughout the entire act and that there be no unprotected contact with the female genitals.

Contraceptive sponges made of polyurethane saturated with a spermicidal substance were introduced in the United States in 1983. The sponge has three effects: (1) it releases the spermicide slowly, (2) it covers the external cervical os, and (3) it absorbs semen. It may be inserted several hours before coitus and need not be changed during repeated episodes of coitus within a 24-hour period. It should be removed 6 hours after intercourse.

The thimble-shaped latex rubber *cervical cap* fits snugly over the normal cervix and is held in place by suction. Additional protection is provided by a spermicide placed within the cap before it is inserted. The cap must be fitted securely; therefore all women cannot use it. It may not be appropriate if the cervix is short or distorted, and it may be difficult to insert and remove. It can be left in place for 2 days, but because of the possible risk of toxic shock syndrome, it should be removed during menses (Fig. 29-3).

Intrauterine devices

The intrauterine device (IUD) is inserted into the uterine cavity by a trained provider and is allowed to remain in place, offering constant protection against pregnancy without need for preparing for each individual coital act. Most IUDs have a fine monofilament thread that protrudes through the cervix into the vagina. Only two types of IUDs are now available: the *Progestasert,* a *T*-shaped device containing a synthetic progesterone that is released slowly, and the *Paragard T 380-A,* a *T*-shaped device, the stem and arms of which are partially covered with copper wire (Fig. 29-4). The copper, which is absorbed slowly by the endometrium, adds to the protective effect of the device itself by altering local enzymes, deoxyribonucleic acid content, glycogen metabolism, and estrogen uptake. The copper T 380-A device must be replaced every 10 years.

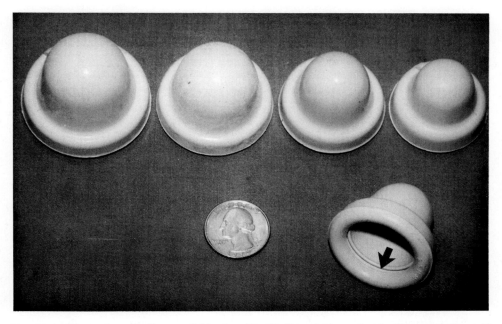

Fig. 29-3. Pictured are the four available sizes (22, 25, 28, and 31 mm inside diameter) of Prentif Cavity-Rim Cervical Cap. Arrow indicates hollow rim that creates suction to hold cap on cervix. (Quarter indicates relative size.) *(From Stenchever MA:* Office gynecology, *ed 2, St Louis, 1996, Mosby–Year Book.)*

Progesterone-containing devices decrease menstrual flow, but they may produce annoying intermenstrual spotting. They also appear to be associated with a higher rate of ectopic pregnancies. An additional disadvantage is that they must be replaced yearly. Complications from IUD usage are often seen following insertion.

The pregnancy rate with IUD usage is 1.5 to 3 pregnancies per 100 woman-years of use. Some pregnancies occur because the patient is not aware that the device has been expelled from the uterus. These accidents can be prevented if the patient feels for the thread, which is attached to the device and comes through the cervical canal into the vagina. If she cannot feel the thread, she should use another form of contraception until she can see her gynecologist. The uterus expels the device in about 10% of women, and in another 10% to 15% it is removed because of a complication or because of a vague concern over the presence of a

foreign body in the uterus. The continuation rate is between 50% and 80% at the end of 1 year.

Although IUDs can be used by either nulliparous or parous women, they are more suitable for the latter. Women who have never been pregnant are more likely to experience unacceptable cramping and bleeding than are those whose uteri have been enlarged by pregnancy. Women who are not motivated enough to use ordinary contraceptive methods consistently, and those in whom oral contraceptives are contraindicated, are suitable candidates for IUDs. Among all contraceptive users, patient satisfaction in current IUD users is the highest.

Contraindications to the use of IUDs include active pelvic infection, acute cervicitis, undiagnosed bleeding, abnormal uterine size or shape, and suspected pregnancy. *Relative contraindications* include recurrent attacks of pelvic infection, multiple sexual partners, severe dysmenorrhea, and

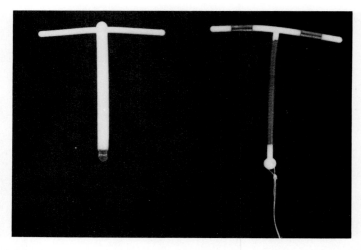

Fig. 29-4. Intrauterine devices (IUDs) currently being marketed in the United States. *Left,* progesterone-releasing IUD; *right,* copper T 380-A. *(From Mishell DR Jr, Stenchever MA, Droegemueller W, Herbst AL:* Comprehensive gynecology, *ed 3, St Louis, 1997, Mosby–Year Book.)*

hypermenorrhea. Intrauterine devices should be used with caution in women with diabetes mellitus, who are prone to develop infections, and in women with valvular heart disease.

The most common complications of IUD usage are perforation of the uterus, intermenstrual spotting, increased menstrual bleeding, increased cramping during menstruation, and infection. Cramping can usually be controlled with prostaglandin inhibitors. Women who have had severe dysmenorrhea that was relieved by oral contraceptives usually do not continue using an IUD unless the pain can be controlled.

Perforation can almost always be prevented by careful selection of patients, care during insertion, and experience. Perforation is more likely to occur with insertion during the first 6 to 8 weeks after delivery than after the tenth. Intraperitoneal IUDs should be removed.

Bacteria are inevitably introduced into the uterus during insertion; hence infection may develop. The patient with a mild, localized infection usually experiences low abdominal discomfort, dyspareunia, thin vaginal discharge, and perhaps low-grade fever for as long as 2 to 3 weeks. The uterus and parametria may be tender, suggesting a low-grade endometritis and cellulitis. They can be treated effectively with a broad spectrum antibiotic.

About 50% of intrauterine pregnancies that occur with an IUD in place are aborted. Removal of the device reduces the abortion rate to 25% or less. When pregnancy is diagnosed, the device should be removed. If the tail is not visible, it may have been drawn upward into the enlarging uterus or extruded before conception. An IUD can be located by sonography if there is a question as to whether it has been expelled. If the device cannot be removed, the patient should be informed of the possibility that serious infection may develop and be given the option of abortion.

Intrauterine devices prevent 97% to 98% of intrauterine pregnancies, but ectopic pregnancies still occur. About 1 in 20 pregnancies in IUD users is extrauterine. Women who are at risk of developing ectopic pregnancies should use another form of contraception if possible.

The method by which IUDs prevent pregnancy is not completely clear. Ovulation continues, and spermatozoa can be recovered from the fallopian tubes, but there is no evidence to suggest that IUDs cause repeated abortions of normally implanted blastocysts. The most likely explanation is that the device creates an intrauterine environment unfavorable for implantation. The local endometrial changes, stromal edema, increased vascularity, and a sterile inflammatory reaction may alter the tissue enough so that it cannot support the blastocyst. In addition, products from the breakdown of inflammatory cells may be toxic to both spermatozoa and blastocysts.

Hormonal contraception

The most popular form of contraception is provided by oral contraceptive agents (birth control pills). Oral contraceptive preparations contain varying amounts of an estrogen, usually *ethinyl estradiol,* and a *progestin,* which usually is a 19-nor derivative of testosterone. The progestational, estrogen, and androgenic effects of the various progestins vary; hence one needs to consider the effects when prescribing oral contraceptives.

Combined oral contraceptives contain both an estrogen and a progestin. The hormones interfere with orderly gonadotropin-releasing hormone release from the hypothalamus, thereby suppressing follicle-stimulating hormone and LH release and inhibiting ovulation. The hormones also have a direct stimulatory effect on the endometrium, so that from 1 to 4 days after the last tablet is taken the endometrium sloughs and bleeds as a result of hormone withdrawal. The bleeding usually is less profuse than that during a normal period and may last only 2 to 3 days. Some women have no bleeding at all.

The contraceptive action is a combined effect of ovulation inhibition, endometrial changes, an alteration in cervical mucus, and perhaps altered tubal function.

The constant daily dose of the estrogen-progestin compound produces changes in the endometrium that are different from those that occur during the normal cycle. The reduction in menstrual and breakthrough bleeding is probably a direct result of the unphysiologic endometrial stimulus; the stroma remains thin, compact, and relatively avascular compared with the normal changes. By altering the ratios and daily doses of estrogen and progestin, one defines whether a birth control pill is a *monophasic, biphasic, or triphasic preparation.* The overall goal is to provide the lowest possible amount of hormone and the highest efficacy with minimal side effects; breakthrough bleeding is the most annoying. In general, monophasic pills are less expensive and are associated with fewer side effects. The low dose pills contain 20 to 35 μg of ethinyl estradiol. There are seven 19-norprogestins in the most commonly used birth control pills. The amount of progestin used in the birth control pill is determined in part by its biologic activity, determined in a bioassay system. One should not be confused by the milligram dose and believe that it is a product with less biopotency. For example, 0.15 mg levonorgestrel is more biologically potent than 1 mg norethindrone. In the past few years there have been three (third generation) progestins: desogestrel, gestodene, and norgestimate. The purported advantages of these progestins are a longer half-life, the significantly greater affinity for the progestin receptor, and minimal to nil affinity for the androgen receptors.

Progestin-only pills, the *minipill,* taken 3 out of 4 weeks, also reduce the risk of pregnancy and may be considered when estrogen administration is contraindicated. The pills are available with either norethindrone or norgestrel. The major contraceptive effects are a result of changes on cervical mucus and the endometrium; inhibition of ovulation is less predictable. The more commonly prescribed birth control pills are seen in Table 29-2.

SIDE EFFECTS. Undesirable side effects are common but fortunately are transient, usually lasting for no more than three or four cycles. They include mild nausea, vomiting, breast engorgement, headache, vertigo, and fluid retention that may result in a weight gain of 3 or more pounds. If these disagreeable side effects do not disappear

Table 29-2. Estrogen and progestin components of oral contraceptives*

Commonly used products	Type	Progestin	Estrogen
BERLEX LABORATORIES			
Tri-Levlen 6/	Triphasic	0.15 mg Levonorgestrel	30 µg Ethinyl estradiol
5/	C	0.075 mg Levonorgestrel	40 µg Ethinyl estradiol
10/		0.125 mg Levonorgestrel	30 µg Ethinyl estradiol
Ovcon-35	C	0.4 mg Norethindrone	35 µg Ethinyl estradiol
Micronor	P	0.35 mg Norethindrone	
Modicon	C	0.5 mg Norethindrone	35 µg Ethinyl estradiol
Ortho-Novum 1/35	C	1 mg Norethindrone	35 µg Ethinyl estradiol
Ortho-Novum 7/7/7	C-Triphasic	0.5 mg Norethindrone	35 µg Ethinyl estradiol
		0.75 mg Norethindrone	35 µg Ethinyl estradiol
		1 mg Norethindrone	35 µg Ethinyl estradiol
Ortho Cyclen	C	0.350 mg Norgestimate	35 µg Ethinyl estradiol
Ortho-Tri-Cyclen	C	0.18 mg Norgestimate	35 µg Ethinyl estradiol
		0.215 mg Norgestimate	35 µg Ethinyl estradiol
		0.250 mg Norgestimate	35 µg Ethinyl estradiol
ORGANON INC.			
Desogen	C	0.15 mg Desogestrel	30 µg Ethinyl estradiol
PARKE-DAVIS			
Loestrin 1/20	C	1 mg Norethindrone acetate	20 µg Ethinyl estradiol
RUGBY LABORATORIES, INC.			
Genora 1/35	C	1 mg Norethindrone	35 µg Ethinyl estradiol
SCHIAPPARELLI SEARLE			
Norethin 1/35E	C	1 mg Norethindrone	35 µg Ethinyl estradiol
SYNTEX LABORATORIES			
Brevicon	C	0.5 mg Norethindrone	35 µg Ethinyl estradiol
Norinyl 1 + 35	C	1 mg Norethindrone	35 µg Ethinyl estradiol
Nor-QD	P	0.35 mg Norethindrone	
Tri-Norinyl 7/	C-Triphasic	0.5 mg Norethindrone	35 µg Ethinyl estradiol
9/		1 mg Norethindrone	35 µg Ethinyl estradiol
5/		0.5 mg Norethindrone	35 µg Ethinyl estradiol
WYETH-AYERST			
Lo-Ovral	C	0.3 mg Norgestrel	30 µg Ethinyl estradiol
Nordette	C	0.15 mg Levonorgestrel	30 µg Ethinyl estradiol
Ovrette	P	75 µg Norgestrel	
Triphasil 6/	C-Triphasic	50 µg Levonorgestrel	40 µg Ethinyl estradiol
5/		75 µg Levonorgestrel	40 µg Ethinyl estradiol
10/		125 µg Levonorgestrel	30 µg Ethinyl estradiol

C, Combination; P, progestin only.
*There are other preparations available; consult the American Hospital Formulary Service, 1997, for a complete list. Most manufacturers include a 21- and 28-day package, sometimes substituting iron for the last 7 days instead of placebo.

spontaneously after a few cycles, one should consider trying another pill with a different hormone ratio. Those pills in which estrogen is dominant are more likely to cause nausea, fluid retention, and breast tenderness than are those with a relatively high progestin content.

Depression, which may be severe and incapacitating, occurs in some women who are taking oral contraceptives. Occasionally it is necessary to discontinue oral contraceptives completely to relieve depression.

The total incidence of breakthrough bleeding is about 8% to 15%, but it occurs more often during the first few cycles than during later cycles. It also occurs more often when progestin-dominant products or those with low estrogen content are used. If the bleeding is slight and occurs only occasionally, and particularly if it consists only of slight spotting during the last few days of pill ingestion, the physician should reassure the patient that it is not harmful and attempt to convince her to ignore it.

The lower the amount of hormone, the less the endometrial stimulation and growth and the greater the possibility of amenorrhea. This concerns both the patient and the physician because of the possibility of pregnancy. Although it is unlikely that one who has taken her pills regularly and fails to menstruate has conceived, some women will not tolerate the uncertainty and will discontinue the method. A pregnancy test should be ordered with the first episode of amenorrhea; if the failure to bleed persists, repeated tests are probably not necessary. Most of the complications are inconsequential when compared to the ease with which pregnancy can be prevented.

CARDIOVASCULAR   DISEASES. No longer is there concern that oral contraceptives increase the risk of cardiovascular diseases; in fact, birth control pills may have a protective effect. Increases in myocardial infarction and cerebrovascular accidents reported during the 1960s and 1970s were based on studies of women who were using formulations containing 50 μg or more of estrogen. Estrogen increases high-density lipo-protein (HDL) cholesterol and decreases low-density lipoprotein (LDL) cholesterol, thereby offering some protection against myocardial infarction. However, the cardioprotective effects of estrogen are much more complicated than influencing HDL metabolism. The progestogens in oral contraceptives have androgenic potential and counteract some of the beneficial effects of estrogen. Some progestogens decrease HDL cholesterol concentrations and increase LDL levels. These undesirable effects are counterbalanced by estrogen, so the net result is no change. The synthetic estrogens in oral contraceptives stimulate an increased liver production of serum globulins. One of these, *angiotensinogen,* may increase angiotensin II in some women and thereby increase blood pressure. Increased blood pressure associated with the use of oral contraceptives is not permanent; the blood pressure returns to its regular level when oral contraceptives are discontinued.

There is no consistent increase in myocardial infarction in women who have used oral contraceptives in the past, and there is no relationship between duration of use and heart attacks.

Recent studies of oral contraceptive users age 20 to 44 revealed no increase in myocardial infarctions or cerebrovascular accidents after 36,248 woman-years of use. The relative risk for venous thrombosis was 0.9. In a later study of women between the ages of 15 and 44, there were no myocardial infarctions, one stroke, and three episodes of venous thrombosis during 36,807 woman-years of use.

Moreover, even in the early studies, increases in heart attacks occurred primarily in older women who smoked more than 15 cigarettes daily and who had preexisting risk factors for coronary artery disease.

The conclusion can be made from these studies that healthy women who do not smoke, even those up to age 50, using low-dose oral contraceptives are not at increased risk of developing strokes or heart attacks. There is a slight increase in venous thromboembolism, but this can be kept at a minimum if only low-dose preparations are used.

There is no indication that oral contraceptives cause diabetes mellitus, and most women with well-controlled disease can take oral contraceptives without deleterious effects.

Women who have had cholestasis and jaundice during pregnancy may respond in the same manner to oral contraceptives. The incidence of cholecystitis and cholelithiasis is almost doubled during the first years of oral contraceptive use. After 4 years, the rate may actually decrease. The most serious complication affecting the liver is the development of benign liver tumors, principally focal nodular hyperplasia and hepatic adenomas. The main danger is from rupture of the tumor with intrahepatic or intraperitoneal hemorrhage and death unless the blood loss is controlled promptly. Malignant liver neoplasms have not been related to the use of oral contraceptives.

There is no evidence to suggest that combined oral contraceptives increase the risk of cancer of the endometrium, breast, or any other organ.

Oral contraceptives actually protect against endometrial and ovarian cancer. Although they do decrease the risk of benign breast disease, there is still controversy as to the relationship between the use of hormonal contraceptives and breast cancer. An increase in cervical neoplasia has been observed after 5 years of usage. Women under 35 years old who smoke cigarettes, have multiple sexual partners, or have a history of sexually transmitted diseases should be monitored carefully with annual Pap smears.

Most women ovulate soon after discontinuing oral contraceptives, but in some there may be a delay of several weeks before ovulation and menstruation are resumed. One percent to 3% are amenorrheic for as long as 6 months. Eventually almost all of those who want to conceive will do so. There is no difference in fertility between those using oral contraceptives and those who use other contraceptive methods. Because of the uncertainty as to when ovulation may resume, women who discontinue oral contraceptives to become pregnant should be advised to use another form of contraception until menstrual periods resume

their normal pattern. There is no increase in spontaneous abortion, chromosomal abnormalities, or congenital defects in women who have used oral contraceptives as compared with those who have not.

Much has been written about the complications related to the use of oral contraceptives, but the advantages, other than protection against pregnancy, have had little publicity. The *noncontraceptive health benefits of oral contraceptives* include decreased menstrual blood loss and less iron-deficiency anemia, regulation of irregular cycles, decreased menstrual discomfort, protection against endometrial adenocarcinoma, reduced incidence of benign breast disease, reduced incidence of ectopic pregnancy, protection against the development of functional ovarian cysts, protection against acute salpingitis, and protection against ovarian cancer.

As a general rule, there is no reason why healthy women below the age of 35 cannot take oral contraceptives, *even though they smoke*. However, stopping tobacco usage should be strongly encouraged. Healthy women between the ages of 35 and 50 can continue to use low-dose oral contraceptives as long as they do not smoke and have no factors that increase the risk of cardiovascular diseases, diabetes, or hypertension.

Each woman taking oral contraceptives should be evaluated before the medication is prescribed and yearly thereafter. The examination should include medical and family history, weight, blood pressure, general physical and pelvic examination, screening cervical cytologic analysis, cervical cultures, an initial rubella screen, and cholesterol assessment.

CONTRAINDICATIONS TO ORAL CONTRACEPTIVES. There are women for whom oral contraceptives should not be prescribed. The *absolute contraindications* include the following:

1. Coronary artery disease, stroke, or thromboembolism either present or in the past
2. Severe hypertension
3. Lupus erythematosus

4. Hemoglobin SS disease
5. Insulin-dependent diabetes with vascular disease
6. Impaired liver function
7. Estrogen-dependent neoplasms and breast cancer
8. Suspected pregnancy
9. Smokers over age 35, particularly obese women

Relative contraindications include the following:

1. History of cholestasis during pregnancy
2. Migraine headaches or headaches associated with oral contraceptive use
3. Depression
4. Seizure disorder

OTHER HORMONE PREPARATIONS.
Medroxyprogesterone acetate (Depo-Provera), when injected intramuscularly in doses of 150 mg every 3 months, inhibits ovulation. Pregnancy rates comparable to those achieved with oral contraceptives have been reported in large numbers of women. The only metabolic effect associated with this preparation is a possible decrease in insulin tolerance and an increase in plasma insulin. Bleeding may occur irregularly during the first few months, but it gradually decreases, and many women become amenorrheic. Weight gain and an unpredictable return in fertility have hindered greater usage. However, it can be the contraceptive of choice for women who find it difficult to take a pill every day.

The slow diffusion of hormone through a silastic delivery system is the basis for an innovative contraceptive technology. *Norplant* consists of six slender silicone rubber capsules that contain levonorgestrel. The match-size capsules are implanted subdermally, usually on the inner surface of the upper portion of the arm, and release hormone at a relatively steady rate over a 5-year period of time. The failure rate is less than 0.1%, and approximately 50% of women continue using the method over 3 years. The most significant difficulty is dealing with abnormal uterine bleeding.

The mechanism of action is similar to progestin-only contraceptives and is multifaceted. The prevention of pregnancy is probably achieved through the inhibition of ovulation, with the thickening of the cervical mucus creating a thin atrophic endometrium that is unfavorable for implantation. Although the delivery system is relatively easy to insert in an ambulatory setting, the removal of these silastic capsules has proved more difficult. There have been a few unfortunate occurrences related to difficult removals, and therefore the method has fallen into disfavor. The basic concept of using a vehicle to release hormone over a practical time frame is applicable to other forms of contraception, and these should be available in the near future.

EMERGENCY CONTRACEPTION. Another method of pregnancy prevention is the use of large doses of hormone after coitus. This should be considered as an emergency measure to be used after unprotected coitus during the fertile period rather than as a regular method of contraception. The medication must be prescribed within 72 hours; the closer to coitus, the greater the effectiveness. The exact mechanism by which postcoital estrogen prevents pregnancy is not yet known, but it does produce a premature fall in corpus luteum progesterone production and changes in the endometrium, which may provide an unacceptable implantation site for the fertilized ovum. In early 1997 the U.S. Food and Drug Administration (FDA) approved six brands of birth control pills that, taken within the prescribed time frame, are 75% effective in preventing pregnancy.

Ovral, two tablets taken initially and then again in 12 hours, is most often prescribed. Because DES ingested by mothers was related to the subsequent development of vaginal adenosis and clear cell carcinoma in their daughters, it is essential that each patient be examined before the drug is prescribed to make certain that she is not already pregnant. Repeat examinations also are essential to make certain the patient did not conceive despite taking the drug. Abortion should be available if pregnancy occurs. Because nausea frequently accompanies this therapy, a prescription for an antiemetic should be included. Also, *RU-486*, an antiprogesterone, has significant potential as a postcoital contraceptive agent.

Surgical contraception

Termination of fertility by a sterilization procedure is the most common form of contraception in the United States. As many as 15 million couples may rely on this method. Elective sterilization is appropriate for women who have completed their childbearing careers and who still have several years of fertility ahead. It may be particularly important for those who cannot use an effective contraceptive method, and it usually is preferable to many years of using oral hormonal contraceptives.

The fallopian tubes can be occluded or severed in conjunction with any indicated abdominal operation or as a primary procedure. This may be accomplished by laparoscopic tubal cautery, by the application of rings or clips, or by removing a segment of each tube through a vaginal or small abdominal incision (minilaparotomy). All of these procedures can be performed in an ambulatory setting. Puerperal sterilization, usually during the first day or two after delivery, is easy and safe and often is an appropriate choice.

The patient should understand that it is unlikely that she will conceive after the operation, but that she is being sterilized (termination of fertility), not castrated (removal of gonads).

Vasectomy can be performed in an outpatient facility with a local anesthetic. There are few complications and a minimal period of disability. Spermatozoa may remain in the reproductive tract for several weeks; consequently, an additional method of contraception should be used until aspermia has been proved. Recanalization occurs in a small percentage of cases, probably less than 5%.

One must always consider the possible emotional effects of permanent elimination of procreative ability. It often is not easy, even for a woman who wants no more children, to relin-

quish her ability to conceive. Men who are somewhat uncertain in their masculine roles may be impotent after vasectomy. These potential effects of sterilization must be explored before the operation is performed.

LEGAL ABORTION

The term *legal abortion* refers to the termination of early pregnancy by a qualified physician in an approved medical facility.

Until the early 1960s termination of pregnancy was considered only when it was likely that the mother would die if she remained pregnant *(therapeutic abortion)*. Such abortions were legal in most states. Abortion was seldom considered because of fetal conditions, even if one could anticipate a fetus being born with a lethal or incapacitating condition, or for social reasons. These abortions were illegal.

Restrictive laws prevented women for whom pregnancy was a personal disaster from obtaining an abortion. They usually had to seek assistance from providers operating illegally, and many developed serious complications or even died as a result of the procedures. Before 1970, when abortion became legal in New York, more than 50% of maternal deaths in New York City followed illegally induced abortion. During the 5-year period from 1955 to 1959, 21% of maternal deaths in Michigan were attributed to illegally induced abortions. During the next 5-year period, 37% of maternal deaths followed abortion.

In January 1973 the U.S. Supreme Court declared all restrictive abortion laws unconstitutional. As a consequence, abortion became legal in all states. The number of illegal abortions and the accompanying deaths fell precipitously after abortion became legal. During the 5-year period from 1975 to 1979, only 17 women died after illegal abortion in the United States.

The decision included directives concerning the performance of abortions, as well as decision making. During the first trimester the decision for abortion can be made by a patient and a physician, but the operation can be performed only by a licensed physician. States usually develop regulations concerning who performs second trimester pregnancy terminations and where they can be done, but the decision for the procedure still rests with the patient and a physician. States may develop regulations for third trimester termination of pregnancy and may even proscribe termination, except to preserve the life and health of the mother. Repeated attempts have been made to reverse the Supreme Court decision and to limit the availability of elective abortion or even to prohibit it. If these attempts are successful, one can anticipate a resurgence of illegal abortions, with the sequelae being pelvic infection and maternal death.

Indications

Therapeutic abortions are performed in women with serious medical diseases that make pregnancy hazardous, in women with fetal conditions that interfere with normal growth and development or that are potentially lethal, and in women with serious psychiatric disorders.

The *maternal medical conditions* for which abortion is most often performed are chronic severe hypertension or renal disease, especially when there is considerable vascular degeneration and reduced renal function; diabetes mellitus, especially when there are associated degenerative vascular changes; and advanced cardiac disease.

Termination of pregnancy can be considered whenever the fetus has little chance of developing normally because of maternal disease such as rubella, when the fetus has been exposed to teratogenic stimuli, or when the fetus is destined to die at an early age from a lethal hereditary condition. Certain chromosomal and metabolic abnormalities that, if present, may influence a decision for abortion can be detected by appropriate amniotic fluid studies early in pregnancy. These procedures are more likely to be performed in the second trimester.

Therapeutic abortion for psychiatric conditions is justified when the pregnancy interferes with necessary psychotherapy or when the psychopathologic condition of the patient and her family is severe enough to suggest that a baby reared in such an atmosphere would have a small chance for normal emotional development.

Elective abortions

The nonmedical reasons for abortion are primarily social or economic, and the decision as to the advisability of terminating pregnancy is one made individually by the woman. Most of these procedures are performed in the first trimester.

Physician responsibility

Physicians who choose to perform elective abortions should counsel patients regarding the advisability of the procedure. The request for the operation should always originate with the patient.

It is obvious that a woman with an undesired pregnancy may think first of termination, without considering other options. Therefore it is essential that a physician not agree to perform an abortion without a thorough review of the situation with the patient. The doctor or a specially trained nurse, social worker, or counselor should discuss with the patient the advantages and disadvantages of keeping the pregnancy. An important aspect to be considered is what effect a baby will have on the patient's life or on members of her family. Abortion is difficult for most women to accept with equanimity; hence counseling, even for those who are adamant concerning interruption, is an important part of the treatment.

The responsibility of physicians in dealing with abortions for medical reasons is somewhat different. They must be able, with the help of appropriate consultants, to evaluate the severity of the systemic disease and to establish the potential risk of permitting the pregnancy to continue. In contrast to elective abortion, physicians may recommend termination for medical reasons. In many instances this is difficult for the patient to accept because she wants the pregnancy.

The need for medical abortions can be reduced by prepregnancy planning. If a condition that contraindicates pregnancy is found, a suitable contraceptive method can be prescribed.

Complications

Complications associated with abortion occur inevitably, but they can be kept at a minimum if the procedures are performed on carefully selected patients by skillful operators in properly equipped facilities. Complications most likely to occur during early abortion are perforation of the uterus, hemorrhage, and infection. Because these complications cannot be foreseen, it is essential that provision be made to treat them promptly when they occur.

The risk of serious complications as a result of abortion during the first 12 gestational weeks for women of all ages is about 1 to 2 per 100,000 procedures. The more advanced the pregnancy when the operation is performed, the greater the risk of serious complications. Uncomplicated induced abortion appears to have little effect on the outcome of subsequent pregnancies.

At best, abortion is an unsatisfactory way of controlling reproduction. In theory, if effective contraceptive methods are used regularly, abortion should not be necessary.

Technique

Blood-typing and a check for Rh antibodies are important preabortion laboratory procedures. Women who are Rh-negative but who have no evidence of isoimmunization should be treated with human anti-D γ-globulin (RhoGAM) to prevent immunization by the fetal red blood cells that enter the maternal bloodstream during abortion.

During the first trimester of pregnancy the uterus can usually be evacuated by dilating the cervix and removing the products of conception by suction curettage. Preoperative use of Laminaria several hours before the uterus is evacuated will soften the cervix and reduce the need for forcible dilatation. Laminaria sticks made of seaweed that absorb water, swell, and gently open the cervix are inserted through the internal os the day before the operation is performed. They are removed just before the uterus is evacuated.

After the twelfth week the safest way to terminate pregnancy is by dilating the cervix and extracting the fetus and placenta with ring forceps and a large curet. This is far more difficult than is suction curettage during the early weeks and should be done only by individuals who are experienced in the technique.

Prostaglandin preparations, given by intraamniotic, intravenous infusion or by intravaginal suppositories, will stimulate uterine contractions at any stage of pregnancy. The placenta is often retained after the fetus is expelled and must be removed surgically.

Progesterone antagonists, which block progesterone receptor sites in the decidua, will induce bleeding in pregnant women within a few days. An additional effect of these substances is to sensitize the uterus to prostaglandins. The available progesterone antagonist, RU-486, plus a prostaglandin preparation, will induce abortion in 95% of women who have been amenorrheic for up to 49 days. It is not available in the United States.

The death rate associated with legal abortion is determined by the stage of pregnancy, the method of induction, and the experience of the operator. Between 1972 and 1978 more than 6 million legal abortions were reported to the Centers for Disease Control. The lowest death rate, 0.5 per 100,000, was for abortions performed on women with pregnancies of 8 weeks' duration or less. The death rate increased progressively to 2.3 at 11 to 12 weeks', 6.7 at 13 to 15 weeks', and 13.9 at 16 to 20 weeks' gestation. During 1983 there were nine maternal deaths following 811,063 legal abortions at all stages of pregnancy.

CRITICAL POINTS

- Unplanned pregnancies in the United States have reached epidemic proportions.
- Birth control pills, tubal sterilization, and condoms are the most common forms of contraception used in the United States.
- The use effectiveness, as opposed to theoretic effectiveness, is defined by the number of pregnancies that occur using a particular method under all clinical circumstances. Greater than 10% pregnancy rates occur with the use of spermicides, periodic abstinence, withdrawal, cervical caps, sponges, diaphragms, and condoms.
- Although in the United States it is used less frequently than other contraceptive methods, the IUD enjoys a high degree of satisfaction with current users. The current evidence does not suggest that there is an increased incidence of pelvic infection in appropriately screened patients using IUDs. Although the overall incidence of pregnancy is significantly reduced with IUD usage, if pregnancy does occur the likelihood of its being an ectopic pregnancy is increased, particularly by a progesterone-containing IUD.
- In the commonly prescribed birth control pills, ethinyl estradiol is the estrogen, and there are seven 19-norsteroids (progestins). Pills are available in monophasic, biphasic, or triphasic preparations in which the amount of progestin varies within the packets depending on the cycle day. A low-dose birth control pill contains from 20 to 35 μg of estrogen.
- Most of the information that has caused concern about the risks associated with the use of birth control pills was obtained from studies of women using formulations containing a higher amount (50 μg) of estrogen. The health risks associated with taking birth control pills are substantially less than those associated with a pregnancy. When patients are counseled about the use of birth control pills, not only should the risks be identified, but the positive aspects of using birth control pills should be listed as well.
- The positive aspects of using birth control pills are reduced flow, less iron-deficiency anemia, less pelvic inflammatory disease, regular cycles, less ectopic pregnancy, less ovarian cysts, less benign breast disease, and a reduction in ovarian and endometrial cancer.
- The FDA has recently approved six preparations for emergency, postcoital contraception. When used within 72 hours, approximately 75% of the pregnancies are prevented.
- Laparoscopic tubal sterilization is the most common female surgical sterilization procedure. This type of sterilization does not increase the risk of medical problems for women in the future.
- The voluntary termination of pregnancy before the period of viability is a legal procedure in the United States. The health care provider should provide accurate information concerning the risk or benefit of the procedure, but the final decision as to whether or not an abortion is performed should remain with the patient. Before the legalization of abortion the incidence of death in women having the procedure illegally was dramatically high. Regardless of the decision the patient makes, she should be offered support and counseling.

When pregnancy is terminated because of a chronic condition such as heart disease, diabetes, or essential hypertension, sterilization should be considered because there is little hope that the condition will improve enough to permit pregnancy in the future.

Patient care following abortion

The patient who has had an uncomplicated elective abortion and little blood loss may be discharged hours after the uterus has been evacuated. Those with serious medical disorders and those in whom intraoperative complications develop should remain in an outpatient facility until they are stabilized. Normal activity may be resumed whenever the patient feels able to carry out her usual duties. Involution usually is complete in 1 month, and menstruation begins 4 to 6 weeks after the abortion has occurred.

The most important aspect of postabortion care is assisting women with their emotional responses, which may occur even in those who have been counseled extensively preoperatively. Although most women have few problems, some experience deep depression. Physicians who perform abortions should encourage patients to express their feelings about the procedure and help them resolve any problem resulting from it.

Questions

1. All of the following preparations have a use effectiveness under 5% *except:*
   A. Combination birth control pill
   B. Intrauterine device
   C. Female sterilization
   D. Depo-Provera
   E. Condom
2. The following conditions are not contraindications to the use of the birth control pills *except:*
   A. Obesity
   B. Smoking less than 15 cigarettes a day
   C. Insulin-dependent diabetes mellitus with vascular disease
   D. Mild stress-related headaches relieved with acetaminophen
   E. Prior history of benign breast disease
3. The noncontraceptive benefits of the birth control pill do not include:
   A. Less vulvovaginitis
   B. Reduction in ovarian and endometrial cancer
   C. Less benign breast disease
   D. Reduced iron-deficiency anemia
   E. Less pelvic inflammatory disease

Answers

1. E
2. C
3. A

Sterilization

APGO LEARNING OBJECTIVE #30

Philip A. Rosenfeld

In deciding to have a sterilization procedure, men and women often seek the advice of their physicians. Providing accurate information will allow patients to make an informed decision regarding this elective surgery.

The student will demonstrate a knowledge of the following:

A. Methods of male and female surgical sterilization
B. Risks and benefits
C. Factors needed to help the patient make informed decisions, including the following:
   1. Potential surgical complications
   2. Failure rates
   3. Reversibility
D. Financial considerations

ROLE OF COUNSELING IN STERILIZATION

Complete and informed counseling is absolutely necessary before any decision is made for permanent sterilization. This must be done at a level understandable to the patient. It is imperative that the physician inform the patient about the advantages and disadvantages, the costs, and the relative safety, both short-term and long-term, for each procedure. The risk/benefit ratio of the procedure must be thoroughly explained and well documented. The patient's present attitude toward future childbearing, posttubal anastomosis, and possible later changes in her personal life must be explained in layman's language. Failure to do so constitutes an injustice on the part of the physician and may lead to later patient apprehension, dissatisfaction, and possible litigation. The possibility of successful reversibility for the man or woman also must be discussed by the provider in great depth.

For a couple, the decision must first be made about which one will undergo the sterilization procedure. There is no doubt that vasectomy un-

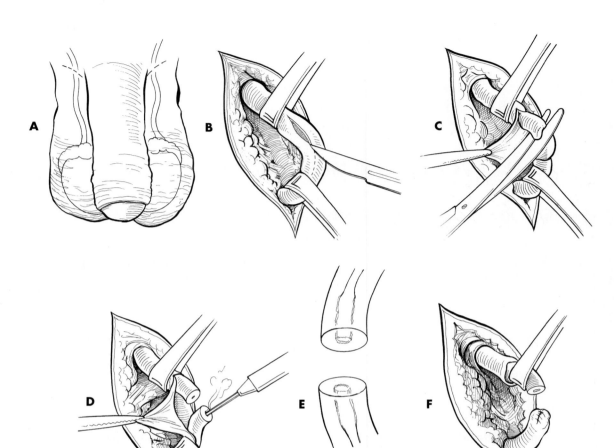

Fig. 30-1. Steps in vasectomy. **A,** Incisions. **B,** Sheath of right vas opened. **C,** Right vas cut. **D,** Fulguration. **E,** Mucosa of lumen destroyed. **F,** Sheath closed over proximal vas.

der local anesthesia is more easily performed than tubal sterilization (Fig. 30-1). Men frequently are reluctant about having such an operation, and it may be left, by default, to the woman to provide permanent contraception.

Male sterilization ordinarily involves simple interruption of the vas deferens through small cutaneous incisions under local anesthesia.

Procedures in women, however, usually encompass general or conduction anesthesia, entrance through the abdominal or vaginal wall, and bilateral interruption of the fallopian tubes. The procedure can be performed vaginally (in a markedly retroflexed uterus) or through a small incision in the abdomen, called a minilaparotomy, either immediately postpartum or as an interval procedure. When done postpartum, the incision usually can be hidden in the umbilical folds. It can also be done later through multiple laparoscopy incisions. Tubal sterilization can be achieved by unipolar or bipolar currents, clips, Silastic bands, or ligation. The unified purpose in any of these methods is to successfully interrupt the flow of the ovum down through the fimbriated end of the tube to meet sperm coming up through the cervix (Figs. 30-2 to 30-5).

FAILURES

Most studies of sterilization report a greater failure rate in women than after vasectomy in men. However, failures can occur on either a short-term or long-term basis. There are approximately 4 failures in every 1000 sterilizations, regardless of the method used.

Cost considerations of comparable procedures in the two sexes favor vasectomy.

RISKS

The incidence of procedure-related mortality per 100,000 procedures was near zero for vasectomy, compared with 4.72 for laparoscopic tubal sterilization and 2.29 for tubal ligations by laparotomy. Long-term mortality was also lower after sterilization in men, but the data for women also include ectopic pregnancies.

The rate of posttubal ectopic pregnancies decreases over successive years. Although the student must always consider the possibility of ectopic gestation when faced with a pregnancy after tubal sterilization, most failures are intrauterine pregnancies. The lifetime risk of an ectopic pregnancy in patients undergoing sterilization is lower than in those who use no contraception at all or who use an intrauterine device; but the risk is higher than in those using condoms, diaphragms, or oral contraceptives.

Some studies suggest an association between male sterilization and prostatic cancer. This has not yet been proved, although sperm antibodies undoubtedly are produced as a result of blockage of the vas deferens. Prostatic cancer probably is more often genetically and age related, these factors being more important than tying off the vas and creating antibodies. In addition, there has been no remarkable increase in prostatic cancer since the beginning of vas deferens ligations.

Complications both minor and major also are more common with tubal sterilization than with vasectomy. Included among the problems are the requirement for intravenous antibiotics, reexploration for hemorrhage, postoperative bowel obstruction, and adhesive disease. Such minor complications as undetermined pain occur more frequently in tubal sterilization patients.

EFFECTS OF STERILIZATION ON CONCOMITANT DISEASE

Women who undergo tubal sterilization should be counseled about the possible effect of interruption of tubal flow on several other pathologic conditions:

1. Prior sterilizations are *not* associated with increased incidence of hysterectomies in married women who have undergone tubal sterilization at age 30 or later. Reported results do not support a biologic connection between tubal sterilization and hysterectomy, and there is no evidence that procedures that coincidentally damaged the mesosalpinx resulted in a higher hysterectomy rate. However, individuals who had menstrual irregularities before the tubal sterilization might return to menstrual irregularities without any oral contraceptives and subsequently might have a hysterectomy. Findings suggest that although physicians may be reluctant to remove the uterus of a fertile young woman, sterilization of either partner lessened the repro-

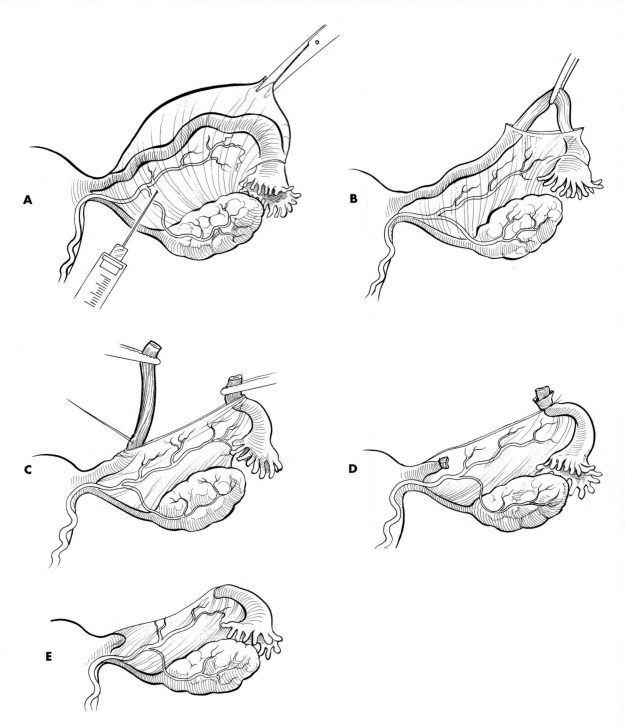

Fig. 30-2. Uchida method of sterilization. **A,** Saline with epinephrine injected below serosa, which becomes inflated locally. Muscular tube, and even blood vessels, can be separated from serosa, which is then cut open. **B,** Muscular tube emerges through opening or is pulled out to form a U shape. **C,** Fimbriated end is untouched, while the end leading to the uterus is stripped of serosa. This can usually be done without damaging blood vessels. **D,** About 5 cm of muscular tube is cut away; the end is buried automatically in serosa. Fimbriated end and serosa opening are closed and tied together. **E,** Blood supply continues normally between ovary and uterus. Hydrosalpinx or adhesion has not been noticed.

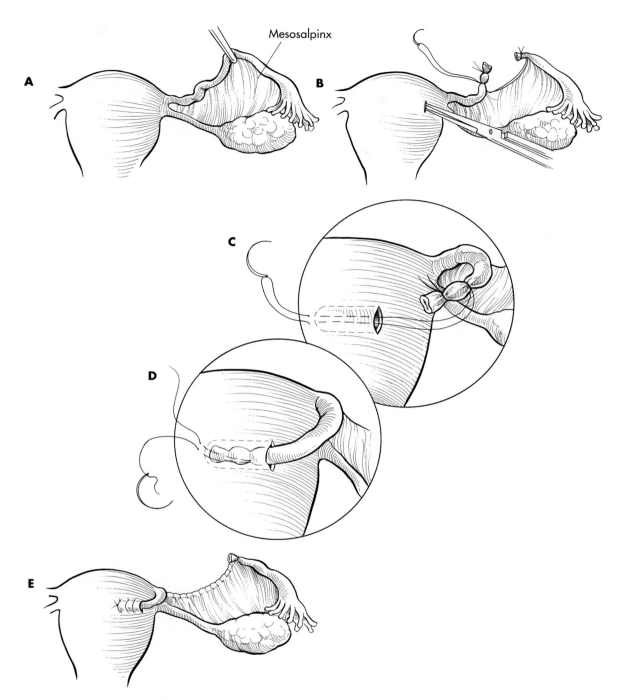

Fig. 30-3. Irving method of sterilization. **A,** Lift and cut oviduct. **B,** Double ligation with gut; one tie is left long for traction (special traction suture); mesosalpinx stripped back. **C,** Special traction suture inserted in tunnel in anterior uterine wall. **D,** Traction suture tied, and proximal tube sutured in tunnel. **E,** Implantation of proximal tubal limb into tunnel in anterior uterine wall.

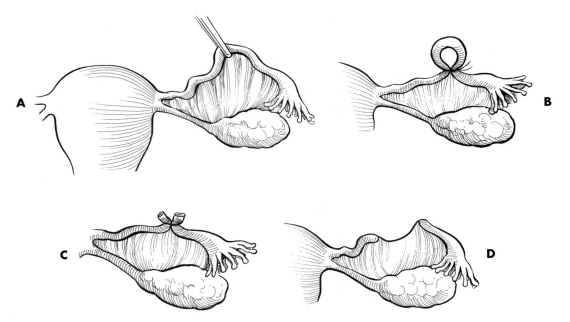

Fig. 30-4. Pomeroy method of sterilization. **A,** Lift. **B,** Ligate. **C,** Section. **D,** Closed ends retract.

ductive value of the uterus and increased the chance that hysterectomy would be chosen.

2. A study adjusted for age, oral contraceptive use, parity, and other ovarian cancer risk factors found a strong reverse relationship between tubal sterilization and ovarian cancer. It was a prospective study with a 12 year follow-up in a large cohort of nurses. The operative mechanism for this protective role in relation to cancer may be the simple reduction in the number of ovulations experienced by the woman. The ovulatory shedding of the epithelial cover of the ovary ends in subsequent invagination of this surface epithelium and has been cited as a possible etiologic factor in the formation of epithelial ovarian cancers.

3. When examining the long-term effect of sterilization on menstrual indexes and pelvic pain, sterilizations are not related to long-term adverse effects on menstrual indexes and do not contribute to noncyclic pelvic pain.

EVALUATION AND FAILURES

After vasectomy, the physician should check male ejaculates regularly for at least 3 months to ascertain whether there has been a complete disappearance of sperm. Radiographic evidence of interrupted fallopian tubes is not necessary, since it is standard practice in postpartum tubal ligations to submit separated portions of each tube for pathologic study. Hysterosalpingographic evidence of tubal sterilization done in the past probably contributed to proximal tubal fistulae via pressure and does not indicate success or failure. Video taping of procedures may well provide an answer in later medicolegal actions. If a woman who has had a tubal ligation misses a menstrual period after having had them fairly routinely, she should report to her physician as quickly as possible to

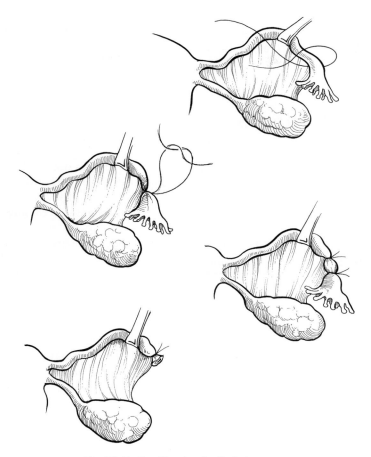

Fig. 30-5. Sterilization by fimbriectomy.

ascertain whether a pregnancy exists and where it is located.

SUMMARY

The student should understand that proper counseling of a patient's desire for permanent sterilization will help prevent later dissatisfaction. Reversal of sterilization in the male—once considered very unlikely—is now successfully done in most institutions. It involves reanastomosis of the tied vas deferens by microscopic surgery. Babies born after such successful procedures are no more likely to be affected by abnormal development, premature labor, ruptured membranes, and so on than are those born to any similar group of patients.

Reversal of female tubal sterilization depends on the original method of sterilization and the amount of normal tube available for reconstruction. Approximately 5 cm of normal tube with normal fimbria are needed for a successful anastomosis and fertility. Therefore procedures such as sequential coagulation of the tube either by unipolar or bipolar technique may not leave the patient with a sufficient remnant of normal tissue to make a reanastomosis successful. If clips and loops are used, which cause less damage to tubes, it is more likely that the tube ends will be successfully rejoined. In-depth counseling of young women should emphasize procedures that leave less tubal destruction. This will allow those who later change their minds about sterilization, whether based on new partners or different relationships, to reverse the sterilization process.

CRITICAL POINTS

- Preoperative counseling is absolutely necessary before any sterilization procedure.
- Advantages of male or female sterilization and their disadvantages need to be fully discussed.
- Possibility of poststerilization ectopic pregnancy along with other failures must be fully explored.
- Successful reversal of female sterilization depends mostly on the length of normal tube remaining.
- Type of sterilization may vary and depends on the preferences of the patient and physician.

Questions

1. Medical studies record that sterilization failures occur more often:
   A. In women
   B. In men
2. Sterilization problems after 30 years of age:
   A. Lead to increased hysterectomies
   B. Do not lead to increased hysterectomies
3. Reversal of sterilization depends on:
   A. Type of procedure performed
   B. Number of children before sterilization
   C. Length of uninvolved tube
   D. Timing of menstrual cycle in which tubal ligation is performed

4. After a male sterilization procedure:
   A. Intercourse is immediately "safe."
   B. No contraception is needed after the first menstrual period.
   C. "Protection" is needed until negative ejaculates have been present for 3 months.

Answers

1. A
2. B
3. C
4. C

Vaginal and vulvar disease

APGO LEARNING OBJECTIVE #31

Joseph B. Buxer

> *Vaginal and vulvar symptoms are frequent patient concerns. To provide appropriate care, the physician must understand the common causes of these problems.*

The student will demonstrate a knowledge of the following:

A. Physiologic changes in normal vaginal discharge

B. Evaluation and management of common vulvar and vaginal diseases, including the following:
   1. Vaginitis caused by bacteria, *Candida, Trichomonas,* viruses, foreign bodies, or atrophy
   2. Vulvitis caused by *Candida,* atrophy, or allergic reaction
   3. Dermatologic conditions of the vulva
   4. Bartholin's gland disease

VAGINAL DISEASE

Physiologic changes in the normal vaginal discharge

Leukorrhea, a term applied to any nonbloody discharge from the vagina, may consist of physiologic secretions or may be produced in response to irritation or infection of the genital organs. A certain amount of vaginal discharge, made up of mucus from the endocervical epithelium, transudate from the vaginal mucosa, and exfoliated vaginal epithelium, is always present but not always obvious to women because these normal secretions are not irritating and usually are not profuse.

The vagina is lined by nonkeratinizing stratified squamous epithelium whose activity, thickness, and glycogen content are controlled by variations in circulating levels of estrogen and progesterone. The pH of vaginal secretions in the normal adult during her reproductive years is between 3.5 and 4.5. The acidity is produced by conversion of cellular glycogen to lactic acid by lactobacilli that are normal vaginal inhabitants, sometimes called Döderlein's bacilli. There are no glands lining the vagina per se.

Before menarche and after menopause—when estrogen production is low—the epithelium is inactive, only a few cell layers thick, and devoid of glycogen. Döderlein's bacilli are absent, and the pH is between 6 and 7. This inactive, unstimulated mucosa is susceptible to infection by organisms such as *Neisseria gonorrhoeae*, whereas the estrogen-stimulated vagina is rarely invaded.

The volume of discharge from the normal vagina varies throughout the menstrual cycle. Early in the cycle, the estrogen level is low, the mucosa is relatively thin and inactive, and there is little secretion from the columnar and cuboidal cells of the endocervix. As estrogen production increases, the vaginal cells proliferate and exfoliate more rapidly, and the endocervical mucosa secretes more and more mucus. Just before ovulation (midcycle), when estrogen production is maximal, cervical mucus is profuse and watery and vaginal desquamation reaches its peak. Many women become aware of a discharge at this time. After ovulation, cervical mucus thickens (a progesterone effect) and the amount of vaginal discharge decreases.

Masters and Johnson were able to demonstrate that the source of vaginal lubrication during sexual excitement is a transudate through the vaginal mucosa from dilated paravaginal venous channels. Vaginal lubrication during sexual excitement is not from endocervical epithelium; secretions from the glands surrounding the introitus play a lesser role than once believed.

Principles of evaluation

Abnormal vaginal discharge is caused by irritation resulting from infection of the vagina or cervix, from atrophy, or even from the presence of a foreign body. Diagnosis of the cause of an abnormal vaginal discharge cannot be made over the phone or even from gross inspection—except, perhaps, if a foreign body is present. Microscopic evaluation is otherwise essential, and pH determination may be helpful.

The "wet prep" is simple and involves less than a minute of examiner time. One drop of normal saline solution at body temperature is dropped onto a Q-tip containing fresh vaginal discharge—which is then touched to a glass slide, covered with a coverslip, and immediately examined under medium magnification with diminished light intensity. A one-cell moving parasite *(Trichomonas vaginalis)* is easily distinguished from a branching structure *(Candida),* a clue cell (bacterial vaginosis), frank pus (cervicitis), or plump parabasal cells (atrophy) (Figs. 31-1 to 31-3).

Trichomonas vaginalis

PATHOGENESIS, SYMPTOMS, AND SIGNS. *T. vaginalis* usually is transmitted by sexual intercourse. However, transmission by the sharing of moist washcloths, sex toys, and other means has been demonstrated. The primary complaint is a vaginal discharge accompanied by an irritating itching or burning sensation.

LABORATORY-DIAGNOSTIC STUDIES. On examination, the vulva and vagina may appear inflamed. Punctate red "strawberry spots" might be pathognomonic but, unfortunately, are rarely seen. Instead, the discharge is abundant, thin, foul-smelling, greenish yellow, and bubbly; and the vaginal pH is greater than 5. The wet prep will show many leukocytes in clumps; at the edge of a clump may be seen a motile cell, slightly larger than a white blood cell, with the flagellum

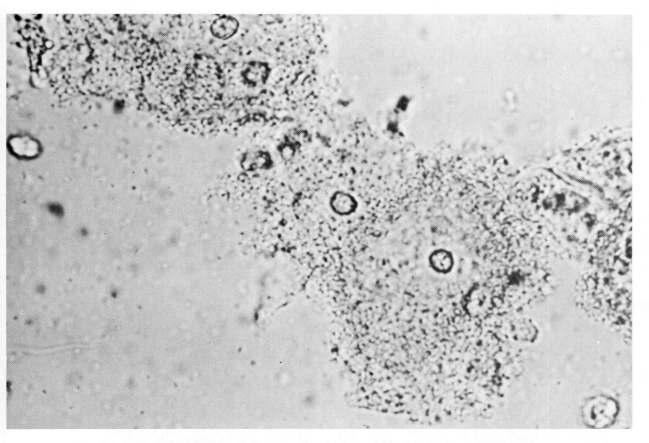

Fig. 31-1. Vaginal epithelial cells from woman with bacterial vaginosis. *(From Holmes KK: Lower genital tract infections in women: cystitis/urethritis, vulvovaginitis, and cervicitis. In Holmes KK, Mardh PA, Sparling PF et al, editors:* Sexually transmitted diseases, *New York, 1984, McGraw-Hill.)*

whipping it into a characteristic head-over-heels tumble.

MANAGEMENT. Metronidazole (Flagyl) is effective when taken orally and will kill the organisms in both men and women. Of course, both partners must be treated so that reinfection from the same partner does not occur. A single dose of 2 g is effective in 90% of cases and is preferred to multiday regimens. For those with treatment failure, repeat therapy, increased dose, or reevaluation of sources of infection and partner compliance may be appropriate. Local therapy in the form of metronidazole vaginal cream is not effective because trichomonads live in both the rectum and the urethra.

Candidiasis

PATHOGENESIS, SYMPTOMS, AND SIGNS. Frequently called "yeast infection" or moniliasis, candidiasis is a very common cause of vulvar irritation that is perceived as itching and is followed by scratching, a raw sensation, superficial skin cracks, erythema, and swelling. It is not

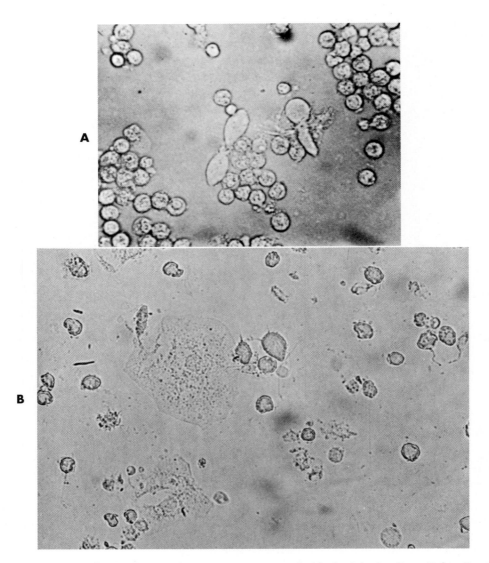

Fig. 31-2. A and **B,** Trichomonads in wet mount prepared with physiologic saline. *(A from Faro S: Trichomoniasis. In Kaufman RH, Faro S, editors:* Benign diseases of the vulva and vagina, *ed 4, St Louis, 1994, Mosby–Year Book.* **B** *from Friedrich EG:* Vulvar disease, *ed 2, Philadelphia, 1983, WB Saunders.)*

usually considered a sexually transmitted disease and seems to be more common during pregnancy (because of elevated vaginal pH), in patients with diabetes (because of increased glycogen in the vaginal epithelium), and after using broad spec-

trum antibiotics (because of loss of vaginal lactobacilli). It is also commonly found in immunosuppressed patients.

The vulva may appear either normal or edematous and inflamed. The vaginal discharge typically

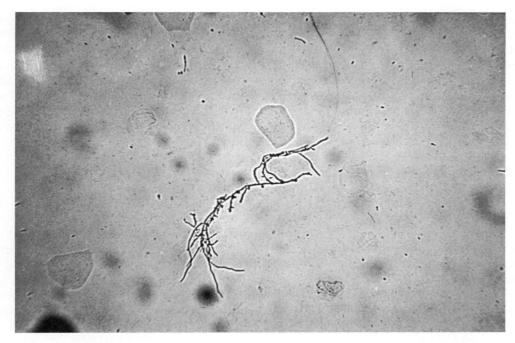

Fig. 31-3. Microscopic appearance of vaginal smear in case of vaginal candidiasis. *(From Merkus JMWM, Bisschop MPJM, Stolte LAM:* Obstet Gynecol Surv *40:495, 1985. Copyright © 1985 by Williams & Wilkins.)*

is thick, white, and in clumps that adhere to the vaginal walls. After prolonged infection there also may be a thin inflammatory exudate. Vaginal pH is slightly above 4.5.

LABORATORY-DIAGNOSTIC STUDIES. Wet prep discloses either few or many pus cells. But the diagnosis is made by seeing the typical mycelia (which look like branching, barren tree limbs) either singly or intertwined like tumbleweed. Spores and budding yeast may be found by experienced examiners, and many advocate the use of a separate slide made by adding a drop or two of 10% potassium hydroxide to a standard wet prep. This clears the slide of both white cells and epithelial cells, which otherwise might obscure the mycelia.

MANAGEMENT. Many very effective local treatments are available for candidiasis, such as miconazole (Monistat) and clotrimazole (Gyne-Lotrimin). Most products are available as both vaginal cream and vaginal suppositories. Either is applied nightly for 3 or 7 days, depending on the concentration selected. Shorter therapy is more convenient and appropriate for the first infection. Ninety percent of patients become asymptomatic.

Frequently, *Candida* organisms are harbored in the oral cavity and the rectum, as well as in the vagina; and these reservoirs may result in recurrent vaginal symptoms by direct contact. Although recurrent candidiasis will necessitate additional work-up, counseling, and innovative therapy, it is very important that reported recurrent symptoms are not just assumed to be recurrent candidiasis. Wet prep confirmation is required until the diagnosis is confirmed.

Bacterial vaginosis

PATHOGENESIS. Bacterial vaginosis has had many different names over the years, from nonspecific vaginitis through *Mycobacterium vaginalis* vaginitis to *Haemophilus vaginalis* vaginitis. Most recently it has been called *Gardnerella vaginalis* because that gram-negative aerobic coccobacillus is nearly always found in association with the condition. However, it is probable that no single organism is responsible. Bacterial vaginosis seems to be more of a condition than a disease and involves the unexplained overgrowth of all anaerobic bacteria in the vagina.

SYMPTOMS AND SIGNS. The patient complains of vulvar itching or burning. Her partner may complain of her disagreeable "fishy" odor, especially after intercourse. There is usually no evidence of inflammation on examination, but there will be an abundant grayish homogeneous discharge with a pH of 5 or more. A drop of 10% potassium hydroxide on a glass slide combined with a drop of discharge produces a characteristic (amine) odor (the "whiff test").

LABORATORY-DIAGNOSTIC STUDIES. The wet prep will show "clue cells," which are vaginal superficial squamous epithelial cells so encrusted with small coccobacilli that the cell borders are obscured. Further examination of the slide shows very few leukocytes (hence the designation "vaginosis" instead of "vaginitis").

MANAGEMENT. Treatment is either local or systemic. Oral metronidazole (Flagyl), 500 mg twice daily for 7 days; clindamycin (Cleocin), 300 mg twice daily for 7 days; or amoxicillin-clavulanic acid (Augmentin), 500 mg 3 times a day for 7 days is effective. Oral metronidazole is by far the least expensive. Metronidazole vaginal cream (Metrogel) applied twice daily for 5 days or 2% cleocin vaginal cream used at night for 7 days is very soothing but rather expensive.

Although there is some evidence that bacterial vaginosis is sexually transmitted, there seems to be no need to treat the sexual partner at first. Many physicians ultimately treat the partner when symptomatic recurrences become frequent.

Bacterial vaginosis during pregnancy has been associated with many complications, including chorioamnionitis, premature rupture of membranes, premature labor, and postpartum endomyometritis. Treatment during pregnancy must be considered.

Atrophy

PATHOGENESIS, SYMPTOMS, AND SIGNS. The pale, thin, dry, smooth epithelium that lines the vagina in estrogen-depleted postmenopausal women is easily traumatized and infected. Patients complain of dryness and dyspareunia, and may even experience some bleeding. It is quite common to have the vaginal speculum cause abrasion and bleeding of the vaginal wall or cervix during a normal gentle examination.

LABORATORY-DIAGNOSTIC STUDIES. Vaginal pH is also elevated in this condition. Wet prep shows many epithelial cells, but few will be normally mature squamous cells with pyknotic nuclei. Some appear as intermediate cells, squamous cells with nonpyknotic nuclei. Most will be large, round, parabasal cells with large nuclei—cells rarely seen in the uninfected vagina under normal hormone control. There may be some white blood cells as well, but few bacteria in the background and no lactobacilli.

MANAGEMENT. Estrogen therapy converts atrophic epithelium into thick, moist, resistant mucosa that is no longer dry or fragile. Oral estrogens are effective, but a more rapid response is achieved with estrogen vaginal cream. One tube of cream is to be used half an applicator high into the vagina every night at bedtime (the cream melts at body temperature and leaks out when the patient is up and about). Maintenance dosage is half an applicator twice a week.

Since vaginal estrogen is absorbed systemically, added progesterone is required for all women with a uterus, as with oral estrogen replacement. Vaginal estrogen may be used for quick response, but oral therapy is more convenient for maintenance and is much less expensive.

Allergy

Many commercial "feminine hygiene" products contain chemicals such as perfumes that can cause local allergic reactions and irritation. If a patient has an irritation without a demonstrable cause, a detailed history may disclose a recent change of soap product or deodorant tampon. Use of the product should be stopped; the irritation is soothed with warm-water sitz baths taken 3 times a day, followed by topical 1% hydrocortisone cream applied gently for 1 week. Then the patient is reexamined. This may be all the treatment needed, but a short course of oral corticosteroids may be used for more severe reactions.

Cervicitis

Cervicitis is another cause of leukorrhea and may be seen on inspection. Wet prep shows only leukocytes, and endocervical cultures for gonococci and *Chlamydia* are required. Initial treatment of the nonpregnant woman with doxycycline, 100 mg twice daily for 7 days, may decrease the discharge. Further therapy must await the culture reports, but in the meantime there should be no intercourse; and the patient must be rechecked in 7 days.

Herpes

Herpes virus vesicles may be seen on the cervix and vaginal walls occasionally. Diagnosis is by tissue culture. Treatment with Zovirax capsules, 200 mg 5 times a day for a week, is recommended for primary disease; but treatment usually is unnecessary for recurrent disease unless recurrences are frequent and symptomatic.

Foreign body

The most common cause for a sudden, profuse, offensive vaginal discharge in an otherwise healthy patient is the "lost" tampon, forgotten for days or weeks since the last period. Although the only treatment needed is removal of the tampon, it must be done precisely as follows:

1. See the patient at the very end of office hours.
2. Have your assistant open a Zip-Lock bag and hold it open between you and the patient's perineum.
3. Gently insert a large vaginal speculum.
4. Grasp the tampon with a ring forceps, but don't squeeze it.
5. Withdraw it rapidly and immediately drop the tampon into the bag.
6. Have the assistant seal the plastic bag instantly because the lost tampon odor is overwhelming and persists for hours.

VULVAR DISEASE

Because the vagina lacks nerve endings that can transmit such sensations as itching or burning, the student must be aware that the frequent complaints that accompany vaginal disorders, such as those already listed, may really be vulvar complaints and may be accompanied by swelling, erythema, and excoriation of the vulvar skin. Unfortunately, many other vulvar disorders produce similar complaints and all necessitate careful evaluation (Fig. 31-4).

Skin irritations that cannot be blamed on a vaginal discharge must be explained otherwise. If after careful examination one is secure that there is no lesion that requires a biopsy, symptomatic treatment with a 0.1% triamcinolone corticosteroid cream applied with fingertip massage may be all that is needed.

The symptoms must disappear and not recur, and the patient must confirm the success of the treatment. Many dangerous vulvar conditions may involve persistent itching or irritation, so one should never refill a first prescription without reexamining the patient. Should symptoms persist, colposcopic examination of the vulva is done without delay, looking specifically for vulvar intraepithelial neoplasia and invasive cancer. These can be diagnosed only by biopsy, and the magnification afforded by the colposcope will disclose the area for biopsy.

The vulvae are covered by skin that is susceptible to any skin disease that can affect other body surfaces. Contact dermatitis and atrophy may be symptomatic; vitiligo is not. Lichen sclerosis is not a premalignant condition, and its cause is unknown. It is found most commonly in postmenopausal women, although it may be seen at any age. Diagnosis is by biopsy, treatment is with 2% testosterone propionate cream gently massaged into the affected areas twice a day.

Hyperplastic lesions (dystrophies) also are diagnosed by biopsy. If there is no atypia, these may be soothed with a mild corticosteroid cream gently massaged into the affected areas twice a day. Carcinoma of the vulva, malignant mela-noma, and Paget's disease also must be diagnosed by biopsy. A biopsy must be obtained with any persistent lesion (Fig. 31-5).

Disorders of Bartholin's glands and ducts

There are two Bartholin's glands, one at the base of each labium majus. These glands drain small amounts of mucus to the surface through a tubular duct. When a duct is plugged with debris it eventually will swell with mucus, resulting in an uncomfortable mass, called a Bartholin's duct cyst, which may reach the size of a golf ball. Treatment is surgical drainage of the duct with an attempt to widen it permanently so that it will not become plugged again. The new duct is established by a small rubber catheter worn until the duct epithelializes or by "marsupialization," a surgical procedure that creates a wide new aperture that one hopes will not close.

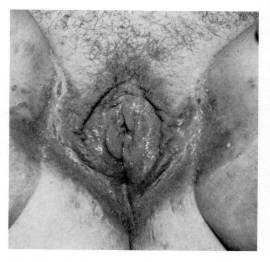

Fig. 31-4. Vulvitis caused by vaginal candidiasis.

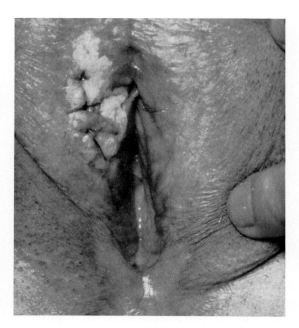

Fig. 31-5. Area of epithelial hyperkeratosis and early cancer.

Unfortunately, the retained secretions may become infected, resulting in a Bartholin's duct abscess. This very painful, debilitating condition necessitates incision and drainage as soon as there is fluctuance. Because permanent repair of the duct is not accomplished in these circumstances, the condition tends to recur.

Infections

The vulvae are covered with skin and are subject to infections common to all skin surfaces. In addition, some infections are specific for vulvar skin, including sexually transmitted diseases. Some of these are listed here, along with a few words about presentation, cause, method of diagnosis, and a suggestion for treatment. More detail will be found in Chapter 32, Sexually Transmitted Diseases.

HERPES. Very painful clusters of vesicles and ulcers are caused by herpes virus type 1 or 2. Herpes is diagnosed by tissue culture and treated symptomatically with an oral antiviral medication (Zovirax).

CONDYLOMATA ACUMINATA. Condylomata acuminata are asymptomatic warts found on examination by the patient. They are caused by a human papillomavirus, commonly type 6 or 11; they are diagnosed by inspection or, if persistent, by biopsy and are treated by local excision or destruction with cryosurgery or laser or a locally applied caustic medication (podophyllin, podophylox, trichloroacetic acid).

MOLLUSCUM CONTAGIOSUM. Molluscum contagiosum are asymptomatic clusters of white papules caused by the molluscum virus. They are diagnosed by inspection, confirmed by microscopic examination revealing molluscum inclusion bodies, and treated by unroofing each papule and touching the inside with a silver nitrate stick.

CHANCROID. An asymptomatic or painful genital ulcer, chancroid is caused by the bacterium *Haemophilus ducreyi* and diagnosed by microscopic examination of an ulcer smear to demonstrate the bacterium. It is treated with an antibiotic (Zithromax).

GRANULOMA INGUINALE (DONOVANOSIS). Granuloma inguinale are subcutaneous nodules that erode to form painless, enlarging, granulomatous ulcers. They are caused by a bacterium, diagnosed by microscopic examination of ulcer scrapings showing Donovan bodies within white blood cells, and treated with an antibiotic (tetracycline).

LYMPHOGRANULOMA VENEREUM. In lymphogranuloma venereum, regional adenopathy and inguinal swelling and abscess for

_ CRITICAL POINTS _

- Cervical infections must be cultured before treatment, although treatment may begin immediately after the cultures are obtained.
- Vaginal infections must be diagnosed by microscopic examination, using the wet prep before any treatment is begun.
- Irritating vulvar lesions must respond very quickly to symptomatic treatment or they must be biopsied.
- A vulvar lesion that is "different" in appearance at presentation must be biopsied before any treatment is started.

mation are caused by a strain of *Chlamydia trachomatis;* diagnosed by the complement fixation test; and treated with an antibiotic (tetracycline).

PRIMARY SYPHILIS. A painless, indurated ulcer, primary syphilis is caused by the spirochete *Treponema pallidum;* it is diagnosed by dark field examination of a smear from the ulcer (early) or serologically (later) and is treated with an antibiotic (penicillin).

PEDICULOSIS PUBIS. With pediculosis pubis, there is intense itching in skin areas covered by pubic hair. The infection is caused by the crab louse and diagnosed by magnifying glass visualization of the louse or its eggs (nits). It is treated with a special cream rinse (permethrin) or shampoo (lindane).

SCABIES. In scabies, intense itching and classic linear burrows in interdigital web spaces, wrists, elbows, anterior axillary folds, periumbilical skin, genitals, buttocks, and sides of the feet are caused by the itch mite *Sarcoptes scabiei.* Scabies is diagnosed by seeing the burrows (5 to 10 mm long) in characteristic distribution and is treated with a lotion (lindane).

Questions

1. A 24-year-old woman has had itching of the vulva, hands, and wrists for 3 weeks. Her boyfriend has had similar symptoms for 2 months. She has several isolated, raised erythematous papules on the labia majora and between the fingers of the right hand. Her most likely diagnosis is:
   A. Herpes simplex
   B. Bacterial vaginosis
   C. Scabies
   D. Candidiasis

2. A 19-year-old woman has had a recurring vulvar irritation for the past year. She has a homogeneous gray discharge with numerous clue cells, a pH greater than 5, and a fishy odor on addition of potassium hydroxide. Her most likely diagnosis is:
   A. Lymphogranuloma venereum
   B. Bacterial vaginosis
   C. Candidiasis
   D. *T. vaginalis* vaginitis

3. A 62-year-old woman with chronic vulvar pruritus has diffusely white, thin, crinkled vulvar epithelium with scattered ecchymoses. Biopsy demonstrates thin epithelium with loss of rete pegs and homogeneity of the dermis. The most appropriate treatment for this condition is:
   A. Topical 2% testosterone propionate cream
   B. Superficial skinning vulvectomy
   C. Laser vaporization of the vulva
   D. Premarin, 0.625 mg orally daily

4. A 31-year-old woman presents with dysuria and a yellowish, frothy, vaginal discharge with a pH of 6.5. Wet prep reveals motile trichomonads. The most cost-effective management for this condition is:
   A. Metrogel, twice daily for 5 days
   B. Metronidazole, 1 g orally for each partner
   C. Metronidazole, 2 g orally for each partner
   D. Metronidazole, 2 g orally for 2 days

Answers

1. C
2. B
3. A
4. C

32

Sexually transmitted diseases

APGO LEARNING OBJECTIVE #32

Joseph B. Buxer

> *To prevent sexually transmitted diseases and minimize their impact on reproductive health, it is necessary to understand their basic epidemiology, diagnosis, and management.*

The student will demonstrate a knowledge of the following:

A. Organisms and methods of transmission
B. Symptoms and physical findings
C. Evaluation and management for each of the following:
   1. Gonorrhea
   2. Chlamydia
   3. Herpes simplex virus infection
   4. Syphilis
   5. Human papillomavirus infection
   6. Human immunodeficiency virus infection
   7. Hepatitis B virus infection
D. Public health concerns, including the following:
   1. Screening programs
   2. Costs
   3. Prevention

Sexually transmitted diseases (STDs) are the infections most frequently encountered by reproductive health professionals. Their long-term sequelae, although unique to each disease, are frequently severe and may be life-threatening. They include such illnesses as tubal occlusion leading to infertility and ectopic pregnancy, neonatal morbidity and mortality from disease transmission to babies during pregnancy and delivery, some internal and external female genital cancers, liver failure, and acquired immunodeficiency syndrome (AIDS). Prevention, so critical in managing these problems for populations at risk, depends entirely on individual behavior. Diagnosis and treatment, although very important, remain secondary to prevention simply because there is no cure for some STDs.

PATHOGENESIS

Bacterial infections include the following:
- Gonorrhea, caused by *Neisseria gonorrhoeae*
- Chlamydia, caused by *Chlamydia trachomatis*
- Chancroid, caused by *Haemophilus ducreyi*
- Granuloma inguinale, caused by *Calymmatobacterium granulomatis*
- Lymphogranuloma venereum, caused by immunotypes L1, L2, and L3 of *C. trachomatis*

Syphilis is caused by a spirochete, *Treponema pallidum.*

Viral infections include the following:
- Acquired immunodeficiency syndrome, caused by the human immunodeficiency virus (HIV)
- Condylomata acuminata, caused by the human papillomavirus (HPV)
- Hepatitis B, caused by the hepatitis B virus (HBV)
- Herpes genitalis, caused by the herpes simplex viruses (HSVs) 1 and 2
- Molluscum contagiosum, caused by the molluscum contagiosum virus

Trichomoniasis is caused by *Trichomonas vaginalis,* a motile protozoan.

The unifying characteristic of these diverse conditions is that each is transmitted by intimate sexual contact; thus all are preventable.

GONORRHEA

Symptoms and signs

Gonorrhea, caused by *N. gonorrhoeae,* a gram-negative diplococcus, is the most commonly reported communicable disease in the United States. One million cases occur each year. Symp-

tomatic men complain of urinary frequency, dysuria, and a purulent urethral discharge. Symptomatic women may have an abnormal vaginal discharge, abnormal uterine bleeding, and dysuria. Many women, however, remain asymptomatic.

Laboratory-diagnostic tests

Diagnosis is made by bacterial culture on a selective medium (Thayer-Martin). This allows for antibiotic susceptibility testing, which is becoming increasingly important as penicillin-resistant and tetracycline-resistant strains spread throughout the world. (Penicillin resistance is achieved by both penicillinase-producing *N. gonorrhoeae* and chromasomally mediated strains.) A presumptive diagnosis, by identifying typical gram-negative intracellular diplococci on Gram stain of a urethral or cervical discharge, is enough to permit immediate definitive treatment. This is particularly acceptable when patient compliance (with instructions not to have intercourse until the diagnosis has been confirmed and all partners have been adequately treated) may be in doubt.

Management

A significant portion of gonorrheal infections are resistant to penicillin, and an alternative antibiotic often must be used. Nearly half of the women with gonococcal infection have coexistent chlamydia infection, which cannot be diagnosed on Gram stain but which, nevertheless, must be treated at the same time. For these reasons, a presumptive diagnosis of gonorrhea (made by examining the Gram stain of a purulent cervical discharge) justifies prompt treatment with 250 mg of ceftriaxone intramuscularly (for gonorrhea) and 100 mg of doxycycline twice daily for 7 days (for chlamydia).

About 40% of untreated women with cervical gonorrhea develop salpingitis. These women are at risk for the sequelae of pelvic inflammatory disease—including pelvic abscess, subsequent ectopic pregnancy, and infertility—and must be adequately treated. Of course, the other 60% also must be treated to prevent the spread of infection to subsequent partners.

CHLAMYDIA

Chlamydia is caused by *C. trachomatis,* an obligate intracellular bacterium that, like a virus, requires tissue culture for laboratory isolation. Genital chlamydia infection is the most common bacterial STD in the United States and is the leading cause of preventable infertility and ectopic pregnancy. Four million new cases occur annually. Because chlamydia is not ordinarily considered a "reportable disease," gonorrhea retains the dubious honor of being the infection most often reported. However, chlamydia has become much more common.

Symptoms, signs, and laboratory-diagnostic tests

Unlike gonorrhea, which is carried either asymptomatically in the endocervix or very symptomatically as salpingo-oophoritis, chlamydia may cause upper genital tract tissue destruction without symptoms and should be considered a chronic infection. Definitive diagnosis is made when an endocervical swab (which contains enough infected endocervical epithelial cells) is inoculated into tissue culture. Presumptive tests, which are much faster, include a monoclonal antibody immunofluorescence assay and an enzyme-linked immunoabsorbent assay.

Management

Treatment is quite inexpensive with doxycycline (a tetracycline), 100 mg twice daily for 7 days, or one of several alternative oral medications. The sequelae of chlamydia are severe and justify screening all patients at risk. They include the expected salpingo-oophoritis complications of ectopic pregnancy and infertility; but, in addition, the pregnant woman may suffer abortion or still-birth, her baby may develop neonatal ophthalmia and pneumonia, and she may develop postpartum endomyometritis.

HERPES SIMPLEX VIRUS INFECTION

Herpes simplex virus infections are caused by HSV types 1 and 2. Although type 2 is more common in genital infections, the types are indistinguishable clinically. Symptomatic primary genital HSV infections affect 200,000 people each year, and recurrent infections are much more common. Nevertheless, most people in the United States who carry this virus (70% of the adult population is HSV-antibody positive) are asymptomatic and will transmit the infection quite innocently.

Symptoms and signs

The HSV lesions start as pruritic vesicles that can appear anywhere on the genitalia. The vesicles then rupture spontaneously, forming shallow painful ulcers that ultimately heal without scarring. The first clinical occurrence may be a true first infection, accompanied by a viremia and severe local symptoms that last about 12 days. Voiding, for example, may become so painful that it is best done while sitting in a tub of warm water.

However, the first clinical occurrence may actually be a recurrence—the first infection having been asymptomatic. This phenomenon is difficult to explain; but it is assumed that when a first clinical occurrence is very mild, circulating antibodies are already present, preventing the viremia and minimizing the symptoms. A true first infection lasts about 12 days. A recurrent outbreak lasts only 5 days. The interval between recurrences is termed *latency* and is what distinguishes one person's illness from another's.

Unfortunately, viral shedding occurs intermittently during latency and is asymptomatic, so the patient does not know when it happens. Symptomatic genital recurrences are 6 times as frequent as oral herpes recurrences, and HSV type 2 genital recurrences are 5 times as frequent as HSV type 1 genital recurrences.

Laboratory-diagnostic tests

Definitive diagnosis is made in tissue culture. There are faster presumptive tests, such as finding giant cells with intranuclear inclusions in a specimen prepared as a Pap smear, or noting increased serologic titers in convalescent sera. Since there is no cure for this disease, only one positive culture is needed to document infection for each patient. Once the diagnosis is made, any typical lesion, or even any typical prodromal symptom that is recognized by the patient, must be assumed to be a recurrence, especially during pregnancy when labor is imminent. Vaginal delivery is not recommended during primary or recurrent disease episodes.

Management

Although there is no cure for HSV infection, there is very helpful treatment available for symptomatic first infections and for patients with frequently recurring disease. The antiviral drug acyclovir, 200 mg 5 times a day, may halve the symptomatic length of a first infection and provide significant relief. Doses of 200 mg 5 times a day will halve the length of recurrent episodes as well, but the disappearance of lesions just 2 days sooner may not be considered cost-effective. However, 200 mg twice a day continuously may eliminate all recurrences and be well worth the cost for patients who experience more than six recurrences each year. This is not a cure, though. This is merely suppression.

SYPHILIS

Syphilis, caused by the spirochete *T. pallidum,* affects 50,000 people each year in the United States. It is found most often among low-income, minor-

ity, heterosexual populations. Congenital syphilis occurs once in 10,000 live births, and its incidence seems associated with the exchange of sex for drugs. The overall incidence of this STD is rising and is now higher than it has been for over 40 years, which is sad because just 50 years ago the introduction of penicillin could have eliminated the disease entirely. Syphilis remains exquisitely sensitive to penicillin.

Symptoms, signs, and laboratory-diagnostic tests

The diagnoses of late latent, tertiary, neurovascular, or cardiovascular syphilis may be made after significant work-up for a myriad of unusual symptoms, or just by serendipity. More important for the generalist, perhaps, are the symptoms of primary and secondary syphilis because these stages are more common, entirely curable, and present an opportunity to prevent the spread of this disease to partners and unborn children.

The classic chancre of primary syphilis is a painless, indurated ulcer located at the site of exposure. The ulcer may be easily found before the serologic screening test for syphilis can turn positive. Therefore dark field examination of a scraping from the ulcer is clearly indicated. Secondary syphilis presents with a variable skin rash that frequently includes the palms of the hands and the soles of the feet. Distinct patches may be seen on mucous membranes, and condylomata lata may be found on the vulva. There may be lymphadenopathy and alopecia as well, and the serologic screening test for syphilis will be positive with a high titer. Latent syphilis, of course, is asymptomatic and is diagnosed by positive serology.

Management

Treatment for primary, secondary, and early latent syphilis of less than 1 year's duration is with a long-acting penicillin called benzathine penicillin G, 2.4 million U intramuscularly, just once. If the patient has latent syphilis of unknown duration, or if more advanced disease is suspected, an infectious disease specialist should be consulted about the required extended work-up and treatment.

Late syphilis and congenital syphilis are both complications of early disease, and both are preventable by early diagnosis and treatment. Sequelae of late syphilis include neurosyphilis (general paresis and tabes dorsalis) and cardiovascular syphilis (thoracic aortic aneurysm and aortic insufficiency).

HUMAN PAPILLOMAVIRUS INFECTION

Human papillomavirus infection is the most prevalent of all STDs. Almost 70 viral deoxyribonucleic acid (DNA) types have been identified so far, about a dozen of which demonstrate predilection for human genitalia. The HPV DNA types are discussed in the literature by number, such as HPV 6, 11, 16, 18, and so on; and each numbered virus presents a unique risk for the development of genital warts, or dysplastic epithelium on the penis, vulva, vagina, cervix and endocervix, or of invasive epithelial cancers. It is assumed that 60% of our adult population has an HPV infection because of the prevalence of HPV DNA in polymerase chain reaction studies.

Genital warts

The physician who manages STDs encounters HPV infections in two very different ways. In the first, the patient presents with obvious genital warts (condylomata acuminata). The virus is transmitted by intimate sexual contact. The HPV types 6 and 11 are most often involved. There are few symptoms and the findings are simply variously sized warts.

Treatment is local removal, by cutting them with a knife or desiccating them with caustic chemicals (podophyllin, podophylox, trichloroacetic acid); by freezing (cryosurgery), coagulating (electrocautery), or vaporizing (laser) them; or by using the immune system to reject (interferon injections) the lesions. The risk of malignant transformation is quite low, and sooner or later local treatment will prevail.

Asymptomatic human papillomavirus infection

The second way a physician encounters HPV infection is through a routine Pap smear report. When cervical cytology is abnormal, and when the lab report suggests either low grade or high grade squamous intraepithelial lesion, it is assumed that HPV infection is present. At this time it is believed that HPV either causes or is a significant cofactor in causing squamous carcinomas of the vulva, vagina, and cervix, and adenocarcinoma of the endocervix by progression through precancers called mild, moderate, and severe dysplasias and carcinomas-in-situ.

The HPV types 16, 18, 31, 33, and 45 are most often involved with precancers of the lower genital tract and transmission is through intimate sexual contact. Early adolescent exposure, multiple sexual partners, and smoking all increase the risk that HPV infection will result in progression to dysplasia and invasive cancer.

There are neither symptoms nor signs for this infection. Virus-caused intraepithelial lesions are microscopic and cannot be seen without magnification (colposcopy). Colposcopy is often used for population screening in Europe; but we rely on Pap smear screening in the United States, with colposcopy used only when indicated.

HUMAN IMMUNODEFICIENCY VIRUS INFECTION

Human immunodeficiency virus infection results in AIDS. The virus is transmitted by intimate sexual contact. Both HIV and HBV, of course, may be transmitted by contaminated needles, blood and blood products, as well as by sexual transmission.

Acquired immunodeficiency syndrome takes years to develop. The STD is infection with HIV. The long-term result of becoming infected with HIV is AIDS, much as the long-term result of becoming infected with the *T. pallidum* spirochete is neurosyphilis.

Shortly after infection with HIV some patients may notice a flu-like illness that resolves in about 2 weeks. The HIV test, which depends on an antibody response to the virus, will remain negative typically for 6 to 12 weeks. This interval between infection and when the test becomes positive is known as the "window period." The CD4 cell count per microliter is normal, between 400 and 1200.

The average interval from infection to AIDS is about 11 years. First there may be a discrete illness with some opportunistic bacterium, virus, fungus, or parasite. Then there is a cascade of illness as the CD4 cell count drops below 200. Kaposi's sarcoma, lymphoma, cervical cancer, and tuberculosis are common. Neurologic complications include dementia, memory loss, alterations in affect and gait, and peripheral neuropathies. This end-stage lasts from just a few months to several years.

There are 2 million Americans infected with HIV; 361,000 have AIDS, and 220,000 have died so far.

HEPATITIS B INFECTION

Hepatitis B virus infection, like HIV, is a viral disease transmitted by contamination with the body fluids of an infected person. Once called serum hepatitis because it seemed most often to follow blood transfusion, HBV is now known to be transmitted by any infected body fluid breaching any skin barrier. This still includes contaminated blood and blood products, of course, but also involves needle punctures and cuts suffered by health care workers or intravenous drug abusers, and intimate sexual contact that results in even micro-scopic tears of epithelial surfaces, such as may occur during receptive anal intercourse. There are 150,000 new cases of heterosexually transmitted HBV infections annually. More than 80% of the male homosexual population is HBV antibody positive.

The role of the HBV carrier is central to the epidemiology of HBV transmission. A carrier is a person who was infected with HBV in the past but, instead of clearing the infection successfully, remained hepatitis B surface antigen (HBsAg) positive. Successfully clearing the infection would leave a patient anti–Hepatitis B surface antibody (HBsAb) positive. This immunoglobulin G antibody grants immunity to subsequent HBV infections. Failing to clear the infection leaves a patient HBsAg positive, in spite of detectable antibody, and thus continually infectious.

Curiously, the likelihood of developing the carrier state varies inversely with the age at which infection occurs. When it is perinatally transmitted to a baby by its carrier mother, HBV infection results in a carrier state in up to 90% of infants; whereas only 10% of acutely infected adults become carriers.

Diagnosis is based on serologic tests for the HBV antigens HBsAg, HBcAg, and HBeAg. Consider "s" as surface antigen; "c" as core antigen; and "e" as, perhaps, an envelope antigen. Each is detectable at a special time during the disease, and its presence and disappearance are used to monitor the process. The serologic pattern of these tests identifies the stage of the infection.

Symptoms start gradually. A flu-like syndrome is followed by fatigue, anorexia, nausea, vomiting, myalgia, malaise, headache, and pharyngitis. After 2 weeks, jaundice is obvious and there is a low-grade fever. About 10% of patients have severe disease with hepatosplenomegaly and lymphadenopathy, and jaundice may persist for 6 weeks while other symptoms slowly resolve. Healing takes up to 3 months. Most patients, nevertheless, recover completely, with only 10%

becoming chronic carriers. There is no known treatment for HBV infection other than supportive care.

There are, however, sequelae to this disease. Almost 10% of young adults become chronic carriers; and a quarter of those progress to HBV-related cirrhosis, which kills 4000 people each year in the United States. Their risk of developing primary liver cancer is 300 times that of the general population, claiming 800 lives in the United States each year. Ninety percent of infants born to carrier mothers are infected with HBV. Ninety percent of these will become chronic carriers, and 25% eventually will succumb to primary hepatocellular carcinoma or cirrhosis.

PUBLIC HEALTH CONCERNS

Screening programs

State, county, and municipal STD clinics screen for all STDs and treat those that are found. They offer treatment and follow-up to all partners as well. Unfortunately, these primary STD clinics reach only those people who are already concerned about the issue. Prenatal care clinics offer STD screening because there may be some risk to a developing fetus. Most women do not consider themselves at risk but are eager to be tested anyway, as part of mothering. Perhaps the greatest opportunity for institutional STD screening takes place at birth control clinics, where patients enter specifically to discuss sexually related issues.

If all three of these opportunities for STD screening were used to maximal advantage, however, there would be no demonstrable change in the incidence of the diseases discussed in this chapter. The greatest number of patient–health care worker interactions in this country occur not in public clinics but in the individual offices of several hundred thousand physicians, most of whom consider themselves primary care physi-

cians. That must be where screening programs achieve significance.

Health care workers who understand the importance of STDs must take every opportunity to educate their patients about STD prevention. It is reasonable to expect even brief professional education to result in patient interest in the concept of STD prevention. This may be followed by a natural curiosity concerning past intimate events and will lead to acceptance of testing for many STDs. But, of even more significance, it may develop an understanding of the need for primary prevention. Since patients don't read our texts, we have the responsibility to interest them in the subject and to provide accurate information.

Costs

The cost of STDs to the U.S. health care system and the national economy is enormous. The volume of wasted assets, both financial and material, is dwarfed only by the weight of human suffering these diseases cause. Most dispiriting, perhaps, is understanding that the whole is truly waste because each disease is preventable.

Can one guess the dollars spent to manage 4 million cases of chlamydia each year? Add the cost of 1 million cases of gonorrhea, 50,000 cases of syphilis, and 150,000 cases of HBV every year. Add, too, 200,000 primary HSV infections each year and many more recurrent infections that require treatment or continuous suppression. Seventy percent of the U.S. population has HSV antibodies. Add, further, 360,000 visits for genital warts and the 10% HPV-generated abnormal Pap smear rate. Sixty percent of the U.S. population is HPV DNA positive.

Finally, consider the potential cost for 2 million HIV-positive Americans, 361,000 of whom have AIDS. All wasted. All preventable. All providers, but especially primary care physicians, must be dedicated to finding and treating STDs. Still more important, they must be dedicated to teaching prevention.

CRITICAL POINTS

- The three most prevalent primary viral infections of the skin of the vulva are genital herpes, condyloma acuminatum, and molluscum contagiosum.
- Condyloma acuminatum is an STD spread by skin-to-skin contact. It is caused by HPV. Auto-inoculation also occurs. It is a highly contagious disease, with 25% to 65% of sexual partners developing the infections.
- Herpes is highly contagious, with 75% of sexual partners contracting the disease. The prevalence of genital herpes is estimated to be between 10 and 30 million cases.
- Nonspecific tests for syphilis, the Venereal Disease Research Laboratory (VDRL) and rapid plasmin reagin, have a 1% false-positive rate. Therefore specific tests—such as the fluorescent treponemal antibody, absorbed (FTA-ABS); hemagglutination treponemal test for syphilis, and microhemagglutination-*T. pallidum*—must be used when a positive, nonspecific test result is encountered.
- After successful treatment of syphilis, the VDRL titer will become nonreactive or, at most, reactive with at least a fourfold titer decline within 1 year. The FTA-ABS may remain reactive indefinitely.
- In middle-class women in the reproductive-age range, bacterial vaginosis represents approximately 50% of vaginitis; candidiasis and *Trichomonas* infection represent approximately 25% each.
- A vaginal pH greater than 5 indicates atrophic vaginitis, bacterial vaginosis, or *Trichomonas* infection, whereas a vaginal pH of less than 4.5 is either a physiologic discharge or fungal.
- Individuals with HIV infection may shed the virus throughout the asymptomatic phase of their disease, which may last for several years. Every year 2% to 10% of these patients will develop AIDS.

Questions

1. One possible consequence of HBV infection is:
   A. Ectopic pregnancy
   B. Cirrhosis of the liver
   C. Acquired immunodeficiency syndrome
   D. Cancer of the cervix
   E. Condylomata lata
2. Treatment for some HPV infections may include:
   A. Benzathine penicillin G 2.5 million U intramuscularly
   B. Doxycycline, 100 mg twice daily for 7 days
   C. Ceftriaxone, 250 mg intramuscularly
   D. Interferon alfa 2-B, 250,000 U subcutaneously
   E. Acyclovir, 200 mg orally 5 times a day
3. The most common presentation of genital HSV 2 is:
   A. Cluster of small pruritic vesicles
   B. Solitary, painless ulcer
   C. Foul-smelling vaginal discharge
   D. Purulent cervical discharge
   E. Swollen, tender inguinal lymph nodes

Answers

1. B
2. D
3. A

33

Salpingitis

APGO LEARNING OBJECTIVE #33

Joseph B. Buxer

The potential impact of acute or chronic salpingitis is significant. Tubal infection may result in chronic pain and infertility. Early recognition and optimal management may help prevent the long-term sequelae of tubal disease.

The student will demonstrate a knowledge of the following:

A. Pathogenesis
B. Common organisms
C. Signs and symptoms
D. Methods of diagnosis
E. Treatment
F. Sequelae, including the following:
   1. Tuboovarian abscess
   2. Chronic salpingitis
   3. Ectopic pregnancy
   4. Infertility

 Salpingitis is a term applied to any infection of the fallopian tubes. It may take the form of severe disease that is acute and life-threatening; it may be chronic, painful, and debilitating; or it may be indolent and virtually asymptomatic.

The common result of all of its forms, however, is the alteration of normal upper genital tract anatomy, leaving it distorted and nonfunctional. Thus, other than preserving life, the physician's prime goal in the treatment of this disease is preventing genital tract destruction and resulting infertility.

PATHOGENESIS

Although the gonococcus is often found in the endocervix of patients with acute salpingitis, it is infrequently cultured from the peritoneal cavity. The gonococcus, therefore, may act only as a pathfinder for the many other bacteria frequently cultured from the purulent exudate at the fimbrial end of a tube. Relatively early in the disease, peritoneal cultures may isolate many different species of bacteria, including gram-positive and gram-negative aerobes and anaerobes. Later, some organisms become dominant and fewer species are isolated. Therefore infections usually involve several organisms.

Chlamydia trachomatis, on the other hand, is frequently cultured from both the endocervix and the fallopian tube fimbria, as well as from peritoneal adhesions. Both gonorrhea and chlamydia are sexually transmitted diseases, and acute salpingo-oophoritis (the ovary is almost always involved in the infection) results from sexual contact with an infected partner. Nevertheless, most bacterial species cultured from the tubes of seriously ill patients are part of the normal flora of the endocervix. It is thought that they are brought to the endosalpinges and ovaries (where they are pathogens) by the sexually transmitted pathfinders.

Most women who harbor gonorrhea and chlamydia in the endocervical canal are asymptomatic; therefore, routine endocervical cultures for each are required to identify carriers. It is not known why some women become severely ill almost immediately and others remain asymptomatic for extended periods, nor is it known what triggers a pathogen's ascent to the upper reproductive tract to create an endometritis and an endosalpingitis. What is apparent, however, is that symptoms of salpingitis secondary to gonorrhea frequently follow a menstrual flow.

The natural history of untreated endosalpingitis includes both destruction of the columnar epithelium that lines the tube and production of a purulent exudate. The fimbria become agglutinated in an attempt to prevent infection from extending to the peritoneal cavity. The resulting distended, pus-filled tube is called a *pyosalpinx.* When pelvic peritonitis follows, bowel and omentum adhere to the tubes in an attempt to keep the infection confined to the pelvis. When that fails, as it does when a localized tubo-ovarian abscess ruptures, generalized peritonitis follows.

Common organisms

Neisseria gonorrhoeae and *C. trachomatis* cause most cases of acute salpingo-oophoritis. Therefore cervical cultures (or antigen detection tests) for these organisms should be the first step in work-up for acute salpingitis. It makes no sense to do cervical cultures for anaerobic bacteria or for gram-negative aerobes, such as *Escherichia coli,* because these are part of the normal flora of the endocervix. Pelvic cavity cultures for anaerobic bacteria and common intestinal organisms are done surgically (laparoscopically) during treatment for advanced disease, such as pelvic abscess. Cultures of peritoneal fluid retrieved by culdocentesis, however, are of little value because of probable vaginal contamination.

Nongonococcal, nonchlamydial bacteria isolated from the upper genital tract include anaerobic gram-positive cocci such as peptostreptococcus; anaerobic gram-negative bacilli of the *Prevotella* group (*bivius, disiens, melaninogenicus,* and so on) and *Bacteroides fragilis;* gram-positive aerobic bacteria such as group B streptococcus and enterococcus; and gram-negative aerobes such as *E. coli, Klebsiella,* and *Gardnerella vaginalis.* The genital tract mycoplasmas, *Mycoplasma hominis* and *Ureaplasma urealyticum,* may be found as well. Salpingo-oophoritis is truly a polymicrobial disease, and understanding this guides therapeutic choices and decisions.

SYMPTOMS AND SIGNS

A patient with early salpingitis usually consults her physician because of symptoms of pelvic discomfort. Her pain is described as mild, achy, bilateral, and generally nonspecific. She may describe a change in the color or quality of her vaginal discharge or perhaps some unexpected mild vaginal bleeding, like the breakthrough bleeding of a birth control pill, or she may describe an unusual discomfort with intercourse. She may also say that she has a new partner.

Signs found on examination occasionally include a low-grade fever and a purulent cervical discharge. More frequently there will be only cervical motion tenderness and adnexal tenderness when the ovaries are gently palpated. Tender, bilateral, adnexal masses are found in more advanced disease.

Severe, advanced salpingo-oophoritis is more likely to bring the patient to a hospital emergency room than to an office. The symptoms of early disease just described, left untreated, have advanced over several days to severe lower abdominal pain, nausea, vomiting, diarrhea, and tenesmus, as well as frequency, dysuria, and urgency. Signs now include fever, tachycardia and dehydration, lower abdominal guarding, and perhaps rebound tenderness—with severe cervical motion tenderness and severe adnexal tenderness when the ovaries are palpated. In fact, the examination may be so uncomfortable that it cannot be completed.

LABORATORY-DIAGNOSTIC STUDIES

Laparoscopic visualization of inflamed and swollen pus-filled fallopian tubes, with purulent exudate oozing from their fimbrial ends and adhesions to adjacent ovaries, bowel, and pelvic sidewalls, is certainly diagnostic of acute salpingo-oophoritis. When Scandinavian investigators discovered that diagnoses made clinically by university faculty gynecologists, then checked by laparoscopy, were wrong 35% of the time, laparoscopy became the "gold standard" for diagnosis. In one third of the cases checked, clinically diagnosed salpingitis had no apparent cause (20%) or was caused by factors other than those identified (15%).

Unfortunately, laparoscopy is major surgery, and it is neither prudent nor possible to subject every patient with suspected salpingitis to this procedure. Laparoscopy is indicated, however, when the diagnosis of salpingitis is in doubt, as it is when there might be an ectopic pregnancy or appendicitis, or even when appropriate antibiotic therapy does not seem to be working.

Most often, however, the attending physician must use mature clinical judgment to unravel an aggregate of symptoms, signs, and laboratory reports, none of which are diagnostic. The physician must decide whether or not to treat the patient for salpingitis long before the cervical cultures for gonorrhea and chlamydia are reported because tissue destruction with salpingitis is relentless and early treatment is much more effective in preserving fertility than late treatment.

Signs that make a physician suspect salpingitis on abdominal examination are bilateral, lower abdominal, direct tenderness; guarding; and rebound tenderness. On pelvic examination the signs include tenderness with motion of the cervix and uterus; and bilateral, adnexal tenderness. Fever over 38° C; a leukocytosis over 10,000 with a left shift; a purulent cervical discharge with gram-negative intracellular diplococci found on Gram stain; and bilateral, tender adnexal masses all suggest salpingitis. Unfortunately, not one of these signs is invariably present, and rarely are all of them found together.

Pelvic peritonitis (salpingo-oophoritis) may be the only peritonitis for which medical management is preferred. Therefore it is critical that surgical emergencies be reasonably ruled out. There should be a quantitative serum beta–human chorionic gonadotropin report of less than 5 mIU/ml and no reason to suspect appendicitis, intraabdominal hemorrhage, or ruptured sigmoid diverticulum. Medical therapy must show significant improvement in the patient's condition within 48 hours or the diagnosis remains in doubt.

Pelvic ultrasonography and computed tomographic scanning may offer some assistance. Ultrasound is particularly useful after regression of a tuboovarian abscess. Laparoscopy was actually contraindicated at one time for use in pelvic infections, and there is still risk of distended bowel perforation when there is generalized peritonitis.

However, laparoscopy is extremely helpful in making the diagnosis; and it seems quite safe in skillful hands, especially during early infectious disease.

MANAGEMENT *Salpingitis*

The initial treatment chosen for a woman suspected of having acute salpingitis depends on how sick she is when first seen. Empiric therapy will be aimed at the two most common organisms of early disease or against the polymicrobial expectation of advanced disease. The drugs chosen for treatment depend on answers to questions such as the following: (1) Is the salpingo-oophoritis early or is a tuboovarian abscess possible? (2) Can the patient tolerate oral medication or is intravenous therapy required? (3) Can the patient be treated safely by repeated office visits or is hospitalization needed?

The patient with recent-onset dyspareunia, mild cervical motion tenderness, mild adnexal tenderness, who can tolerate oral medication, but who is, nevertheless, suspected of early salpingitis must have cervical cultures taken for gonorrhea and chlamydia and requires treatment for those two pathogens. It is not necessary to wait for the culture reports. Drugs of choice change over time, both because of the introduction of more effective medications with fewer side effects and because of the emergence of bacterial resistance. Ceftriaxone, 250 mg intramuscularly, will successfully treat uncomplicated gonorrhea; and 7 days of oral doxycycline, 100 mg twice daily, will successfully treat early chlamydial infection.

When a decision is made for outpatient therapy and the patient is sent home, several significant assumptions are made: (1) that she will take all her medicine as directed; (2) that the medicine will be effective; and (3) that she will abstain from sexual contact and not be immediately reinfected by the same partner. The patient must be reevaluated within 24 to 48 hours. If she is not getting better by then, the diagnosis is in doubt.

The patient who comes to the emergency room with fever, dehydration, anorexia, vomiting, and signs of peritonitis cannot be treated at home and must be hospitalized, hydrated, and treated with appropriate parenteral antibiotics. The infection must now be assumed to be advanced and polymicrobial. There will be no peritoneal cultures to work with unless the patient goes to surgery. However, at least two sets of aerobic-anaerobic blood cultures are appropriate for patients with high spiking fevers.

Which bacteria are treated? Gonorrhea and chlamydia are obvious. In addition, the anaerobic gram-negative bacilli of the *Bacteroides* group, gram-positive anaerobes such as peptostreptococcus, gram-negative aerobic bacilli such as *E. coli,* and perhaps gram-positive aerobes such as group B streptococcus and enterococcus must be remembered. Unfortunately, there is no single antibiotic that can reliably do it all. Until there is, one must work with the concepts of multiple drug therapy.

The 1991 Centers for Disease Control (CDC) recommendations for inpatient management of salpingo-oophoritis included a combination of cefotetan, 2 g intravenously, and doxycycline, 100 mg intravenously, each one given every 12 hours. The clinician must remain flexible regarding therapy, however, because bacteria may become resistant; less expensive treatment may become available; and CDC recommendations are updated about every 3 years.

Classic triple therapy consists of ampicillin, clindamycin, and gentamicin. Ampicillin is effective therapy for gram-positive cocci, both aerobes and anaerobes; gentamicin remains effective against most Enterobacteriaceae (aerobic gram-negative rods); and clindamycin covers the anaerobic gram-negative rods. Although not the drug of choice for chlamydia, clindamycin is still quite effective.

The physician can easily be overwhelmed by the number of available extended spectrum penicillins, with and without penicillinase inhibitors, the generations of cephalosporins, the cephalexins, aminoglycosides, quinolones, macrolides, and, of course, the tetracyclines and chloramphenicol. Rather than attempt to remember the unique pharmacologies of literally dozens of drugs, the physician should try to remember basic principles. The goals are to stop tissue destruction and reduce pain. Which bacteria are most likely to be involved with the working diagnosis? There are families of appropriate antibiotics. Which are safe and tolerated by the patient? Whatever antibiotic combinations are recommended in the future, the germs that cause salpingitis will probably remain the same.

SEQUELAE OF SALPINGITIS

Tuboovarian abscess

A tuboovarian abscess (TOA) forms when the body attempts to localize untreated or ineffectively treated salpingitis by walling it off. Although the attempt may be lifesaving, it is always at the cost of severe tissue destruction and normal reproductive function. Early, accurate diagnosis of acute salpingitis and effective treatment with appropriate antibiotics are crucial in preventing this natural phenomenon.

A TOA is suspected when a patient with salpingitis is found to have an adnexal swelling or mass. Abscesses, frequently bilateral, are indistinguishable from tuboovarian complexes (TOCs) by palpation. A TOA is an accumulation of inflammatory cells and bacteria in a newly created space. A TOC is the agglutination and adherence of infected structures into a space-occupying mass without walled-off pus. The difference between the two is that a TOC seems to respond more easily to antibiotic therapy than does a TOA, perhaps because some antibiotics (aminoglycosides) are rendered ineffective in the anaerobic, low-pH environment of a walled-off cavity lacking a blood supply.

TOCs usually respond to appropriate antibiotics, and about half of TOAs also respond. Defi-

nite improvement in both symptoms and signs must be seen within 72 hours of therapy or the diagnosis must be confirmed surgically. A TOC confirmed by laparoscopy may be cultured and medical management adjusted and continued. A TOA confirmed by laparoscopy that does not respond to medical treatment is best removed or adequately drained. Total abdominal hysterectomy and bilateral salpingo-oophorectomy, once mandatory, are no longer required. Unilateral excision of a TOA may be all that is needed. A ruptured TOA, of course, is a surgical emergency necessitating stabilization of a patient in septic shock, laparotomy, removal of the ruptured abscess, and peritoneal lavage.

Chronic salpingitis

The most important consequences of acute salpingitis are the chronic sequelae. Chronic pelvic pain is debilitating and depressing and is much more common in women who have had salpingo-oophoritis. Unfortunately, the relationship between salpingitis and chronic pelvic pain has neither been investigated nor characterized properly.

Nevertheless, scar tissue may be more easily reinfected and less reliably cleared of disease. Adhesions may fix tissues that are normally mobile, and stretching these adhesions may cause pain. An ovary, bound to the pelvic sidewall by adhesions, may hurt during ovulation; and the use of an oral contraceptive to induce gonadal quiescence may both eliminate the pain and aid in its diagnosis. Lysing adhesions laparoscopically—which restores normal relationships and mobility to the tubes, ovaries, and intestine—may succeed in relieving pain.

Ectopic pregnancy

Ectopic pregnancy remains a potentially lethal complication of attempting childbirth. It is a common consequence of the tissue damage caused by salpingitis and an even more common consequence of the attempt to repair that damage surgically. The tube may be mobile enough to capture the egg and allow fertilization. However, with extensive destruction of both the ciliated epithelium and the muscularis of the tube (both are supposed to help move a zygote along)—and with extensive scarring of the endosalpinx, dividing it into myriad blind sacs—it is no wonder that one third of surgically repaired postsalpingitis pregnancies are unable to reach the uterine cavity. (For additional information see Chapter 10, Ectopic Pregnancy.)

Infertility

Infertility as a result of inflammatory damage is caused by peritubal and paraovarian adhesions that interfere with the normal, dynamic tuboovarian relationships. The most sensitive targets of tissue destruction are the ampulla and fimbria of the tubes. Results range from phimosis and fimbrial agglutination to the classic retort-shaped hydrosalpinx that falls posterolaterally below the ovary and is stuck there by webs of adhesions.

Investigators claim that severe salpingitis, even tuboovarian complexes, when aggressively managed medically, can result in successful pregnancies in 33% of women who attempt to become pregnant. But this means that 67% of women who wish to become pregnant after severe salpingo-oophoritis are unsuccessful. Nevertheless, the majority of women with a single bout of less serious salpingitis remain fertile, with only about 15% of women infertile after one episode of salpingitis, about 30% after two, and about 60% after three. In most cases fertility is not restored by surgery, and in vitro fertilization becomes an expensive and often last resort.

Chronic salpingitis can be a terrible disease and its consequences are debilitating, disabling, and even fatal. The student who has had no experience with the illness (even by its other names, such as salpingo-oophoritis or pelvic inflamma-

tory disease [PID]) may wonder how frequently the average primary care physician, such as a family doctor or a generalist obstetrician-gynecologist, encounters the illness in a normal practice. Unfortunately, the true incidence is unknown, partly because it is not a reportable disease (except when there is a positive culture for gonorrhea, which is reportable); partly because most early cases are seen in an ambulatory setting and are not accurately counted; and partly because a significant portion of infections are "silent," asymptomatically destroying reproductive tissue and function and first discovered at surgery done for an ectopic pregnancy or as part of an infertility work-up. The best estimate we have is that 1.5 million episodes occur annually in the United States. This results in 350,000 hospitalizations each year for PID. One in seven women of reproductive age in the United States reports having been treated for PID. Tubal factor infertility occurs in 20% of known PID patients, 7 times as many as in the non-PID population. Ectopic pregnancy is 10 times as likely to happen to a patient who had PID than to one who did not.

Chronic pelvic pain, dyspareunia, pelvic adhesions, and other inflammatory residua, often necessitating surgical intervention, occur in 20% of cases. In addition, tuboovarian abscess, the major early complication of acute salpingo-oophoritis, occurs in 10% of patients hospitalized with acute PID, amounting to 35,000 TOAs in the United States each year.

Sexually transmitted disease is common in the United States, and the primary care physician must deal with it, in its many forms, daily. Most important is early diagnosis, at a time when complaints are vague. Careful bimanual pelvic examination is the only way to find the signs that lead to early treatment. The term "pelvic deferred" should not appear in the chart, especially when a woman of reproductive age complains of low abdominal pain. The possibility of salpingitis should always be considered.

CRITICAL POINTS

- Early salpingitis most often involves *N. gonorrhoeae, C. trachomatis,* or both.
- Late salpingitis most often involves anaerobic bacteria, as well as *C. trachomatis, E. coli,* and any bacteria normally found in the endocervix.
- The gold standard for diagnosis of PID is laparoscopy.
- Treatment may be ambulatory in early disease and inpatient for advanced disease.
- Sequelae of salpingitis include chronic pain, infertility, and ectopic pregnancy.

Questions

1. The most frequent symptom of acute salpingitis is:
   A. Urinary frequency
   B. Pelvic discomfort
   C. Nausea and vomiting
   D. Abnormal bleeding
   E. Purulent vaginal discharge
2. When using clinical symptoms and signs to diagnose acute salpingitis, the percentage of false-positives is approximately:
   A. 10%
   B. 25%
   C. 35%
   D. 45%
   E. 50%
3. The most accurate method of diagnosing acute PID is:
   A. History
   B. Pelvic examination
   C. Vaginal probe ultrasound
   D. Severity of leukocytosis
   E. Diagnostic laparoscopy

4. A 16-year-old girl who has never been pregnant complains of bilateral lower abdominal pain of 6 days' duration. The pain started immediately after her menstrual flow ended. Her temperature is 38° C and she has a tender left adnexal thickening. The diagnosis is acute salpingo-oophoritis. Optimal treatment for this patient is:
   A. Outpatient treatment with intramuscular cefotetan and oral doxycycline
   B. Oral doxycycline
   C. Intramuscular procaine penicillin
   D. Inpatient treatment with intravenous cefotetan and doxycycline
   E. Inpatient treatment with intravenous cefotetan

Answers

1. B
2. C
3. E
4. D

34

Pelvic relaxation

APGO LEARNING OBJECTIVE #34

Philip A. Rosenfeld

Patients with conditions of pelvic relaxation and urinary incontinence may come to medical attention in various ways. To identify those who would benefit from therapy, the student should be familiar with the types of pelvic relaxation and incontinence and the approach to the patient with symptoms suggestive of these problems.

The student will demonstrate a knowledge of the following:
A. Predisposing factors
B. Anatomic changes
C. Signs and symptoms
D. Initial approach to the patient and options for therapy for each of the following conditions:
  1. Cystocele
  2. Rectocele
  3. Vaginal or uterine prolapse
  4. Urinary incontinence

PATHOGENESIS

Delancey has stated that, "There has been little stimulus to study genital prolapse because empirically derived operations are available that are somewhat successful in treating these conditions." Understanding pelvic floor support principles will help the beginning student. This support basically consists of two large muscle groups: the pubococcygeus and, more important, the levator ani. The levator ani muscles close off the pelvic floor so that structures above them rest on their upper surface (Fig. 34-1). Pelvic floor relaxation

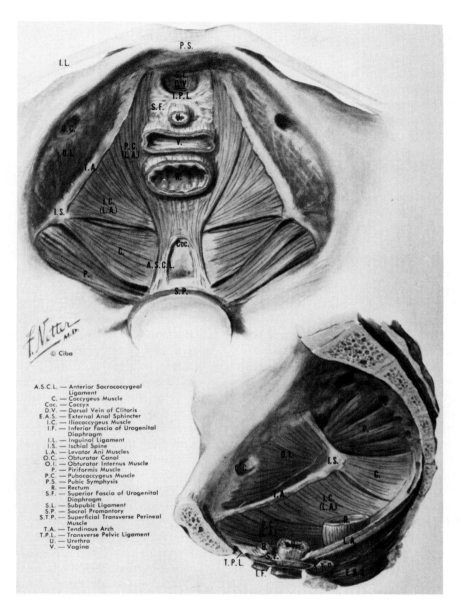

Fig. 34-1. Muscles within pelvic cavity. *(Copyright © 1954, 1965 by CIBA Pharmaceutical Company. Division of CIBA-GEIGY Corporation. Reprinted with permission from* The CIBA collection of medical illustrations, *illustrated by Frank H. Netter, M.D. All rights reserved.)*

involving these two muscle groups is found to some degree in 50% of parous women, but is significant in fewer than half this number. To quote Thiede, "At least half of the gynecological operations performed on elderly women are related to pelvic floor dysfunctions and since the number of women over 50, approximately 36,000,000, is growing, pelvic floor dysfunction in only 10% of them would constitute 3.6 million women and a major health care need."

Each patient's symptoms and complaints are distinct, and one female organ may protrude to a greater degree than another. Often the examining physician finds more than one specific organ involved. In the early days of obstetric care, the second stage (complete dilatation of the cervix) was shortened by the application of forceps and the almost universal episiotomy. It was believed at that time that there would be *ultimately* less postreproductive pelvic relaxation and protrusion of the affected organs. However, today there are fewer forceps applications and many fewer episiotomies. Consequently, the obstetrics of today may lead to greater muscle and support tearing and an increased need for postmenopausal operative repairs. This thinking has not yet been borne out. If one adds the diminution of elasticity of tissues promoted by aging and the concomitant lack of estrogen to previous pelvic muscle tears, it is understandable why women could develop a prolapse of one or more pelvic organs. The diminished blood supply and weakening of connective tissue plus the replacement of supporting muscle by fat also contribute to weakened pelvic structures; on the other hand, with each individual delivering fewer children, and with a more liberal use of sterilization, the physician may well see fewer cases of prolapse in the future.

SYMPTOMS AND SIGNS

The symptoms and signs of pelvic relaxation depend on the anatomic site affected. For example, a

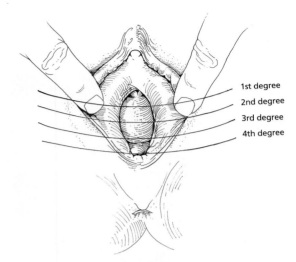

1st degree
2nd degree
3rd degree
4th degree

Fig. 34-2. Evaluation of cystoceles.

cystocele is a prolapse of the bladder into the anterior portion of the vagina. The extent of that prolapse can be measured by manually depressing the posterior vaginal wall and asking the patient to perform a Valsalva's maneuver (Fig. 34-2). Any relaxation greater than normal yet not down to the midportion is considered a first degree prolapse. If the patient's bladder comes to the imaginary line at the midportion of the vagina, it is considered a second degree prolapse. Any prolapse beyond that but not all the way to the posterior vaginal wall constitutes a third degree prolapse. A fourth degree prolapse is defined as the bladder filling the entire vagina with or without downward pressure.

The presence of a cystocele suggests that bladder emptying becomes inefficient because the bladder is no longer an abdominal organ. Therefore the symptoms seen might be those of recurrent urinary tract infection. Because an acute angle with the urethra is possible (unless the urethra also is prolapsed), the patient with a pure cystocele ordinarily would not be incontinent of urine. However, if the urethra is prolapsed into the anterior vaginal vault, there is descent of the urethrovesical angle so that it is no longer intraab-

Table 34-1. Types and causes of persistent urinary incontinence

Type	Definition	Common causes	Primary treatment
Urgency	Leakage of urine (usually larger volumes) because of inability to delay voiding after sensation of bladder fullness is perceived	Unstable bladder, isolated or associated with the following: 　Local genitourinary condition (e.g., cystitis, urethritis, tumors, stones, diverticula, mild outflow obstruction) 　Central nervous system disorders (e.g., stroke, dementia, parkinsonism, spinal cord injury)	Bladder relaxants (e.g., Ditropan) Estrogen (if atrophic vaginitis or urethritis is present) Training procedures Surgical removal of obstructing or irritating lesions
Stress	Involuntary loss of urine (usually small amounts) with increases in intra-abdominal pressure	Weakness and laxity of pelvic floor musculature Bladder outlet or urethral sphincter weakness	Pelvic floor (Kegel) exercises α-Adrenergic agonists, estrogen, bladder neck suspension
Overflow	Leakage of urine (usually small amounts) resulting from mechanical forces on an overdistended bladder	Anatomic obstruction by prostate, stricture, cystocele Acontractile bladder caused by diabetes or spinal cord injury Neurogenic (detrusor-sphincter dyssynergia)	Surgical removal of obstruction Intermittent catheterization Indwelling catheter
Functional	Urinary leakage associated with impairment of cognitive or physical functioning, psychologic unwillingness, or environmental barriers to toilet	Severe dementia or other neurologic disorders Psychologic conditions such as depression, anger, regression, or hostility Inaccessible toilets or toilet substitutes Unavailable caregivers	Habit training and scheduled toileting Incontinence undergarments, pads External collection devices Environmental manipulations

Modified from Kane RL, Ouslander JG, Abrass IB: *Essentials of clinical geriatrics*, ed 3, New York, 1994, McGraw-Hill.

dominal. The patient then has a type of incontinence designated *stress incontinence.* This means that the stresses of coughing, sneezing, lifting, and pushing render the patient's internal sphincter ineffective; and she loses a small amount of urine.

Urinary incontinence (Table 34-1) also may be seen in overflow, where the residual urine approaches the bladder capacity of 400 ml and the patient never effectively empties this organ. In a type of urinary incontinence known as *urgency incontinence,* spontaneous muscular contractions of the bladder occur involuntarily. These patients unfortunately may be subjected to this incontinence on the way to the bathroom and lose a great deal of urine at one time, unlike the patient with stress incontinence.

Continuous involuntary urinary loss points toward a fistula, with leakage coming as a result of many factors, most of them postoperative.

A *rectocele* is a herniation of the rectum into the posterior vagina and is demonstrated similarly to the cystocele, where the examiner's fingers are used to hold up the bladder while the examiner asks the patient to push down (Valsalva's maneuver). Patients with minimal rectocele complain of very few symptoms other than occasional pressure. If the rectocele becomes large, stool coming down the rectosigmoid is caught in the outpocketing of the rectum into the vagina; to have a bowel movement, these patients may need to push this rectocele back deliberately by inserting their fingers into the vagina.

The *enterocele* is the only true herniation in the pelvis. It is termed a "true" herniation because small bowel comes into the vagina and the sac is covered internally by peritoneum. Neither the cystocele nor the rectocele does this.

LABORATORY-DIAGNOSTIC STUDIES

As noted, cystocele and rectocele are demonstrated by using Valsalva's maneuver. An enterocele is best demonstrated while the patient is awake and the examiner is pushing down manually on any rectocele. The patient is then asked to do Valsalva's maneuver. If a bulge comes down *above* the rectum from the top of the vagina or behind the cervix, it is considered an enterocele.

Uterine prolapse is documented by placing the patient in stirrups in the lithotomy position and asking her to perform the Valsalva's maneuver. If the cervix comes to the introitus, there is first degree prolapse; if it comes beyond the introitus, it is considered second degree prolapse. A complete prolapse (procidentia) occurs as the cervix and part of the lower uterine segment come out into the vagina. The cervix and/or vagina in procidentia may be irritated or eroded from rubbing on the patient's underwear or inner thighs. The symptom of this kind of relaxation is pelvic pressure. Prolapse of the uterus ordinarily is preceded by retroversion or retroflexion of the uterus, in which the long axis of the uterus is tilted toward the sacral promontory. Usually with procidentia the cervix is somewhat elongated.

Testing for the type of incontinence most properly is done down through channel cystometry. Cystoscopy may accompany this work-up for completeness.

MANAGEMENT

Depending on the patient's symptoms, operative procedures, usually done through the vagina, are tailored to correct all of the deficiencies, even those anticipated and not yet present. Obviously, each patient must be told all the options for her repair. The physician must be sure that options and success rates are explained. The ability to correct incontinence depends not only on the patient's tissue factors, but also on the choice of procedure and the surgical skills of the gynecologist.

With minimal relaxation of the pelvic floor, Kegel exercises (purposeful squeezing of the pubococcygeus muscles) may provide a temporary solution. If the pelvic relaxation is extreme and the patient is unwilling or unable to undergo surgical correction, a pessary designed for a specific situation may be inserted, periodically removed, washed, and put into place again (Fig. 34-3). Occasionally the uterine cervix alone is prolapsed, and the fundus or body of the uterus remains well supported. Although cervical amputations were once done for this condition, most patients today undergo vaginal hysterectomy. The operator must realize that most of the symptoms in this prolapse are cervical and not fundal. The surgical approach must be modified to accommodate these findings.

If the uterus has already been removed and the patient has prolapse of the vagina, the surgical skill of the individual surgeon will determine which corrective procedure is needed—especially if

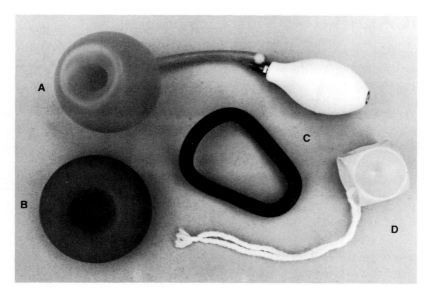

Fig. 34-3. Examples of pessaries (*A,* Inflatable; *B,* donut; *C,* Smith-Hodge; *D,* cube-type). *(From Mishell DR Jr et al:* Comprehensive gynecology, *ed 3, St Louis, 1997, Mosby–Year Book.)*

the vagina is to be left functional for sexual intercourse.

Individuals may have the vagina suspended either to the sacrum or to the anterior abdominal wall, although this latter procedure is anatomically unsatisfactory. In recent times Nichols perfected an operative procedure that secures the sides of the prolapsed vaginal wall to the sacrospinous ligament. When any of these procedures is done, sexual intercourse remains possible.

If the uterus is present but prolapsed, and intercourse is not wanted, a LeFort procedure may be accomplished with minimal blood loss. Invagination of the vagina surrounding the cervix and uterus is done in a way that resembles turning a paper bag inside-out. If no uterus is present and the vault alone is prolapsed, a colpocleisis may be accomplished with removal of the mucosa of the vagina and an actual closing of the submucosa. This results in a shortened or absent vagina in patients who do not desire coitus.

Well over 150 operations are now available to attempt correction of sphincter looseness and the incontinence it causes. Therefore no one operation is considered ideal. The range of operations can be broadly divided into those that repair the endopelvic fascia only (a Kelly plication) and those considered suburethral or paraurethral sling procedures (Pereya or Stamey). Other retropubic urethral procedures are done in the space of Retzius (the Marshall-Marchetti-Krantz [MMK] procedure or Burch method). The laparoscopic approach is beginning to be perfected.

Most patients with residual urine or urgency incontinence can be helped by antispasmodic drugs that relax the involuntary contractile nature of the bladder muscles.

Recurrent incontinence after attempted surgical correction may require sling operations and self-catheterization. This suggests the presence of a "pipe stem" urethra with rigidity. Urologists now perform more and more primary slings.

Any operative correction is at best only 80% satisfactory. The retropubic urethropexy operations (MMK, Burch, or Tenagho) are considered to be the longest lasting.

CRITICAL POINTS

- An understanding of pelvic floor structure and support is necessary.
- Weakened pelvic support occurs as a result of childbirth, aging, and estrogen diminution.
- Prolapse of a support-weakened bladder is called a cystocele.
- Protrusion of the rectum into the vagina with difficult defecation is a rectocele.
- An enterocele involves bowel prolapse via the posterior cul-de-sac and is the only true pelvic hernia.
- Sacrospinal ligament fixation will preserve coital ability.
- Many operations exist for correction of stress incontinence of urine.

Questions

1. The predominant symptom of a cystocele is:
   A. Loss of urine with stress
   B. Nocturnal enuresis
   C. Constipation
   D. Recurrent urinary tract infections
2. The only true hernia in the pelvis is:
   A. Cystocele
   B. Rectocele
   C. Urethrocele
   D. Enterocele
3. Urgency incontinence is noted by:
   A. Loss of a large amount of urine
   B. Loss of a small amount of urine
   C. Loss of urine with coughing, sneezing, and so on
   D. Bed wetting
4. Kegel exercises involve:
   A. Abdominal muscle tension
   B. Pubococcygeus muscle squeezing
   C. Insertion of a Foley catheter
5. Overflow incontinence means:
   A. An empty bladder
   B. Inefficient emptying of the bladder with large residual
   C. Loss of urine involuntarily
   D. Nocturnal enuresis

Answers

1. D
2. D
3. A
4. B
5. B

Endometriosis and adenomyosis

APGO LEARNING OBJECTIVE #35

John H. Mattox

> *Endometriosis and adenomyosis are common problems of women of reproductive age. This chronic problem may result in pelvic pain, infertility, and menstrual dysfunction.*

The student will demonstrate a knowledge of the following:
A. Theories of pathogenesis
B. Symptoms and physical findings
C. Common sites of implants
D. Methods of diagnosis

ENDOMETRIOSIS

Endometriosis is the abnormal growth of endometrial tissue outside the uterine cavity. The disease was first mentioned in the medical literature in 1860 by the renowned Viennese pathologist, von Rokitansky. The observations of Sampson in the 1920s focused on one of the current major theories of the origin of the disease and documented its histologic variability. Whether aberrant endometrial tissue is located on the serosal surface of the peritoneal structures or the ovary *(endometriosis)*, or in the wall of the myometrium *(adenomyosis)*, functioning endometrial tissue that responds to ovarian hormones, predominantly estrogen, is the prerequisite for the genesis and maintenance of this condition. Therefore it is rarely encountered before menarche and usually becomes quiescent after menopause.

It is estimated that between 1% and 2% of the female population has endometriosis, and many physicians believe that the incidence is increasing. Characteristic lesions can be recognized during at least 5% of pelvic operations and in 30% of women with infertility; frequently it is an unexpected finding. Some women may have asymptomatic endometriosis; it is more likely to be problematic in the third and fourth decades of life.

Pathogenesis

No single hypothesis can explain all of the varied clinical presentations seen with endometriosis. The possible explanations include several theories: (1) coelomic metaplasia; (2) retrograde menstruation; (3) blood or lymph dissemination; (4) immunologic induction; and (5) combinations of these.

According to the metaplasia theory, undifferentiated coelomic epithelial cells, similar to those from which the paramesonephric ducts are formed, remain dormant on the peritoneal surface until the ovaries begin to function. They respond to cyclic stimulation by ovarian estrogen and progesterone, in a manner similar to that of normal endometrial cells, and eventually can be identified as definite lesions on the peritoneal surface. The longer cyclic stimulation and withdrawal persist without a break, such as that provided by pregnancy, the larger the lesions can become.

Sampson's investigations indicate that endometriosis can be caused by retrograde transport of menstrual fluid from the uterus through the tubes during menstruation. Blood often can be seen in the cul-de-sac, and endometrial tissue can be identified in the tubal lumen in women who undergo surgery during menstruation. The typical lesions of endometriosis can be produced in primates by diverting the menstrual flow into the peritoneal cavity. Endometriosis also occurs in young women with congenital obstructing defects in the cervix or vagina, which are associated with reflux menstruation into the peritoneal cavity.

Another theory suggests that an "inciting substance" in the menstrual fluid entering the peritoneal cavity could induce the formation of endometrial glands and stroma in undifferentiated mesenchyme. This would explain the location of the lesions in the ovary and the cul-de-sac, the areas first affected by reflux menstruation.

The theory that an immune complex in menstrual fluid induces change in certain susceptible individuals, resulting in endometriosis, is more plausible than is the single hypothesis of the growth of transplanted endometrial cells. Endometrial cells from menstrual discharge usually do not grow in tissue culture, so it is difficult to accept cell transplantation as the sole factor in the development of a condition as common as endometriosis.

Heredity may be a factor in the development of endometriosis. Simpson and colleagues conducted focused interviews with 123 women who had been treated for endometriosis. The incidence of the condition in female siblings over age 18 years (5.8%), mother (8.1%), and first-degree relatives (6.9%) was considerably higher than that in the husbands' female relatives (1%) and mothers (0.9%). The precise genetic mechanism is not known.

Gross pathologic findings

The gross appearance of endometriosis is variable, depending on the stage of the disease and the length of time it has existed. Minimal lesions appear as bluish red spots, possibly surrounded by a ring of puckered scar tissue scattered over the pelvic peritoneal surfaces. Each of these small foci may grow as a result of repeated cyclic stimulation; the larger lesions are known as *endometriomas* (Fig. 35-1). As endometriomas continue to grow they coalesce and, with scar tissue, may completely obliterate the cul-de-sac. The tubes and ovaries become densely adherent to the posterior surfaces of the broad ligaments, and in more advanced cases the rectosigmoid adheres to the posterior surface of the uterus, further immobilizing the adnexal structures (Fig. 35-2). A "window-like" defect in the peritoneum can be a result of endometriosis. Eventually, the entire pelvis may be filled with a solid mass of agglutinated structures that may be completely obscured by adherent bowel and omentum.

The adhesions produced in response to the lesions are dense and firm and can be separated only by sharp dissection. As the planes are opened, thick brown fluid escapes. This fluid consists of old blood and cellular debris formed within the endometrioma. The blood may be the irritant that initiates the peritoneal reaction, which is eventually responsible for the dense scarring.

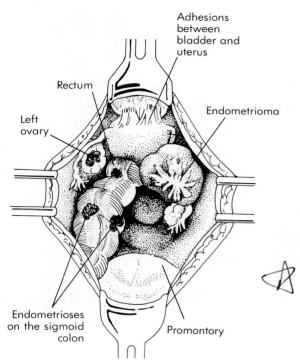

Adhesions
between
bladder and
uterus

Rectum

Left
ovary

Endometrioma

Endometrioses
on the sigmoid
colon

Promontory

Fig. 35-1. Advanced endometriosis with lesions and adhesions on various pelvic structures.

Ovarian involvement varies from small cystic collections to a single loculated structure, which may measure as much as 10 cm in diameter, an *ovarian endometrioma*. Other lesions such as hemorrhage into an ovarian cyst or a corpus luteum cyst can form the "chocolate cyst" and be confused with ovarian endometriomas. Whenever possible, an exact diagnosis should be made before a definitive operative procedure is performed because the treatment of each of these lesions is different.

The rectosigmoid colon and urinary tract may be involved. The lesions are on the peritoneal surface and rarely penetrate the entire thickness of the wall. Occasionally the vagina, cervix, episiotomy scars, laparotomy scars, umbilicus, round ligaments, lungs, and extremities are sites of endometrial implants.

A typical lesion of endometriosis contains glands and stroma like those of endometrium in its normal location (Fig. 35-2). Repeated episodes of bleeding within a lesion may produce enough pressure atrophy to destroy the glandular epithelium, leaving only the stroma and hemosiderin-containing macrophages. Usually a considerable amount of fibrous tissue surrounds the older lesions. During pregnancy lesions usually exhibit a typical decidual reaction.

A classification system developed by a committee of what is now the American Society for Reproductive Medicine (ASRM) is simple and informative. Points are accumulated for each of several aspects of the lesions as they are seen through the laparoscope or at laparotomy (Fig. 35-3).

Symptoms *Endometriosis*

The most common symptoms are: (1) pelvic pain; (2) abnormal uterine bleeding; and (3) infertility. Lower abdominal and pelvic pain in some form is the most common symptom of endometriosis. The cycling ectopic endometrium bleeds in conjunction with the normal menstrual flow; but the blood is contained within the involved organ or affected tissue, distending it and the surrounding peritoneum. Pain is most severe in areas of peritoneal scarring, which are put under tension as the lesions expand during the bleeding phase.

Dysmenorrhea is a common symptom, but dysmenorrhea in women is not always a result of endometriosis. Most women who have had painful periods since menarche (primary dysmenorrhea) do not often have endometriosis; the pain caused by endometriosis appears at a later time (secondary dysmenorrhea).

Pelvic pain that increases in severity with the onset of menses is postulated to be indicative of endometriosis, whereas the dysmenorrhea that is relieved as menses progress is less likely to be caused by endometriosis. Although it is interesting to try to establish this clinical correlation, the character of the menstrual pain is not sufficiently

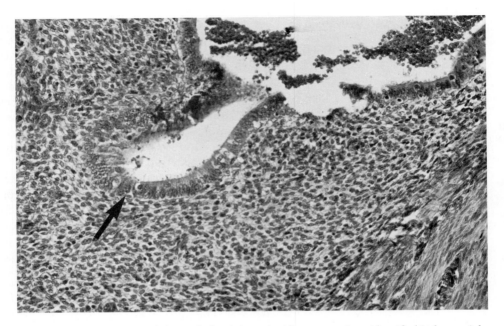

Fig. 35-2. Adenomyosis. Endometrial gland *(center)* with myometrium identified in lower right corner.

discriminatory to exclude the diagnosis of endometriosis. *Rectal tenesmus* and *dyspareunia* are common and severe before and during menstruation if there is considerable involvement in the cul-de-sac and uterosacral ligaments. Most women are free from pain during the first half of the cycle.

A disturbing feature of endometriosis is that significant disease can be encountered without much symptomatology; severe pelvic pain can occur in some women with minimal endometriosis.

Abnormal uterine bleeding may occur in women with endometriosis. It most often results from a considerable amount of ovarian destruction by advanced lesions and may not exhibit a characteristic pattern.

Many women with endometriosis are *infertile*. It is easy to understand why this occurs when the lesions are so extensive that the tubes and ovaries are immobilized by, or even buried within, the masses of endometriosis. The mechanism of infertility is not obvious when there are only scattered lesions that do not appear to disturb tubal or ovarian function.

Several theories based on experimental findings have been proposed to explain infertility coexisting with endometriosis in the absence of a mechanical factor. It has been postulated that an autoimmune response is triggered in some women when endometriotic tissue is phagocytized and absorbed by the host; this results in the rejection of the embryo or disrupted sperm transport. Another theory involves the existence of the luteinized unruptured follicle syndrome. It is postulated that the ovarian follicle fails to release the ovum despite the occurrence of the biochemical changes that are associated with ovulation. Increased prostanoids have been identified in some women with endometriosis, and their presence might alter tubal smooth muscle activity, thus compromising ovum transport. Another possibility is that increased numbers of macrophages in the peritoneal cavity phagocytize spermatozoa.

Patient's Name _____ Date_____

Stage I (Minimal) - 1-5
Stage II (Mild) - 6-15
Stage III (Moderate) - 16-40
Stage IV (Severe) - >40
Total_____

Laparoscopy_____ Laparotomy_____ Photography_____
Recommended Treatment_____
_____
Prognosis_____

PERITONEUM	ENDOMETRIOSIS	<1cm	1-3cm	>3cm
	Superficial	1	2	4
	Deep	2	4	6
OVARY	R Superficial	1	2	4
	Deep	4	16	20
	L Superficial	1	2	4
	Deep	4	16	20

	POSTERIOR CULDESAC OBLITERATION	Partial	Complete
		4	40

	ADHESIONS	<1/3 Enclosure	1/3-2/3 Enclosure	>2/3 Enclosure
OVARY	R Filmy	1	2	4
	Dense	4	8	16
	L Filmy	1	2	4
	Dense	4	8	16
TUBE	R Filmy	1	2	4
	Dense	4*	8*	16
	L Filmy	1	2	4
	Dense	4*	8*	16

*If the fimbriated end of the fallopian tube is completely enclosed, change the point assignment to 16.

Additional Endometriosis: _____

Associated Pathology: _____

To Be Used with Normal
Tubes and Ovaries

L   R

To Be Used with Abnormal
Tubes and/or Ovaries

L   R

Fig. 35-3. Classification of endometriosis. *(From the American Society for Reproductive Medicine: Revised American Fertility Society classification of endometriosis, Fertil Steril 43:351, 1984. Reproduced with the permission of the publisher, the American Society for Reproductive Medicine.)*

Although it is rare, *malignant transformation* in endometriosis does occur. Sampson carefully described the qualifying criteria. These endometrioid cancers are usually adenocarcinoma and are more likely to be observed in an ovarian endometrioma. Therapy is similar to that for other ovarian malignancy.

Physical findings

There are also certain findings on pelvic examination that should raise suspicion: (1) a fixed retroflexed uterine corpus; (2) extreme uterosacral ligament tenderness with nodularity; (3) bilateral fixed tender masses in the adnexa; and (4) tender thickening of the rectal-vaginal septum. These findings have a significant association with pelvic endometriosis.

Endometriosis can be diagnosed with certainty only by direct inspection, and optimally by microscopic examination of the lesions. In some instances, histologic confirmation is impossible because both glands and stroma have been destroyed as the lesions enlarge. In this event the only remaining suggestions of endometriosis may be deposits of hemosiderin.

Differential diagnosis

It is difficult to diagnose endometriosis accurately by history and physical examination alone. Small lesions, particularly those involving the tubes and ovaries, cannot be felt; and even those in the cul-de-sac may be missed. Endometriosis can be confused with other pelvic conditions.

PELVIC INFECTION. The lesions that most often simulate endometriosis are those that follow repeated attacks of salpingo-oophoritis. Both conditions may cause pain before and during menstruation and dyspareunia. The tubes and ovaries adhere to the posterior leaves of the broad ligaments and in the cul-de-sac in both. The residua of recurrent salpingitis are smoother as compared with a fixed nodular mass of endometriosis involving the uterosacral ligaments and the cul-de-sac.

The history often is helpful. There is nothing in the history of a patient with endometriosis that is similar to that of recurrent attacks of acute salpingo-oophoritis; the latter is often associated with fever.

OVARIAN CARCINOMA. Cul-de-sac nodularity may on occasion resemble ovarian carcinoma. Endometriosis usually is associated with dysmenorrhea, and pelvic examination is painful. Women with ovarian cancer usually are older; there is no associated increase in dysmenorrhea; symptoms usually are minimal and may consist only of vague gastrointestinal discomfort, and the pelvic examination often produces no pain.

BENIGN OVARIAN NEOPLASMS. An endometrioma of the ovary cannot be distinguished from a primary benign ovarian neoplasm by pelvic examination alone. Direct laparoscopic inspection and biopsy of the enlarged ovary are necessary.

URINARY TRACT LESIONS. Urinary tract endometriosis is suggested in women with cyclic or intermittent hematuria. This is an unusual symptom and occurs only if an endometrial lesion penetrates the bladder wall. The ureters usually are involved in extrinsic lesions, which constrict rather than penetrate. These may eventually constrict the ureter completely.

BOWEL LESIONS. Cyclic dyschezia or hematochezia is an uncommon symptom of endometriosis and usually reflects bowel mucosal involvement. Any lesion visualized at sigmoidoscopy should be biopsied. On barium enema extraluminal disfiguration or annular constriction can be seen when pelvic endometriosis involves the colon.

Laboratory tests

It would be of enormous benefit to be able to diagnose, as well as monitor, women with serologic testing. Unfortunately, no such assay exists.

CA-125, a cell surface antigen, can be detected by radioimmunoassay in the serum of many patients with endometriosis; however, it does not have any clinical use at this time. Although the erythrocyte sedimentation rate or leukocyte count may be slightly elevated, particularly with an acute painful episode, these tests are not particularly helpful in the management of women with endometriosis.

Treatment

The symptoms associated with endometriosis can be relieved by surgery or a variety of hormone regimens. The treatment one chooses for a specific patient is determined by several factors: (1) her age; (2) the severity of symptoms; (3) the extent of the disease; (4) whether she wishes to become pregnant, and, if so, whether now or in the future (Table 35-1).

GENERAL PRINCIPLES

- Not every woman needs therapy. *Expectant management* is a term that has been used to characterize the woman who is not interested in conceiving, whose minimal endometriosis is causing no menstrual disturbance, and who has little or no discomfort.
- Whether or not infertile patients with minimal endometriosis (ASRM stage I) require therapy is currently debatable.
- Conservative surgery is definitely more successful for moderate and severe endometriosis when improving fertility is the major objective.
- Hormonal therapy usually is administered for at least 6 months.
- Ovarian endometriomas larger than 2 cm in diameter are not permanently responsive to medical therapy.
- In spite of appropriate hormonal or conservative surgical therapy, a conservative estimate of recurrence over 7 years is approximately 15%.

SPECIFIC THERAPY.

Conservative operations are those in which the most important goals are to reduce the severity of the symptoms and to retain or improve fertility. A *conservative* approach

---

Table 35-1. Possible therapies for endometriosis

I. Surgical
  A. Conservative
    1. Laparoscopy with electrocautery or laser vaporization of lesions
    2. Removal of specific lesions and possible uterine suspension with presacral neurectomy
  B. Definitive
    1. Abdominal hysterectomy
    2. Salpingo-oophorectomy if diseased
    3. Bowel resection rarely
II. Hormonal
  A. Progestin-dominant birth control pills
    1. Cyclically
    2. Continuous
  B. Progestin (medroxyprogesterone)
    1. Intramuscular (Depo-Provera)
    2. Oral
  C. Attenuated androgen (danazol)
  D. GnRH analog (Synarel, Lupron)
III. Combined medical and surgical treatment

GnRH, Gonadotropin-releasing hormone.

---

includes resection or destruction by cautery or laser of most or all visible endometriosis, freeing tubes and ovaries that are immobilized by disease or adhesions, removing an extensively damaged tube and ovary if the other is reasonably normal, freeing and suspending a retrodisplaced uterus that is bound down in the posterior cul-de-sac, and presacral neurectomy to relieve dysmenorrhea. *Definitive surgery* is used when the major goal is to relieve pain. These procedures are appropriate for women who have no desire for pregnancy or when the endometriosis is so extensive that preservation or restoration of fertility is impossible. Frequently these patients have been unsuccessfully treated with medicine or laser surgery. The operation most often performed is hysterectomy, bilateral salpingo-oophorectomy, and resection of as much disease as possible.

Hormone therapy eliminates the repeated cyclic variations in ovarian estrogen and progesterone that stimulate periodic growth and disintegration of the ectopic endometrium. Hormone therapy includes the following: cyclic low-dose combined oral contraceptives, which produce minimal endometrial growth and scant withdrawal bleeding; continuous high-dose estrogen-progestogen combinations to produce a pseudopregnancy state in which uterine and ectopic endometrium is converted to decidua, which eventually undergoes necrosis; and long-acting progestogens, which also produce decidualization, necrosis of the endometrium, and amenorrhea.

Danazol, an attenuated androgen, can produce a pseudomenopausal state by interfering with gonadotropin secretion and steroidogenesis. By inhibiting the secretion of estrogen and progesterone, the reproductive tissues and the endometriosis undergo atrophic change. The side effects—weight gain, hot flashes, and oily complexion—can be disagreeable, albeit temporary. The dose varies from 400 to 800 mg daily, and the medication is expensive.

The use of gonadotropin-releasing hormone (GnRH) agonists may be an important adjunct to treat this disease. By down-regulating (see Chapter 7, Intrapartum Care) the gonadotrope, follicle-stimulating hormone and luteinizing hormone are inhibited. In the absence of ovarian stimulation, E_2 declines to postmenopausal levels, a milieu that cannot sustain endometriosis. The GnRH agonists are gradually becoming primary therapy and are usually prescribed in the more difficult cases. Daily self-administration is required for some agonists, but a monthly depot preparation is available. Osteoporosis has been reported in women using these analogs for 6 months or longer.

SPECIAL CONSIDERATIONS. The major concern for young women who want to delay pregnancy is to preserve fertility by limiting further growth of the lesions. Creation of a pseudopregnancy state with continuous use of a birth control pill controls the growth of en-

dometriosis, although probably less effectively than with danazol. A product containing norgestrel can be given daily, although other progestin-dominant preparations also are effective. This produces a decidual change and eventually necrosis in the ectopic endometrium, and presumably limits its growth. Breakthrough bleeding is controlled by increasing the daily dose when spotting occurs.

A possible approach is to use cyclic low-dose oral contraceptives. Endometrial stimulation is minimal, and bleeding is scant; this may serve to inhibit the growth of ectopic endometrium. Low-dose oral contraceptives may be considered for young women with family histories of endometriosis and as a treatment of dysmenorrhea.

Women with endometriosis who are also infertile require special consideration. The major goal in treatment is to improve fertility; hence oral contraceptives and the production of pseudopregnancy states usually should not be considered.

The women benefit most from conservative surgical procedures designed to remove as much endometriosis as possible and to correct endometriosis-induced scarring that reduces fertility. Uterine suspension may be performed if the uterus is adherent in cul-de-sac endometriosis, and presacral neurectomy to relieve dysmenorrhea. Pregnancy rates from 30% to 90% have been reported after surgical procedures depending on the stage of the disease.

Ordinarily, hormone therapy should not be used after surgery, even though a few small areas of endometriosis are left. Because most conceptions occur during the first 12 to 15 months after surgery, the patient should be given an opportunity to use this time without suppressing ovulation. Medication may be prescribed later for patients who do not conceive or for those whose lesions recur after surgery.

A long-acting progestogen such as medroxyprogesterone (Depo-Provera) in doses sufficient to produce and maintain amenorrhea is effective in relieving pain. Because anovulation and amen-

Table 35-2. Clinical differentiation of endometriosis and adenomyosis

	Endometriosis	Adenomyosis
Approximate age when symptomatic	25-35 yr	40-50 yr
Parous	Sometimes	Usually
Symptoms	Usually	Sometimes
Abnormal uterine bleeding	Yes	Yes
Dysmenorrhea	Yes	Yes
Infertility	Yes	No
Pelvic pain	Yes	Yes
Responsive to hormone therapy	Yes	No
Responsive to conservative surgery	Yes	No
Requires hysterectomy	Sometimes	Usually

orrhea sometimes persist for many months after it is discontinued, this drug should not be used in women who may want to become pregnant quickly.

Surgery is indicated for reasons other than relieving symptoms or improving fertility. An operation is indicated whenever one or both ovaries are larger than 5 cm in diameter, regardless of the age of the patient and even though she is known to have endometriosis. Ovarian endometriosis rarely produces symptoms, but it is impossible to differentiate them from ovarian neoplasms by pelvic examination alone. Oophorectomy is not often necessary, even for large ovarian endometriomas. Individual cysts can be dissected out of the normal stroma. One usually can preserve enough ovarian tissue for normal hormone secretion and even pregnancy.

Endometriosis of the rectosigmoid can cause partial or complete bowel obstruction. Bowel resection is appropriate if the lesion cannot be differentiated from cancer or whenever there is significant narrowing of the bowel lumen.

ADENOMYOSIS

Adenomyosis, a benign uterine condition in which endometrial glands and stroma are found deep in the myometrium, is often considered to be a form of endometriosis. The disorders probably are not related but only share histologic similarity. The frequency with which adenomyosis is diagnosed depends largely on how many sections of uterine wall are studied. By definition, the ectopic endometrium is located 2.5 mm (a single low power) below the basal layer of endometrium. The reported incidence varies from about 10% to about 90% of all hysterectomies. It is diagnosed most often in women between the ages of 40 and 50 (Table 35-2).

The pathogenesis is not entirely clear, but adenomyosis is related in some way to estrogen stimulation or possibly the breakdown of the endometrial basement membrane during delivery. The cells in the basal portions of the endometrial glands grow downward between the myometrial muscle bundles and may lose their connection to the uterine cavity. The lesions usually are diffuse, with patches of endometrial tissue scattered throughout the entire thickness of the uterine wall. The process may be extensive enough to enlarge the uterus, but not often beyond a size comparable to a pregnancy of 8 to 10 weeks. Occasionally, the process may be more circumscribed, with the formation of a distinct nodule, an *adenomyoma,* but this formation is much less common than is diffuse involvement.

Adenomyosis is often associated with uterine fibroids. The most frequently reported symptoms are colicky secondary dysmenorrhea and abnormal bleeding, but many women with adenomyosis have no symptoms.

The diagnosis is suspected in a woman over 40 who complains of increasingly severe dysmenorrhea and excessive bleeding and whose uterus is enlarged and tender, particularly during menstrual flow.

Hormone therapy relieves the pain of ordinary dysmenorrhea and that associated with endometriosis, but these preparations have little effect on the pain associated with adenomyosis.

The only uniformly successful treatment for adenomyosis is hysterectomy. However, an operation will not be necessary if menopause can be expected to occur soon and if the pelvic pain can be controlled. The symptoms will usually disappear after ovarian hormone secretion ceases.

CRITICAL POINTS

- The etiologic factors of endometriosis include retrograde menstruation, metaplasia, vascular metastasis, immunologic defects, and a genetic predisposition.
- Classic symptoms of endometriosis are cyclic pelvic pain, dysmenorrhea, and infertility. However, some patients with endometriosis are asymptomatic.
- A most significant physical finding of endometriosis is a fixed retroverted uterus with thickening and tenderness posterior to the uterus. The classic abnormality of endometriosis is tender nodularity of the uterosacral ligaments.
- Therapy must be tailored to the degree of symptomatology, the patient's age, and her desire to maintain fertility.
- Symptomatic adenomyosis occurs primarily in parous women over the age of 40. The classic symptoms are secondary dysmenorrhea and abnormal uterine bleeding. The most common physical sign is a diffusely enlarged uterus that is particularly tender during menstruation.
- Hysterectomy often is necessary to treat adenomyosis.

Questions

1. The most likely cause of endometriosis is:
   A. Coelomic metaplasia
   B. A combination of theories
   C. Retrograde menstruation
   D. Immunologic deficiency
   E. Vascular spread of endometrial fragments
2. Physical findings not associated with endometriosis are:
   A. Bilateral ovarian masses
   B. Fixed retroversion of the uterus

C. Uterosacral implants
D. Uterine enlargement
E. Periadnexal adhesions

3. A 19-year-old single female with symptomatic stage 1 (minimal) endometriosis requests therapy. She should be advised to:
   A. Use birth control pills
   B. Undergo laparoscopic laser ablation of the lesions
   C. Take GnRH agonist therapy
   D. Wait until the disease or her symptoms increase
   E. Consider a combination of medical and surgical therapy

Answers

1. B
2. D
3. A

36 Chronic pelvic pain

APGO LEARNING OBJECTIVE #36

Philip A. Rosenfeld

> *Manifestations of a heterogeneous group of pelvic disorders may have serious sequelae if not recognized.*

The student will demonstrate a knowledge of the following:

A. Definition of chronic pelvic pain
B. Incidence and etiology
C. Clinical manifestations
D. Diagnostic procedures
E. Physiologic component
F. Management

Chronic pelvic pain (CPP) may be a frustrating illness for both the patient and the treating physician. Although CPP is probably responsible for 10% of all gynecologic office visits, its definition eludes the usual terse terms used in medicine. Forty percent of all laparoscopies are done for CPP, and 12% of all hysterectomies are done for similar complaints. Yet obstetricians-gynecologists still have not agreed on an acceptable explanation for the etiology and ultimate treatment of this condition.

A consensus of authors defines CPP as pain in the area of the pelvis, noncyclic, in the same location, and lasting a minimum of 6 months. Some suggest adding to this list the failure to respond to the usual mild analgesics and the requirement for many office visits.

The patient must determine how painful the condition is, where it is located, and how she responds to certain treatment offerings.

PATHOGENESIS

Pelvic pain in the premenarcheal patient is unlikely to have gynecologic origins. The patient with multiple partners has a much greater chance of acquiring sexually transmitted diseases (STDs), with CPP resulting from an inflammatory response. Some authors suggest the "PQRST" system to assess this pain. "P" stands for that which provokes or palliates the pain,

"Q" for its quality, "R" for region and radiation, "S" for severity, and "T" for time of duration and/or occurrence.

The source of this pain may range from a small ovarian cyst to massive adhesions within the abdomen, either from endometriosis or from pelvic inflammatory disease (PID). Observers have argued for years over whether or not adhesions actually cause pain. There has been complete disagreement concerning why individuals with massive adhesions, mostly caused by endometriosis, may have no pain; and those with a few specks of endometriosis and a few burned-out scarred areas may be in great distress.

Because of this lack of definite findings, CPP patients are often shuffled from physician to physician, ultimately undergoing multiple surgical procedures followed by increasing disability and incomplete or unsatisfactory results. These patients should be thoroughly studied.

SYMPTOMS AND SIGNS

The history must include questions about menstruation, parity, regularity of flow, and sexual activity. It also must include an inquiry about possible sexual abuse because this has been implicated as a possible recall mechanism. Such abuse certainly plays some part in the onset of CPP.

The timing of the onset of pain is important. Pains occurring in the middle of the cycle ordinarily are related to ovulation. Those late in the cycle probably are hormonally related (i.e., progesterone-influenced). Those beginning at the period's end suggest infection. Disproportionate pain at menses may suggest endometriosis or, if early in menarche, could represent an outflow tract obstructive phenomenon.

These patients typically miss days at school or work. They may report they are totally incapacitated for part of their lives.

LABORATORY-DIAGNOSTIC STUDIES

Diagnosis of CPP should be one of elimination after a very complete work-up with appropriate diagnostic studies. The usual office diagnostic studies must be done. These include not only the history but also a complete physical examination; pelvic examination; Pap smear; and tests for syphilis, chlamydia, and gonorrhea. The complete blood count with differential usually is normal. Other diagnostic tests, including liver function, electrolytes, and lipid studies, also are usually performed.

An attempt to accurately map the areas of pain localization over the lower abdomen may be made. This assures the physician that the locale remains the same over ensuing months.

An interested physician who will relate quietly to the patient is absolutely necessary if the patient is to be convinced that her best interests are being served, especially patients with CPP. The patient should be approached in stepwise fashion. An interview, physical examination, and a 1-hour pain-mapping session are done initially with a clinical psychologist. An attempt is made to determine whether the patient uses pain to avoid particular jobs or to avoid sexual intercourse. Questions may include the following:

Do you avoid working in the kitchen because leaning against the counter causes pain?

Have you stopped doing aerobic exercises because jarring creates pain?

Have you stopped sexual intercourse because it is the sole cause of the pain?

It is also important to watch the woman while she walks to the examining room. This can give a clue about possible neurologic, muscular, or skeletal problems consistent with pelvic pathology.

One suggested source of pelvic pain is the increased peritoneal secretion of prostaglandins. Prostaglandin metabolites have been considered etiologically because increased amounts of this substance in the peritoneal fluid can cause uterine contractions, uterine ischemia, and perhaps sensitization of pain fibers. Pelvic adhesions, as previously noted, probably cause pain only when these viscus-peritoneal adhesions are twisted or rotated to change their length or tension. Nearly two thirds of all laparoscopies for pelvic pain find some abnormalities, but whether these abnormalities cause the pelvic pain is problematic. Obvious relief of symptoms by operative laparoscopy points to such a causative factor, but some women respond positively with *only* reassurance and no operative dissection at laparoscopy.

Can pelvic pain result from ovarian sources? Cysts that have not leaked and caused adhesive response nor undergone torsion nor are ovarian remnants of previous surgery probably do not cause pelvic pain, even though the ovary may subsequently become cystic. Uterine leiomyomas do not cause pain unless they undergo degeneration or protrude through the cervix with an attempt to abort. Pelvic varicosities were once widely considered a cause of CPP, and uterine suspensions were performed to correct them. These operations probably were to no avail.

In 1987 Schoen suggested that psychic energy is unconsciously converted to physical symptoms as an ego defense mechanism, accounting for many of the symptoms of CPP. Psychologic evaluation by trained personnel to uncover possible deep-seated emotional problems may be helpful, but is certainly risky unless the patient is well prepared by the physician for such inquiry.

MANAGEMENT

It is important that such a patient be treated kindly and with a great deal of understanding. Although the history and physical examination may not lead to a definitive diagnosis, the patient's complaints are real and must be treated accordingly.

A frustrated patient and physician often meet in the operating room with a preoperative diagnosis of CPP. Unless this is truly a diagnostic procedure (not hysteroscopy, but more often laparoscopy), such a diagnosis is totally inappropriate. After repeated office visits, the ineffective use of medications, and nonspecific findings both historically and physically, the physician may well be left with the one remaining alternative—diagnostic laparoscopy.

In 1984 Slocum reported nearly 90% improvement with the injection of dermatome trigger points using local anesthetics with or without steroids.

Once the decision has been made to do a laparoscopy, what are the usual findings? In 1993 Howard stated that more than one half of women with abnormal laparoscopy findings had had a normal preoperative pelvic examination. Data from Kresh and colleagues on 100 consecutive patients found adhesions in 51% and endometriosis in 32% of patients. They acknowledged that adhesions were found in 14% of the control individuals, but suggested that adhesions in the control group were different. The control group had fine adhesions with no restriction of organ mobility, whereas those in the CPP group were denser, tighter, and had restricted mobility and expansibility of the involved organs. Multicenter studies and various individual reports appear to show that CPP patients have approximately twice the incidence of laparoscopically detected pathology as "normal women." These pathologic conditions include endometriosis, postoperative adhesions, and adhesive disease after pelvic inflammatory processes.

The relationship between the patient and her physician must be ongoing. However, the physician should not hesitate to bring in adjuvant personnel, especially from the field of psychiatry, to elucidate any underlying psychologic condition. Some would also include an anesthesiologist trained in pain relief. The gynecologist must be supportive and answer questions as fully as possible and appropriate, but must not fall into the easy trap of giving repetitive prescriptions first for nonsteroidal antiinflammatory agents and ultimately for narcotic drugs, thus creating an addicted individual. *Reassurance is foremost.* The psychologist's main role is to investigate the psychosexual convolutions of this long-standing disease process.

Presacral neurectomy—the operative removal of the cord nerves at the T-11, T-12 at the sacral promontory—may or may not help. A so-called LUNA procedure, in which there is *laser uterosacral nerve ablation*, may be satisfactory temporarily. The use of trigger point injections already has been noted.

Total abdominal hysterectomy with or without bilateral oophorectomy is not appropriate unless another pathologic condition exists. Fortunately, on some occasions, simple reassurance alone has helped some patients.

CRITICAL POINTS

- Forty percent of all laparoscopies and 12% of hysterectomies are done for pelvic pain.
- Multiple sexual partners may lead to STDs, PID, and CPP.
- Diagnosis of CPP depends on the length of disability and on failure to ascertain other causes.
- About two thirds of laparoscopies done for pelvic pain find some abnormality, such as adhesive disease.
- Reassurance and understanding are a significant part of physician treatment.

Questions

1. Chronic pelvic pain is defined as:
   A. Pain in the same location for at least 6 months
   B. Pain that varies in location for less than 30 days
   C. Pain that responds to mild analgesics and varies in location
   D. Pain that is cyclic and present for more than 30 days
2. One suggested cause of pelvic pain is:
   A. Chronic anovulation
   B. Secretion of increased prostaglandins into the peritoneal cavity
   C. Coital positioning
   D. Method of contraception
3. Suspected causes of pelvic pain include:
   A. Ovarian cysts
   B. Fibromyoma uteri
   C. Pelvic varicosities
   D. Pelvic adhesions of unknown etiology
4. Successful treatment of CPP may include:
   A. Abdominal hysterectomy
   B. Bilateral salpingo-oophorectomy
   C. Uterosacral ligament nerve ablation
   D. Uterine suspension

Answers

1. A
2. B
3. D
4. C

37

Disorders of the breasts

APGO LEARNING OBJECTIVE #37

Philip A. Rosenfeld

Breast cancer is among the leading causes of death in women. Every physician should understand the basic approach to evaluating the common symptoms associated with the breast.

The student will demonstrate a knowledge of the following:

A. Standards of surveillance of an adult woman, including breast self-examination, physical examination, and mammography
B. Diagnostic approach to a woman with a chief complaint of a breast mass, nipple discharge, or breast pain
C. History and physical findings that may suggest the following abnormalities:
   1. Interductal papilloma
   2. Fibrocystic change
   3. Fibroadenoma
   4. Carcinoma
   5. Mastitis
D. How to teach a woman to perform breast self-examination

PATHOGENESIS

Basic anatomy and physiology

As outlined by Marchant, the breasts are of ectodermal origin and make their appearance as early as the thirty-fifth day of embryonic life. The epithelial ridge that eventually forms the breast undergoes a series of alterations to form functioning units, including the lactiferous ducts and alveoli. Infant breast tissue may hypertrophy after delivery when there is increased cellular activity because of estrogen crossing the placental barrier. The breast thereafter remains dormant until puberty. The pubarcheal development of the breast or *thelarche* occurs over a period of several years. This growth results from an increase of estrogen and growth hormone. Estrogen receptors depend on prolactin for increased ductal development. Progesterone is required for complete alveolar development. Gonadotropin-releasing hormone stimulates prolactin, potentiated by estrogen.

The functioning units of the breast include the alveoli, the lactiferous ducts, and their supporting tissue. During pregnancy there are obvious increased levels of estrogen, progesterone, and placental lactogen. These produce active growth of the breast in preparation for nursing. It is, however, the decreased secretion of estrogen after delivery and the suppression of prolactin-inhibiting factor (PIF) by sucking that increases the prolactin level and increases the mother's lactation. Human milk as now understood produces excellent growth for the newborn, and lactation and nursing should be encouraged.

Sucking causes an increase in prolactin but also increases thyroid-stimulating hormone (TSH) and oxytocin. Thyroid-releasing hormone (TRH) increases both prolactin and TSH levels. Bromocriptine (dopamine or PIF) was formerly used to suppress postpartum lactation but is no longer prescribed because the drug may cause hypertension, seizures, strokes, or myocardial infarctions. Continued breast-feeding acts as a contraceptive because it suppresses ovulation, but sexual activity should be considered safe only for 10 weeks after delivery because only during this period does the prolactin sufficiently suppress gonadotropin levels.

Anatomic abnormalities

Abnormalities in breast development during thelarche should be recognized by the student, including the normal formation of "breast buds." If these buds are misdiagnosed as threatening lumps and are injudiciously removed by an overly eager surgeon, further breast development will be markedly curtailed and hypodevelopment of that specific breast occurs. Unilateral overdevelopment of the breast is not uncommon and should not be disturbed. Large or hypertrophied breast tissue should be surgically excised when such hypertrophy promotes rounded shoulders and poor posture. This should be explained to the patient in great detail. Corrective operations should be performed by someone who understands both the physiology and the likely cosmetic effects of such surgery.

SPECIFIC DISORDERS OF THE BREAST

Benign breast disease

Benign breast diseases include mild hyperplasia (less than four epithelial cells deep); fibroadenoma and fibrosis; ductal ectasia; squamous metaplasia; and mastitis, either inflammatory or periductal. Women with these findings are at no more risk for invasive cancer than are comparable women with no breast biopsies. Findings that put the woman at a slightly increased risk (1.5 to 2 times) include moderate hyperplasia and papilloma with a fibrovascular core. Those with a definitely increased risk (5 times) include ductal or lobular atypical hyperplasia (a borderline lesion).

The term "fibrocystic disease" should be eliminated from our medical literature and certainly never used on a medical form. There have been denials of hospitalization and surgical coverage by insurance companies that interpret fibrocystic disease as a premalignant lesion and withhold payment to individuals because they have a "pre-existing" condition. "Fibrocystic changes" is the preferable term and does not imply an underlying disease process.

Inappropriate lactation syndrome: galactorrhea

Galactorrhea may be characterized as follows: (1) occurs more than 6 (or 12) months postpartum; (2) comes from one or both breasts; and (3) possibly is accompanied by amenorrhea. The causes of galactorrhea include increased estrogen levels (produced by decreasing PIF). However, this

PIF = prolactin inhibiting factor

has become rare since the new oral contraceptives were developed. Prolonged sucking (even in an adoptive parent) may induce galactorrhea by decreasing PIF and increasing prolactin levels. Viral infections such as herpes zoster simulate sucking by affecting the sensory arc. Over 100 drugs may decrease PIF; most of these are phenothiazine derivatives. Stress may also decrease PIF, or the patient might have a pituitary stalk lesion that interferes with PIF flow. A hypothyroid condition can induce galactorrhea by reflexively increasing TRH, which increases prolactin levels.

Increased prolactin levels occasionally result from lung or renal tumors or leiomyomas, but these are quite unusual causes. The Albright form of galactorrhea has an accompanying intracellar tumor. Chiari-Frommel syndrome occurs with an antecedent pregnancy and persistent lactation, whereas del Castillo's syndrome has no antecedent pregnancy but a spontaneous onset and persistence of lactation. Only 33% of hyperprolactinomas are associated with galactorrhea.

Sheehan's postpartum intrapituitary hemorrhage is a syndrome that can first be suspected by the absence of lactation. Sheehan's syndrome should be considered in a patient with massive intrapartum blood loss.

Nipple discharge and breast pain

Nipple discharges are worrisome. Such discharges may result from drugs taken, mostly tranquilizers and some oral contraceptives, or from stimulation of the breast by the patient or the patient's partner. If the discharge is bilateral, this should be noted. The student must carefully describe and document the origin of such discharge, its color, and how it can be demonstrated (on the bra, after a shower, and so on). Bloody or serosanguineous discharges necessitate investigation. Routine Pap smears of these discharges tend to be worthless. Further investigation of the duct system should be done at mammography with additional techniques.

Breast pain (mastalgia) sometimes is difficult to explain. It may result purely from the size of the breasts and their dependency when bra support is poor. This must be noted and an attempt made to correct the situation with a more supportive bra. Careful physical examination may determine the cause of pain, but it is also important at this time that the physician restate to the patient the technical aspects of self-examination of the breast.

Present-day treatment of mastalgia consists of the antigonadotropin Danocrine or the antiestrogen tamoxifen. Neither are satisfactory, and both have side effects. Methyltestosterone may be given short trials.

Breast cancer

Breast cancer is the second leading cause of cancer death after lung cancer. Close to 150,000 cases of breast cancer are discovered in women each year. One half of breast cancers occur in women over 65 years of age. Although the most common sign of cancer of the breast is finding a lump, the increasing use of mammography (no longer Xerox but now x-ray) has provided the most promising way to discover a small cancer at a time when it is most easily "curable."

Genetic involvement in breast cancer is quite apparent, and patients who have first-degree relatives with premenopausal or bilateral breast cancer have a 50-50 chance of developing breast cancer. A fatty diet, alcoholic beverages, smoking, and female hormones have all been thought to be causative. Multiple cohort studies have not indicated a direct connection between hormone replacement and breast cancer, but a negative mammogram is necessary before hormone replacement is begun. Estrogen itself may cause increased growth of a nidus of breast cancer but is not believed to be a causative agent de novo. Most researchers believe that former users of estrogen are not at increased risk for cancer of the breast but that present users may be. This also seems to be

Table 37-1. Breast self-examination

1. Lie down and put a pillow under your right shoulder. Place your right arm behind your head.
2. Use the finger pads of your three middle fingers on your left hand to feel for lumps or thickening. Your finger pads are the top third of each finger.
3. Press firmly enough to know how each breast feels. If you are not sure how hard to press, ask your health care provider. Or try to copy the way your health care provider uses the finger pads during a breast exam. Learn what your breasts feel like most of the time. A firm ridge in the lower curve of each breast is normal.
4. Move around the breast in a set way. You can choose either the circle, the up and down line, or the wedge. (See Fig. 37-1.) Do it the same way every time. It will help you to make sure that you have gone over the entire breast area, and to remember how your breast feels.

As outlined by the American Cancer Society.

true with some of the other estrogen-dependent carcinomas.

Breast cancer is a systemic disease. Oophorectomized women have a decreased risk of breast cancer. Obese women have a greater risk, perhaps because there is more free serum estrogen estradiol and a lower serum hormone binding globulin level.

DIAGNOSTIC STUDIES

SELF-EXAMINATION. Most breast lumps (90%) are discovered by the patient during self-examination. Thus the student must understand how to instruct each patient in monthly examination of her breasts (Table 37-1).

Patient self-examination is best done after a menstrual period and perhaps while in the shower, where wetness may aid in palpation (Fig. 37-1).

MAMMOGRAPHY. There is a 3-year to 5-year lag "between the earliest possible tumor detection by mammography and the point where a tumor becomes palpable," so routine mammography is recommended. The 5-year survival rate in patients in whom the cancer was discovered by self-examination is only 50%, but the 5-year survival rate in patients where the cancer was discovered by mammography is 98%. Frazer and colleagues found a 10-year survival rate of 96% in patients

whose cancer was discovered before the breast tumor exceeded 0.5 cm in diameter.

Various organizations have suggested time schedules for mammography. The American Cancer Society, in its 1995 recommendations, stated that all women between 35 and 40 should have a baseline mammogram. After the age of 40, mammography should be done on a yearly basis. How long the studies should be continued thereafter is still a question.

If the patient has a first-degree relative with carcinoma of the breast, the baseline mammogram should be done at an earlier age, perhaps as early as 25. The mammographer may, however, report difficulty in assessing possible tumors because of the denseness of the breast tissue in younger patients.

The risk of cancer of the breast as a result of repeated mammography has been vastly overstated. Broadbent and Reed reported that one would need 100 yearly mammograms to increase the rate of cancer of the breast by 1%, and that would only raise it from 7% to 8%.

In a questionnaire sent to 30 physicians in the Sacramento area, only 23% correctly identified the 5-year survival rate with mammographically discovered "minimal" breast cancers (98%). However, 73% of the same physicians did know that the radiation dose received from mammography is correctly only one third of that from a single x-ray study of the abdomen.

The practical use of mammography is to detect *nonpalpable cancer*. Tumors double their size every 100 days. It takes 10 years for one malignant cell to continue doubling to reach the size of 1 cm, those ordinarily found by the patient. More than five calcifications found in a mammography cluster are associated with cancer in about 25% of cases.

There is an extremely high benefit/risk ratio using mammography as a means of early detection. Major risk factors that can substantially increase an individual woman's chances of breast cancer are age (it increases rapidly from 25 to 50 years of age, after which it continues to increase but at a slower rate), a family history of breast cancer, and the presence of some forms of benign breast disease.

Biopsy. The standard approach to a patient with a breast mass should be to determine whether it is benign or malignant. One cannot rely on either negative mammography or a "benign feel" to a breast mass to determine its potential malignancy. A surgical biopsy is the ultimate confirmation. Off-handed dismissal of an unexplored breast mass obviously shortens patient survival if such a mass is cancerous. In this litigious society, it will provide much evidence for testimony against the physician. It is better to have confirming examinations by surgeons to ascertain the best procedural approach.

When one finds a dominant lump, the physician must obtain a negative pathology report before the patient can be assured that her mass is benign. These lumps sometimes evade surgical investigation, and needle localization by the radiologist is needed. This means radiologically "pointing out" the lesion to the surgeon. The excised sample is sent for pathologic study with the needle in place to be sure that the exact area designated was removed.

Fine needle aspiration and other methods. Before any excisional biopsy the obstetrician-gynecologist may try fine needle aspiration of the breast. This technique involves a 22-gauge or 23-gauge needle and no local anesthesia. Aspiration obtains not histologic tissue but cells for the detection of cancer. Cyst fluid obtained by needle aspiration is probably worthless for cytologic identification of carcinoma, and cysts are considered benign unless they recur or persist through the next menstrual period. If the fluid is blood or if no fluid is obtained, an open biopsy should be recommended. Fine needle aspiration technique is easily learned and obviously is most helpful when the cytologic results obtained are positive. Ultrasound is not advised as a screen-

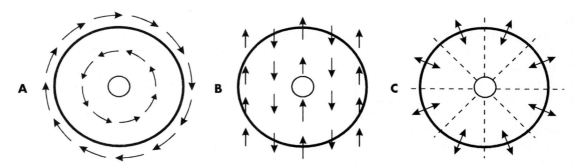

Fig. 37-1. Method of breast self-examination. Patient can choose either the circle **(A),** the up and down line **(B),** or the wedge **(C).**

ing technique, but it does show cysts of the breast more clearly than x-ray mammography.

Older methods, such as thermography, should not be used.

MANAGEMENT: SURGERY. The lymph nodes are the key to surgery, and the patient's prognosis depends on the presence or absence of positive nodes. For example, 10 years postoperatively, 75% of patients whose nodes originally were negative continue free of disease, whereas only 25% of patients with positive nodes are disease-free.

The kinds of surgery now done and the types of drugs used for chemotherapy are changing radically. Radical mastectomy with muscle removal and an empty chest wall is no longer done because the survival rate has not been found to improve with such drastic surgery. More modified radical procedures with node samplings are now performed. The antiestrogen tamoxifen is recommended not only when there are estrogen receptors in the carcinomatous tissue but also in the treatment of all carcinomas of the breast. Lumpectomies with radiation are often performed, depending on the cancer's spread.

First-degree relatives of these patients ultimately may be given prophylactic tamoxifen. A word of caution is necessary since the estrogen antagonistic factor in tamoxifen is accompanied by an estrogen agonistic factor that may stimulate a hyperplastic reaction in the endometrium. Such treated individuals must be routinely biopsied for atypical hyperplasia. This is done via endometrial sampling or by ultrasound measurement of the endometrium.

Cosmetic surgery may not improve the survival rate, but it certainly allows the patient to live a more normal life. Cytoxin and methotrexate are used in addition to tamoxifen in therapy for breast cancer, depending on each individual case and the physician's preference.

BREAST CANCER AND PREGNANCY. The student must understand that pregnancy and breast cancer are specifically antagonistic conditions. The age at first pregnancy is important. If the mother is over 35, she has 3 times the risk of breast cancer of a mother less than 18 years old. Examination of the breast should not be delayed because the patient is pregnant. It is important to determine whether the masses felt in the pregnant breast are truly benign. If chemotherapy is necessary for cancer of the breast, it can be given safely after the first trimester of pregnancy. The radical procedures previously done in pregnancy are usually no longer done.

CRITICAL POINTS

- About 150,000 new cases of breast cancer are discovered each year.
- Mammography done on a routine basis is the most efficient way to discover early nonpalpable cancers.
- Fibrocystic *disease* is *not* premalignant; the term should not be used on records.
- Surgery is needed to confirm or rule out the benign nature of breast lesions.

Questions

1. The percentage of breast lumps discovered by *the patient* is estimated at:

A. Less than 5%
B. 25%
C. 50%
D. 90%

2. Mammography in the young (less than
   30 years old) patient may be undesirable
   because:
   A. Density of breast tissue makes radio-
      graphs difficult to read.
   B. Radiation in a young patient is too
      dangerous.
   C. Breasts in young women do not show
      lumps.
3. Fibrocystic disease is:
   A. A precancerous lesion
   B. A term not to be used
   C. More common in grand multiparas
   D. Ordinarily just found in menopausal
      women

4. Breast buds indicate:
   A. Impending carcinoma
   B. Lumps that need to be immediately
      removed
   C. Developing breasts that must be left
      alone
   D. Müllerian abnormalities elsewhere

Answers

1. D
2. A
3. B
4. C

38

Gynecologic procedures

APGO LEARNING OBJECTIVE #38

Philip A. Rosenfeld

The evaluation and management of gynecologic problems frequently necessitates diagnostic and therapeutic surgical procedures. Understanding the risks and benefits of such procedures is important.

In counseling patients about their options for treatment and the reasons for having the procedures performed, the student will demonstrate a knowledge of the following:

A. Definition
B. Indications
C. Risks
D. Contraindications
E. Financial considerations
F. Language useful in describing the procedure to a patient for each of the following:
   1. Colposcopy and cervical biopsy
   2. Cone biopsy
   3. Cryotherapy
   4. Culdocentesis
   5. Dilatation and curettage
   6. Electrosurgical excision of the cervix
   7. Endometrial biopsy
   8. Hysterectomy
   9. Hysterosalpingography
   10. Hysteroscopy
   11. Laparoscopy
   12. Laser vaporization
   13. Mammography
   14. Needle aspiration of breast mass
   15. Pelvic ultrasonography
   16. Pregnancy termination
   17. Vulvar biopsy

The student should understand the language used to explain anticipated procedures, the alternatives, and the risks to the patient. Procedures that necessitate general anesthesia (i.e., hysterectomy and laparoscopy) increase mortality risk to approximately 1 in 10,000.

It is important that the patient have a clear understanding of what surgery is proposed. Not only the complications but also the *alternatives* and *prognosis* of each surgical procedure must be explained. This is obviously important when individuals are being advised to have nonemergency procedures (i.e., those that are not treating life-threatening conditions and are therefore somewhat elective). It is also necessary that the patient be told what the chances are that the proposed surgical procedure may make her condition worse.

Besides a complete history of the present illness, its length, and its involvement with other organs, each patient must have a complete physical. It must be determined which methods previously have failed to improve the condition.

COLPOSCOPY AND CERVICAL BIOPSY

The ordinary screening method for cervical cancer is the Pap smear. However, since nearly 25% of Pap smears are false-negative, occasionally it is necessary that the cervix be visualized microscopically. This becomes mandatory when the patient has an abnormal Pap smear.

Through the use of a colposcope (a binocular cervical microscope) the *squamocolumnar junction,* the seat of reserve cell changes leading to cervical cancer, is magnified and studied following the addition of 3% to 5% acetic acid. This chemical will change the refractory index of the cells, making the surface epithelium more visible to the physician. The acetic acid usually is in the form of vinegar, has a dehydrating effect, and accentuates the nuclear/cytoplasmic ratio.

The entire *transformation zone* should be fully visualized. This transformation zone comprises all tissue between the original and the current squamocolumnar junction. Unless the patient is pregnant, an endocervical curettage also should be performed and biopsies taken in any areas that appear abnormal. If surface epithelium is properly biopsied, minimal bleeding is encountered and can easily be controlled with some protein precipitant like ferric subsulfate (Monsels) or silver nitrate. There are no contraindications to this pro-

cedure unless the patient is pregnant; then the endocervical scraping is omitted and the number of biopsies minimized. Depending on the findings of this colposcopy and cervical biopsy procedure, further therapy of cervical neoplasia may be indicated.

A *cone biopsy* is done when preinvasive cervical lesions are quite extensive. It is also done when there is widespread glandular involvement. This conization or removal of a "cone-shaped" piece of tissue, where the large size is usually on the ectocervix, can be adequately performed either with a scalpel (cold knife cone) or a carbon dioxide laser. By doing this wider, deeper procedure the risk of bleeding increases, both at the time of the removal of the cone and for some time postoperatively when sutures or eschars disintegrate. This later bleeding can become quite worrisome and infrequently necessitates more surgery, sometimes including an emergency hysterectomy. Ordinarily, preemptive suturing of the cervix, especially in the 3 o'clock and 9 o'clock position where the descending branches of the uterine vessels come down the exocervix, will facilitate obtaining this conization and minimize bleeding. The raw bed of endocervical tissue following the cone ordinarily can be cauterized and/or sutured. The conization is designed not only to prove the absence of invasive disease of the cervix, but also to serve as a curative measure, especially when all margins are free of dysplastic cells.

More recently, a loop electrical excision procedure (LEEP) or loop excision of transformation zone (LETZ) procedure has been done, using a thin wire and an electrosurgical cautery. This thin wire technique, as an office procedure under local anesthesia, will remove the same amount of affected tissue as a conization and does not necessitate hospitalization.

Cervical stenosis may be produced by cone biopsy if the external or internal os heals in a closed fashion. Stenosis may present as external amenorrhea and cyclic pain, and can necessitate cervical dilatation to release the menstrual blood. A scarred cervix may be suspected in labor when the cervix fails to dilate normally. If the cervical canal is cut too deep an *incompetent cervix* may result in the second trimester, with laborless dilatation of the cervix and midtrimester fetal wastage.

CRYOSURGERY

The cryosurgical unit consisting of either a carbon dioxide or nitrogen oxide tank connected to a probe will freeze and thaw the affected cervix in a manner similar to the methods just discussed. The student must explain to the patient that cryosurgical destruction of the affected area does not remove any tissue for pathologic study. Therefore the physician must have a clear-cut understanding that there are no cells buried below the surface that will emerge later as a carcinoma. The cryosurgical technique is painless and less costly than the other methods described, but it will result in a watery discharge as the dehydrated, desiccated cells slough. This may last for several weeks and can be annoying. One further difficulty with the cryosurgical technique is that the squamocolumnar junction (that area to be most carefully followed) is reestablished higher in the canal, not down on the surface area where it can be studied more easily as it can following laser and LEEP procedures. Cryosurgical technique is still used because the instrumentation is relatively inexpensive and the technique is easily performed in an ambulatory setting. It is ordinarily done in low-grade intraepithelial neoplasia where further pathologic specimens are not considered mandatory.

CULDOCENTESIS

To perform culdocentesis, an 18-gauge spinal length needle is inserted quickly into the posterior cul-de-sac (dependent position of the pelvis) (Fig. 38-1) between the uterosacral ligaments. With a tenaculum placed on the posterior lip, the cervix is

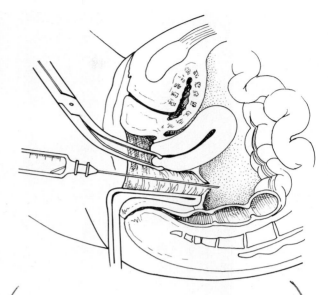

Fig. 38-1. Culdocentesis. An 18-gauge needle, with attached syringe, is being inserted into cul-de-sac.

pulled anteriorly and outwardly; the needle with syringe is introduced into an area where any collection of fluid can be at least partly removed and studied. Though culdocentesis is used primarily for the diagnosis of ectopic pregnancy, it also can be used to obtain cultures in patients with pelvic inflammatory disease (PID). The pus obtained can be studied by Gram smear and culture. Because the inflamed peritoneum is painful in these patients, culdocentesis is not ordinarily done in patients with PID.

Even when a ruptured or leaking ectopic pregnancy is suspected, culdocentesis is often not used because of newer, more rapid and accurate methods to measure human chorionic gonadotropin levels and because of the availability of ultrasound. For eccyesis (ectopic), the material in the attached syringe contains blood that will not clot. More properly, this is previously clotted blood, not unclotted blood because the fibrinogen already has been used up. This finding indicates that there has been some leak of blood from the tube or, less likely, from another source, including

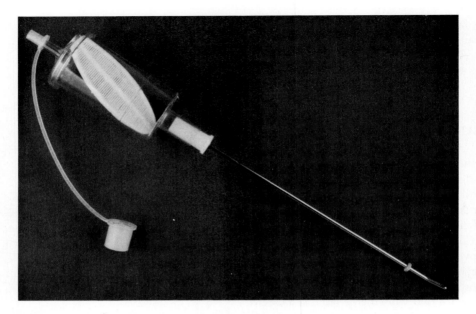

Fig. 38-2. Endometrial biopsy suction curet; there are several types available. Curet is attached to pump producing negative suction. Uterine cavity depth is determined since curet is calibrated in centimeters. Sample obtained is collected in tissue trap. Preprocedure tranquilizer or paracervical block can reduce discomfort and should be used as necessary.

hemorrhagic cyst of the ovary. The hematocrit of this previously clotted blood should exceed 15% to be significant.

Such a procedure can be performed either in the operating room or in the office if the patient is put in semi-Fowler's position a short while beforehand in order to accumulate fluid in the posterior cul-de-sac.

DILATATION AND CURETTAGE

Dilatation and curettage (D&C) ordinarily is done to determine and examine the contents of the uterine cavity and frequently the endocervical canal (Fig. 38-2). If the fertility status of the endometrium is the only pathologic report desired, a small suction biopsy from the anterior uterine wall can be obtained in an outpatient setting. Diagnostic D&Cs are seldom done under general anesthesia because the reliability of specimens

obtained by office procedures are rarely questioned today when done properly. Wherever the operation is performed, tissue for diagnosis is obtained from the endometrial cavity in a purposely random manner to sample all areas. Once the endometrium has been properly curetted a smaller curet may be used to obtain a separate endocervical canal specimen. The D&C is the most often performed gynecologic procedure and is more diagnostic than curative. It does not cure irregular intermenstrual bleeding. However, the tissue microscopic diagnosis can be intelligently used by the provider to decide on proper therapy.

ELECTROSURGICAL EXCISION OF THE CERVIX

Electrosurgical excision of the cervix was mentioned previously with the LEEP or LETZ procedure. Previously, a larger wire and hotter current were used to clear chronic cystic cervicitis when the cervix contained a multitude of nabothian cysts. This procedure is no longer done.

ENDOMETRIAL BIOPSY

An endometrial biopsy ordinarily is performed to determine either endometrial maturation or the presence or absence of endometrial hyperplasia and/or carcinoma of the endometrium. The procedure is similar to the D&C but, as noted, does not necessitate as complete a curetting to obtain the required sample.

HYSTERECTOMY

Hysterectomy is the most commonly performed major gynecologic procedure in women who have benign conditions. A *total hysterectomy* means that the cervix is removed along with the fundus of the uterus (the adnexa are not included). The cervix sometimes may be left in place (supracervical hysterectomy) because of operative technical difficulties, but this necessitates careful following of possible cervical changes with frequent Pap smears, colposcopy, and so on. The ovaries normally are conserved in women under 40 years. Ovaries are removed in older women, and ordinarily hormone replacement therapy is initiated. Without a uterus, estrogen replacement alone is sufficient; but if the patient has a uterus, progesterone should be added to offset possible estrogen-produced endometrial hyperplasia. The hysterectomy can be performed either abdominally or vaginally; but ordinarily the uterus is not removed vaginally in women with large pelvic masses, a history of previous infection, a narrow subpubic arch, without prolapse of the uterus, or when there is a suspicion of malignancy.

Vaginal hysterectomy is the method of choice for the removal of a uterus in a parous woman whose uterine size does not exceed a comparable 12-week size in pregnancy. Vaginal hysterectomy also may include the removal of the ovaries through the vagina, or they may have been disconnected and dropped in the cul-de-sac by previous laparoscopy during the first phase of that operation. In the United States, about 30% of the approximately 600,000 hysterectomies each year are done via the vaginal route; the remaining 70% are performed abdominally.

Within recent times a third method of removing the uterus, *laparoscopic-assisted vaginal hysterectomy,* has become popular. Uterine-supporting tissues are released through the laparoscope, and the remaining portion of the procedure with delivery of the uterus is finalized through the vaginal route. The minimal number and small size of incisions involved in this latter procedure ordinarily lets the patient go home sooner and with less blood loss.

With all hysterectomies the two most common complications are hemorrhage and infection. The hemorrhage may appear intraoperatively or may occur later. Infection may be in the wound or through the previously opened vagina and sometimes necessitates large doses of antibiotics and a prolonged hospital stay. Other complications—including injury to bladder, rectum, ureters, and large blood vessels—occasionally are encountered and must be included in warnings given to the patient before her consent and decision for this major surgery. The patient must be told that both reproductive and menstrual functions of the uterus will no longer exist and that hormone replacement will be necessary if the ovaries are simultaneously removed.

HYSTEROSALPINGOGRAPHY

Hysterosalpingography is ordinarily part of an infertility work-up to determine the contour of the uterus and the patency of the tubes. An oil-base or water-base dye is inserted through the cervix, and the diagnosis of irregular uterine cavity (Fig. 38-3) or blocked or distorted fallopian tubes is made fluoroscopically. This procedure also can

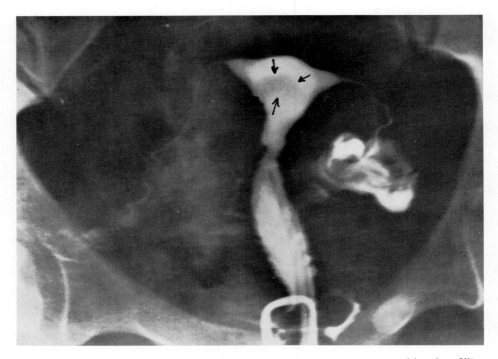

Fig. 38-3. Hysterogram showing submucous myoma. Uterine cavity is normal but has filling defect. Two previous curettages failed to disclose tumor.

be used to determine the presence of submucous fibroids and polyps by reducing the amount of dye injected into the uterine cavity. This latter technique has been replaced, for the most part, by hysteroscopy. Hysterosalpingography also is useful in diagnosing intrauterine scarring. However, the definitive diagnosis and treatment of this condition are also best made through the hysteroscope.

HYSTEROSCOPY

As indicated, transcervical visualization of the uterine cavity and the cornual openings is done using an endoscopic instrument at least 5 mm in diameter. Larger instruments are available for operative procedures. Hysteroscopy can be

done as an outpatient procedure with paracervical anesthesia.

The hysteroscope can be used to diagnose infertility; when a cause is found it can be corrected if a resectoscope is added to such combined operative procedures. For example, if a septate uterus is discovered the septum may be divided with scissors, laser, or resectoscope. Hysteroscopy may be used to remove an intrauterine device (IUD) after the string has become invisible to the examiner. The procedure also can be used to remove cervical polyps or to sample a suspected endometrial neoplasm. The distending medium may be carbon dioxide or some liquid whose intake and outflow can be accurately measured, thus preventing pulmonary edema and hypernatremia. Lenses of hysteroscopes ordinarily have a 30° angle. Their use in outpatients may make unnecessary approximately 70% of hospital admissions for the diagnoses mentioned previously.

LAPAROSCOPY

In laparoscopy a telescopic tube approximately 6 to 10 mm in diameter is inserted through an infraumbilical incision, primarily to study the pelvic organs. The usual distending medium is carbon dioxide, although a newer technique exists that allows insertion without gaseous distention. During the examination several other instruments may be inserted in other parts of the lower abdomen to be used in the diagnosis and possible treatment of pelvic pain. The scope is also used to assess PID and infertility where operative management may be attempted later. The student already has become aware of the use of laparoscopy in vaginal hysterectomy. One of the most promising, newer uses for laparoscopy is not only in the diagnosis of ectopic pregnancy, but also in its therapy. By instrumentation through various sites, trophoblastic material may be removed from the tube and tubal surgery by laparotomy avoided.

In sterilization procedures the laparoscope is used to interrupt both fallopian tubes, either by Silastic bands or metal clips, or by unipolar or bipolar cautery. Adhesions may be treated through the laparoscope.

These laparoscopic procedures, when done by knowledgeable physicians, will markedly shorten both the hospital stay and the patient's postoperative recovery. Such dangers as vascular, bowel, and viscus perforations must be explained to the patient before a decision is made. Procedures for sterilization should be carefully presented and the failure rate of approximately of 1 in 250 procedures documented and explained to the patient.

The laparoscope is now being used by surgeons in other specialties to remove gall bladders, resect bowel, repair hernias, and biopsy such organs as the liver under direct vision.

LASER VAPORIZATION

Lasers used in previous times include the carbon dioxide, potassium titanyl phosphate, and yttrium aluminum garnet. Future lasers including the excimer are now incorporated in certain surgical procedures. However, the workhorse of gynecology will probably remain the carbon dioxide laser, which can be used both intraabdominally and externally. In addition to its use in infertility within the abdomen for fulguration of endometriosis, the laser can be used outside the abdomen for conization of the cervix and for vaporization of lesions caused by the human papillomavirus (HPV). Such condylomata can be destroyed if the procedure is carefully done, but the patient must be counseled that this procedure is *not* curative because HPV travels between visible lesions with impunity.

Skill is required for the vaporization of such external lesions as condylomata and certainly in those cases where vulvar intraepithelial features are found. Suitable biopsies must be done before laser destruction.

MAMMOGRAPHY

Mammography is the best screening device now available for the detection of breast cancer. Lesions smaller than those ordinarily discovered by the physician or patient by palpation can be picked up by mammograms read by a qualified radiologist. The anxious patient should know that repeated mammography will not increase her chances of breast cancer by additional radiation. Statistics indicate that 100 yearly mammograms would be necessary to increase the patient's risk of carcinoma of the breast by 1%.

Most recommendations include baseline mammography in women between 35 and 40 years old, with mammogram every 18 months to 2 years from 40 to 50 and yearly mammograms after age 50. So far physicians have not agreed about frequency in older patients. Ultrasound of the breasts is used primarily to distinguish cysts. The patient must be told that self-examination, routine breast examination by a physician, and mammography combine to make up good diagnostic care with regard to breast cancer.

When the mammography reveals an abnormality not palpable, one option is to localize the lesion mammographically and do a biopsy. Stereotaxic needle biopsy is now replacing excisional biopsy.

NEEDLE ASPIRATION OF A BREAST MASS

Needle aspiration of breast tissue has gained some popularity among physicians. The main objections center around the strong possibility that the results of a needle aspiration may represent a sampling error and miss the lesion. Some experts believe that needle aspiration is useful only when positive and that a palpable mass with a negative needle aspiration is an unfinished diagnosis that needs immediate clarification. Fine needle aspiration can be done in the physician's office without local anesthesia. It is done with a 23-gauge or 24-gauge spinal needle, quickly inserted directly into a suspected mass as it is rendered immobile by the other examining hand. Occasionally a needle is used to localize the site of a proposed biopsy. When the area is confirmed radiographically, the patient is sent to the operating room and the correct removal of specimen is again confirmed radiographically before sending the biopsy to pathology for definitive diagnosis. These fine needle aspirations give a cytologic answer, not a histologic one. The patient must realize that only an open biopsy will give sufficient tissue for the pathologist to render a definite histologic diagnosis.

PELVIC ULTRASONOGRAPHY

Pelvic ultrasonography may now be done both abdominally (as originally conceived) and vaginally (using a special intravaginal 5-MHz probe). Placing the probe closer to the ovaries and tubes through the vagina has helped the ultrasonographer make a diagnosis of ectopic pregnancy earlier in its life span. The procedure also can be used in infertility patients to estimate follicle number and size.

Abdominal ultrasonography (usually a 3-MHz probe) is used obstetrically to evaluate the condition and age of the fetus. In gynecology ovarian cysts and their specific nature, leiomyomata of the uterus, and other pelvic cystic structures can be evaluated correctly via ultrasound. In abdominal ultrasound, a large volume of urine in the bladder will help visualization of the pelvic organs. This filling of the bladder is not necessary when the ultrasonographic probe is inserted through the vagina.

The patient should be assured there is no danger in ultrasonography but that the information acquired is only a part of the general inquiry and

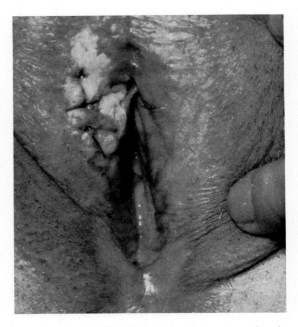

Fig. 38-4. Area of epithelial hyperkeratosis and early cancer.

laboratory studies needed before a definitive diagnosis may be made. The skill of the ultrasonographer is very important to the diagnostic results and must be taken into account by the referring physician.

PREGNANCY TERMINATION

Depending on federal, state, and city laws and on local hospital regulations, pregnancies may be voluntarily terminated—usually up to 20 weeks' gestation. Such terminations may be done in a physician's office by suction extraction to remove trophoblastic tissue and products of conception, or the patient may require dilatation and evacuation in an operating room if the fetus is of a greater gestational age. Instillation of materials into the amniotic sac is done in later stages of gestation to induce the patient to go into labor and deliver the dead fetus. Both the patient and the physician must understand the rationale for termination of pregnancy and that infection, hemorrhage, perforation, and occasional operative missing of the fetus (especially early) have been reported. Many terminations, especially later in gestation, are done today because of genetic abnormalities. Technical skill in the performance of such terminations is an obvious requirement.

The student must understand that any patient who requests termination or requires a termination for medical reasons undergoes a deep psychologic adjustment. Treatment of that portion of the process must not be neglected.

VULVAR BIOPSY

Lesions that fail to heal, are questionable, or are recurrent (Fig. 38-4) may be removed by a vulvar biopsy. Most carcinomas of the vulva have been present for a long time, and the diagnosis ultimately is made by a much-delayed biopsy of the vulva. These procedures may be done with a dermal punch of about 4 mm, in which a tube of superficial tissue can be removed under local anesthesia. It usually requires no postoperative suturing. This can be done rather painlessly on an outpatient basis. The biopsy result will correctly point to further therapy. Such a procedure may be curative, but usually is only diagnostic.

CRITICAL POINTS

- One must thoroughly counsel patients on procedures proposed, alternative therapy, and possible adverse outcomes.
- Practitioners must have a fundamental understanding of all of the common gynecologic procedures.
- The decision regarding the appropriateness of an operative procedure is made after a thorough clinical assessment of, and discussion with, the patient.
- Hysterectomy is the most common gynecologic procedure performed. The vaginal route, if technically feasible, is preferred for patients with benign disease.

Questions

1. What percentage of Pap smears are considered to be false-negative in most labs?
   A. Less than 5%
   B. 75%
   C. 25%
   D. 50%
2. When extensive preinvasive cells are found by colposcopy, the next logical step is:
   A. Hysterectomy
   B. Laser ablation of transformation zone
   C. Cryosurgery
   D. Cone biopsy
3. Culdocentesis is the:
   A. Insertion of a needle in the cul-de-sac
   B. Incision and drainage of a pelvic abscess
   C. Laparoscopic examination of the cul-de-sac
   D. Removal of a gall bladder
4. A "lost" IUD can best be located by:
   A. Culdocentesis
   B. Hysteroscopy
   C. Laparoscopy
   D. Colonoscopy

Answers

1. C
2. D
3. A
4. B

IV

Reproductive endocrinology, infertility, and related topics

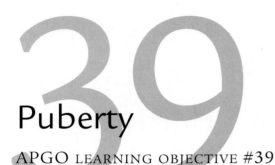

Puberty

APGO LEARNING OBJECTIVE #39

P. Coney

The maturation of the reproductive system at the time of puberty is accompanied by physical and emotional changes that are part of this normal transition. To provide appropriate care and counseling, the physician must have an understanding of the normal sequence of puberty and recognize deviation from the norm.

The student will demonstrate a knowledge of the following:

A. Normal puberty, including the following:
   1. Physiologic events that take place in the hypothalamic-pituitary-ovarian axis and their target organs
   2. Sequence of and expected ages at which these changes occur
   3. Psychologic aspects
B. Abnormal puberty, including the following:
   1. Characteristics, causes, and diagnostic approach to evaluate the cause
   2. True precocious puberty, pseudo-precocious puberty, and delayed puberty

Puberty is synonymous with sexual maturation. It is characterized by a series of timely endocrine and physical changes in growth and appearance of secondary sex characteristics. In the United States, 95% of girls will develop signs of puberty between the ages of 8 and 13. The average age of culmination of these events, menarche, is 12.8 years for the American girl. Nutritional and socioeconomic conditions, genetics, and general health status influence the onset and progression of pubertal development. The purpose of this dynamic period is the attainment of full reproductive competence.

NEUROENDOCRINOLOGY OF PUBERTY

The prepubertal years are characterized by increasing hormone production. In infancy, circulating concentrations of gonadotropins and sex steroid hormones are comparable to adult levels. Levels fall progressively to very low and almost undetectable levels by age 6 to 8. During this period of low gonadotropin and hormone concentrations, all stages of follicular development can be demonstrated in the prepubertal ovary, as well as a constant rate of atresia. As the girl ages toward 8 to 9 years, the number of follicles that progress in size to the graafian stage increases. Concomitant with the progression of follicular size, the mean concentrations of gonadotropins and estrogen increase. Mean ovarian weight also increases. At approximately age 8 to 9, levels of gonadotropins and estrogen become detectable. A marked increase in estrogen occurs between ages 11 and 12.

The hypothalamus controls secretion of gonadotropins and sex steroid hormones by its influence on the anterior pituitary gland. Reproductive function is thus controlled by gonadotropin-releasing hormone (GnRH), which is secreted by the hypothalamus into the portal system, which connects the anterior pituitary to the median eminence. The GnRH is a decapeptide that was characterized structurally in 1971. The new ability to synthesize GnRH was used to elucidate our understanding of hypothalamic control of reproduction. Once in the portal system, GnRH is transported to the anterior pituitary. The secretion of GnRH is pulsatile and periodic, occurring every 60 to 90 minutes. Pulsatile secretion of GnRH causes *up-regulation* of GnRH receptors in the medial basal region of the hypothalamus, resulting in increased secretion of GnRH. This action on the pituitary results in episodic secretion of follicle-stimulating hormone (FSH) and luteinizing hormone (LH), which regulate function of the ovary. A slower secretory rate results in infrequent pulses, which causes amenorrhea or anovulation. A faster or continuous secretory rate results in *down-regulation* or a refractory state of pituitary response, leading to anovulation and amenorrhea. Evidence that supports GnRH as the mediator of hypothalamic, pituitary, and ovarian regulation of reproduction includes the following: (1) intravenous administration of GnRH initiates puberty in hypogonadal subjects; (2) chronic administration of GnRH abolishes the endocrine and physical changes associated with puberty; and (3) episodic increases in FSH and LH occur nocturnally in girls just before puberty.

What specific event initiates puberty is not known. What maintains the hypothalamus in a suppressive mode before the onset of puberty is not known. At about age 8, the central inhibition of hypothalamic GnRH secretion is abolished and the endocrinologic changes of puberty are initiated. Pro-opiomelanocortin and the neurotransmitters aspartate and glutamate have been implicated, but the exact role of each is not clear. The negative feedback inhibition on the hypothalamus is removed, and increased hypothalamic secretion of GnRH results. The pituitary increases its secretion of FSH and LH. Indirect evidence suggests that sex hormones, particularly estrogen, mediate the feedback mechanism just before puberty, as in the period after puberty. Physiologic regulation of secretion of GnRH, FSH, and LH is influenced by sex steroid hormones and other ovarian factors (inhibin, activin, and follistatin). Gonads, however, are not necessary for activation of the hypothalamic-pituitary system in the initiation of puberty.

DEVELOPMENT OF SECONDARY SEX CHARACTERISTICS

Secondary sex characteristics are induced by hormones from the adrenal gland and the ovary (Fig.

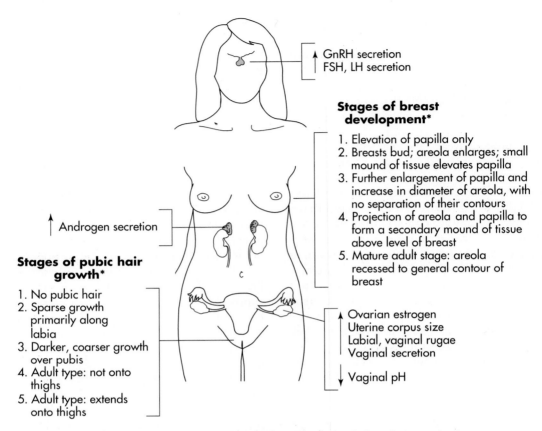

Stages of breast development*

1. Elevation of papilla only
2. Breasts bud; areola enlarges; small mound of tissue elevates papilla
3. Further enlargement of papilla and increase in diameter of areola, with no separation of their contours
4. Projection of areola and papilla to form a secondary mound of tissue above level of breast
5. Mature adult stage: areola recessed to general contour of breast

GnRH secretion
FSH, LH secretion

Androgen secretion

Stages of pubic hair growth*

1. No pubic hair
2. Sparse growth primarily along labia
3. Darker, coarser growth over pubis
4. Adult type: not onto thighs
5. Adult type: extends onto thighs

Ovarian estrogen
Uterine corpus size
Labial, vaginal rugae
Vaginal secretion

Vaginal pH

* Marshall-Tanner classification of pubertal development of breast and pubic hair growth

Fig. 39-1. Major events in normal pubertal development.

39-1). The first sign of female sexual development is thelarche, or breast development. Pubarche, the appearance of pubic hair, follows thelarche by about 6 months. Adrenarche is marked by an increase in androgen secretion and occurs shortly after thelarche. Generally, pubic hair must appear before the Tanner stage 5 of breast development (Fig. 39-1). Pubic hair is unlikely to appear before initiation of thelarche. Most often, breast development equals pubic hair development. The Marshall-Tanner classification system (Fig. 39-2) of breast development and pubic hair growth during the pubertal period is universally accepted as the standard for assessment. Axillary hair ap-

pears during Tanner stages 3 to 4 of breast development. African-American girls develop secondary sex characteristics sooner than do white American girls.

GROWTH AND BODY COMPOSITION

Growth hormone secretion is increased with puberty. Sex steroid secretion is responsible for the increase in growth hormone secretion. Growth hormone and sex steroids are responsible for acceleration of linear growth, or the growth spurt

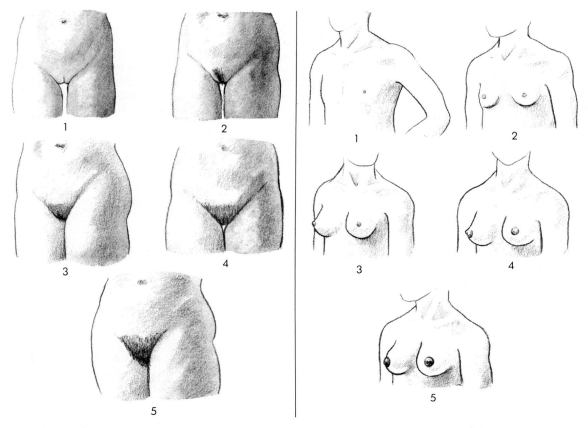

Fig. 39-2. Standards for pubic hair and breast stages. Stage 1 is the least developed; stage 5 represents adult development. *(Redrawn from Tanner JM: Growth and endocrinology of the adolescent. In Gardner L, editor: Endocrine and genetic diseases of childhood, ed 2, Philadelphia, 1975, WB Saunders.)*

observed in puberty. Peak height velocity for the female is attained early in the pubertal process. Bone age is better correlated with menarche and the onset of secondary sex development than is chronologic age. Bone age can be determined from radiographs of the hand, elbow, and knee. Bone age, height, and chronologic age are used to predict final adult height. Osseous maturation is more advanced in females than in males of the same chronologic age. Skeletal age is an index of maturity. Cumulative growth charts are used for comparison. Height can be compared among peers, but adults will not achieve the same height at the same maturity. Boys and girls have equal lean body mass, skeletal mass, and body fat before puberty. After puberty, boys have 1.5 times more lean body and skeletal mass than girls, and girls have 2 times more body fat than boys.

MENARCHE

Menarche, the onset of menstruation, is the true biologic marker of puberty. It generally occurs about 4 years after the appearance of thelarche. As a result of estrogen secretion, vaginal secretions increase and the vaginal pH is reduced. The vaginal mucosa thickens and becomes rugated, a sign of vaginal mucosa cornification by estrogen. The labia also protrude, thicken, and become rugated.

Table 39-1. Causes of delayed puberty

Constitutional	Miscellaneous conditions
Central nervous system disorders	Idiopathic hypopituitary dwarfism
Tumors (adenomas, craniopharyngiomas, germinomas)	Gonadal dysgenesis
Inflammatory lesions	Anorexia nervosa
Vascular lesions	Hyperprolactinemia
Irradiation	Hypothyroidism
Developmental defects (septo-optic dysplasia, dysraphism, cleft palate, holoprosencephaly)	Laurence-Moon syndrome
	Prader-Willi syndrome
Isolated gonadotropin deficiency	Cushing's disease
Histiocytosis X	Congenital adrenal hyperplasia
	Chronic illness

The uterus increases in size and lengthens. The mean weight of the ovaries also increases. A critical body weight is believed to be important in the onset of menarche. Body weight is not believed to be as critical as the percentage of body fat, which should be in the range of 17% to 22%. The menstrual cycle is an expression of the concerted actions of the hypothalamus, pituitary, and ovary that lead to functional changes in the reproductive tract. The physical changes are noted in the appearance of the girl. The end result is reproductive capability.

A wide range of individual differences may be observed in normal pubertal development. The real issues concern whether the age of initiation of puberty and the progression of pubertal events are normal.

PATHOPHYSIOLOGY OF PUBERTY

There are two categories of pathophysiologic puberty: *delayed puberty* and *precocious puberty*.

Delayed puberty

Failure of menarche by age 16 and failure of thelarche by age 13 constitute a diagnosis of delayed puberty. Diagnostic considerations include constitutional, or idiopathic, delay and conditions that cause hypogandotropic hypogonadism and hypergonadotropic hypogonadism (Table 39-1).

EVALUATION. Approximately 0.4% of normal girls will have delayed puberty of the constitutional variety. The first step in evaluating them is to obtain a thorough history to elicit all symptoms of chronic illness, nutritional status, and family history for age of onset of puberty in both parents. Physical examination should document height, weight, linear growth for age, and pubertal milestones achieved. Assay of gonadotropins, FSH, LH, karyotype, thyroxine, prolactin, and estrogen levels are indicated if clinical findings warrant. Response to GnRH is useful in diagnosing gonadotropin deficiency.

MANAGEMENT. It is important to determine whether the patient represents a normal, delayed variant or if an extensive evaluation is warranted. The constitutional type often experiences spontaneous onset and progression of puberty. Reassurance is all that is required. In other cases, the underlying disorder or disease is treated and, where indicated, steroid hormone replacement is provided.

Table 39-2. Causes of precocious puberty

Central precocious puberty	Pseudoprecocious puberty	Incomplete precocious puberty
Idiopathic	Ovarian disease	Exogenous sex steroids
Central nervous system disease	Tumors (granulosa cell, lipoid germ cell)	Adrenal tumors
Congenital defects or malformations	Cysts	Ovarian cysts
Tumors (craniopharyngiomas, gliomas, ependymomas, dysgerminomas)	Adrenal gland disease	Ovarian tumors (arrhenoblastoma, lipoid)
Space-occupying lesions (cysts)	Tumors	Congenital adrenal hyperplasia
Trauma (head)	Hyperplasia	Vaginal trauma, foreign body, or infection
Infection (abscess, encephalitis, meningitis, granulomas)	Primary hypothyroidism	
Irradiation	McCune-Albright syndrome	
Neurofibromatosis		
Prader-Willi syndrome		
Tuberous sclerosis		
Hydrocephalus		
Hypothalamic hamartomas		
McCune-Albright syndrome		

Precocious puberty

The appearance of secondary sex characteristics in girls under age 9 is considered precocious. When there is premature activation of cyclic hypothalamic and pituitary function with sex steroid secretion, follicular maturation, and ovulation, the diagnosis is central or true precocious puberty. Pseudoprecocious puberty is the presence of secondary sex characteristics in the absence of pituitary gonadotropin secretion, follicular maturation, and ovulation. In the isosexual form, the sex characteristics are consistent with the genetic sex. In the heterosexual form, the sex changes are consistent with the opposite genetic sex, virilizing in the girl. Incomplete precocious puberty is isolated, partial pubertal development, thelarche, pubarche, or menarche.

Even though the clinical signs are similar, it is important to distinguish the different types of precocious puberty (Table 39-2). Treatment,

causes, clinical course, and prognosis for all types are different.

EVALUATION. The history is extremely important. It should include questions about use or ingestion of exogenous steroids. These can be ingredients of medicinal preparations, creams, and cosmetics. Behavioral changes, particularly seizure activity, should be documented. Careful dating of pubertal events or lack thereof should be done: breast development, pubic hair growth, vaginal bleeding, and cyclicity. A family history for pubertal abnormalities, history of infections, and trauma also should be taken.

Careful physical and abdominopelvic examination should be performed. The skin should be examined for café-au-lait spots, hirsutism, and acne. Check carefully for cranial nerve deficits and skeletal deformity. Radiographic evaluation for bone age, and computed tomography or magnetic resonance imaging of the hypothalamic-pituitary and abdominopelvic regions, may be necessary.

Biochemical evaluation of thyroid, gonadotropin, and sex steroid hormones also may be useful.

MANAGEMENT. The aim of therapy for precocious puberty is to arrest and, if possible, regress the secondary sex characteristics and decrease growth velocity. In central precocious puberty, gonadotropin levels must be reduced and steroidogenesis inhibited. Agents used include medroxyprogesterone intramuscularly or orally, and GnRH analogues. When used continuously, a prepubertal state of endocrine function is achieved. When organic disease is the cause of precocious puberty, the underlying disorder is treated.

CRITICAL POINTS

- Puberty in females is characterized by specific developmental stages on the basis of somatic signs, degree of breast development, amount of pubic hair, and onset of menstruation.
- If a girl at 13 years of age is without evidence of secondary sex characteristics, or if the stages of puberty do not progress within 5 years, evaluation should be done and treatment given if indicated.
- Presumption of diagnosis for disordered sexual development can be obtained from findings in the history and physical examination.

Questions

1. An 8-year-old girl has a 6-month history of pubic hair growth. She has no history of vaginal bleeding or accelerated growth. Breast development is Tanner stage 1. Which of the following is the most likely diagnosis?
   A. Central precocious puberty
   B. Isosexual precocious puberty
   C. Heterosexual precocious puberty
   D. Incomplete precocious puberty
   E. Pseudoprecocious puberty
2. The primary endocrine event that precedes development of secondary sex characteristics in puberty is:
   A. Increase in concentration of portal GnRH
   B. Decrease in concentration of portal GnRH
   C. Increase in portal dopamine
   D. Increase in portal estrogen
   E. Decrease in portal androgen

3. Successful treatment of central precocious puberty is accomplished with agents whose mechanism of action is which of the following?
   A. Adrenal gland suppression
   B. Anterior pituitary suppression
   C. Thyroid gland suppression
   D. Anterior pituitary activation
   E. Adrenal gland activation
4. Which of the following is the most common cause of delayed puberty?
   A. Central nervous system disease
   B. Chronic illness
   C. Constitutional
   D. Adrenal hyperplasia
   E. Ovarian tumor

Answers

1. D
2. A
3. B
4. C

40

Amenorrhea

APGO LEARNING OBJECTIVE #40

P. Coney

The absence of normal menstrual bleeding may represent physical, endocrinologic, or psychologic problems. A systematic approach for the evaluation of this complaint will aid in the timely determination of its cause.

The student will demonstrate a knowledge of the following:

A. Definitions of primary amenorrhea, secondary amenorrhea, and oligomenorrhea
B. Causes of amenorrhea
C. Approach to evaluate a patient with amenorrhea
D. Treatment options

Amenorrhea is inappropriate absence of menstruation. Amenorrhea is appropriate during pregnancy and at menopause. It is a common symptom that often is not associated with major disease. It can, however, be caused by disorders of the hypothalamus, pituitary, adrenal cortex, ovary, or uterus, or by chronic illness (Table 40-1). Amenorrhea is classified into *primary* and *secondary* forms. Primary amenorrhea is failure of onset of menstruation by age 16. Secondary amenorrhea is cessation of menstruation after a period of normal, spontaneous, and regular menstruation, generally 3 months. The distinction between the two has merit because of the often significant organ dysfunction that can give rise to primary amenorrhea and the psychologic impact on the young woman that accompanies failure of menstruation. *Oligomenorrhea* is infrequent menstruation, more a prolongation of cycles (45 days or more), but with some degree of predictability and regularity.

Table 40-1. Causes of amenorrhea

	Primary amenorrhea	Secondary amenorrhea
Anatomic	Vaginal agenesis or Müllerian agenesis Imperforate hymen Atrophy or destruction (infection, irradiation, surgery)	Atrophy or destruction (infection, irradiation, surgery) Hypothalamus or pituitary isolated GnRH deficiency Tumor (adenoma, glioma, craniopharyngioma) Hyperprolactinemia Eating disorders Marked shifts in weight Stress Strenuous exercise Psychotropic medication Drug addiction Sheehan's syndrome
Adrenal cortex		Congenital adrenal hyperplasia Hormone-secreting tumor Addison's disease Cushing's syndrome
Ovary	Gonadal dysgenesis	Hormone-secreting tumor Halban's syndrome Polycystic ovarian disease Premature ovarian failure
Miscellaneous	Hypothyroidism	Hypothyroidism

GnRH, Gonadotropin-releasing hormone.

PRIMARY AMENORRHEA

Diagnostic considerations

An evaluation is warranted when menarche fails to occur by age 16 or when secondary sex characteristics fail to develop by age 13. Approximately 20% of adolescents who present with primary amenorrhea will have some variant of uterovaginal agenesis. The diagnoses to be considered include the Mayer-Rokitansky-Küster-Hauser syndrome, androgen insensitivity syndrome, müllerian dysgenesis in varying degrees, imperforate hymen, and transverse vaginal septum.

The *Mayer-Rokitansky-Küster-Hauser syndrome* is agenesis of the vagina and uterus. The external genitalia, fallopian tubes, and ovaries develop normally. This is the most common form of congenital absence of the vagina. Thirty percent of these patients will have an abnormality of the renal tract, either a single or solitary pelvic kidney; 10% to 12% will have skeletal, rib cage, and spinal deformities. In all patients with vaginal agenesis, there is less than a 10% chance that a uterus is present. If there is a uterus, it is often hypoplastic with cervical dysgenesis and requires removal. If the uterus is functional, the patient often will have a pelvic mass. The history reveals a period of cyclic, abdominal pain.

Androgen insensitivity results from a deficiency of the cytoplasmic androgen receptor. The deficiency can be complete or incomplete, and this will determine the clinical picture. The classic and complete form of androgen insensitivity is *testicular feminization.* Classically, the patient presents with primary amenorrhea. Examination reveals an absence of axillary and pubic hair. Breast development is complete. The external genitalia appear normal except that the vagina can be only a dimple or shortened, ending in a blind pouch. The gonads often can be palpated in the labia or found in the inguinal canal or abdominal cavity. These patients are psychologic and phenotypic females. The genotype is 46 XY male. This disorder is thought to be inherited by an X-linked recessive mode. Androgen levels are in the male range, but the individual is unable to respond to the hormone message because of the lack of receptor activity. Luteinizing hormone (LH) and follicle-stimulating hormone (FSH) levels are in the male range. The intraabdominal location of the gonads with a Y chromosome increases the propensity for malignancy in these patients. The longer the gonads are left in place, the greater the risk of malignancy. Consequently, gonadectomy is recommended.

Counseling is an important aspect of care in patients with uterovaginal agenesis. It should be done as soon as the diagnosis is certain, with appropriate steps taken to provide psychiatric care if needed. The lack of fertility potential for these patients is particularly traumatic. Vaginoplasty will allow satisfactory sexual function but not pregnancy.

Imperforate hymen and low, complete or suprahymenal septa will result in obstruction of blood flow. The ovaries, uterus, and cervix are normal; and menstruation occurs at the appropriate time. Blood is retained and—depending on the length of time the problem goes unrecognized—hematometra, hematosalpinx, and hematocolpos can occur (Figs. 40-1 and 40-2). The patient will report episodic but cyclic abdominopelvic pain. Examination of the vagina and rectum readily confirms the diagnosis. A simple cruciate incision will correct the defect of imperforate hymen. Vaginal septa require complete surgical removal. The incidence of endometriosis is high in women with these types of obstructive congenital defects.

Müllerian dysgenesis and anomalies can present in several forms: uterine hypoplasia, cervical agenesis, double uterus with rudimentary horn, or obstructed hemivagina. Laparoscopy, ultrasonography, and hysterosalpingography usually are needed to pinpoint the diagnosis.

Another 35% of patients with primary amenorrhea will have congenital gonadal failure as a result of *gonadal dysgenesis.* Gonadal dysgenesis is a chromosomal disorder in which gonadal differentiation fails. The gonads are represented by a streak of tissue. Gonadal dysgenesis is further classified into mixed and pure varieties. Mixed gonadal dysgenesis is streak gonads with dysgenetic testicular elements. Usually there is a streak on one side and a dysgenetic testis on the other side. The presentation spans a spectrum of external genital appearance of phenotypic female to phenotypic male. Pure gonadal dysgenesis is streak gonads with either a 46 XX or 46 XY genotype; it constitutes about 40% of cases seen. Other forms of gonadal dysgenesis include X chromosome monosomy (Turner's syndrome) and structural X chromosome abnormalities (isochromosome [i]Xq, del[Xp],del[Xq], translocations).

The most common (40%) karyotype associated with gonadal dysgenesis is X chromosome monosomy, or Turner's syndrome. Features of Turner's syndrome are numerous, and often referred to as "stigmata." The most common are short stature, webbed neck, cubitus valgus, shield chest, high-arched palate, and low-set ears. Not every stigma is present in every case. The only consistent features are short stature and primary amenorrhea with sexual infantilism. Other anomalies commonly observed in patients with Turner's syndrome include cardiac abnormalities, particularly coarctation of the aorta, renal anomalies, skeletal abnormalities, inflammatory

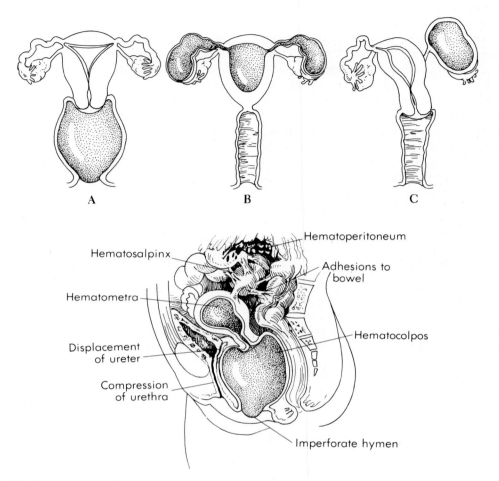

Fig. 40-1. A, Imperforate hymen; hematocolpos. **B,** Congenital atresia of cervix; hematometra; bilateral hematosalpinx. **C,** Uterus bicornis unicollis; lateral hematometra in blind, rudimentary form.

bowel disease, chronic otitis media, and lymphatic abnormalities.

Mosaicism (Table 40-2) is found in patients with gonadal dysgenesis. Mean adult height is normal or greater in this group. Somatic anomalies occur less frequently than in the X monosomy group. Some will undergo breast development and even menstruate.

Deletions of the long and short arm of the X chromosome usually result in short stature and some Turner's syndrome stigmata. Isochromo-

some for the X long arm is the most common of the structural abnormalities of X. These patients have streak gonads, short stature, and Turner's syndrome stigmata.

Patients with pure gonadal dysgenesis have streak gonads and primary amenorrhea. XX gonadal dysgenesis patients have normal stature, and stigmata of Turner's syndrome are absent. Patients with XY (Swyer syndrome) gonadal dysgenesis (like XX) have normal stature, streak gonads, and no Turner's syndrome stigmata. These

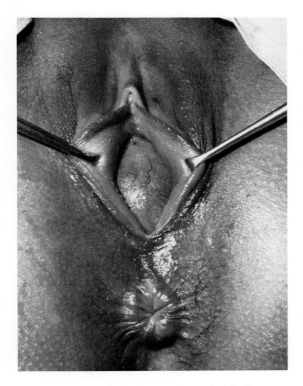

Fig. 40-2. Imperforate hymen distended by hemato-colpos.

patients are at risk to develop gonadoblastomas or dysgerminomas because of the Y chromosome. The risk, unlike testicular feminization, is high in the first and second decades of life. The streak gonads of these patients should be removed as soon as the diagnosis is made.

The diagnosis of gonadal dysgenesis is based initially on gonadotropin levels followed by chromosomal analysis (Table 40-2). Chromatin buccal smears are no longer used for diagnosis because patients with mosaicism and structural X abnormalities (20%) will be missed. In these patients, gonadal dysgenesis represents primary and complete ovarian failure. There is preservation of müllerian structures; thus the fallopian tubes and uterus are normal as well as the vagina.

Again, counseling and education of the patient about her diagnosis is crucial. More often than not, the patient desires induction of puberty to avoid problems of self-esteem and peer pressure. This benefit outweighs the risk of any potential adverse effect of low-dose estrogen and progesterone on growth potential. The issue of reproduction should be discussed. In these patients, unlike those with androgen insensitivity, pregnancy and childbirth can occur with donor oocytes and assisted reproduction techniques.

The remainder of patients with primary amenorrhea will have hypogonadotropic hypogonadism, chronic illness, and possibly pituitary neoplasms (Table 40-1). The most common cause of hypogonadotropic hypogonadism is isolated gonadotropin-releasing hormone (GnRH) deficiency, *Kallmann's syndrome.* It is autosomal dominant inherited. Anosmia or hyposmia and congenital deafness are associated with this disorder. There is decreased or absent secretion of GnRH by the hypothalamus. There is tremendous heterogeneity of gonadotropin deficiency in these patients, and the disorder is difficult to distinguish from physiologic delay in puberty. These patients do respond to GnRH therapy.

Prepubertal hypothyroidism will cause delay in puberty. A common cause of primary hypothyroidism is chronic autoimmune thyroiditis. Hypothyroidism can also have profound effects on growth. The effects on growth and sexual maturation are reversed with replacement therapy. Other causes of primary amenorrhea include infection and irradiation of the pelvis. Tuberculosis is a common cause of primary amenorrhea in underdeveloped countries.

SECONDARY AMENORRHEA

Diagnostic considerations

Secondary amenorrhea may affect a large number of women at some time during their reproductive years. It often takes 1 to 2 years for adolescents to establish a regular and cyclic pattern of menstruation after menarche. During this time, menstruation can be absent, infrequent, or too frequent. Secondary amenorrhea is gradual or

Table 40-2. Features of gonadal dysgenesis

Feature	X chromosome monosomy	Structural X abnormalities	Mixed gonadal dysgenesis	Pure gonadal dysgenesis
				Swyer
FSH, LH	Elevated	Elevated	Elevated	Elevated
Karyotype	XO	[i]Xq, del[Xp], del[Xq],etc., translocations	45 X/46 XY 45 X/46 XX/46 XY	46 XX 46 XY
Stature	Short	Short	Normal to tall	Normal to tall
Inheritance	Sporadic	Sporadic	Sporadic	AR X-linked
Secondary sex characteristics	None	None	Can be masculine	None
Stigmata*	Yes	Yes or no	None	None
Malignant degeneration of germ elements	No	No	Yes	Yes
Intelligence	Normal	Normal	Normal	Normal
Uterus and vagina	Yes	Yes	Yes	Yes
External genitalia	Phenotypic female	Phenotypic female	Phenotypic female to ambiguous	Phenotypic female

FSH, Follicle-stimulating hormone; LH, luteinizing hormone.
*Clinical features associated with Turner's syndrome.

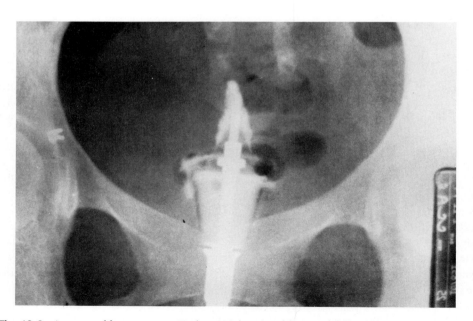

Fig. 40-3. Attempted hysterogram. Endometrial cavity obliterated following postpartum curettage. Cannula tip is at cervicouterine junction, and no endometrial cavity is visualized.

abrupt cessation of menses after menarche. Generally, if menses are absent for 3 months or more, investigation is in order. A rigid protocol is not necessary to evaluate these patients.

Pregnancy testing should be the first step in evaluating a patient with secondary amenorrhea. Detection of urinary β–human chorionic gonadotropin is quick, simple, and reliable. If negative, further evaluation should be determined by history and clinical findings. The most common uterine cause is *Asherman's syndrome.* This syndrome is due to partial or total endometrial obliteration by synechiae or adhesions. It always follows a surgical curettage for postpartum hemorrhage or abortion. The diagnosis is suspected with history, failure to sound the cervical os, and absence of bleeding following progesterone withdrawal. Hysterosalpingography and hysteroscopy confirm the diagnosis (Fig. 40-3). Multiple irregular filling defects are noted in a small-capacity uterus on radiography. Adhesions are visualized with hysteroscopy. Treatment is hysteroscopic lysis of adhesions followed by oral estrogen administration to regenerate the endometrium.

In the absence of pregnancy and uterine factors, the most common causes of secondary amenorrhea are hypogonadotropic hypogonadism and adrenal and ovarian dysfunction. Hypogonadotropic hypogonadism can result from pituitary and hypothalamic dysfunction. Pituitary tumors, most commonly adenoma and craniopharyngioma, can cause amenorrhea. Tumors, medications, and trauma also can cause hyperprolactinemia, which can lead to amenorrhea. Some uncommon causes of hyperprolactinemia include empty-sella syndrome and renal disease. Measurement of prolactin is simple and should always be done. Suspected tumor can be accurately diagnosed with computed tomography or magnetic resonance imaging of the pituitary. Failure of secretion of GnRH in the periodic, 60 to 90 minute pulses with appropriate amplitude can result from psychogenic stress, eating disorders, marked shifts in weight, or illicit and psychotropic drug

usage. The degree of disruption of GnRH secretion is reflected in the menstrual pattern and can range from oligoovulation to anovulation to amenorrhea.

Adrenal causes of amenorrhea result from hypersecretion of androgens as observed in congenital adrenal hyperplasia (CAH) and Cushing's syndrome. The excess androgens affect ovulation by initiating inappropriate feedback on the hypothalamus, thus affecting GnRH secretion and pituitary secretion of gonadotropins. In its classic form CAH is seen in the newborn and in infancy. In reproductive-age women, an attenuated form is seen. The patient may experience amenorrhea shortly after menarche, associated with acne, weight gain, and hirsutism. Measurement of the androgens testosterone, dehydroepiandrosterone sulfate, and 17-hydroxyprogesterone will confirm the diagnosis.

Ovarian causes of amenorrhea include persistent corpus luteum cysts (Halban's syndrome), premature ovarian failure, and polycystic ovarian disease. The period of amenorrhea with persistent

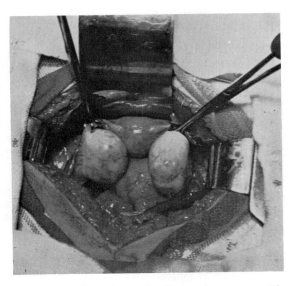

Fig. 40-4. Polycystic ovaries in young woman with polycystic ovarian syndrome.

corpus luteum cyst is short-term, followed by irregular bleeding. Premature ovarian failure can occur at any time up to age 35. The most common causes are idiopathic, followed by genetic and autoimmune disease. The patients are diagnosed by elevated gonadotropin levels. Polycystic ovarian disease is a condition of large, multicystic ovaries that generally are anovulatory (Fig. 40-4). The central cause of polycystic ovaries is hyperandrogenemia, the source of which can be adrenal and/or ovarian. There is associated hirsutism and obesity.

The hyperandrogenemia exerts inappropriate feedback on the hypothalamus and pituitary, resulting in large, polycystic, and anovulatory ovaries. Diagnosis is made by history, measurement of gonadotropins and androgens, pelvic examination, and sonography of the ovaries. Hyperthecosis is another ovarian condition in which the ovaries secrete large quantities of androgens. Signs of masculinization are more pronounced in hyperthecosis. Diagnosis can be confirmed only by microscopic analysis of ovarian tissue.

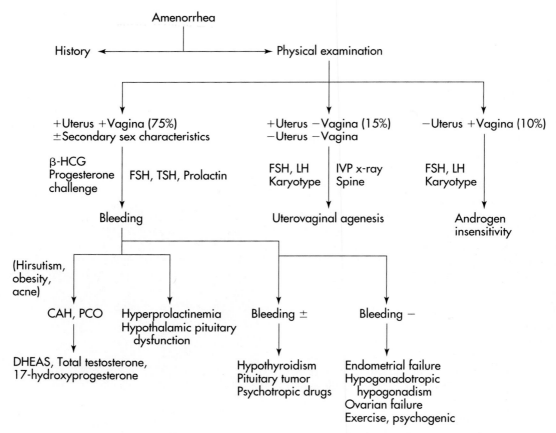

Fig. 40-5. Diagnostic considerations for amenorrhea. β-*HCG,* Beta–human chorionic gonadotropin; *FSH,* follicle-stimulating hormone; *TSH,* thyrotropin-stimulating hormone; *CAH,* congenital adrenal hyperplasia; *PCO,* polycystic ovaries; *DHEAS,* dehydroepiandrosterone sulfate; *IVP,* intravenous pyelogram; *LH,* luteinizing hormone.

MANAGEMENT

The history and physical examination are extremely important in the management of amenorrhea. The history should include chronology of pubertal events, menstrual patterns, life-style practices (eating habits, athletic training, aerobics), drug and medication usage, symptoms of chronic illness, congenital anomalies, central nervous system trauma, headaches, and visual disturbances. The physical examination should pay special attention to stature, weight, presence, pattern and quantity of body hair, breast development, lactation, pigmentation, and cushingoid features. Pelvic examination should be detailed, with documentation of presence and absence of vagina, uterus, and pelvic and adnexal masses.

Laboratory and radiologic investigation should be directed by pertinent history and clinical findings. An algorithm (Fig. 40-5) may be useful, but need not be followed rigidly, depending on the history and findings of the examination. Withdrawal bleeding after progesterone challenge implies estrogen levels sufficient to prime the endometrium and the presence of an unobstructed outflow tract. Minimal laboratory evaluation should include measurement of gonadotropins, FSH, LH, prolactin, and thyroid hormones.

Treatment depends on the diagnosis. Where possible, therapy specific for the disorder is recommended. Patients with primary amenorrhea are most likely to have the most serious causes. Psychologic sequelae can be severe. Counseling and education are important in comprehensive and successful management of these patients. In most patients with secondary amenorrhea, the cause will be chronic anovulation. Therapy is almost always directed to the patient's desires. If pregnancy is desired, ovulation induction is warranted. If cyclic menses are desired, regulation can be achieved with oral contraceptives and cyclic progesterone. All patients with amenorrhea and hypoestrogenism should receive hormone replacement therapy in the form of continuous estrogen and cyclic progesterone if a uterus is present. Surgical therapy for vaginoplasty is often delayed until late adolescence or when sexual function is desired.

CRITICAL POINTS

- Amenorrhea is either a state of chronic anovulation or the result of genetic and anatomic abnormalities.
- It is important to distinguish between dysfunctions involving the hypothalamic-pituitary-ovarian-uterine axis and dysfunctions outside this system.
- Treatment should be tailored to the patient's desires regarding development of secondary sex characteristics, pregnancy, and menstrual cycles.

Questions

1. The most common cause of secondary amenorrhea in the reproductive-age female is:
   A. Uterovaginal agenesis
   B. Chronic anovulation
   C. Androgen insensitivity
   D. Transverse septa
   E. Congenital adrenal hyperplasia
2. The most common cause of ovarian failure as a result of genetic aberration in primary amenorrhea is:
   A. Mixed gonadal dysgenesis
   B. Pure gonadal dysgenesis
   C. X monosomy
   D. Swyer syndrome
   E. Testicular feminization
3. A 32-year-old gravida II para II was delivered of a term, healthy infant. Placental separation was delayed, requiring manual removal. Hemorrhage followed, and dilatation and curettage was performed. She has failed to menstruate since the procedure. She fails to bleed after progesterone withdrawal. The diagnosis is best made by:
   A. Ultrasound of the uterus
   B. Hysteroscopy
   C. Dilatation and curettage
   D. Fluoroscopy of the uterus
   E. Laparoscopy
4. Which of the following genetic causes of primary amenorrhea is associated with the highest and earliest risk of malignant degeneration of the gonad?
   A. 46 XX
   B. 46 XY (Swyer syndrome)
   C. 46 XY (androgen insensitivity)
   D. 46 XX/45 X0
   E. 46,X,i(Xq)

Answers

1. B
2. C
3. B
4. B

Hirsutism and virilism

P. Coney

The signs and symptoms of androgen excess in a woman may cause anxiety and may represent serious underlying disease.

The student will demonstrate a knowledge of the following:

A. Normal variations in secondary sex characteristics
B. Definitions of hirsutism and virilism
C. Causes of hirsutism and virilism
D. Basic evaluation of the patient with hirsutism or virilism

Hirsutism is excessive hair growth in a woman in areas where hair does not normally grow. It is essentially a male-like pattern of hair growth on the face, trunk, limbs, extremities, lower abdomen, and pubis. Approximately 10% of U.S. women will manifest hirsutism, and about 90% of hirsute women have a disturbance in androgen production (increased) or androgen metabolism that can range from mild to severe. The cosmetic embarrassment of hirsutism is what motivates patients to seek evaluation and therapy. Although hirsutism can be caused by functional disorders, it is important to eliminate any serious underlying organic disease as the cause. In the absence of disturbances in androgen production and metabolism, hirsutism is commonly familial or racial and is best termed *hypertrichosis*. Hirsutism is rare in some races (Mongolians, Africans, and Eskimos), common in descendants of Mediterranean and Mexican origin, and uncommon in descendants of Nordic ancestry. This results from a genetic difference in the sensitivity of the epidermal (hair follicle) appendages. Hirsutism often is accompanied by acne and seborrhea.

Virilism is hirsutism plus signs of masculinization: clitoromegaly, temporal hair recession or male pattern balding, deep voice, male muscular pattern, excessive facial hair (moustache, beard), and excessive body hair (extremities, male escutcheon). Virilism is always associated with hyperandrogenemia.

PATHOGENESIS

Androgen metabolism

Testosterone is the major circulating androgen and is produced by the testicles and adrenal glands in men at a rate of 2.5 to 11 mg/day. In women, androgens normally are secreted by the ovary and adrenal cortex. The adrenal cortex contributes about 10% of the testosterone in men and 25% of that in women. The remainder is derived from the ovary (25%) and from peripheral conversion from androstenedione (50%). Testosterone is reduced in the target cell to its α-reduced derivative, dihydrotestosterone (DHT). The DHT is further reduced to α-androstane-3α 17β-diol (3α-diol) in the target tissue, particularly the hair follicle. The DHT and 3α-diol are more active than testosterone, and their levels reflect androgen action at the target tissues.

Approximately 99% of circulating testosterone is bound to serum proteins, primarily sex hormone binding globulin (SHBG) (78%), which is under the positive control of estrogen and the negative control of androgens. Consequently, 1% of circulating testosterone is free and represents the biologically important fraction of blood androgens; it correlates with clinical androgenicity. Dihydrotestosterone has 20 times the potency of testosterone, which is 5 to 10 times more potent than androstenedione. The weaker androgens, dehydroepiandrosterone (DHEA), its sulfate (DHEAS), and androstenedione, are mainly of adrenal origin. Both DHEA and DHEAS appear to stimulate activity of the sebaceous gland. More than 95% of DHEA is derived from the adrenal gland. Since the sulfate moiety, DHEAS, has a longer half life than DHEA, it is the assay of choice and represents the index of adrenal androgen secretion.

Increases in androgen secretion occur throughout the menstrual cycle in women, peaking at the preovulatory and luteal phases. Levels of 17-hydroxyprogesterone (17-OHP) rise during the

Table 41-1. Mean plasma concentrations of androgens in normal women

Steroid	Mean (range: ng/dl)
Androstenedione (A)	160 (90-290)
Testosterone	40 (30-80)
DHEAS	170 μg/dl
Androstenediol	80 (73-90)
17-OHP	
Early follicular	<50
Late follicular	<150
Midluteal	<200
Postmenopausal	<20

A, Circadian fluctuation; DHEAS, dehydroepiandrosterone sulfate; 17-OHP, 17-hydroxyprogesterone.

menstrual cycle and are most reflective of corpus luteum activity. In the follicular phase of the cycle, 17-OHP is derived from the conversion of 17α-hydroxypregnenolone, which is primarily from the adrenal gland.

Androgens play a critical role in steroid biosynthesis in women (Table 41-1). Estrogens are synthesized from either androstenedione or testosterone as immediate precursors. When the daily production rate of androgens increases by 1 mg in a woman, hirsutism usually is manifest. When testosterone levels increase elevenfold, signs of virilism will be present. Increased glandular secretion, extraglandular production, or peripheral biotransformation causes increased concentrations of androgens. Despite the increased production rates, SHBG is depressed, resulting in increased intrahepatic metabolic clearance rates. More circulating testosterone is derived (75%) from direct glandular secretion than from peripheral conversion in hirsute women. Over-

Table 41-2. Causes of hirsutism and virilism

	Functional	Neoplasms	Miscellaneous
Adrenal	Congenital adrenal hyper-plasia	Carcinoma Adenoma	
Ovarian	Polycystic ovarian disease Hyperthecosis Stromal hyperplasia	Arrhenoblastoma, luteoma, lipoid cell, hilus cell, Sertoli Leydig cell (all uncommon)	

Other	Acanthosis nigricans
	Insulin resistance
	Hyperprolactinemia
	Idiopathic hypothyroidism
	Acromegaly
	Cushing's disease
	Ectopic ACTH syndrome
			Drugs
			  Phenytoin
			  Minoxidil
			  Cyclosporine

ACTH, Adrenocorticotropic hormone.

whelmingly, androgen excess in women is derived from abnormal adrenal or ovarian function (Table 41-2).

Normally, hair growth increases physiologically in adolescence. Facial hair increases in postmenopausal women and generally disappears from other areas of the body. Abrupt or excessive hair growth is not a characteristic of women aged 20 to 40 years unless there is an underlying disturbance in androgen production or metabolism. Hirsutism also is observed in other endocrinologic disorders, such as hyperprolactinemia and acromegaly, caused by excesses of prolactin and growth hormone.

The ovary is the most common source of excess androgens in women, followed by the adrenal gland. The excess androgen level is often modest, and these patients are categorized as having polycystic ovarian disease disorder. Ovarian hyperandrogenism is perhaps an end result of a number of disease processes or pathogenic mechanisms. Second to functional excess secretion of androgens, unusual but important causes of aberrations in androgen synthesis and metabolism resulting in hirsutism include adrenal hyperplasia, insulin resistance, hyperprolactinemia, and hyperthecosis.

SIGNS AND SYMPTOMS

Patients present with excessive testosterone, polycystic ovaries, menstrual abnormalities, hirsutism, and sometimes virilism. Acanthosis nigricans is characterized by hyperkeratotic, hyperpigmented skin lesions located mostly in skin folds. The hyperandrogenism, insulin resistance, and acanthosis nigricans (HAIR-AN) syndrome describes this correlation with insulin resistance presumably caused by defects in insulin receptors or the presence of autoantibodies to the insulin receptor. There is evidence of glucose intolerance with subsequent risks of diabetes mellitus, atherosclerosis, and hypertension.

There is resistance of the target cell to insulin action, which coexists with the skin lesions (type A insulin resistance). Aspects of the disease that remain unknown are the cause of the receptor defect and the nature of the link to ovarian disease and the features observed.

Ovarian hyperthecosis was first described in 1943 and is characterized by the presence of islands of luteinized thecal cells in the ovarian stroma unassociated with follicles. It is distinguished from the polycystic ovarian disease syndrome by higher testosterone levels, normal follicle-stimulating hormone (FSH) and luteinizing hormone (LH) levels, and evidence of hyperinsulinism. Patients may be virilized. The cause is unknown. Patients with hyperthecosis do not have clinical features of acanthosis nigricans.

LABORATORY-DIAGNOSTIC TESTS

The first step in the evaluation is to obtain a careful history that includes the chronology of hair growth, whether the hair growth is abrupt in onset or long-standing, and whether there is a history of excessive hair growth in relatives. It is also important to eliminate drug intake as a source of excess androgen. Such drugs include testosterone and testosterone-related agents, progestational agents, glucocorticoids, minoxidil, diazoxide, and phenytoin (Table 41-2).

The next step is to perform a physical examination. This should include determination of the extent of hair growth and some clinical impression of the extent of androgen excess. The method for assessing hair growth developed by Ferriman and Gallwey is the standard for the assessment of hirsutism (Table 41-3). Signs of hyperkeratosis should be sought in areas of skin folds, the neck, and the axillae. Since all sites are not consistently involved in everyone, it is desirable to study a number of sites. Hair growth is scored according to the sum of the gradings on the body. This system records hair growth in "hormonal" sites. When this system is used, a score of 8 or greater is definitely abnormal. This provides a semiquantitative assessment for diagnosis and is helpful when following the effectiveness of drug therapy. Signs of virilism should be noted (clitoromegaly, deepening voice, hair loss, temporal recession of hairline) that suggest a tumor in the adrenal glands or ovary.

Positive correlations have been made between insulin and androgen levels. Hyperinsulinemia may cause hyperandrogenemia and vice versa. Consequently, in women with hyperandrogenemia, abnormalities in insulin action should be explored.

Late-onset congenital adrenal hyperplasia appears to affect 1% to 6% of hyperandrogenic women. Screening and diagnostic criteria are not well established or standardized. If hypertension is observed, specific measurements of deoxycortisol or derivatives are indicated. Basal follicular levels of 17-OHP can be predictive in 80% of hyperandrogenic patients with 21-hydroxylase deficiency. Levels above 150 ng/ml are highly predictive of an abnormal adrenal stimulation test result. The adrenal gland is stimulated with 1 mg of Cortrosyn intravenously, and 17-OHP is measured 30 minutes later.

Elevated levels of prolactin are correlated with elevated DHEAS levels. Treatment of the hyperprolactinemia results in a decrease in DHEAS. The incidence of elevated prolactin and DHEAS levels is reported to be as high as 30% in patients with hyperandrogenemia.

A significant number of patients will have abnormal levels of androgens arising from either the adrenal gland or the ovary. The diagnosis of hyperandrogenism, however, may prove complex at times; and certain parameters are more sensitive than others. No single test can predict all cases of altered androgen metabolism. An attempt should be made to identify the source of hyperandrogenism so that appropriate management techniques can be developed (Fig. 41-1). Which tests to obtain are determined by clinical findings. Most patients will be more concerned about the cosmetic alteration than the underlying cause for the alterations.

Table 41-3. Definition of hair gradings at each of 11 sites*

Site	Grade	Definition
1. Upper lip	1	Few hairs at outer margin
	2	Small moustache
	3	Large moustache
	4	Larger moustache
2. Chin	1	Few scattered hairs
	2	Small concentration of hairs
	3 and 4	Covered completely
3. Chest	1	Circumareolar hairs
	2	Midline hair also
	3	Fusion, ¾ covered
	4	Covered completely
4. Upper back	1	Few scattered hairs
	2	More but scattered
	3 and 4	Covered completely
5. Lower back	1	Sacral tuft of hair
	2	Some lateral extension
	3	¾ covered
	4	Covered completely
6. Upper abdomen	1	Few midline hairs
	2	More, midline
	3 and 4	Half and fully covered
7. Lower abdomen	1	Few midline hairs
	2	Midline streak
	3	Midline band
	4	Inverted V growth
8. Arm	1	Sparse growth; <¼
	2	More, incomplete
	3 and 4	Covered completely
9. Forearm	1, 2, 3, 4	Complete cover of dorsal surface; light and heavy growth
10. Thigh	1, 2, 3, 4	As for arm
11. Leg	1, 2, 3, 4	As for arm

Modified from Ferriman D, Gallwey JD: Clinical assessment of body hair growth in women, *J Clin Endocrinol Metab* 21: 1440, 1961.
*Grade 0 at all sites indicates absence of terminal hair.

Initial laboratory evaluation should include levels of total testosterone, DHEAS, and 17-OHP. If T and DHEAS levels are modestly elevated (less than 200 ng/dl [1.0 ng/ml] and less than 800 ng/dl, respectively), a tumor is unlikely. The 17-OHP level will be elevated (greater than 200 ng/dl, follicular phase of cycle) if there is nonclassic congenital adrenal hyperplasia, and adrenal stimulation should be performed to determine the severity and to confirm the diagnosis. Additional studies can be obtained to differentiate general adrenal or ovarian hyperfunction, such as that involving cortisol, FSH, or LH (Fig. 41-1). Hyperandrogenism of ovarian origin is often associated

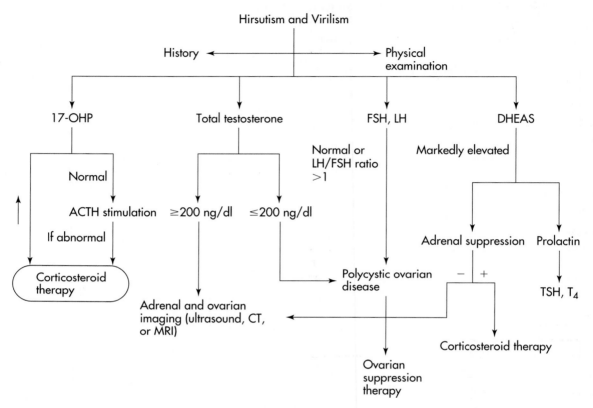

Fig. 41-1. Steps in evaluation of hirsutism and virilism. *17-OHP,* 17-Hydroxyprogesterone; *ACTH,* adrenocorticotropin hormone; *CT,* computed tomography; *MRI,* magnetic resonance imaging; *FSH,* follicle-stimulating hormone; *LH,* luteinizing hormone; *DHEAS,* dehydroepiandrosterone sulfate; *TSH,* thyrotropin-stimulating hormone; T_4, thyroxine.

Table 41-4. Treatment strategies for hirsutism

Agent	Target action
Antiandrogens	Hair follicle: competes and binds with androgen receptor
Oral contraceptives, progestins, corticosteroids, gonadotropin-releasing hormone agonists	Testosterone production: suppress pituitary, ovarian, or adrenal secretion of androgens
Depilatories, electrolysis	Hair follicle: removal of hair

with dysrhythmic secretion of LH and FSH, resulting in an increased ratio (greater than 1). In the presence of markedly elevated androgens and/or signs of virilism, ultrasonography and computed tomographic scans of the adrenal glands and ovaries are indicated. Further testing might include fasting blood glucose and insulin levels.

Hyperandrogenism can be demonstrated in approximately 50% of patients with hirsutism. When the total testosterone level is not elevated, the free testosterone level often is. The level of SHBG is decreased as a consequence of increased production rates of testosterone and increased metabolic clearance rates. Increased activity of 5α-reductase can be detected by measuring levels of 3α-diol. These tests need not be part of the screening process but will demonstrate abnormalities in androgen production, transport, and end-organ activity when other tests are negative. Although many cases of hyperandrogenemia have a mixed source, both adrenal and ovary, most cases are of ovarian origin. The diagnosis of idiopathic hirsutism is reserved for patients in whom elevated androgen production cannot be demonstrated.

MANAGEMENT

Identification of the source of excess androgen production certainly simplifies management.

Drug therapy is directed toward decreasing androgen secretion, increasing plasma androgen binding capacity, and decreasing peripheral metabolism at the hair follicles (Table 41-4). Women who do not have ovarian or adrenal neoplasms or other endocrinologic disorders (i.e., the majority of women) will require therapy to alleviate the cosmetic embarrassment of excess hair growth and acne, which affect the majority. Patients who desire fertility should have an infertility evaluation and appropriate therapy.

Oral contraceptives and corticosteroids are all effective in treating hirsutism resulting from functional causes. Antiandrogens include spironolactone and cimetidine; spironolactone is the more effective agent. Antiandrogens act by competing with testosterone for the androgen receptor at the target cell. Oral contraceptives act by inhibiting pituitary gonadotropins for ovarian suppression and by increasing SHBG levels to increase the binding of plasma testosterone. Corticosteroids inhibit the adrenal secretion of androgens. Gonadotropin-releasing hormone agonists inhibit ovarian activity by down-regulation of pituitary gonadotropin secretion.

Combination therapy is often desirable and more effective. Local measures (electrolysis, bleaching, depilatories) should be used after hormonal therapy has reduced the rate of hair growth, usually in 3 to 6 months. The use of lower maintenance doses of medication can then be evaluated.

CRITICAL POINTS

- Hirsutism can be a distressing symptom for which patients seek advice and therapy.
- The patient may be most concerned with the cosmetic change, but serious endocrine disease of diverse etiology can exist.
- When virilism is present, the physician must consider tumors of the adrenal or ovary; these necessitate prompt diagnostic work-up.
- Hirsutism is most frequently associated with chronic anovulation and an ovarian source of excess androgen.
- The goal of treatment is to target the pathogenic sites of hyperandrogenism.

Questions

1. In the absence of signs of virilism, which of the following sources is the most common in mild to moderate hirsutism?
   A. Thyroid
   B. Adrenal
   C. Ovary
   D. Pituitary
   E. Lung
2. The androgen responsible for intracellular processing of androgenic expression is:
   A. Androsterone
   B. Androstenedione
   C. Dihydrotestosterone
   D. Testosterone
   E. Dehydroepiandrosterone
3. Antiandrogens effectively diminish the rate of hair growth through which of the following actions?
   A. Ovarian suppression of androgen secretion
   B. Adrenal suppression of androstenedione secretion
   C. Pituitary suppression of gonadotropin secretion
   D. Competition for binding of the androgen receptor
   E. Competition for binding of the progesterone receptor
4. In patients with hirsutism caused by polycystic ovarian disease, the most effective therapeutic combination is:
   A. Electrolysis and progestins
   B. Corticosteroids and depilatories
   C. Antiandrogens and oral contraceptives
   D. Oral contraceptives and progestins
   E. Electrolysis and corticosteroids

Answers

1. C
2. C
3. D
4. C

Normal and abnormal uterine bleeding

APGO LEARNING OBJECTIVE #42

John H. Mattox

> *The occurrence of bleeding at times other than with expected menses is a common event. Accurate diagnosis of abnormal uterine bleeding is necessary for appropriate management.*

The student will demonstrate a knowledge of the following:

A. Endocrinology and physiology of the normal menstrual cycle
B. Definitions of abnormal uterine bleeding and dysfunctional uterine bleeding
C. Causes of abnormal uterine bleeding
D. Evaluation and diagnosis
E. Management

NORMAL UTERINE BLEEDING

Menstruation is the periodic discharge of blood and disintegrating endometrium after a normal ovulatory cycle. Normal menstrual cycles are composed of two phases, depending on the point of reference: a *follicular* (ovary) or *proliferative* (endometrium) *phase,* which begins with the first day of menstrual flow and culminates in ovulation, and a *luteal* (ovary) or *secretory* (endometrium) *phase,* which ends with the onset of menstruation.

Overview of the menstrual cycle

• Normal menstruation depends mainly on the functional integrity of three endocrine sites: the hypothalamus, the anterior pituitary gland, and the granulosa-theca cells of the ovary. They are often referred to as the *hypothalamic-pituitary-ovarian axis.* The process is precisely coordinated, but stimuli from the cerebral cortex mediated through the hypothalamus can influence menstrual function. Examples are cessation of periods and irregular menstruation associated with fear of pregnancy, emotional crises, exercise, or rapid weight change.

A neurochemical transmitter known as *gonadotropin-releasing hormone* (GnRH), which is produced in the hypothalamus, is secreted in a pulsatile fashion into the capillary plexus from the median eminence (*arcuate nucleus*) and is carried through the portal vessels to the anterior lobe of the pituitary gland, the *adenohypophysis*. The result of its neurohormonal action is the production and pulsatile release of the gonadotropins, follicle-stimulating hormone (FSH), and luteinizing hormone (LH) from the anterior pituitary cells. These hormones are transmitted to the ovary, where they stimulate follicle development and ovulation. The characteristic cyclic pattern of FSH and LH secretion during the normal menstrual cycle is governed predominantly by cyclic changes in ovarian estrogen and progesterone secretion (Fig. 42-1).

The principal modulator of hypothalamic-pituitary activity is estradiol (E_2), which along with inhibin has a strong negative feedback relationship with FSH. Ovarian steroidogenesis is at a minimum during the first few days of a menstrual cycle (Fig. 42-2). The initial growth of the follicle is stimulated by growth factor(s). Low concentration of E_2 triggers secretion of GnRH, with a consequent release of FSH and LH. These hormones stimulate follicle growth by increasing E_2 production. The increase in E_2, in conjunction with a rising concentration of FSH, increases the number of FSH receptors and results in granulosa cell proliferation. Intraovarian and circulating E_2 rises more steeply during the latter part of the follicular phase, reaching a maximum just before ovulation. The rising estrogen concentration inhibits FSH secretion; a dramatic increase then acts on the hypothalamic-pituitary system and stimulates LH and, to a lesser extent, FSH release (positive feedback). Estradiol triggers the midcycle surge of LH, which must be precisely timed to induce ovulation. The secretion of LH continues at a lower level. Its principal function is to support the growth of the corpus luteum. The secretion of progesterone increases rapidly after ovulation, and there is a concurrent but lesser increase in estrogen production. High levels of progesterone are maintained until about day 23 or 24 of the cycle, when the corpus luteum begins to regress if the ovum has not been fertilized. The withdrawal of hormonal support of E_2 and progesterone to the endometrium is followed by its disintegration and menstruation. The low concentration of ovarian hormones permits the cycle to be reinitiated.

HORMONES OF MENSTRUATION

THE HYPOTHALAMUS. *Gonadotropin-releasing hormone* is a decapeptide that is produced and secreted in the hypothalamus by special neuronal tissue in the region of the median eminence. It is secreted in a pulsatile fashion, becoming circhoral (about every 60 minutes) around the time of ovulation but less frequent during the luteal phase. The half-life of GnRH is several minutes. Although exact control mechanisms have not yet been fully elucidated, there are certain neuromodulators that are known to affect the secretory patterns of GnRH.

 Endogenous opioids suppress LH secretion, presumably because of the direct effect on the GnRH neurons. Catecholamines play a major role in the control of GnRH secretion. Dopamine generally inhibits LH secretion, whereas norepinephrine—via α-receptors—stimulates LH secretion. The exact interrelationship of the centrally located aminergic, opioidergic, and petidergic neurons and their control is unclear.

THE ANTERIOR PITUITARY. The exquisite timing of gonadotropin secretion is of paramount importance to a normal menstrual cycle. The *gonadotropes* are pituitary cells that are responsible for the synthesis, storage, and release of FSH and LH. Most of the pituitary gonadotropes produce both hormones. However, the cell population is heterogeneous, and some cells predominantly release one hormone or the other. The anterior pituitary is part of an endocrine unit called the *hypothalamic-hypophyseal complex,* which is subjected to numerous "messages" that result in secretion of gonadotropin hormones. The amplitude and the frequency of hormone release are determined by altering the sensitivity of the hypothalamic-hypophyseal complex by making it more sensitive or less sensitive to incoming stimuli. The negative feedback response of E_2 on

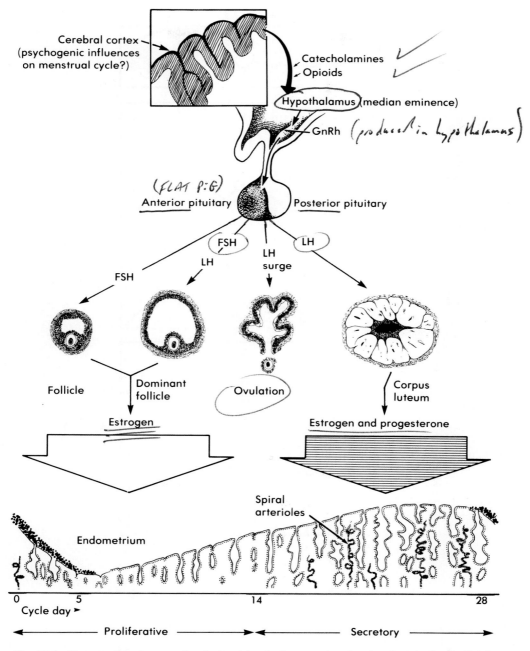

Fig. 42-1. Hormonal and anatomic relationships during menstrual cycle. There is also feedback from ovarian hormones estradiol and progesterone to pituitary and hypothalamus.

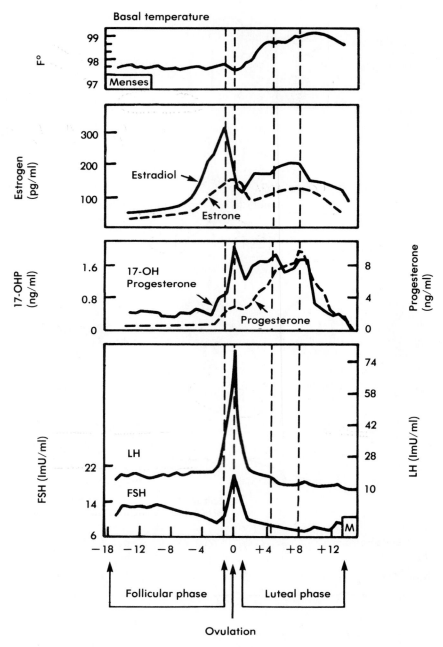

Fig. 42-2. Means of serum FSH, LH, estrone, E_2, progesterone, and 17-hydroxyprogesterone *(17-OHP)* during normal menstrual cycle.

Ant. Pituitary

FSH and LH secretion predominates during most of the menstrual cycle. At the time of ovulation, the positive feedback response (E_2 stimulating LH and FSH secretion) is the key event that ultimately results in ovum release. This stimulatory response is unique to the hypothalamic-pituitary-ovarian axis.

Follicle-stimulating hormone and LH are glycoproteins that have similar α-subunits and different β-subunits and a somewhat similar molecular weight, 33,000 and 28,000, respectively. The half-life of these hormones is contingent on the amount of sialic acid in the molecule and is approximately 4 hours for FSH and 1 hour for LH.

THE OVARY. Estradiol and estrone (E_1) are elaborated by the ovary, and there is an ongoing dynamic interconversion of E_1 to E_2 and vice versa. During the reproductive years the net result favors E_2 secretion; it has the greater biologic potency and plays a more significant role in modulating and effecting the normal menstrual cycle. *Estrogens* are 18-carbon compounds that circulate bound to sex steroid–binding globulin. They are inactivated at a relatively rapid rate by the liver and are excreted in conjugated forms as glucuronates and sulfates via the urine predominantly and by the feces to a lesser extent. Estrogens are secreted as a result of the interaction of the ovarian theca and granulosa cells; the latter aromatize the androgens, androstenedione, and testosterone to E_2. The positive-feedback response requires that E_2 concentration be at least 200 pg/ml for 48 hours to trigger the LH surge.

The biologically active estrogens have an important maturational effect on the genital tissues; they also bring about the feminine habitus and stimulate growth of the ductal system of the breasts. Estrogens also play a role in long-bone growth and epiphyseal closure. The absence of estrogen after menopause predisposes women to osteoporosis and genital and breast atrophy, as well as cardiovascular disease.

Knowledge of the role of intraovarian hormones in controlling events of the menstrual cycle continues to expand. Several protein hormones have been identified. Inhibin, a peptide synthesized by the granulosa cells, is secreted into the follicular fluid and ultimately can be measured in the peripheral circulation. Follicle-stimulating hormone stimulates the production of inhibin, which in turn feeds back to reduce FSH levels. The secretion of inhibin also appears to be under paracrine control. A major role of inhibin is postulated to be that of ensuring that a dominant follicle is formed by reducing the available FSH to the cohort of follicles in that cycle.

Progesterone is a 21-carbon compound that is secreted by the luteinized granulosa cells of the corpus luteum and is found predominantly in the latter half of the cycle. Serum concentration of at least 3 ng/ml is found in an ovulatory cycle. The plateau of its secretory pattern is reached about 7 days after ovulation and reaches levels of greater than 10 ng/ml. Just before ovulation, there is a small increase in progesterone that enhances pituitary sensitivity and is necessary for an optimal LH surge. For tissues to be sensitive to the action of progesterone, they must first have been exposed to estrogen, which induces progesterone receptors.

The primary reproductive function of progesterone is to induce secretory activity in the endometrial glands, thereby preparing the endometrium to receive a fertilized ovum. Its other biologic effects include desensitizing the myometrium to oxytocic activity, altering the histologic appearance of the vagina, inhibiting the secretory activity of the cervical glands, stimulating development of the alveolar system of the breasts, and, because of its thermogenic property, causing the increase in basal body temperature following ovulation.

STRUCTURAL CHANGES.

THE OVARY. At the time menstruation is taking place, recruitment of a number of primordial ovarian follicles, stimulated primarily by FSH, is initiated and continues for 5 days; LH stimulation also is required. The dominant follicle is then selected, although it cannot be grossly identified for 2 to 3 more days. The increased production of

E$_2$ resulting from the increase of both FSH receptors and granulosa cells is responsible for the process of selection. The ova that are excluded regress under the influence of intraovarian androgen production to under atresia. As the dominant follicle evolves, its lining granulosa cells become more cuboidal and multilayered, and a central cavity, the *antrum,* becomes filled with a transudate, *liquor folliculi.* The oocyte, surrounded by its own granulosa cells, awaits release. Follicle growth and volume can be determined by ultrasound. The mean diameter before rupture is 19.5 mm, with a range between 18 and 25 mm. However, there may be variation from cycle to cycle in the same woman. As a result of positive feedback, the LH surge, ovulation follows in 28 to 36 hours. The LH spike also facilitates the resumption of meiosis of the oocyte, the luteinization of the granulosa cells, and the synthesis of prostaglandins required for the rhexis of the follicular wall and extrusion of the oocyte.

The rupture of the follicle is attended by capillary bleeding. The blood replaces the spilled follicular fluid, and a corpus hemorrhagicum is formed. Through the continued action of LH, the granulosa cells become luteinized, and a corpus luteum results. The corpus luteum continues to grow and function, aided by the pulsatile secretion of LH, until about day 23 or 24 of the cycle, when it begins to regress. If the ovum, which was discharged at the time of ovulation, is fertilized, this regression does not take place; the corpus luteum continues to function as the corpus luteum of pregnancy, being maintained by the "LH effect" of human chorionic gonadotropin (HCG). In the absence of pregnancy the corpus luteum becomes progressively less sensitive to LH stimulation. As the corpus luteum regresses, it becomes hyalinized and has a characteristic convoluted structure that can been seen histologically, the *corpus albicans.*

THE UTERUS. The cervical mucosa, the myometrium, and the blood vessels of the uterus are all influenced by the cyclic changes in the levels of the hormones of ovary, but the endometrium shows the most dramatic effect of the influence of estrogen and progesterone. The changes are divided into three phases.

Proliferative phase. Immediately after menstruation the endometrium is thin, the epithelium is cuboidal, and the glands are straight and narrow. The stroma is compact. This stage lasts until the ninth day of the cycle. The continued stimulatory effect of estrogen brings about an increased thickness of the mucosa during the late proliferative phase. The epithelium becomes columnar. As the phase progresses, the stroma becomes looser, more abundant, and more vascular. This phase lasts until about day 14 of the menstrual cycle (Fig. 42-3).

Secretory phase. During the postovulatory premenstrual stage, the progesterone from the corpus luteum stimulates the proliferative endometrium to exhibit secretory activity. The mucosa becomes thick and velvety. The glands become widened and assume a corkscrew pattern, and the stroma becomes edematous and loose. Early in the secretory phase the nuclei appear to move away from the basement membrane, leaving a characteristic area of *subnuclear vacuolization.* Secretion within the lumen of the glands is maximal by day 25 (Fig. 42-4). Special staining techniques reveal that secretions are rich in glycogen.

By carefully examining the endometrial architecture with the use of well-defined criteria developed by Noyes, Hertig, and Rock, it is possible to monitor the progressive maturation. These dating criteria are used to assist with the diagnosis of the luteal phase defect.

If the ovum is fertilized during the cycle and the corpus luteum persists, this phase progresses to the formation of the *decidua,* the endometrium of pregnancy.

Menstrual (bleeding) phase. The decline in E$_2$ and progesterone initiates the process of menstruation. Following ovarian steroid decline, the height of the endometrium diminishes, with a subsequent reduction in blood flow and vascular stasis. The spiral arterioles play a special role in menstruation by undergoing rhythmic vasoconstriction and relaxation. Ischemia is followed by tissue breakdown with cellular migration from

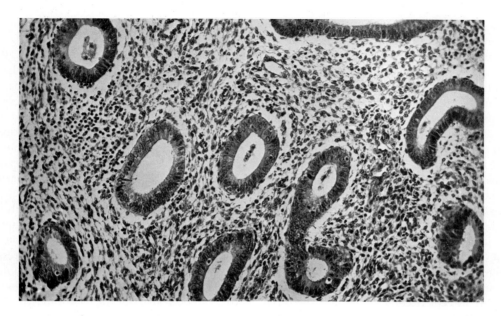

Fig. 42-3. Proliferative endometrium. Increase in number and size of glands and compact stroma. Although some glands are elongated, they are not tortuous. (×197.)

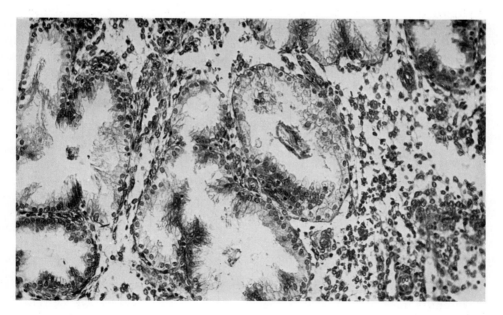

Fig. 42-4. Secretory endometrium. Stroma is scanty and loose, and dilated tortuous glands show intraluminal tufting and secretory activity. (×220.)

the vascular bed; subsequently, enzymatic destruction of the endometrium occurs. The separation along the endometrial surface occurs between the layers basalis and the spongiosa and compacta, the latter two being discarded. Concomitantly, small vessels are being "plugged" with thrombin, and the growth of a new endometrial surface is being stimulated by estrogen. The entire event is relatively precise and uniform, occurring over the entire endometrial surface.

Concentration of prostaglandin $F_{2\alpha}$ increases throughout the menstrual cycle; the highest amounts are measured at the time of menstrual flow. This potent vasoconstrictor probably plays a key role in initiating spiral arteriolar spasm.

THE CERVICAL MUCUS. In the immediate postmenstrual phase, the cervical mucus is scant, viscid, and opaque. During the follicular phase the columnar cells become taller, and the cervical glands begin to secrete increasing quantities of thin, clear, watery mucus that exhibits the physical properties of *spinnbarkeit* (the ability to form long, thin threads) and *arborization* (fern pattern formed). These changes are a result of estrogen stimulation. After ovulation, under the influence of increasing progesterone production, the cervical mucus gradually returns to the postmenstrual phase.

THE VAGINA. The adult vaginal epithelium is composed of three stratified layers of squamous cells that shed representative cells reflecting the state of hormonal stimulation (Fig. 42-5). In a hematoxylin and eosin–prepared vaginal smear, cells from these layers can be identified. The *superficial cell,* the most mature cell, is large and flattened and is usually an eosinophilic staining cell with a small dark nucleus. The layer below the superficial cells, the *intermediate cell* layer, is made up of medium-sized basophilic cells. The parabasal cell is a more immature cell and has a larger nucleus-to-cytoplasm ratio. These cells are not usually seen in the vaginal epithelial profile of a woman in the reproductive age range unless infection has aided in the denudation of the surface. The predominance of basal cells is seen in the absence of estrogen stimulation.

CLINICAL ASPECTS OF NORMAL MENSTRUATION. The length of the menstrual cycle and the duration and amount of flow vary considerably among normal women, but pronounced deviations from the accepted norms should suggest the possibility of functional or anatomic abnormality. Clinically significant characteristics of menses are the age at onset, periodicity, duration, amount of flow, character of flow, and associated symptoms.

AGE AT ONSET. The first period usually occurs at about 12 years of age, but menses may appear at age 9 or may be delayed until age 16 without being considered abnormal. Many factors are responsible for this wide variation. The most significant are race, heredity, general health, nutritional status, and body mass of the individual girl. Periods that start before the age of 9 years define *precocious puberty*. Menses delayed past the age of 16 years define *primary amenorrhea*.

Ranges between 25 and 34 days may be considered normal. The postovulatory phase is constant at 14 ± 2 days, whereas the preovulatory interval may be as short as 3 or 4 days or as long as 21 days. Cycles shorter than 3 weeks or longer than 5 weeks may indicate some disturbance of ovulation. Patients with short cycles are said to have *polymenorrhea*. If the cycle intervals are unusually long (45 to 60 days), the condition is designated as *oligomenorrhea*.

DURATION. The usual length of flow is 5 ± 2 days, but periods may last as long as 8 days or stop after 2 days and yet be within normal limits. Extremely short or scant periods are designated as *hypomenorrhea*, and unusually long or profuse menses are referred to as *hypermenorrhea*.

AMOUNT OF FLOW. The amount of blood lost at each period varies greatly. The average is about 40 ± 20 ml. A loss of more than 80 ml is considered abnormal but may not be reflective of an ovulatory disorder.

ASSOCIATED SYMPTOMS. A characteristic group of symptoms may appear several days be-

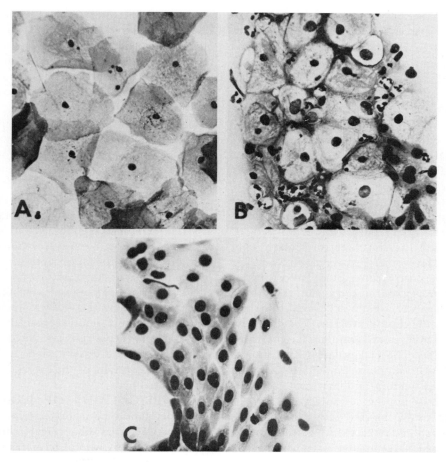

Fig. 42-5. A, Cornified (superficial cells, strong estrogen effect). **B,** Intermediate cells and parabasal cells, smaller rounder cells with large nuclei, associated with progesterone influence. **C,** Clump of basal cells, vaguely outlined with large nuclei, indicating lack of estrogen. *(From Riley G: Endocrinology of the climacteric,* Clin Obstet Gynecol *7:432, 1964.)*

fore the menstrual flow. These symptoms, which include weight gain, edema, breast fullness and discomfort, heaviness of the legs, and irritability or depression, are referred to as *molimina.* An exaggeration of these symptoms is usually termed *premenstrual syndrome.* Even though menstruation is a normal function and should be free from disturbing symptoms, most women experience some degree of discomfort during the period of bleeding. A sense of weight in the pelvic region, mild backache, and cramping are such common complaints that they may be considered normal accompaniments of menses. Pain that becomes more severe and rhythmic characterizes *dysmenorrhea.*

HYGIENE OF MENSTRUATION. Women need not restrict their usual daily routine in any way during the menstrual flow; this includes work, social, and athletic activities. Many couples abstain from sexual intercourse during menstruation because of aesthetic reasons. A daily bath or shower is not only permissible but most helpful in eliminating the characteristic odor that is sometimes present during the menstrual period.

Perineal pads have been used for many years to absorb the menstrual discharge, but currently the majority of women use intravaginal tampons. Their safety is not entirely absolute or universal. A relatively rare acute infection, *toxic shock syndrome* (TSS), although limited to neither women nor menses, occurs far more often in women specifically at the time of the menstrual period or shortly thereafter. Toxic shock syndrome has also been reported in women using a diaphragm and the contraceptive sponge. The risk is higher for women between ages 15 and 24 and during the postpartum period. The organism involved is *Staphylococcus aureus;* an endotoxin produced by this bacterium is believed to be responsible for the clinical problem. The illness is characterized by fever, rash, myalgia, fatigue, nausea, and emesis; TSS can progress into shock, coma, and death. Tampons should be changed at least every 4 to 6 hours, and intermittent rather than regular use appears advantageous; for example, tampons may be used during the day, but external pads should replace them at night. Also, external minipads can be used when the flow is scant.

ABNORMAL UTERINE BLEEDING

Excessive or inappropriately timed bleeding through the vagina is one of the most common symptoms encountered by the practitioner who provides health care for women. Abnormal bleeding can be the harbinger of serious pelvic disease or can denote a relatively minor problem. The source of the bleeding can be any of several sites along the menstrual outflow tract. Therefore a thorough and systematic examination is required in every patient who has this complaint. Blood loss of more than 80 ml during a period is called *hypermenorrhea,* whereas a condition marked by

too-frequent bleeding episodes (cycles less than 21 days) is *polymenorrhea.* Abnormal uterine bleeding between periods is *metrorrhagia.* Another common term for excessive uterine bleeding is *menorrhagia.* These descriptive terms characterize the patient's symptoms and should not be used as the diagnosis.

Etiologic factors

Most abnormal uterine bleeding is caused by a complication of pregnancy, a tumor, or hormonal dysfunction. The last term is used to characterize a disorder of the hypothalamic-pituitary-ovarian axis that acts on the endometrium to produce abnormal bleeding. Women receiving exogenous hormone therapy for contraception, for estrogen-progestin replacement, or as treatment for certain endocrine disorders may experience abnormal endometrial shedding as a bothersome side effect. Less commonly, a serious constitutional illness such as chronic hepatitis is associated with abnormal bleeding. The classification in Table 42-1 provides an overview of the causes of abnormal uterine bleeding.

COMPLICATIONS OF PREGNANCY. Pregnancy should be suspected when women of reproductive age have abnormal bleeding. Threatened, complete, or incomplete abortions are by far the most common complications of pregnancy associated with bleeding. Other less common causes are ectopic pregnancy and gestational trophoblastic disease. All of these topics are discussed in other chapters.

ORGANIC LESIONS. Uterine leiomyomas, particularly those of the submucous type, are the genital tract lesions that most often cause abnormal bleeding in women who are not pregnant. Other entities include carcinoma of the vagina, cervix, uterus, and ovaries; adenomyosis; endometriosis; and chronic salpingo-oophoritis with extensive ovarian destruction. These are discussed in other chapters.

Endometrial polyps may cause intermenstrual staining and postmenopausal bleeding, as well as menorrhagia and hypermenorrhea. Because pol-

> ### Table 42-1. Causes of abnormal uterine bleeding
>
> I. Complications of pregnancy
> II. Organic lesions
>   A. Endocervical or endometrial polyp
>   B. Cervical malignancy
>   C. Benign leiomyoma or malignant uterine tumors
>   D. Chronic endometritis
>   E. Adenomyosis
>   F. Endometriosis
>   G. Salpingo-oophoritis
>   H. Ovarian tumors
>   1. Nonneoplastic cysts
>   a. Follicular
>   b. Corpus luteal
>   2. Functioning stromal tumors (granulosa-theca cell type)
> III. Trauma (intrauterine device)
> IV. Hormonal disorders
>   A. Menstrual cycle
>   1. Anovulatory
>   2. Ovulatory
>   B. Exogenous
>   1. Hormone replacement therapy
>   2. Contraceptive therapy
> V. Constitutional diseases
>   A. Disorders of coagulation
>   B. Liver disease
>   C. Leukemia
>   D. Anticoagulant therapy
>   E. Thyroid disorders
>   F. Adrenal disorders

yps generally do not cause an appreciable enlargement of the uterus, they are frequently overlooked. Endocervical polyps protruding from the os may cause spotting following coitus.

DYSFUNCTIONAL UTERINE BLEEDING

DEFINITION. Dysfunctional uterine bleeding is abnormal endometrial bleeding caused by an endocrine dysfunction related to the circulating levels of the ovarian steroid hormones, estrogen and progesterone. The clinical manifestation is bleeding abnormal in amount, duration, or timing in a woman of reproductive age. When this diagnosis is given, it is assumed that the physician has ruled out organic causes of abnormal uterine bleeding.

INCIDENCE. Dysfunctional uterine bleeding may occur at any age between menarche and menopause. It is encountered most frequently at the two extremes of menstrual life, when disturbances of ovarian function are most common. More than 50% of dysfunctional bleeding occurs in premenopausal women 40 to 50 years of age, about 20% occurs during adolescence, and the remaining 30% is found at other times during the reproductive period. About 85% of cases are associated with *anovulation*.

PATHOPHYSIOLOGY. Dysfunctional uterine bleeding reflects a disturbance in the critical sequential hypothalamic-pituitary-ovarian interaction essential for ovulation, normal corpus luteum function, and normal endometrial growth and development. Bleeding associated with anovulation is caused by unopposed estrogen effects on the endometrium that result in "breakthrough bleeding" or by relative declines in circulating estrogens, causing "estrogen withdrawal bleeding."

If there is a deficiency of progesterone following ovulation, there may be abnormal bleeding, a *luteal phase defect*. If the corpus luteum fails to regress appropriately and progesterone continues to be secreted, progesterone breakthrough bleeding occurs. Somewhat related is the chronic administration of a long-acting progestin, medroxyprogesterone acetate. Abnormal endometrial bleeding occurs in the absence of sufficient estrogen to maintain a structurally sound endometrium. An atrophic endometrium is formed that is subject to breakdown, resulting in bleeding. Ovarian dysfunction may be caused by a primary defect or pathologic lesion within the ovary itself, or it may be a result of malfunction of other endocrine glands, notably the hypothalamus, pituitary, and thyroid. Anovulatory cycles tend to be self-perpetuating. When the ovary is unresponsive, as is the case in the aging gland of the perimenopausal woman, follicles fail to develop and ovulate, despite increased gonadotropin stimulation. Conversely, if the ovaries are healthy and responsive, the defect in ovulation may be a result of inadequate gonadotropin secretion secondary to hypothalamic-pituitary dysfunction. In either case the result is the same—absence of progesterone secretion. The granulosa-theca cell complex continues to secrete variable quantities of estrogen. This continued secretion causes a relative excess of estrogen that results in bleeding from the endometrium.

PATHOLOGIC FINDINGS OF THE ENDOMETRIUM. Dysfunctional bleeding is often associated with hyperplastic endometrium, a result of long-standing, unopposed estrogen stimulation. It also may occur with normal-appearing proliferative endometrium.

Hyperplastic endometrium with dysfunctional bleeding characteristically is thickened and may be polypoid, but in some cases it may appear to be normal. Microscopically, the typical picture is that of benign cystic (Swiss cheese) hyperplasia (Fig. 42-6). There is great disparity in the size and shape of the glands; the epithelium is cuboidal or columnar with deeply stained nuclei, and usually there is no evidence of secretion. In a small percentage of patients an adenomatous pattern is seen (Fig. 42-7).

Rarely, dysfunctional bleeding occurs with "mixed" endometrium, showing estrogen and progestational changes. In these instances the cycle is regular; but the bleeding period is prolonged, and the flow is irregular. This is called *irregular shedding*, a term that denotes asynchronous prolongation of shrinking, shedding, and involution of the endometrium rather than the rapid disintegrative process during the normal cycle.

CONSTITUTIONAL DISEASES. Although constitutional causes are uncommon, they must be considered, particularly in a woman with continued, recurrent episodes of abnormal uterine bleeding. Constitutional diseases most likely to cause uterine bleeding—such as thrombocytopenia, factor VIII deficiency, and leukemia—

Table 42-2. Diagnosis of abnormal uterine bleeding

Problem-oriented history
General physical and pelvic examination
Hemoglobin
Serum HCG
Assessment of the endometrium
Other hormone studies as indicated

HCG, Human chorionic gonadotropin.

---

interfere with the blood-clotting mechanism. Hypothyroidism has been shown to induce a secondary factor VIII deficiency, which may be responsible for the bleeding problem.

Management

An accurate diagnosis must be made before one can treat abnormal bleeding effectively. This requires that the physician be thoroughly aware of what constitutes normal bleeding and acceptable variations from the norm. The ultimate goal is to determine the cause of all cases of prolonged, excessive, or irregular flow. A general approach that can be applied to the assessment of most women with abnormal bleeding is found in Table 42-2. When this outline is followed, several factors such as the age of the patient, the chronicity or recurrence of the problem, and the patient's risk of genital tract malignancy must be considered. Also, some specialized studies such as hysteroscopy or hysterosalpingography may be helpful in diagnosing certain problems that might otherwise have been overlooked.

ADOLESCENCE

DIAGNOSIS. In girls, abnormal bleeding is almost always caused by a disturbance of ovarian function that results in anovulation. It occurs because of immaturity of the hypothalamic-pituitary axis with a lack of appropriate ovarian

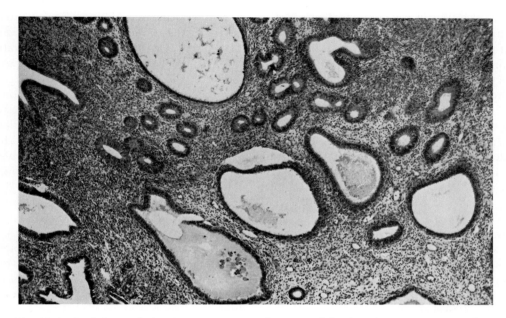

Fig. 42-6. Cystic hyperplasia. Note nonsecretory character of glands and great variation in their size, resembling holes in Swiss cheese. (×60.)

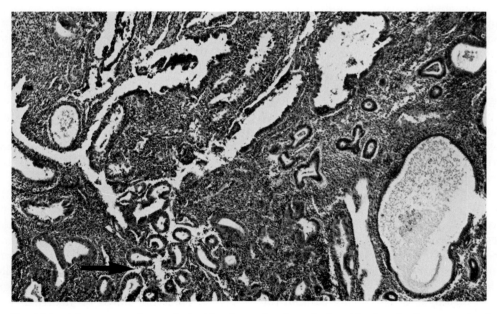

Fig. 42-7. Adenomatous hyperplasia. Glands are closely packed and back-to-back as a result of extraluminal budding. (×60.)

stimulation and positive estradiol feedback. However, clinical observation suggests that fewer than 20% of postpubertal females remain anovulatory for more than 5 years after menarche.

The possibility of pregnancy, blood dyscrasia, or malignancy must be kept in mind. Adenocarcinoma of the vagina or cervix has been described in young women who were exposed to diethylstilbestrol in utero. If an acute hemorrhage occurs in the adolescent, particularly with the first menstrual flow, a blood dyscrasia or more serious illness should be suspected. Usually, a careful history and pelvic exam will rule out the more serious conditions.

Classens and Cowell found that 28% of 79 adolescents hospitalized at the Toronto Hospital for Sick Children from 1971 through 1980 had an underlying coagulation disorder; 10% had other pathologic conditions.

In the adolescent, a gentle rectal examination may suffice to evaluate the pelvic structures. The use of pelvic sonography also can be considered. If the uterus and adnexa cannot be assessed readily, the physician should consider examining the patient under general anesthesia.

When ordering a complete blood count, interpretation of the red blood cell indexes should not be overlooked. A serum ferritin level may be helpful in diagnosing iron deficiency anemia. If a clotting disorder is seriously considered, a platelet count, partial thromboplastin time, prothrombin time, and bleeding time will assist in making the diagnosis.

As the risk of malignancy is remote in the adolescent, endometrial curettage is rarely necessary. It may be required and can be useful in temporarily controlling acute hemorrhage in selected cases.

THERAPY. Because most dysfunctional uterine bleeding in this age group occurs because of abnormal hormonal stimulation of the endometrium, it usually can be effectively controlled by endocrine therapy. The underlying issue in the anovulatory patient is unopposed estrogen. This effect on the endometrium can be combated by a combined progestin-estrogen contraceptive agent or cyclic progestin therapy. Oral administration of one of the progestin-dominant oral contraceptive steroids for 3 to 6 months usually will regularize uterine bleeding. Periodic administration of a progesterone such as oral medroxyprogesterone acetate, 5 mg daily for 14 days/month, will eliminate the endometrial hyperplasia caused by unopposed estrogen stimulation and will regulate uterine bleeding; *this is not an effective contraceptive agent.*

On occasion it will be necessary to control an acute episode of bleeding; conjugated estrogens administered intravenously, 25 mg every 4 hours for 24 hours, or a progestin-dominant oral contraceptive steroid, one tablet every 6 hours for 3 to 4 days, usually will control the acute bleeding. After the acute episode has been controlled, combined estrogen-progestin oral contraceptives should be continued cyclically for 3 to 6 months. Progesterone therapy alone, orally or intramuscularly, is not optimal therapy for controlling acute bleeding.

Bed rest, increasing oral fluid intake if a curettage is not contemplated, and oral iron replacement therapy are additional measures that should be instituted. In adolescents who have a particularly heavy flow, it is prudent to continue iron therapy. If significant blood volume depletion occurs as a result of the heavy bleeding that cannot be controlled by hormone therapy, and if the patient is developing volume replacement and shock, dilatation and curettage should be considered.

CHILDBEARING PERIOD

DIAGNOSIS. In reproductive-age women complications of pregnancy, pelvic infections, endometriosis, leiomyomas, and neoplasia are more likely causes of irregular bleeding. Particularly appropriate questions to be asked are as follows: Is there intermenstrual bleeding or staining? (Suspect endometrial polyp or malignancy.) Does bleeding occur after coitus? (Suspect cervical neo-

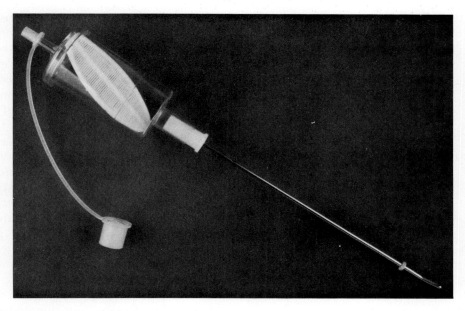

Fig. 42-8. Endometrial biopsy suction curet. Several types are available. Curet is attached to pump, producing negative suction. Uterine cavity depth is determined (curet is calibrated in centimeters). Sample obtained is collected in tissue trap. Preprocedure tranquilizer or paracervical block can reduce discomfort and should be used as necessary.

plasia.) Have there been any recent periods of amenorrhea? (Suspect pregnancy or oligoovulation.) Is the patient taking any estrogen hormones? (Suspect endometrial hyperplasia.)

Women in this age range are less likely to have an unrecognized coagulopathy than are adolescents. However, hypothyroidism is more likely, and measurement of the serum thyroid-stimulating hormone level may be helpful. Also, for any woman with a disorder of ovulation, a serum prolactin test should be ordered. Because uterine malignancy is uncommon in women under 30, an endometrial sampling is not required routinely. If the physician has any reason to be suspicious of malignancy or a precursor, an in-office or outpatient endometrial sampling using an aspiration curet usually will be sufficient (Fig. 42-8). In dealing with recalcitrant or recurrent dysfunctional bleeding, a hysterogram can be a valuable aid. Endometrial polyps and submucous myomas can

be diagnosed by this procedure (Figs. 42-9 and 42-10). Hysteroscopy often can provide additional diagnostic information. Its advantages include allowing one to perform a directed biopsy, to identify and remove endometrial polyps, and to perform lysis of intrauterine adhesions. Uterine curettage generally should be viewed as a diagnostic, not a therapeutic, procedure; it does not in itself correct the factors responsible for anovulation. Curettage is best performed premenstrually or at the time of bleeding if it is acyclic; this will indicate whether or not there is a progesterone effect.

THERAPY. In the patient with dysfunctional bleeding, if no contraindications exist, cyclic hormone therapy with a combination estrogen-progestin medication may be tried for 3 to 6 months. In the patient who has a long-standing history of oligoovulation or anovulation, cyclic progesterone therapy—medroxyprogesterone, 5

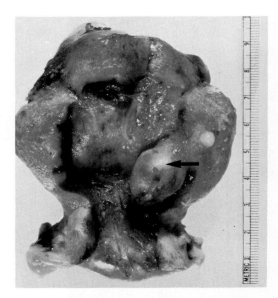

Fig. 42-9. Pedunculated submucous myoma. Uterus is normal size. Diagnosis can be made by hysterogram. (See Fig. 42-10.)

mg, or norethindrone acetate, 5 mg, for 14 days each month—should eliminate estrogen-induced endometrial hyperplasia and should produce regular withdrawal bleeding episodes. Medroxyprogesterone acetate also has a more favorable effect on serum lipids than do the 19 nonsteroids. It is seldom necessary to remove the uterus because of dysfunctional bleeding. However, hysterectomy may be indicated if the bleeding cannot be controlled by hormone therapy or if there is a contraindication to such therapy. Some patients are unable to tolerate endocrine treatment because of side effects related to the medication; other women prefer hysterectomy to many years of hormonal therapy.

Nonsteroidal antiinflammatory drugs have been shown to be effective in reducing uterine menstrual flow in women who have regular, ovulatory, but excessive menses. It is ineffective in controlling anovulatory bleeding. An oral iron preparation should be administered if the patient gives a history of heavy flow; her iron stores may be depleted, but her hemoglobin may not yet have decreased enough to permit a diagnosis of anemia.

Greenberg noted that menorrhagia may be accompanied by depression. He diagnosed mild-to-moderate depression in 31 of 50 women being considered for hysterectomy because of excessive uterine flow.

The severity of blood loss with excessive but regular uterine bleeding correlates poorly with the patient's history of how many tampons or maxipads are required to contain the flow. Chimbira, Anderson, and Turnbull also found that endometrial surface area did not prognosticate the severity of flow: the larger uterine cavity, 46 cm^2, produced a mean loss of 85 ml; however, the largest mean loss, 525 ml, was found with a uterine surface area of 26 cm^2.

Endometrial ablation with laser or a resectoscope has been used to reduce uterine bleeding in the absence of uterine pathology.

PERIMENOPAUSAL PERIOD. The assessment of women with abnormal bleeding during the climacteric (perimenopausal period) is similar to that of women in the childbearing years. However, sampling the endometrium should be part of the routine evaluation in this group. If the bleeding cannot be controlled easily with cyclic progestin therapy or if the patient cannot tolerate the medication, hysterectomy should be considered. The risks and benefits of estrogen replacement therapy in women over 40 must be considered when discussing any surgical treatment with the patient.

The patient with postmenopausal bleeding should be considered to have precancerous or malignant disease until proved otherwise. However, such benign lesions as atrophic endometritis and cervical polyps are more frequent causes of postmenopausal bleeding. Uterine curettage is essential in the study of patients in this age group. Although endometrial hyperplasia may be the result of unopposed endogenous estrogen production, particularly in an obese woman be-

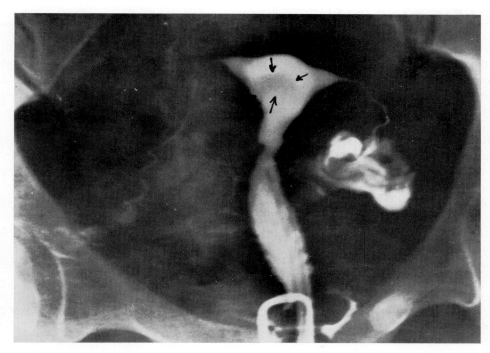

Fig. 42-10. Hysterogram showing submucous myoma. Uterine cavity is normal but has filling defect. Two previous curettages failed to disclose tumor.

cause of the conversion of androstenedione to estrone, the patient should still be thoroughly questioned to determine whether she is taking estrogen. Digoxin also has been reported as having estrogenic activity and has been associated with endometrial hyperplasia. The rare possibility of an ovarian estrogen-producing tumor also must be considered. It is particularly important in this age group for the physician to search for an explanation of why there is excessive estrogen production at a time when it should be waning.

If anemia is diagnosed, other sources of blood loss such as colon cancer should be considered, and appropriate screening advised. Hypothyroidism is more common in this age group, and the evaluation of thyroid function should be considered a routine measure every 5 years.

THERAPY. The treatment of irregular bleeding in postmenopausal women consists mainly of treating pathologic conditions of the uterus and ovaries. Endocrine therapy is less likely to be appropriate; however, cyclic progestin therapy (medroxyprogesterone, 5 mg daily for 14 days/ month) may be tried after malignancy has been excluded.

Progesterone prevents the replenishment of estrogen receptors in the endometrial cells and thereby reduces the growth effect of estrogen. It also facilitates the intracellular conversion of estradiol to estrone, a weaker estrogen. This cellular effect is related more to the length of time progesterone is administered.

If there are no medical contraindications, birth control pills can be used in nonsmokers under the age of 50.

CRITICAL POINTS

- For a normal menstrual cycle to occur, the pulsatile and highly regulated secretion of GnRH is required. The coordination of this secretion is impacted by the hormonal messages from the brain, neurotransmitters, and neuromodulators, as well as the feedback from the other parts of the axis, the anterior pituitary (FSH and LH), and the ovary (E_2 and progesterone).
- Although during most of a normal menstrual cycle the negative feedback (predominantly from the ovary) coordinates the cycle, it is the positive feedback from E_2 that is responsible for the LH surge; this event is the unique hallmark of the hypothalmic-pituitary-ovarian axis.
- After pelvic and systemic disease have been excluded, the major cause of dysfunctional uterine bleeding in adolescent and perimenopausal patients is a disorder of ovulation.
- In women with excessive uterine flow (menorrhagia) the standard evaluation is a serum HCG, hemoglobin, endometrial sampling, and possibly hysteroscopy or hysterography.
- In women with excessive uterine flow, even when associated with small leiomyomas, bleeding can be reduced significantly with the use of nonsteroidal antiinflammatory medications.
- Dilatation and curettage can be used to control hemorrhage, but this procedure does *not* treat the underlying disorder.
- In patients with oligoovulatory or anovulatory bleeding, cyclic progestin therapy is effective; oral contraceptive steroids can also be used in reproductive-age women who need a method of contraception.
- Hysterectomy is used only after all conservative measures have been tried without success.

Questions

1. For a normal menstrual cycle to occur, there must be:
   A. Pulsatile secretion into the portal vessels
   B. The stimulation of the granulosa cells by FSH enhanced by E_2
   C. The triggering of the LH surge by E_2, which induces the event of ovulation
   D. The secretion of progesterone after ovulation, which results in the secretory changes in the endometrium
   E. All of the above

2. In an adolescent who is brought to the emergency room with acute uterine bleeding, anemia, and hypovolemic shock, the practitioner should be very concerned about:
   A. Blood dyscrasia
   B. Leiomyomas
   C. Cervical polyp
   D. Hypothyroidism
   E. An ovarian malignancy

3. A woman in the reproductive age range has a 3-month history of irregular uterine bleeding. All the tests listed are appropriate to order initially *except*:
   A. Hemoglobin
   B. Serum HCG

C. Liver function studies

D. Endometrial biopsy

E. Antinuclear antibodies

4. In treating a 32-year-old patient with anovulatory uterine bleeding, the following treatment would *not* be indicated:

A. Cyclic progestin therapy

B. Birth control pills

C. Nonsteroidal antiinflammatories

D. Conjugated estrogens and progesterone

E. Clomiphene

Answers

1. E
2. A
3. C
4. D

Dysmenorrhea

APGO LEARNING OBJECTIVE #43

P. Coney

> *Dysmenorrhea is often the impetus for women to seek health care. Effective treatment is available and based on accurate diagnosis.*

The student will be able to do the following:
A. Define *primary* and *secondary* dysmenorrhea
B. Understand the causes of dysmenorrhea
C. Outline management options for dysmenorrhea

Dysmenorrhea is painful menstruation and is the most common of all gynecologic symptoms. It often is accompanied by a constellation of symptoms that can include—in addition to crampy, pelvic pain—nausea, vomiting, diarrhea, and constipation often severe enough to necessitate confinement to bed. The symptoms characteristically begin and end with the menses. Dysmenorrhea affects some 70% of cycling women; and, in 10% to 20%, the symptoms are severe and disabling. It may be preceded by weight gain, breast pain and fullness, irritability, depression, headache, fatigue and mood swings—symptoms most commonly associated with the premenstrual syndrome.

The first step in evaluation of the patient with dysmenorrhea is a detailed history, followed by pelvic and rectovaginal examinations. The pain is crampy, midline, and pelvic; it radiates to the back and lower extremities. It is most severe the first two days of menstruation. In rare cases, syncope and collapse may occur. It is important to listen to the patient tell about the nature of her pain, associated systemic symptoms, and the degree of disability. One must take her seriously.

PRIMARY DYSMENORRHEA

Primary dysmenorrhea is a diagnosis of exclusion in any pelvic pathology. The severity of primary dysmenorrhea should never be underestimated. It can be incapacitating. The onset occurs relatively early after the onset of regular, cyclic menses. A family history in patients' mothers is common. It is generally observed that primary dysmenorrhea affects women who are cycling and presumably ovulatory.

The association between dysmenorrhea and prostaglandins is well established. Although ubiquitous, activity of the microsomal enzyme, prostaglandin synthetase, is very high in the uterus. Prostaglandin levels increase in the uterine endometrium sixfold in the late luteal phase of the menstrual cycle. Prostaglandin levels are higher in women with dysmenorrhea than in asymptomatic women. Levels increase in response to declining levels of estrogen and progesterone. Lysosomal enzymes hydrolyze phospholipids from the cell membranes of desquamated endometrium. These phospholipids serve as precursors for arachidonic acid, the precursor of prostaglandin biosynthesis, particularly prostaglandin $F_{2\alpha}$. The parent prostaglandin compounds, E and F, are products of the metabolism of prostaglandins of the G and H series known as endoperoxides. Prostaglandins E_2 and $F_{2\alpha}$ are highly active biologically. The potent vasoconstrictive action of these agents leads to tissue ischemia, endometrial desquamation, bleeding, and hypercontractility of the uterine muscle. Excessive levels of prostaglandins increase myometrial contractions and reduce uterine blood flow, resulting in ischemia of the uterine muscle and increased stimulation of autonomic pain fibers in the uterus. In women with dysmenorrhea, prostaglandins cause elevated uterine basal tone, increased frequency of contractions, and an incoordinate contractile pattern. Very similar symptoms occur when prostaglandins are used to induce uterine hypercontractility in abortion and labor, lending support to the role of prostaglandins as the primary mediator of menstrual pain. Because prostaglandins in minute quantities exert activity on the intestines, ovaries, uterus, blood vessels, and stomach, a wide range of symptoms may be observed clinically.

SECONDARY DYSMENORRHEA

Secondary dysmenorrhea is caused by organic, pelvic pathology. The onset occurs many years after menarche. It is important to distinguish between the two types of dysmenorrhea because treatment depends on the nature of the underlying pathology in secondary dysmenorrhea and on interruption of the functional etiologic mechanisms in primary dysmenorrhea.

Common pelvic causes of dysmenorrhea include adhesions, infection, endometriosis, adenomyosis, pelvic congestion syndrome, and anatomic defects that cause obstruction to blood flow: cervical stenosis, vaginal septa, imperforate hymen, and noncommunicating horn of the uterus. These disorders are discussed in detail elsewhere in this text. The exact mechanism of dysmenorrhea resulting from these disorders is unclear. Often the patient with pelvic pain syndrome is difficult to distinguish from others with pure dysmenorrhea, except that the pain is not limited to the time of menses. Ultrasound, the hysterosalpingogram, hysteroscopy, and laparoscopy have improved the chances of making an accurate diagnosis. Such accuracy is critical because treatment of the primary disease is essential in eradicating the dysmenorrhea.

MANAGEMENT

Although prostaglandin mediation of pain is the physiologic basis for the primary disorder, there can often be an associated psychologic component. Recurrent pain may lead to negative and neurotic behavior. Although mild symptoms often necessitate nothing more than reassurance, moderate to severe primary dysmenorrhea should be managed with medical therapy. Therapy is directed toward suppression of ovulation and inhibition of prostaglandin production. The hormonal contraceptives, oral (contraceptive pills) and injectable (medroxyprogesterone acetate), effectively suppress ovulation. Endometrial growth and development are decreased, and prostaglandin synthesis and release also are decreased, leading to reduced menstrual fluid volume. Primary dysmenorrhea generally responds to medical therapy.

Nonsteroidal antiinflammatory drugs (NSAIDs) (Table 43-1) will inhibit prostaglandin production and reduce intrauterine pressure, pain, and bleeding. Clinical trials have proved that NSAIDs are effective in the management of primary dysmenorrhea and should replace nonspecific analgesics. Peptic ulcer disease and hypersensitivity to aspirin are contraindications for the use of NSAIDs. Side effects to NSAIDs include bronchospasm, gastrointestinal distress, and hypersensitivity. Occasionally, dizziness, hearing and visual disturbances, seizures, and blood dyscrasias may occur. Supportive therapies in the form of exercise, biofeedback, antispasmodics, diuretics, and acupuncture have been shown to be helpful. In cases of extreme psychologic and behavioral dysfunction associated with dysmenorrhea, psychiatric consultation should be offered.

Combination therapy, hormonal and NSAIDs, can be very effective. If dysmenorrhea is resistant to therapy and there is a negative pelvic examination, laparoscopy is indicated to detect pelvic pathology.

Table 43-1. Nonsteroidal antiinflammatory drugs for the treatment of dysmenorrhea

Agent	Brand name	Dosage
Naproxen	Naprosyn	Initial dose, 500 mg; 250 mg every 6-8 hr
Naproxen sodium	Anaprox	Initial dose, 550 mg; 275 mg every 6-8 hr
Ibuprofen	Motrin	400 mg every 4-6 hr
Meclofenamate sodium	Meclomen	50-100 mg every 4-6 hr
Mefenamic acid	Ponstel	Initial dose, 500 mg; 250 mg every 6-8 hr
Ketoprofen	Orudis	25-50 mg every 6-8 hr
Ketorolac tromethamine	Toradol	10 mg every 4 hr

CRITICAL POINTS

- Symptoms of dysmenorrhea can range from mild to severe and can cause significant incapacitation.
- Primary dysmenorrhea is a disorder of excessive uterine prostaglandin production.
- Secondary dysmenorrhea is caused by a wide variety of pelvic diseases.
- Detailed management most often results in alleviation of the symptoms and normal function for the patient.

Questions

1. Menstrual cramps are caused by uterine hypercontractility. The mechanism of pain is mediated by which of the following actions of prostaglandins?
   A. Blood vessel vasoconstriction
   B. Blood vessel vasodilatation
   C. Smooth muscle relaxation
   D. Decreased uterine bleeding
   E. Decreased endometrial growth

2. A 19-year-old woman has complaints of excessive bleeding and pain with menses for 6 months. Intermenstrual bleeding occurs intermittently. She experienced menarche at age 12. She takes no medications. Pelvic examination reveals a 6-cm adnexal mass. The next appropriate step in the management of this patient is:
   A. Ibuprofen, 400 mg orally every 6 hours as needed
   B. Cyclic oral contraceptive for 2 months
   C. Observation and reexamination in 2 months

D. Hematocrit determination
E. Ultrasound examination of pelvis

3. A sexually active 15-year-old presents with a 1-year history of cyclic menstrual pain. The pain is midline, crampy, radiates to the back and lower extremities, and is worse during the first 2 days of menses. She often experiences nausea, vomiting, and diarrhea, necessitating days missed from school. Pelvic and rectovaginal examinations are negative. The best management option for this patient is:
   A. Oral contraceptive and NSAID therapy
   B. Oral contraceptive therapy
   C. Prostaglandin inhibitor therapy
   D. Psychiatric consultation
   E. Reassurance and antiemetics

Answers

1. A
2. E
3. A

Climacteric

APGO LEARNING OBJECTIVE #44

P. Coney

Women spend as much as one third of their lives in the postmenopausal years. Understanding the physical and emotional changes caused by estrogen depletion is important for all physicians who provide health care for women. Methods to minimize the effects of estrogen deprivation can enhance longevity and improve the physical, emotional, and sexual quality of a woman's life.

The student will demonstrate a knowledge of the following:

A. Description of the physiologic changes in the hypothalamic-pituitary-ovarian axis
B. Symptoms and physical findings associated with hypoestrogenism
C. Long-term changes associated with hypoestrogenism
D. Management of climacteric
E. Risks and benefits of estrogen therapy

Menopause is the cessation of menstruation. It is a natural and inevitable event in a woman's life. The menopausal state is characterized by marked decline in circulating estrogen levels compared with the reproductive years. It can occur abruptly, as with surgical removal of the ovaries; spontaneously, at the average age of 50 for women in the United States; or prematurely, in women under 35 years of age. Climacteric describes a constellation of signs and symptoms the woman may experience in the years leading up to menopause and for years after it. The interval is variable, reflecting declining ovarian function.

ENDOCRINOPATHY

The ovary ages by gradual depletion of primordial follicles. During the reproductive years, more than 90% of circulating estrogen is derived from the follicles destined to ovulate each month. In the absence of follicles, estrogen levels drop precipitately. The ovary continues endocrine function by secreting androgens that are converted primarily to estrogens peripherally. The negative feedback of estrogen on the pituitary is abolished; pituitary gonadotropins rise (greater than 40 mIU) and remain elevated.

Symptoms most commonly experienced during climacteric include fatigue, headache, irritability, insomnia, depression, loss of sense of well-being, and hot flushes. The hot flush, which can last from a few minutes up to 30 minutes, is classic for menopause. The sensation of heat is mostly about the head, neck, and upper torso. Palpitations and sweating often follow the hot flush. There is increased skin temperature and arterial vasodilatation. Long-term side effects from menopause include osteoporosis, increased risk of cardiovascular disease, and atrophic changes of the genital tract.

OSTEOPOROSIS AND MENOPAUSE

Osteoporosis is a deterioration of bone strength secondary to loss of bone mass. The condition is gradual, accelerated in many women after menopause, and progressive. Loss of bone mass occurs most dramatically within the first 3 years after menopause. Bone formation rate, conversion of osteoclasts to osteoblasts, is enhanced by estrogen. In the absence of estrogen the resorption rate, the conversion of osteoprogenitor cells to osteoclasts, is accelerated. Many factors may increase the risk for osteoporosis, including age, small skeletal frame, amenorrhea, corticosteroid therapy, thyrotoxicosis, inactivity, heredity, cigarette smoking, steroid use, and diet. The decline in bone mass related to menopause begins at menopause, is related to estrogen deficiency, and continues. Postmenopausal women lose bone at a rate of 1% to 3% per year. Skeletal fractures, disability, and death can follow. Bone loss is noted first in trabecular bone (vertebrae) and later in cortical bone (hips, extremities). Fractures become evident in the seventh and later decades of life. The incidence rates of bone fracture are highest in Scandinavia and England, intermediate in Asia, and lowest in Africa.

Several prospective studies of estrogen use in postmenopausal women have been done with up to 15 years of follow-up, and all of them show convincingly that estrogen administration will prevent bone loss when compared with placebo or control populations. When started within 3 years after the last menstrual period, there is 3% to 8% gain in bone; there was no change in bone mass when estrogen was started after 6 years. Without estrogen replacement, loss of bone mass can be as high as 11%. Osteoporosis-related skeletal fracture is also significantly lower in estrogen-treated women.

CORONARY HEART DISEASE AND MENOPAUSE

In the Western world, coronary heart disease (CHD) is the major cause of death in both men and women. The CHD mortality is lower in women before menopause than in men, but after menopause mortality exponentially rises to approach that of men. Presumably, this trend is associated with hormonal changes of the ovary. The CHD risk is substantially increased in young women after spontaneous and surgically induced menopause. Hysterectomy, with or without oophorectomy, predisposes to CHD.

A tremendous amount of experimental evidence exists to support a beneficial or protective effect of estrogen replacement against CHD. Nearly all reports are observational. Many are retrospective rather than prospective. Others are prospective cohort studies. Apart from this, there appears to be consistency in the suggestion that cardiovascular benefits derive from estrogen therapy. The exact magnitude of the associated protection is not clear. Cardiovascular disease has declined over the past 20 years by nearly 30%. This decline has been attributed to improved medical care and life-style changes, particularly reduced cigarette smoking. Cigarette smoking has decreased in men by 26%, but by only 8% in women, since the mid-1960s. A marked decline in cardiovascular disease mortality in women is consistent with the increased use of estrogen replacement in that interim.

In 1983 the Lipid Research Clinics program reported the all-cause mortality in estrogen users to be half that of nonusers. The one gadfly report was from the Framingham study, which did not suggest any such cardiovascular benefits. Actually, prospective evaluation of postmenopausal morbidity found that estrogen use was associated with an increased incidence of stroke and CHD, despite a more favorable cardiovascular risk profile in the estrogen users. There was some interaction with cigarette smoking (seemed to enhance) and coronary risk with estrogen use. It is not difficult to conclude from current studies that estrogen replacement therapy probably confers protection against ischemic heart disease and stroke. Overviews of more than 30 reports estimate the reduction in CHD risk by estrogen therapy in the range of 44%.

Data suggest that high density lipoprotein (HDL) cholesterol levels might be the biologic mechanism by which estrogen confers protection. Sex hormones are known to alter lipid profiles. Within months after menopause, serum concentrations of total cholesterol rise by 6%, low density lipoprotein (LDL) cholesterol by 11%, and triglycerides by 9%, with a gradual fall in HDL cholesterol. Treatment with oral estrogen lowers total serum cholesterol and LDL cholesterol and raises HDL. Transdermal estrogen therapy reduces total cholesterol and LDL cholesterol, but HDL cholesterol levels are unchanged. These changes are consistent with improved cardiovascular disease risk profile.

Estrogen users have lower vessel occlusion scores than nonusers. In one report, the odds ratio estimate of the risk of coronary artery occlusion for estrogen users relative to nonusers was 0.4 after adjustment for age, smoking, diabetes, cholesterol level, and hypertension (which is statistically significant). In monkeys, endothelial cell turnover of leukocyte adhesion to the endothelium is enhanced by sex hormones, which inhibit development of atheroma. This may reduce LDL uptake by the arterial wall and increase LDL degradation. Arterial blood flow is improved by estrogen to vascular beds, and estrogen may act directly on vessel walls to induce vasodilatation.

GENITAL TRACT AND BODY CHANGES AND MENOPAUSE

Menopause is often diagnosed retrospectively after a period of amenorrhea. Because the decline in ovarian function usually is gradual, a minority of women will experience menstrual irregularity leading up to menopause—from prolonged and heavy menses to intermenstrual bleeding.

Menopause is associated with regression of the reproductive organs. The cervix shortens. Vaginal atrophic changes are common. The vaginal mucosa becomes thinner, has diminished lubricative response, and is easily traumatized. Sexual response also can diminish with decline in estrogen levels. Dyspareunia and nonspecific vaginitis are common. Epithelia lining the bladder and urethra undergo atrophic changes, resulting in increases in cystitis, urinary frequency, and incontinence. Breasts can decrease in size. The epidermis thins, and skin loses some elasticity. There is generally loss of axillary and pubic hair, with an increase in facial hair. The psychologic impact along with the affective symptomatology can represent major crisis and distress for the woman. But there is clear improvement in all areas of affective symptomatology in women treated with estrogen.

MANAGEMENT

Indications for hormone replacement therapy in menopause include vasomotor instability, genital tract atrophy, and prevention of osteoporosis and cardiovascular disease. Estrogen is available in several formulations for estrogen replacement therapy in the menopausal woman (Table 44-1). These formulations obviously vary in their effectiveness for any given woman. The goal of therapy is to achieve the greatest benefit with the lowest dose. For this reason, natural estrogens (Table 44-1), not synthetic estrogens, are sufficient for the therapeutic and preventive goals of estrogen therapy. Circulating levels of estrogen are achieved comparable to the early to midfollicular levels in the premenopausal state. When more potent or synthetic formulations are used the risk of side effects is increased.

The oral route is the most popular and the easiest route to dose. The lower doses of transdermal estrogens have proved sufficient to reduce osteoporosis. The schedule of dosing is estrogen given daily and the progestin given daily or cyclically. When given cyclically, the progestin is given

for 10 to 12 days every month in doses of 5 to 10 mg. When given daily with the estrogen, progestin is given in doses of 2.5 to 5 mg. The uterine bleeding that automatically follows with progestin therapy is often undesirable and accounts for the high rates of noncompliance or failure of estrogen replacement therapy.

Women who have an intact uterus and who use estrogen unopposed with progestin have an eight-fold increased risk of developing endometrial cancer. It is axiomatic that a large number of women who use estrogen require opposition with progesterone because of their intact uterus and the risk of developing endometrial cancer. Does opposed estrogen therapy with progestin nullify this protective effect against CHD? Some progestins have adverse effects on lipoprotein metabolism. Treatment with 19-nortestosterone derivatives will block the estrogen-induced increase in HDL in a dose and duration fashion. The alteration is much less with 17-hydroxyprogesterone derivatives. Recent reports suggest a beneficial lowering of LDL (by 23%) with conjugated estrogen and medroxyprogesterone acetate. Favorable lipid patterns also have been reported in women who use continuous low-dosage progestin and cyclic estrogen for 3 years.

Contraindications to estrogen replacement therapy include a history of deep venous thrombosis, estrogen-dependent neoplasia, and liver dysfunction. Many epidemiologic studies and metaanalyses have been done to investigate the relationship of exogenous estrogen and the incidence of breast cancer. The conclusions to date show that estrogen does not significantly affect the risk of breast cancer. The balance of risk versus benefit is always carefully reviewed in patients who may have contraindications.

The patient should have periodic examinations during climacteric to receive education regarding the physiologic changes of aging and menopause. An estrogen-only regimen may be given to women who have had hysterectomy. When progestin is administered, the continuous

Table 44-1. Natural estrogen formulations

Formulation	Daily dose (mg)
17β-Estradiol	0.05-2
Conjugated equine estrogens	0.3-2.5
Piperazine estrone sulfate	0.3-5
Micronized estradiol	1-2
Estrogen creams	0.05-3

combined regimen usually will result in break-through bleeding during the first few months of therapy. The cyclic regimen will result in cyclic monthly withdrawal bleeding. The patient should receive instructions about diet, exercise, and hormonal therapy. Intervention may be necessary before a cessation of menses during the time of waning ovarian function.

CRITICAL POINTS

- Aging in a woman brings endocrine changes that affect behavioral, structural, and functional processes.
- A real decline in estrogen secretion is characteristic of the menopausal ovary, but androgens are continually secreted.
- A woman's general health and disease status is related to estrogen levels, particularly affective discomfort, osteoporosis, and coronary artery disease.
- In the absence of contraindications to estrogen replacement therapy, estrogen and modified life-style practices can improve the quality of life in the aging woman.

Questions

1. The incidence of endometrial cancer can be reduced in the patient taking estrogen replacement by which of the following actions?
   A. Detecting vaginal atrophy
   B. Administering calcium with estrogen
   C. Performing endometrial biopsy at frequent intervals
   D. Opposing estrogen with progestin
   E. Down-regulating with gonadotropin-releasing hormone

2. The bulk of bone mass loss occurs within which of the following time intervals following menopause?
   A. First 3 years
   B. First 3 months
   C. Second decade
   D. First 6 years
   E. First year

3. The reductive influence of estrogen on which of the following lipid fractions is most critical in reducing CHD risk?
   A. High density lipoprotein
   B. Triglyceride
   C. Low density lipoprotein
   D. Cholesterol
   E. Lipoprotein

4. The most appropriate first step in treating a menopausal woman with vaginal itching is to:
   A. Examine for specific vaginal flora
   B. Administer metronidazole orally
   C. Administer Mycostatin topically
   D. Administer estrogen cream topically
   E. Examine for a foreign body

Answers

1. D
2. A
3. C
4. A

45

Infertility

APGO LEARNING OBJECTIVE #45

John H. Mattox

The evaluation and management of an infertile couple necessitates both an understanding of the processes of conception and embryogenesis and sensitivity toward the emotional stress that can result.

The student will demonstrate a knowledge of the following:
A. Definition
B. Causes
C. Evaluation and management

From the beginning of recorded time the problem of the barren marriage has played a major role in the lives of humans. Many ancient religious rites and social practices are concerned specifically with fertility and sterility. Magic potions and incantations still are used by some primitive peoples to enhance the reproductive capacity of newlywed couples.

A frequently quoted estimate is that 1 out of every 6 couples in the United States is involuntarily childless, and there is concern that the problem is getting worse. The fertility rate, the number of live births per 1000 women of childbearing age (15 to 45 years), has declined over recent decades; and today many women are delaying childbearing. The number of women who have their first child when they are over 30 is increasing.

Concomitantly, the knowledge of reproductive physiology has improved, serving to increase therapeutic opportunities in such areas as ovulation induction, microsurgery, and in vitro fertilization.

To maintain an appropriate perspective of reproductive biology, it should be recalled how inefficient the human reproductive process is. Approximately 40% of fertilized ova are lost. The generally accepted incidence of clinically recognized spontaneous abortion is 15%; approximately 7% of infants are born prematurely; and 3% to 4% have a major or minor anomaly.

DEFINITIONS

Infertility can be diagnosed if a woman has not been able to conceive during a period of 1 year of unprotected intercourse. Monthly *fecundability* (conception rate) is approximately 20%, but this is age-dependent. More than 60% of normal couples who have unprotected coitus regularly will conceive within 6 months, about 90% within 1 year. The remainder will be pregnant by the end of the second year.

Infertility is considered to be *primary* if conception has never occurred; it is *secondary* if there has been at least one prior pregnancy. *Sterility* means that conception is impossible and that the causative factor is irremediable; this word is used infrequently.

ESSENTIAL FACTORS FOR REPRODUCTION

Normal fertility depends on many factors in both the man and the woman. It is appropriate to consider the couple as the "biologic unit" of reproduction. The man must produce a sufficient number of normal, motile spermatozoa that can enter the urethra through patent pathways to be ejaculated and deposited at the appropriate time for fertilization. After deposition, the male gametes must be able to penetrate and be sustained in the cervical mucus. Following *capacitation* and *acrosomal reaction,* the preparation of the spermatozoa for fertilization, they must ascend through the uterine cavity into the fallopian tube to meet the ovum.

The female must produce a healthy fertilizable ovum that enters the fallopian tube and becomes fertilized within a period of hours. The conceptus must be transported through the tubal lumen to the uterine cavity. There, it must implant itself in endometrium that has been prepared to receive it. The embryo must grow and develop normally. This entire process takes about 5 days.

Although human sperm can exist for long periods of time in the upper genital tract of the woman, they are thought to maintain their fertilization potential for only about 48 hours. It is believed that a healthy ovum can be fertilized over a period of 24 hours.

If any one of these essential processes is defective or impeded, infertility may result.

CAUSES

Although it is usually the woman of an infertile couple who consults the physician first, it is obvious that she is not necessarily totally responsible for infertility. A male factor is either the sole cause or is an important contributing cause in about 40% of infertile couples (Table 45-1).

In the available literature these estimates vary from clinic to clinic. In approximately 10% to 15% of couples, several factors are responsible, and this increases patient frustration and makes therapy more complex.

Male factors

FAULTY SPERMATOGENESIS AND INSEMINATION. Like ovulation, the production of male gametes depends not only on the integration of hormone signals along the hypothalamic pituitary-gonadal axis but also on intragonadal hormone action. The intratesticular

---

Table 45-1. Cause of infertility (%)

Male factor	40
Female factor	50
Tubal factor	25
Ovulatory disorder	20
Cervical factor	5
Miscellaneous	5
Unknown	5

concentration of androgens and the relationship to specialized androgen-binding proteins is critical. The entire process from the formation of the primitive germ cell to the ejaculation of viable motile sperm takes approximately 3 months.

Faulty spermatogenesis may be the result of a number of congenital or acquired causes, some of which may be apparent after taking a history and performing a physical examination. However, a significant number of infertile men have no clear antecedent information or genital abnormalities that would indicate a cause. About 25% of infertile men will demonstrate oligozoospermia (less than 20 million spermatozoa per ml); the cause is elusive, and therapy in this group of patients is disappointing. If severe oligozoospermia (less than 5 million sperm per ml), azoospermia (no sperm), or aspermia (no semen produced) is identified, more extensive assessment should be considered, including appropriate hormone studies, chromosomal analysis, and perhaps testicular biopsy.

A unilateral or bilateral undescended testis, regardless of the time of correction, can result in semen quality lower than that produced by normal men. Significant trauma, which could result in a break in continuity of the testicular tubule structure, can result in the formation of antisperm antibodies. Although mumps orchitis experienced before puberty does not appear to affect spermatogenesis, orchitis after puberty is not unusual and can seriously damage fertility. A history of infection, such as nonspecific urethritis and chronic prostatitis, or prior genital tract surgery—such as a hydrocelectomy, repair of testicular torsion, or herniorrhaphy—have all been associated with defective semen production.

Men with gonadal dysgenesis (Klinefelter's syndrome) may produce no sperm even though their Leydig cells are normal. Hypogonadotropic hypogonadism with anosmia (Kallmann's syndrome) and severe hypothyroidism are both associated with azoospermia. Certain medications may have a deleterious effect on sperm production. Men exposed to diethylstilbestrol (DES) in utero may have structural abnormalities of the ejaculatory system, as well as deficient spermatogenesis. Nitrofurantoin has been associated with deficient sperm production, and certain medicines to treat hypertension can result in impotence. Excessive use of alcohol, nicotine, or marijuana can significantly alter the production of sperm. Severe pyrexia has resulted in transient oligozoospermia. Although great emphasis has been placed on the role of high scrotal temperature induced by constrictive underwear or long, hot baths, it is unlikely that these habits in moderation significantly hamper fertilizing capability. A varicocele, coiling of the venous plexus around the testes, has been assigned a major etiologic role in infertility. Although it is clear that reduced sperm motility may be observed and ultimately corrected following varicocelectomy, fertility is not necessarily improved. Therefore the etiologic role of the varicocele remains unclear. Although sperm count, motility, and morphology are important, sperm function is even more so. Simply, can the sperm traverse the female genital tract and fertilize an ovum?

Cervical mucus penetration and other problems can be assessed by postcoital exam. The sperm penetration assay evaluates human sperm penetration of specially prepared zona-free hamster ova. Cases have been described of infertile men whose sperm concentration and motility were normal but whose sperm were unable to penetrate hamster ova. Impotence, whether induced by medication or by psychogenic causes, obviously will prohibit pregnancy. The number of spermatozoa and the volume of the ejaculate are definitely decreased with frequent (daily or greater) coitus. Optimal timing, which allows for the replenishment of healthy sperm and adequate seminal plasma, is approximately 48 hours. Severe hypospadias or obstruction caused by scarring of the epididymis, vas deferens, or urethra following infection also may interfere with insemination. The most frequent organism is *Neis-*

seria gonorrhoeae. If the penis is abnormally short, buried in fat, or malformed, emission may take place out of the vagina. Premature ejaculation may produce the same results. In the woman, dyspareunia, vaginismus, or an intact hymen may prevent intromission and a normal deposition of the ejaculate.

Female factors

TUBAL FACTOR. The fallopian tube is not merely a conduit. Although tubal patency is essential for fertility, the ascent of spermatozoa and the passage of fertilized ova require physiologic support. Tubal obstruction, either partial or complete, has been a cause of infertility in about 25% of women who fail to conceive. Although tubal closure is more likely to be caused by endosalpingitis that can be gonococcal, chlamydial, or polymicrobial in origin, congenital anomalies also are a possibility. Tubal infertility is increased following appendicitis, particularly if rupture has taken place and there has been pelvic surgery, particularly ovarian wedge resection. Peritubal scarring and immobilization of this structure can occur with endometriosis or perisalpingitis associated with a puerperal infection. Mucosal damage and fimbrial compromise, as well as the kinking and mobilization that occur from perisalpingeal involvement, can occur following infection.

After a clinically documented episode of salpingitis, a woman has an 11% to 12% chance of being infertile. After two episodes the figure increases to 23%; after three or more episodes it is 54.3%. It has been estimated that nearly 300,000 women in the United States have been rendered sterile by salpingitis as of the year 1990.

DISORDERS OF OVULATION. An abnormality of ovulation is responsible for infertility in approximately 20% to 25% of women. The finely orchestrated events resulting in the development of a normal ovum, its periodic extrusion from the follicle, and the cyclic secretion of adequate amounts of estrogen and progesterone by the corpus luteum are essential for normal fertility. In all cases of anovulation or oligoovulation, the underlying endocrine disorder is an altered hypothalmic-pituitary-ovarian interrelationship. Women who have complete absence of ovarian function as in gonadal dysgenesis or premature ovarian failure from whatever cause can be considered to be sterile, but with the possibility of donor ovum or a donor embryo these patients may have children. Although ovarian androgen excess (polycystic ovary syndrome) is a relatively common cause of infertility, hypothyroidism is not. Hyperprolactinemia, either tumor-related or non–tumor-related, usually produces anovulation. For a more thorough description of the disorders of ovulation, see Chapter 42, Abnormal Uterine Bleeding. Luteal phase deficiency, which is found in 2% to 3% of infertile couples, is discussed in Chapter 11, Spontaneous Abortion.

CERVICAL FACTOR. Abnormalities in the structure or the function of the cervix are present in 5% of infertile couples. Obstructive lesions of the cervix such as large polyps, pedunculated leiomyomas, congenital atresia, or stenosis following cauterization or cryotherapy may interfere with ascent of spermatozoa. Alterations in the cervical mucus can be the result of a hormonal deficiency, a chronic infection, or medication. It is in the preovulatory cervical mucus that the sperm must undergo the process of capacitation. It is believed that certain bacteria are lethal to spermatozoa. Whether chlamydial infection plays any role when present in the endocervix remains to be determined.

As ovulation approaches and the peak of estrogen production is reached, the cervical mucus secretion is increased and can be copious. Some women find this annoying. The mucus is thin, clear, and can be drawn into threads 10 to 12 cm long—*spinnbarkheit.* Very few vaginal epithelial or white blood cells can be seen at this time; if the mucus is allowed to dry on a slide, a pronounced ferning pattern is evident. The cervix not only is a source of mucus production but also forms a reservoir in which sperm can live for many hours after deposition and from which they can be dispatched to the upper tract to penetrate an egg. It is this concept of the reservoir that represents the basis for the postcoital test.

UTERINE FACTOR. Malformations, malpositions, and tumors of the uterus do not often interfere with conception, but they occasionally may be a factor in faulty nidation and early abortion. A movable, nontender retrodisplacement of the uterus is not a factor in infertility; most of the time this should be considered a normal finding. Submucous myomas may obstruct the uterine ends of the tube and thus prevent fertilization, or they may distort the uterine cavity and interfere with nidation. Women who were exposed to DES while in utero may have characteristic cervical, uterine, and tubal deformities that can interfere with conception and lead to abortion, ectopic pregnancy, or premature labor.

Miscellaneous factors

Chronic infections, debilitating diseases, and severe nutritional deficiencies may alter the function of both male and female gonads and thus reduce fertility. Advancing age also may play a role; in women, fertility reaches a peak between 20 and 30 years of age and then slowly declines until menopause. Anovulatory cycles are common in the premenopausal period.

It has long been recognized that impotence, premature ejaculation, vaginismus, and dyspareunia are likely to be associated with psychologic dysfunction. An example is repeated failure to have intercourse during the fertile period because of recurrent minor illness; because the woman or man is "too tired"; or even because of periodic dyspareunia, vaginismus, or impotence. Other causes for impotence must be sought; use of prescription drugs should be reviewed, and the prolactin level should be evaluated.

Both men and women can develop antibodies against the numerous antigens in seminal fluid and spermatozoa, but the exact mechanism whereby antisperm antibodies result in infertility is unclear. The fact that antibodies can be detected in serum does not mean that they are responsible for infertility; women and men with antisperm antibodies can achieve a pregnancy. The higher the titer of sperm antibodies, the more plausible the diagnosis of "immune infertility" becomes. Only a small percentage of cases of unexplained infertility may be caused by antisperm antibodies.

INVESTIGATION OF THE INFERTILE COUPLE

The investigation of infertility must be conducted systematically, according to a planned program, and within a brief time frame. Because multiple factors commonly are present, a full study of both partners should be carried out, even when conditions that obviously would impair fertility are detected early in the investigation. Both husband and wife must be interested in the solution of their common problem. The plan of study, the time, and expense involved should be explained to them during the first interview to ensure full cooperation and to prevent future misunderstandings.

The physician must not only be prepared to conduct the basic medical investigation but also be willing to expend the time and energy to deal with the couple's emotional distress. These patients—usually the women more than the men—can be frustrated, angry, and depressed. On occasion, psychotherapy should be recommended. The basic studies usually can be completed within 3 or 4 months.

History

The form in Fig. 45-1 is a useful guideline in obtaining important fertility information.

Physical examination

A complete general physical and genital examination should be performed on each partner.

WOMAN

Age: Race: Religion:
Occupation:
Years of marriage: Previous Marriage
Duration of involuntary infertility:
Past history   *Present history*
1. Medical   1. General
   Sexually transmitted disease   Habits
   Endometriosis   Diet
   Tumors   Work and health status
   Other medical problems   Menstrual cycle
2. Surgical   2. Sexual
   Pelvic operations   Contraception
   Appendectomy   Frequency of coitus
3. Obstetrics   Postcoital practices
   Prior pregnancies, including   Libido
      ectopics and abortions   3. Personal
   Previous infertility evaluation   Motivation for childbearing
4. Menstrual history   Attitude toward partner
                                     Career aspirations

MAN

Age: Race: Religion:
Occupation:
Years of marriage: Previous Marriage
Past history   *Present history*
1. Medical   1. General
   Sexually transmitted infection   Diet
   Mumps orchitis   Bathing habits
   Varicocele   Work and health status
2. Surgical   Medications and drugs
   Herniorrhaphy   2. Sexual
   Hydrocele   Frequency of coitus and technique used
   Orchiopexy   Premature ejaculation
   Injury to genitals   Adequacy of erection
                                     Timing of coitus
                                  3. Personal
                                     Motivation for childbearing
                                     Attitude toward partner
                                     Career aspirations

Fig. 45-1. Infertility history.

Evaluation of the semen

A complete semen analysis and study of the effects of cervical secretions on sperm motility and survival will provide the basic information necessary for evaluating the man. A single analysis may be inconclusive because sperm count varies from day to day and is dependent on emotional, physical, and sexual activity. Two specimens at monthly intervals usually are examined.

SEMEN ANALYSIS. The specimen should be collected by ejaculation into a clean, wide-mouth, screw-top plastic container after masturbation following a 2- or 3-day period of abstinence from intercourse. Couples who cannot accept this method can collect the semen in a specialized condom. The specimen should be transported to the laboratory within 1 hour of emission. No particular precaution need be taken to control its temperature, except that excessive heat and cold should be avoided.

Following are the standards for normal male semen analysis as determined by the World Health Organization:

Volume	2 to 6 ml
pH	7 to 8
Viscosity	Liquefaction within 30 minutes
Sperm concentration	20 to 250 million/ml
Sperm motility	Greater than 50% within 1 hour of collection
Mobility (quality of motility)	3 to 4 hr +
Morphology	Greater than 50% normal sperm

In addition, there should be no significant sperm agglutination or pyospermia. Special staining is required to differentiate leukocytes and immature sperm.

Hysterosalpinogram

The usual test for the study of tubal patency is dependent on the injection of a radiopaque substance through the cervicouterine canal, uterus, and tubes into the peritoneal cavity. If properly

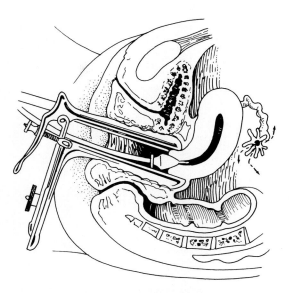

Fig. 45-2. Hysterosalpingography. Sagittal section showing technique. Contrast medium flows through intrauterine cannula and out through tubes, the cervix being closed by a rubber stopper.

performed, the tests provide accurate information concerning tubal structure and should, unless contraindicated, be included as a part of every infertility study. The assumption sometimes is made that tubal patency is equivalent to normal function. These two characteristics are not necessarily the same.

Tests for patency should never be performed in the presence of acute infections of the vagina, cervix, or tubes, or during any episode of uterine bleeding since the contrast medium may enter the open blood vessels. If pregnancy is suspected, tests for tubal patency should be delayed until the diagnosis can be definitely eliminated.

With this test for patency, the site of tubal obstruction can be located accurately; and valuable information concerning the presence of such tubal abnormalities as hydrosalpinx or fixation from adhesions is provided. It also is possible to demonstrate small submucous fibroids or other congenital or acquired defects that may be present in the uterine cavity (Figs. 45-2 and 45-3).

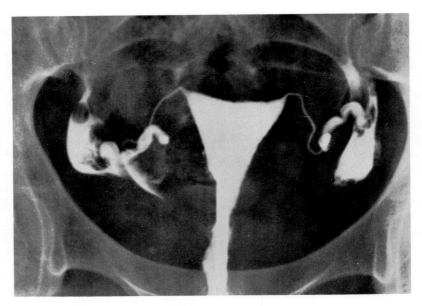

Fig. 45-3. Normal hysterosalpingogram showing passage of radiopaque material through fimbriated ends of tubes.

If the hysterosalpingogram is normal, the patient has about a 75% chance of having normal pelvic structures and no peritubal involvement. To replace this valuable test by laparoscopy and dye instillation as a routine initial approach negates the diagnostic effect and the therapeutic value, increases the risk to the patient, and is not cost-effective.

In general, water-soluble media are preferable to oil-soluble types because they are absorbed rapidly from the peritoneal cavity. A small amount of medium is injected under fluoroscopic control to fill the normal uterine cavity without distending it. This may reveal small irregularities that would be obscured by a larger amount. Additional contrast medium, which should distend the uterus and flow through the tubes, is then injected.

Laparoscopy

Direct observation of the passage of indigo blue dye from the uterus through the fimbriated ends of the tubes is possible with the laparoscope and may be used to determine tubal patency by those experienced in the use of the instruments. An added advantage of this method is that it provides an opportunity for direct visualization of the pelvic structures, supplementing other methods for evaluating normalcy.

Disorders of ovulation

The production of normal ova and their release from the ovary, as well as their pick-up by the fallopian tube, are primary requirements for female fertility. Documentation of when ovulation occurs is an important part of an infertility investigation. Most clinical tests used to assess ovulation are indirect and determine more specifically whether or not progesterone is secreted in significant concentrations.

Ovulation probably is occurring if the basal body temperature curve is typically biphasic with a sustained rise of at least 0.6° F during the last 2 weeks of the cycle. Luteal phase deficiency can be suspected if the thermal rise is maintained for less than 11 days. A serum progesterone obtained around 10 days following a positive urinary luteinizing hormone (LH) detection kit reading should be greater than 10 ng/ml. A concentration of at least 3 ng/ml suggests that ovulation has occurred.

An endometrial biopsy performed late in the luteal phase, cycle day 24 to 26, can determine whether changes in the glands, stroma, and vasculature correspond to the cycle day when the sample was obtained. Normally there is agreement between the histologic dating and the menstrual cycle timing ± 2 days. If progesterone secretion is inadequate, lag in endometrial development will be greater than 2 days.

Ovulation predictor kits can be purchased over-the-counter by the patient. Using an immunocolorimetric assay for LH in the urine, the LH surge can be identified. Using the most accurate kits, ovulation will occur in approximately 24 hours in 88% of women. These kits assist in timing of coitus, diagnostic testing, and certain therapies.

Cervical factor evaluation

After fertility potential in the husband has been established by semen analysis, it becomes necessary to determine the effect of the vaginal and cervical secretions on the activity of the sperm. Spermatozoa can penetrate the cervical mucus during a period of only 24 to 72 hours in the entire menstrual cycle. This occurs in the ovulatory phase of the cycle when the mucus is copious, thin, watery, and exhibits maximal spinnbarkheit and arborization.

The postcoital test (PCT) of cervical mucus provides information concerning the number of spermatozoa that have entered the cervical canal and the percentage that retain their motility in the cervical mucus, but it gives minimal information about the adequacy of the semen specimen. Therefore it is not a substitute for semen analysis. It is essential that the PCT be performed when secretions are optimal for sperm penetration and survival; the day before ovulation is most appropriate. The test can be correctly interpreted only at the end of the cycle to ascertain that the timing of the examination was appropriate. Urinary LH predictor kits have greatly facilitated the timing of this test.

The patient is instructed to report for examination about 6 to 8 hours after coitus; she is told not to use a precoital lubricant or a postcoital douche. At least 2 days' abstinence before the test is desirable. Endocervical mucus is aspirated and the material is examined for clarity, viscosity, and spinnbarkheit. The specimen is then spread on a clean glass slide and examined for the presence of sperm and, after it has dried, for arborization of the mucus. The cervical environment is clearly normal if there are 10 or more highly motile spermatozoa. The most common explanation for a poor postcoital examination is that the specimen was obtained at the wrong time.

TREATMENT

The treatment of infertility often begins with the first consultation, although no specific therapeutic program can be outlined until all data obtained from the complete investigation of the couple have been analyzed and correlated. A significant percentage of women conceive after the initial visit or after assessment of tubal patency. Grant reported "spontaneous" cures of primary infertility in 35% of 1415 patients. Similar results were obtained in 1166 women with secondary infertility.

Failure of insemination

Obvious abnormalities such as an intact hymen, developmental defects, or obesity should be corrected if possible. If failure of insemination occurs because of penile abnormalities, therapeutic insemination with the husband's semen should be considered. Impotence, vaginismus, and dyspareunia are seldom of organic origin, and psychotherapy usually is necessary for their correction. Faulty sexual techniques can be corrected by discussing the coital technique with both partners and suggesting necessary modifications.

Coitus every 36 hours during the period starting 3 days before and ending 2 days after the anticipated time of ovulation should cover minor deviations from the expected ovulatory pattern. If temperatures are being recorded, the couple should have intercourse on the day the temperature falls and the day after. Timing coitus using urinary LH readings can enhance fertility.

Failure of spermatogenesis because of destructive testicular disease cannot be improved, and the inability to transport the sperm because of occlusion in the ductal system is difficult to correct surgically. Any documented infection of the male reproductive system should receive appropriate antibiotic therapy.

Cervical infections should be eradicated, and the cervix returned to as normal a state as possible. The treatment of benign disease of the cervix is discussed in Chapter 49, Cervical Disease and Neoplasia.

Viscous cervical mucus, which can interfere with the ascent of the sperm through the cervical canal, may be the result of a diminished effect or production of estrogen. Intrauterine insemination (IUI) using the partner's ejaculate is the most effective initial therapy if cervical mucus deficit seems to be the cause.

THERAPEUTIC INSEMINATION. Therapeutic or artificial insemination refers to the artificial injection of semen into the cervical canal. It is termed *homologous* insemination if the husband's semen is used and *therapeutic* donor insemination if the semen is from a donor other than the husband.

Homologous insemination is indicated if the husband is normally fertile but is unable to ejaculate the semen over the cervix because of obesity or a penile defect. If a cervical abnormality appears to prevent the invasion of a sufficient number of sperm, IUI with processed ejaculate has proved successful. Neither type of insemination should be considered unless a reasonable study of the woman proves her to be free from defects that might be partly responsible for the failure to conceive, nor without the express written consent of both partners.

Insemination with the husband's semen presents no legal problem, but heterologous insemination involves a great many emotional, ethical, legal, and religious considerations. If the male partner is solely responsible for the failure to conceive, the couple can be offered adoption, insemination, or an intracytoplasmic sperm injection as part of an in vitro fertilization cycle.

Healthy donors with physical characteristics and a blood type compatible with that of the infertile husband should be selected. Donors should be screened thoroughly for infection, including acquired immunodeficiency syndrome, chlamydia, hepatitis, and other sexually transmitted diseases. A complete genetic history and a physical examination are necessary. Routine karyotyping is not productive and is unnecessary. In February 1988 the standard for therapeutic donor insemination was changed from fresh to quarantined frozen and thawed ejaculate because of the potential for human immunodeficiency virus transmission. Frozen ejaculate can be purchased commercially, and the specimens are more costly.

Tubal abnormalities

Although restoration of tubal patency often is equated with restoring tubal function, that is not necessarily the case. Attempts to force open diseased and damaged tubes with the use of contrast media, antibiotic preparations, or adrenal cortical substances have been uniformly unsuccessful and place the patient at risk for developing a serious tubal infection. Surgical procedures are preferred, but the results have not been spectacular. The outcome of tuboplasty is determined by the cause of the occlusion, the extent of the damage, and the experience of the surgeon. It is easier to restore patency in tubes that have been occluded by a sterilizing operation, tubal reversal, than in those that have been damaged by infection. With microsurgical techniques, reversal of sterilization can result in pregnancy rates as high as 65%. If pregnancy occurs following tubal surgery, the patient should be monitored *closely* because her chances of having a tubal pregnancy are increased.

Selective tubal cannulization under fluoroscopic guidance is a new technique that may avert any need for a major tubal operation in patients with cornual occlusion.

Disorders of ovulation

Women who have ovarian failure, as evidenced by at least two serum follicle-stimulating hormone (FSH) levels in the menopausal range, are sterile. Such patients would include those with gonadal dysgenesis (Turner's syndrome) and premature ovarian failure. There is no known way to restore ovarian function. However, it is possible to use donor ova and the partner's ejaculate and, after in vitro fertilization, effect zygote transfer into the patient's uterus, which has been appropriately stimulated by estrogen and progesterone. Women who are oligomenorrheic or amenorrheic should be thoroughly evaluated to determine the etiology of these conditions before the institution of any therapy. This assessment is discussed in detail in Chapter 40, Amenorrhea.

More often the cause of the ovulatory disturbance is related to hypothalamic-pituitary dysfunction, and clomiphene is the initial drug of choice. This medication sends a "message" of estrogen deficiency at the level of the hypothalamus by preventing the replenishment of estrogen receptors; it also activates the negative feedback relationship between estrogen and gonadotropins. Because of the perceived reduction in estradiol, gonadotropin-releasing hormone is secreted, stimulating the release of FSH and LH.

Clomiphene is available as a 50-mg tablet (Clomid, Serophene, or generic) and is administered initially 5 days each cycle after uterine bleeding that either occurs spontaneously or is induced by progesterone. Most of the pregnancies occur after three consecutive ovulatory cycles, and the incidence of side effects is low. This drug should not be used in women who have hepatic disease and should be discontinued in those who experience scotomata and severe ovarian hyperstimulation while taking it. Clomiphene is of minimal value in women who are estrogen-deficient.

If a pregnancy does not occur within three to six ovulatory cycles, other fertility factors should be assessed or reassessed. Individuals with polycystic ovary syndrome are often hyperresponsive to clomiphene, and a smaller dose may be required initially to induce ovulation.

Luteal phase defects can be treated by supplementing the deficiency of progesterone. Some clinicians use clomiphene because enhancing follicular development will result in normal corpus luteum function and progesterone output. Others prefer progesterone vaginal suppositories, 25 mg twice a day, or progesterone in oil, 12.5 mg intramuscularly once a day. Treatment is started 2 days after ovulation and is continued until menstruation.

As a general rule, individuals who do not respond to clomiphene therapy are candidates for menotropin therapy (Pergonal, Humegon), which contains equivalent amounts of FSH and LH, 75 IU per ampule, and is administered parenterally. This medication is expensive and needs to be monitored closely by individuals familiar with its usage. Human chorionic gonadotropin is administered to simulate the LH surge after the ovarian follicles are stimulated and a dominant follicle is developed. Ovarian hyperstimulation, multiple pregnancies, and an increased number of spontaneous abortions are a few of the complications. Before instituting this therapy, other causes of infertility should be eliminated.

Miscellaneous factors

Uterine myomas are rarely responsible for the failure to conceive, and myomectomy is seldom indicated to improve fertility. If the myomas obstruct the cornual ends of the tubes or distort the endometrial cavity, removal should be considered if no other cause of infertility can be found. *Congenital fusion defects* of the müllerian system, that is, bicornuate and septate uterus, rarely cause infertility; spontaneous abortion and premature labor are more characteristic problems with these developmental anomalies. However, it is reasonable to consider *metroplasty,* a uterine reconstruction, if no other cause of infertility can be identified. It must be remembered, though, that approximately 10% of women with a uterine anomaly will have a luteal phase defect and that this should be excluded before any surgery is performed.

Infertility caused by development of antisperm antibodies does not occur often. Condom therapy for several months has been shown to reduce antibody concentrations but has not necessarily resulted in a greater number of pregnancies than in those individuals who are left untreated. Cyclic corticosteroid therapy for the male or female who is producing antisperm antibodies has resulted in higher pregnancy rates, but the use of these drugs can produce some serious complications. Superovulation with IUI has also been suggested and is the preferred initial therapy.

Although in vitro fertilization and embryo transfer (IVF-ET) is a form of therapy that was initially developed to treat women with obstructive tubal disease, it is clear that the indications are expanding. In some IVF centers severe oligozoospermia, disorders of ovulation, immune infertility, and unexplained fertility are considered reasonable indications after all other therapies have failed. Gamete intrafallopian transfer (GIFT) is a procedure wherein eggs and sperm are replaced into healthy-appearing tubes at laparoscopy. Pregnancy rates tend to be higher than in IVF-ET, but no direct prospectively controlled study has been conducted.

Emotional care

Couples with an infertility problem usually are depressed and anxious and have decreased libido. Referral to a counselor, an appropriate support group, or RESOLVE (a national lay group that provides information and support to couples with infertility problems), and, occasionally, psychotherapy will be helpful. Although it is obvious to the practitioner that the couple is under significant stress during the fertility evaluation, the dis-

CRITICAL POINTS

- Infertility applies to a couple that has been attempting to achieve pregnancy after 1 year of unprotected intercourse. If a pregnancy has never occurred, it is considered to be primary.
- The cause of infertility is found approximately half of the time in the man. Among the factors responsible for female infertility are tubal disease, disorders of ovulation, and problems with the cervix. The infertility evaluation consists of a thorough history and physical examination on both the male and female partner; five basic tests are ordered: semen analysis, hysterosalpingogram, postcoital examination, timed endometrial biopsy, and a diagnostic laparoscopy with chromopertubation.
- Approximately 10% of the time multiple factors are involved that need to be treated concomitantly to optimize therapy.
- Couples with infertility experience significant emotional distress, and management of psychosocial problems should be incorporated into the treatment plan.

tress does not seem to have any bearing on the couple's ability to function as parents when pregnancy is achieved.

Although adoption remains a theoretic option, few infants are available; thus other therapeutic modalities should be pursued as long as it is emotionally and financially feasible for the couple to do so.

Questions

1. In a young, healthy woman in the reproductive age range, the most likely cause of infertility is:
   A. An abnormal semen analysis
   B. A disorder of ovulation
   C. Uterine fibroids
   D. A cervical factor
   E. An immune infertility
2. The least informative test in the initial diagnostic assessment of a young couple with infertility is:
   A. A semen analysis
   B. Hysterosalpingogram
   C. A timed endometrial biopsy
   D. Antisperm antibodies
   E. Cervical cultures for gonorrhea and chlamydia
3. The following values are considered appropriate for a normal semen analysis *except:*
   A. A sperm count of greater than 20 million/ml
   B. A semen volume of 2 to 6 ml
   C. Greater than 80% normal forms
   D. Greater than 50% motility
   E. Complete liquefaction within 60 minutes

Answers

1. B
2. D
3. C

46

Premenstrual syndrome

APGO LEARNING OBJECTIVE #46

John H. Mattox

> *Premenstrual syndrome involves physical and emotional discomfort and may affect interpersonal relationships. Effective management of this condition necessitates an understanding of symptoms and diagnostic methods.*

The student will demonstrate a knowledge of the following:

A. Definition
B. Theories of cause
C. Methods of diagnosis

The manifestations of premenstrual syndrome (PMS) were first described by Frank in 1931. He suggested that women who demonstrated edema, weight gain, and emotional disturbances before the onset of menstruation had a premenstrual disease caused by excess estrogen. In 1953 Dalton and other investigators suggested that women with these symptoms should be categorized under the heading *PMS*. The symptoms now attributed to this condition number well over 50 and are outlined in Moos' menstrual distress questionnaire. This questionnaire is divided into eight categories, with symptoms related to (1) pain, (2) concentration, (3) behavioral change, (4) autonomic reactions, (5) water retention, (6) negative affect, (7) arousal, and (8) control.

Premenstrual tension has been recognized for over 50 years. Only recently, though, has there been concentrated interest in the constellation of symptoms because women have become more involved in jobs outside the home and are assuming many responsible positions in the work force. When severe, premenstrual symptoms may sometimes prevent women from attaining their best level of performance. In addition, PMS has occasionally been used as a legal defense in criminal cases involving charges such as murder. A great deal has been written in both the lay and professional press because of the renewed interest in this area.

Most women experience some changes in body sensation and mood before the onset of menstrual flow *(molimina).* For some women, the number and the severity of the symptoms are so extreme that they comprise a medical disorder. Otherwise healthy women experience one or more of these symptoms in a mild-to-moderate form. The incidence of PMS has been reported in 5% to 95% of populations studied; 2% to 3% of women of childbearing age have severe PMS. It has been suggested that about 5 to 6 million women experience severe symptoms each month in the United States. Fortunately, threatening symptoms such as homicidal or suicidal ideation occur only in a very small percentage of women. The *Diagnostic and Statistical Manual of Psychiatry, DSM IV,* 1995, lists criteria that must be met to make the diagnosis of premenstrual dysphoric disorder (PDD). This classification has added more objectivity and organization to a somewhat elusive disorder; however, the commonly used abbreviation *PMS* will continue. Finally, it is important to differentiate PDD from a concurrent or underlying affective disorder (e.g., depression, which is the most common of such disorders).

ETIOLOGIC FACTORS

The postulated etiologic factors involved in PMS are insufficient progesterone, excess estrogen, abnormal fluid retention, nutritional problems, glucose metabolism, and abnormalities of opioid or serotonin. The exact cause of premenstrual tension is unknown, but its cyclic nature and timing suggest that there is a hormonal dysfunction in women who experience the symptoms. Progesterone insufficiency results in a relative estrogen excess. It has also been shown that PMS is more apt to occur in women with endometriosis or luteal phase defect, which may explain why the symptoms appear as long as a week before the onset of menstruation, when progesterone levels are usually high.

Fluid retention

In the past, fluid retention was believed to precipitate the various manifestations of PMS, and diuretics were used as part of the clinical management. Studies assessing weight change, sodium exchange, and total body water have failed to uncover a pattern of fluid retention in most women with PMS. Aldosterone levels are not significantly elevated. Progesterone does, however, affect the renin-angiotensin-aldosterone mechanism and water metabolism by inducing a temporary natriuresis followed by fluid retention.

Nutrition and exercise

A great deal of emphasis has been placed on proper nutrition and the importance of exercise in reducing PMS. Deficiencies in vitamin B_6 (pyridoxine), vitamin D, and calcium have been suggested as a cause of PMS, although the supporting data are questionable. It has also been suggested that pyridoxine affects the biosynthesis of brain catecholamines that regulate mood behavior. Hypoglycemia may also invoke symptoms of PMS. The relationship between the amount of carbohydrates and protein in the diet may be important. Some studies have suggested that the reduction of carbohydrates and the increase of protein may be beneficial.

Hyperprolactinemia

Hyperprolactinemia has been cited by some researchers as another possible cause of PMS. However, some studies do not indicate that women with PMS have elevated prolactin levels. In addition, women with hyperprolactinemia rarely have symptoms of PMS.

Endogenous opioids

More recently, Reid and Yen have suggested that an endogenous opiate peptide may be responsible for the symptoms of PMS in some women, especially those with the depressive symptoms. Opiate peptides do affect the amount of gonadotropin secretion and produce changes in the concentration of luteinizing hormone. Direct measurement of β-endorphin concentrations in the portal hypophyseal blood of the rhesus monkey has revealed that levels of opiate peptides are high during the midluteal phase and undetectable at the onset of menstruation. These authors postulate that progesterone, acting either alone or in combination with estrogen, can increase central endogenous opiate peptide activity. They further suggest that this may trigger the subsequent neuroendocrine manifestations of PMS. Finally, a deficiency of serotonin has been postulated as an etiologic factor in PMS primarily because a significant number of patients report improvement with serotonin uptake inhibitors.

SYMPTOMS

Headache, nervous irritability, insomnia, and crying spells are the most common manifestations of premenstrual tension. Many women complain of backache, lower abdominal pain, and tender or painful breasts as well. These symptoms usually appear about 7 to 10 days before the period is due, and they gradually increase in intensity. Usually they disappear once the menstrual flow is well established. A weight gain of 1 to 3 kg (2 to 6½ lb) during the premenstrual phase is common. Generalized edema and diminished urine output occur frequently. Rapid loss of weight gained and marked diuresis usually follow the onset of menstruation, along with regression of the other symptoms. The physician should also consider other possible diagnoses, including chronic depression (which may become aggravated before menstruation) and manic depressive illness.

MANAGEMENT

Women who suffer from PMS may experience irritability, depression, fatigue, edema, breast discomfort, and the other symptoms associated with the syndrome for quite some time before they consult a physician. Frequently, when women first seek medical help, they inform providers of feeling that they are "going crazy." It would be helpful for physicians to inquire about the symptoms of PMS every time they take a menstrual history. Such information provides a more complete picture of the patient. Frequently, the early diagnosis of patients with PMS can prevent many emotional difficulties within the home and on the job.

Once symptoms characterizing PMS are identified, the patient should be reassured that she is not becoming "psychotic" and that measures can be taken to help her. Early in the management of the patient, it is usually helpful to bring any immediate family members into a discussion concerning the symptoms.

It is essential to have the patient keep a daily diary about her symptoms and behavior, recording the predominant symptoms and rating the intensity (1 = least severe to 4 = most severe) (Fig. 46-1). She should be told that PMS is a common disorder of women in their childbearing years, that the symptoms usually disappear at menopause, and that there are a number of things that can be done to alleviate the symptoms. Some suggested studies are seen in Table 46-1. With treatment, the patient will learn to cope with her

Table 46-1 Suggested studies

Condition	Appropriate evaluation
Hypothyroidism	Thyroid-stimulating hormone
Hypoglycemia or diabetes mellitus	Glucose tolerance test
Anemia	Hemoglobin; red cell indices
Lupus erythematosus	Double-stranded deoxyribonucleic acid
Severe mood changes not limited to the luteal phase	Psychiatric consultation

Name: _____ Age: _____ Month: _____

MENSES GRADING	SYMPTOM GRADING
1- None	1- None
2- Slight	2- Slight
3- Moderate	3- Moderate, present and interferes with activities
4- Heavy/clots	4- Severe, disabling, unable to function

CYCLE DAY

1 2 3 4 5 6 7 8 9 10 11 12 13 14 15 16 17 18 19 20 21 22 23 24 25 26 27 28 29 30 31

Menses = X

SYMPTOMS

Nervousness
Mood swings
Irritability
Anxiety

Weight gain
Swelling of extremities
Breast tenderness
Bloating

Headache
Increased appetite
Heart pounding or racing
Fatigue
Dizziness or faintness

Depression
Forgetfulness
Crying
Inability to concentrate
Insomnia

Weight in lb (early AM)

Basal body temperature (°F)

.9
.8
98.6
.4
.2
.0

Fig. 46-1. Premenstrual syndrome diary.

symptoms in a more effective manner. She should be taught the importance of a good exercise program, such as walking regularly for 20 to 30 minutes 3 times per week, and she should be put on an appropriate diet. The elimination of tobacco and caffeine is beneficial to most patients. A diet that is low in carbohydrates but contains a reasonable amount of protein, vegetables, and fruit helps other women. Protein should be obtained primarily from fish rather than from red meat. Pyridoxine in doses of 100 to 400 mg/day has been recommended, but well-controlled studies are not available.

Progesterone in pharmacologic amounts, administered by suppository or intramuscularly, has been recommended by Dalton. In large doses progesterone does inhibit smooth muscle contractions and is a central nervous system depressant. Substituted progesterone (medroxyprogesterone acetate) and the 19 norsteroids (the progestins in oral contraceptives) are not "pure" progesterones. Unfortunately, initial placebo-controlled studies have not been promising; progesterone is no more effective than a placebo.

In women with severe breast pain (cyclic mastodynia) and swelling, bromocriptine or danazol has proved to be helpful. However, these medications should not be necessary for most patients. Some patients report improvement of their symptoms with oral contraceptives. This form of therapy can be used in patients up to age 50 and who need contraception, have associated dysmenorrhea, and have no existing medical contraindication. In addition, prostaglandin inhibitors such as mefenamic acid, 250 mg, and naproxen sodium, 275 mg, taken orally every 4 to 6 hours may relieve not only dysmenorrhea but symptoms of PMS as well. Unfortunately, diuretics are probably the most frequently used medication in the treatment of PMS. Although there is very little evidence of major fluid retention with this syndrome, spironolactone, 25 mg taken orally 2 times a day, may be prescribed the week before menstruation when edema is severe. Gonadotropin-releasing hormone analogs have been proved effective but are very costly for continuous use. Selective serotonin reuptake inhibitors (SSRI) have proved efficacious in treating PDD. Surprisingly, daily SSRI treatment for the last 2 weeks of the cycle has been effective. Most experience has been gained with fluoxetine (Prozac). Again, large-scale, well-designed studies are lacking. Anxiolytics have also been effective, with alprazolam (Xanax) (0.25 mg taken orally 2 times a day) recommended as a trial therapy after the evaluation is complete.

Certainly, patients showing marked alteration in mood swings with manic and/or severe depressive symptoms, as well as those exhib-

CRITICAL POINTS

- Premenstrual syndrome—or, more correctly, premenstrual dysphoric disorder—is a constellation of symptoms so severe that they interfere with a woman's daily life.
- The etiology of PDD has not been clearly identified. The diagnosis is contingent on the severe symptoms occurring during the luteal phase, with relief following menses; the best way to document the changes is with a PMS questionnaire. The most appropriate therapy is achieved by spending time with the patient and by treating the major symptom or symptoms associated with the problem (as identified by the diary); the majority of patients experience significant improvement in the (true) cases of PMS.
- Atypical symptoms or behaviors on the part of the patient indicate the need for a psychiatric consultation.

iting psychotic behavior, should have a psychiatric evaluation before treatment. Tricyclic antidepressants have not been effective in treating PMS.

In summary, PMS encompasses a number of symptoms that women experience before the menstrual period; control of these symptoms is clearly important. Patients who are prone to the syndrome should first be evaluated carefully. They should maintain a diary, itemizing their symptoms for a number of cycles. They should be reassured that they are not psychotic and that their symptoms are brought about by hormonal changes affecting the body from PMS, so that the family can provide strong emotional support. With appropriate changes in life-style—which might include the start of an exercise program, a balanced diet, certain drug therapies, and the support of an understanding physician who may recommend family-centered therapy—most women with PMS can be helped significantly.

Question

1. All of the following statements concerning PMS are true *except:*
   A. There is a constellation of symptoms that are so severe that they interfere with daily life.
   B. Virtually all women experience molimina, but less than 5% have severe PMS.
   C. The cause is believed to be a deficiency in progesterone.
   D. Appropriate laboratory studies to include would be a hemoglobin, thyroid-stimulating hormone, and glucose tolerance test.
   E. The most effective form of psychologic and medical management necessitates the use of a PMS diary.

Answer

1. C

V

Neoplasia

Gestational trophoblastic neoplasia

APGO LEARNING OBJECTIVE #47

Joanna M. Cain

> *Gestational trophoblastic neoplasia is important because of its malignant potential and the associated risks of morbidity and mortality.*

The student will demonstrate a knowledge of the following:
A. Symptoms and physical findings suggestive of gestational trophoblastic neoplasia
B. Methods used to confirm the diagnosis of gestational trophoblastic neoplasia
C. Approach to the management and follow-up of patients with gestational trophoblastic neoplasia

Gestational trophoblastic neoplasms are diseases related to malignant degeneration of trophoblastic tissue. There is a continuum from the most benign form, hydatidiform mole, to the most malignant form, choriocarcinoma. These are pathologic descriptions, however; and now that the tumor marker β–human chorionic gonadotropin (β-HCG) can be measured, the malignant potential or activity of these tumors is derived from the levels of HCG.

RISK FACTORS AND SYMPTOMS

The relationship of nationality or race on the incidence of these diseases is not clear. Many Asian countries have a high incidence, possibly related to diet. Age is also a significant factor. The development of hydatidiform mole is 10 times more common in women over the age of 45. The woman's partner also may contribute because the chromosomal pattern of moles is most commonly 46 XX, derived completely from paternal origin. Finally, a history of a previous hydatidiform mole increases the risk of a future molar pregnancy to 2% to 3%.

Since this class of neoplasia is derived from trophoblastic tissue and is associated with elevated levels of HCG, it is logical to assume that many of the characteristics of pregnancy are associated with the disease process. Careful documentation of previous pregnancies and the date of the last menstrual period are important, both for the more malignant diseases, which are associated with a previous delivery, and for most cases of gestational trophoblastic disease (GTD), which may be identified by the presence of a uterus larger than would be expected from the date of the last menstruation. Approximately 50% will be larger. Because the implantation of this abnormal trophoblastic tissue is not secure, one of the hallmarks of GTD is bleeding in the second trimester. Furthermore, vesicles may be passed with or without associated bleeding. Often women with these symptoms are referred with a diagnosis of threatened abortion or incomplete abortion. One third of women with GTD will have nausea and vomiting that is earlier and more severe than expected in a normal gestation, and 15% will have abdominal pain associated with large ovarian theca-lutein cysts stimulated by the elevated HCG. Symptoms of preeclampsia in the second trimester (headache, swelling feet, weight gain, blood pressure elevation) are highly suggestive of GTD. Rarely, symptoms of hyperthyroidism (possibly related to binding of the HCG molecule to the thyroid-stimulating hormone receptor site) are associated with this disease.

PHYSICAL EXAMINATION

Elevated blood pressure, pedal edema, and other signs of preeclampsia need to be looked for in the physical examination. As noted previously, the uterus is often larger than expected. The ovaries also may be palpable. If so, they should be handled very gently because rupture of the large theca-lutein cysts, while very rare, is associated with life-threatening hemorrhage. Examination of the vagina and cervix should proceed only after ultrasound diagnosis in the mid- to late second trimester. A differential diagnosis of bleeding in the second trimester includes vasa previa and placenta previa, in which a primary vaginal examination would not be appropriate. Vaginal and cervical examination may establish a diagnosis by revealing the presence of the classic vesicles (Fig. 47-1). A

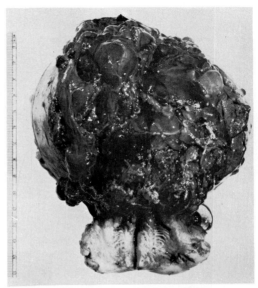

Fig. 47-1. Hydatidiform mole at approximately 100 days' gestation. Note uneffaced, undilated cervix with deep molar penetration into myometrium. Patient is a 43-year-old primigravida.

rare type of hydatidiform mole, partial mole, is associated with the presence of a fetus and a genotype that is often triploid. However, multiple malformations are associated with these gestations, and the management of the life-threatening molar placenta takes precedence.

DIAGNOSIS

The two most important methods in diagnosis are ultrasound of the uterus and ovaries and measurement of serum HCG. The characteristic pattern, when present, cannot be confused with normal pregnancy (Fig. 47-2). The pattern during early molar pregnancy may be less distinctive because the cysts are smaller. A repeat examination in 2 to 3 weeks usually clarifies the diagnosis.

Assays for HCG may be helpful in suspected GTD because the serum concentration of HCG usually is much higher than during comparable

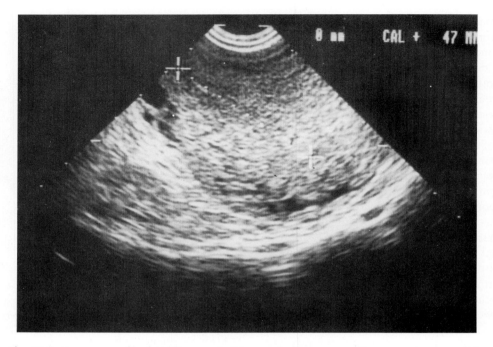

Fig. 47-2. Sonogram of hydatidiform mole. The mottled, snowstormlike appearance caused by cystic villi is typical and distinct from an intrauterine pregnancy.

stages of normal pregnancy. This alone is not a reliable diagnostic measure, however, because the levels at the time of peak secretion in normally pregnant women, at about 60 to 70 days' gestation, may be in a range consistent with a mole. Normal serum values of HCG rise during early normal pregnancy and reach about 50,000 mIU/ml by 45 days and a maximum of as much as 600,000 mIU/ml at about 60 days. The titer then decreases rapidly and is rarely above 20,000 mIU/ml after 100 days' gestation. These levels are slightly higher in multiple pregnancies. Values for hydatidiform mole often reach 1.5 to 2 million mIU/ml but can be less if the mole is regressing.

Because of potential confusion in early pregnancy, both ultrasound and HCG studies are important to the diagnosis. Additionally, clinical assessment of risk factors, symptoms, and physical findings aid in early diagnosis. Older methods of diagnosis such as amniography or flat plate films of the abdomen generally are not used today because of the sensitivity of ultrasound and HCG studies.

MANAGEMENT

Initial management should include evacuation of the uterus. Suction curettage is the primary method, even when the uterus has enlarged beyond the size expected for a 20-week gestation. Suction is preferable to a standard curettage because the uterus can be emptied more rapidly and the wall is less likely to be injured or perforated. Oxytocin infusion is often used after the suction curettage is partially completed to decrease the likelihood of bleeding by contraction of the uterine wall. Careful curettage of the uterine wall with a large, sharp curet completes the operation. Hysterotomy is not used for evacuation. In some cases, if the woman does not wish further childbearing, hysterectomy—with or without prophy-

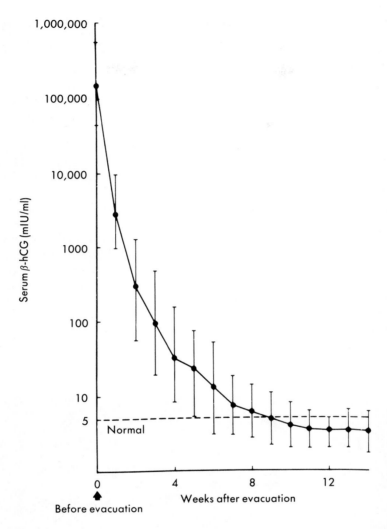

Fig. 47-3. Regression curve for HCG after evacuation of hydatidiform mole. *(From Morrow CP, Kletzky OA, Disaia PJ et al:* Am J Obstet Gynecol *128:424, 1977.)*

lactic chemotherapy—may be considered for primary management. In women with ovarian enlargement and theca-lutein cysts, the cysts are not treated surgically but merely followed. They will regress with the falling HCG.

As many as 10% of women develop acute pulmonary complications during or after curettage. This is thought to be initiated by embolization with trophoblastic tissue and/or fluid overload

associated with pregnancy-induced hypertension and hyperthyroidism. The classic symptoms are hypoxia, tachycardia, and tachypnea.

Follow-up

After evacuation of complete hydatidiform moles, 15% to 25% of women will develop persistent disease. For the partial mole (associated with a fetus) the risk is less, about 10%. The risk of malignancy warrants careful follow-up to identify patients who require further treatment. Before modern chemotherapy, the mortality rate with persistent GTD approached 85% within a year of diagnosis.

Standard follow-up is predicated on two factors. First, the uterus should return to its normal size within 4 to 6 weeks, and bleeding should cease within 1 week. Second, the β subunit of HCG should fall steadily at a regular rate (Fig. 47-3).

Physical examination for uterine involution and decrease in ovarian masses, if present, should occur every 2 weeks until the uterus has returned to normal size. If there is significant delay in resolution and the HCG is slow to resolve, a second evaluation and curettage may be indicated.

The quantitative β subunit of HCG must be measured weekly by radioimmunoassay until two consecutive negative levels are reached. Sixty percent to 80% of women will have nondetectable levels by 8 weeks after evacuation. Regression to nondetectable levels can, however, take as long as 6 months. Monthly levels should be measured for 1 year after a normal level is reached. Levels that plateau or elevate necessitate further investigation for potential metastatic or persistent GTD. Standard pregnancy tests are not adequate for following patients because even the most sensitive will not detect the low levels of HCG that may be present with residual disease.

A chest radiograph should be obtained after the mole is evacuated to evaluate for pulmonary metastases, and the study should be repeated as warranted by abnormal findings during follow-up.

An effective contraceptive method is strongly encouraged during the follow-up period of 1 year. A new pregnancy obviously would raise concerns about the emergence of disease. Low-dose oral contraceptives do not interfere with the interpretation of HCG assays, nor do they increase the risk of trophoblastic disease.

If the uterine size and β-HCG return to normal, no active treatment is necessary.

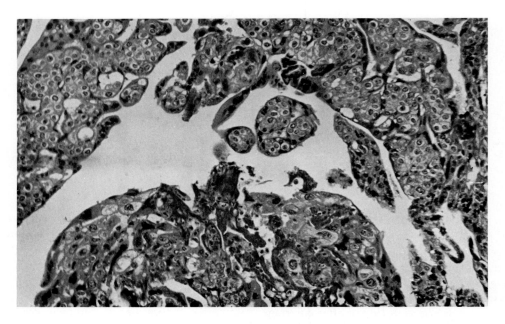

Fig. 47-4. Section through viable choriocarcinoma. Neoplastic trophoblastic cells are of both syncytial and Langhans' type. There is no necrosis or hemorrhage in this field.

TREATMENT

Invasive mole and choriocarcinoma (Fig. 47-4) are the pathologic subtypes most often associated with persistent or elevating β-HCG during follow-up of a hydatidiform mole. Of the most aggressive subtype, choriocarcinoma, 50% were preceded by a mole. Twenty-five percent develop following abortion and 25% following delivery at term or after an ectopic pregnancy. Regardless of the pathology, however, the management is predicated by estimates of high or low risk for persistence (Fig. 47-3).

When a diagnosis of persistent and/or metastatic disease is made, evaluation by chest radiography, head and abdominal computed tomographic scan, and possibly spinal tap for CSF β-HCG is initiated. Additionally, complete blood cell count, liver function studies, and electrolyte and thyroid studies are performed. The classification into low-risk or high-risk categories established by the evaluation determines the chemotherapy protocol.

Women in low-risk categories can be treated with single-agent chemotherapy. The drugs most often used are methotrexate and actinomycin D (dactinomycin). Methotrexate, a folic acid analogue that interferes with normal cell metabolism, was the first drug to eradicate abnormal trophoblast effectively. The disease can be completely eradicated in almost every patient with localized or low-risk metastatic disease.

Women in high-risk categories require aggressive multiagent chemotherapy. Even with this extensive and widely disseminated disease, 80% to 90% of women respond to treatment. The most serious sites for treatment are liver and brain metastases, which often receive concurrent radiation and chemotherapy. The outcome for all women with GTD depends heavily on the initial management and therapy. The best results, especially in high-risk patients, are obtained when women with gestational trophoblastic neoplasms are treated in centers equipped with the necessary diagnostic facilities and staffed by expert personnel experienced in managing this disease.

Follow-up after treatment for persistent or metastatic disease

Following successful treatment, prolonged observation is necessary. Tests should be appropriate to the sites of metastatic disease identified. For example, women with pulmonary metastases should have serial follow-up chest radiographs. The pulmonary lesions usually regress slowly but should disappear completely. A general rule for the first year of follow-up is monthly β-HCG studies and physical examination every 3 months.

CRITICAL POINTS

- Classic presentation includes uterine bleeding, severe nausea and vomiting, and uterine size larger than expected in a woman who is pregnant.
- Other, more rare symptoms include ovarian enlargement, hyperthyroidism, and pregnancy-induced hypertension.
- The genetic composition of hydatidiform mole usually is entirely paternal in origin.
- Diagnosis is based on elevation of β-HCG beyond normal pregnancy values and ultrasound pattern consistent with mole.
- Treatment is uterine evacuation and careful serial follow-up of β-HCG.
- Persistent or metastatic disease necessitates careful evaluation and then selection of chemotherapy regimen.

Questions

1. The genetic composition of trophoblastic disease is:
   A. Equally derived from maternal and paternal chromosomes
   B. Derived entirely from maternal chromosomal material
   C. Entirely derived from paternal chromosomal material
   D. Derived from mature endometrial cell
2. A 22-year-old woman is seen for a physical exam. She reports a pregnancy loss 2 months previously and continued vaginal spotting since. The next step in management is:
   A. Pelvic ultrasound examination
   B. Chest x-ray
   C. Chest, abdomen, and pelvic computed tomographic scan
   D. Hysteroscopy
3. An 18-year-old primigravida, status post–induced abortion I, is seen in follow-up for changes consistent with hydatidiform mole seen on her pathology specimen at the time of an induced abortion. She is not symptomatic. The best follow-up plan is a β-HCG drawn:

A. Every other week until three are normal, then stop
B. Every week until two are normal, then every month for 1 year
C. Every month until two are normal, then every 6 months for 5 years
D. Every 2 weeks for 2 times, then every 2 months for 6 times

4. A 40-year-old woman has bleeding at 12 weeks' gestational age. An ultrasound is consistent with a molar pregnancy. The best management for this patient is:
   A. Close monitoring of HCG after evacuation
   B. Methotrexate before evacuation
   C. Actinomycin D after evacuation
   D. Birth control pills to suppress the ovaries before evacuation

Answers

1. C
2. A
3. B
4. A

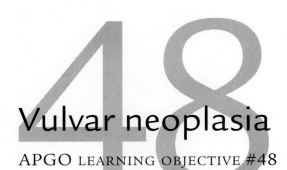

Vulvar neoplasia

APGO LEARNING OBJECTIVE #48

Joanna M. Cain

Improper evaluation of vulvar symptoms often delays treatment of vulvar neoplasia. Early recognition and diagnosis will improve outcome and may avoid the need for extensive surgery.

The student will demonstrate a knowledge of the following:
A. Characteristics of the typical patient who is at risk for vulvar neoplasia
B. Methods of diagnosis
C. Management of the patient with vulvar symptoms

Vulvar cancer is for the most part a curable disease, but this depends on the patient and the health care giver's education and attention to vulvar symptoms. Patients often give a history of extensive self-treatment before they seek medical care. Attention to vulvar symptoms by health care givers requires physical examination of the vulvar area and often biopsy to establish a diagnosis. Since vulvar cancer can mimic many benign lesions, recognition of invasive disease can be difficult and a high index of suspicion is appropriate.

Treatment without examination is not appropriate for vulvar disease. Improvement in survival of women with vulvar cancer depends on early diagnosis and can only be further improved by careful patient education and improved early diagnosis of these cancers.

RISK FACTORS AND SYMPTOMS

Vulvar carcinoma is most frequently encountered in women between the ages of 60 and 79. Fewer than 15% are under 40. Invasive cancer is more common in the older age ranges, and carcinoma in situ occurs most often in the younger age ranges. Association with human papillomavirus and a history of concurrent or past vulvar or cervical carcinoma in situ or invasive disease are higher risk features. In addition, smoking may correlate with a higher incidence of both carcinoma in situ and invasive disease. The involvement of carcinogens in the initiation of this disease is well illustrated by its increased incidence in Wales and other coal mining areas, where coal tars are suspected to be involved. Vulvar cancer is not known to be an inherited disease.

The symptoms produced by vulvar disease, whether benign or malignant, include pruritus and local irritation and pain. Bleeding is more commonly associated with invasive disease but can occur with benign disease as well. The finding of a mass effect in the area often suggests extensive malignant involvement of the vulva.

DIFFERENTIAL DIAGNOSIS

White lesions of the vulva include a variety of diagnoses that have little relationship to each other except for their white appearance. These lesions vary from simple primary or secondary loss or absence of pigment to hyperplastic lesions that may be primarily benign but conceal an invasive cancer (Fig. 48-1). Hyperplastic dystrophies and lichen sclerosis are two vulvar abnormalities that can be difficult to differentiate from invasive carcinoma. The axiom of diagnosis is vulvar biopsy at initial diagnosis and a low threshold for biopsy on follow-up examination if the area fails to respond or if it changes in comparison to the surrounding areas.

Pigmented lesions can vary from benign nevi to pigmented, elevated carcinoma in situ to malignant melanoma. The more irregular the surface or perimeter and the more thickened or friable the lesion, the more it necessitates biopsy for diagnosis. A pigmented lesion that enlarges rapidly may be a melanoma. It is not possible to tell from simple viewing of a lesion whether there is malignant potential or not (Fig. 48-2).

Ulcers also must be differentiated from their benign counterparts. Certainly the ulcers associated with infectious diseases such as herpes have a classic presentation and resolution. If ulcers fail to follow the classic pattern, a biopsy is warranted.

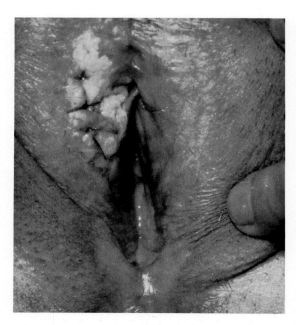

Fig. 48-1. Area of epithelial hyperkeratosis and early cancer.

Finally, presentation of condylomatous lesions of the vulva associated with human papillomavirus are increasingly common, especially in younger women. In older women the new presentation of condylomatous lesions necessitates a biopsy. In younger women, biopsy may initially be optional, but failure to resolve promptly after therapy necessitates biopsy.

Multifocal disease is common with benign diagnoses and carcinoma in situ. Unifocal disease is more common with invasive disease. Multifocal disease warrants more than one biopsy, although selection of the most suspicious area is appropriate.

DIAGNOSIS

Biopsy of the lesion is required for diagnosis. Tissue should be obtained from obviously ulcerated and abnormal areas with an attempt to include normal tissue and a depth of tissue that will

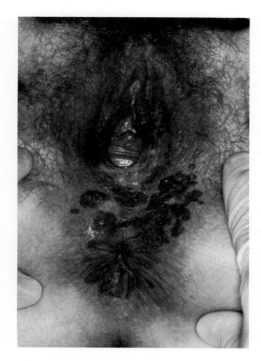

Fig. 48-2. Multiple areas of pigmented carcinoma in situ.

allow estimates of invasion. As noted previously, multiple lesions will necessitate multiple biopsies for the most accurate evaluation.

Biopsy of the vulva is a simple procedure easily accomplished in the ambulatory setting. A Keye's punch is most often used after cleaning and numbing the skin. This allows a core biopsy 3 to 7 mm in diameter, which can then be carefully raised and incised at the base with iris scissors. Local cauterization with silver nitrate usually is adequate for any bleeding following biopsy.

PATHOLOGY AND TREATMENT

Most invasive cancers of the vulva are squamous. Ten percent to 15% of invasive cancers are other cell types, including melanomas, adenocarcinomas, and sarcomas. These are rare types that often

Table 48-1. International Federation of Gynecology and Obstetrics staging system for vulvar cancer

TUMOR	
T1	≤2 cm
2	>2 cm
3	Spread to lower urethra, vagina, anus
4	Involving upper urethra, bladder, rectum, fixed to bone

NODE STATUS	
N0	Negative nodes
1	Unilateral regional node metastasis
2	Bilateral regional node metastasis

METASTASES	
M0	No metastases
1	Distant metastases (including pelvic nodes)

Stage I	T1 N0 M0
Stage II	T2 N0 M0
Stage III	T1 2 N1 M0
	T3 N0 1 M0
Stage IVA	T1 2 3 N2 M0
	T4 Any N M0
Stage IVB	Any T Any N M1

necessitate a different pattern of treatment and should be managed at cancer treatment centers by physicians with extensive experience with vulvar malignancy.

Carcinoma in situ of the vulva is successfully treated by local excision, laser ablation, and occasionally by topical chemotherapy. The choice of treatment depends on the lesion size and location.

Based on clinical examination, an International Federation of Gynecology and Obstetrics (FIGO) and primary tumor, regional nodes, and metastasis (TNM) stage (Table 48-1) is assigned. Small local lesions can be cured by surgery (Fig.

48-1). The extent of the surgery is predicated by the size of the lesion, the depth of invasion, and the location in the vulva. Some early unilateral lesions, for example, are appropriately treated by radical unilateral vulvectomy with or without concurrent node dissection. The survival rate is significantly influenced by the stage of the disease. The most common stages, I and II, have a 90%,

5-year survival rate that is higher for negative nodes and lower for positive nodes (decreasing with the number of positive nodes). For stage III the survival rate is 40%, but drops to only 25% for stage IV disease. For locally advanced disease, an alternative to surgical treatment is radiation and chemotherapy with a 50%, 5-year survival in this highly selected population.

CRITICAL POINTS

- Delays in diagnosis of vulvar malignancy may result in a higher stage of disease at diagnosis and decreased survival rates.
- Vulvar cancer is most common in older women.
- Vulvar cancer can mimic other benign lesions and can be differentiated only by biopsy.
- Squamous carcinoma is the most common cell type.
- Therapy is primarily surgical except for very advanced disease.

Questions

1. A 62-year-old woman is seen for a 3-month history of vulvar itching. She has been very healthy and has no history of previous cancers. Her 26-year-old daughter has both herpes and papillomavirus. This patient's highest risk factor for vulvar cancer is:
   A. Age
   B. Family history of sexually transmitted disease
   C. General health
   D. Itching
2. A 22-year-old pregnant woman is seen at 18 weeks' gestational age with new onset of condylomatous lesions. She has a history of carcinoma in situ of the cervix treated by cone biopsy 1 year previously. She smokes one pack of cigarettes per day. Examination reveals multiple slightly pigmented papillary lesions of both labia majora. The most likely diagnosis on biopsy is:

   A. Carcinoma in situ
   B. Invasive squamous carcinoma
   C. Malignant melanoma
   D. Invasive adenocarcinoma
3. A 53-year-old woman with biopsy-proved squamous carcinoma of the vulva is seen for consultation to plan treatment. She has a 1-cm lesion on the right labium majus. She has no palpable groin nodes. The most appropriate treatment for this patient is:
   A. Surgery alone
   B. Radiation plus surgery
   C. Radiation plus chemotherapy
   D. Radiation alone

Answers

1. A
2. A
3. A

49

Cervical disease and neoplasia

APGO LEARNING OBJECTIVE #49

Joanna M. Cain

Detection and treatment of preinvasive cervical lesions reduces the medical and social costs, as well as the mortality, associated with carcinoma of the cervix.

The student will demonstrate a knowledge of the following:

A. Symptoms and physical findings of cervicitis and neoplasia
B. Management of the patient with an abnormal Pap smear
C. Histologic categories
D. Risk factors
E. Course of cervical neoplastic disease
F. International Federation of Gynecology and Obstetrics staging
G. Indications for screening

Cervical cancer is a disease that has been significantly decreased because of an effective screening test—the Pap smear. Further decreases in its incidence will require reduced exposure of women to risk factors and a better understanding of the multifaceted nature of its oncogenesis.

RISK FACTORS AND PRESENTATION

Most cervical cancer (80%) is squamous in origin and is dependent on the presence of multiple risk factors. The ethnic background of women was associated with the disease in the past, but more recent figures show an increasing trend in young white women and a decreasing trend in black women. The most prominent among the risk factors is the presence of human papillomavirus (HPV), particularly certain subtypes such as 16 and 18. The direct effect of the virus on oncogenesis is unknown, but it is best conceptualized as making a hostile environment for normal deoxyribonucleic (DNA) repair. Obviously, other factors that impair a cell's ability to repair DNA and provide normal metabolic support will increase damage to the cell and oncogenesis, including nutritional deficiencies (chronic alcoholism and low folate and retinoic acid levels). Other factors related to cervical cancer are cigarette smoking and immunosuppression (human immunodeficiency virus [HIV] and chronic corticosteroid use are examples). Also, increasing intervals between Pap smears (greater than 3 years) is associated with a higher incidence of invasive cervical cancers.

Classic risk factors—early first intercourse, marriage or conception at an early age, and multiple sexual partners—are markers for increased exposure to various viruses, as well as signs of increased risk-taking behavior in some women, and may be correlated with increases in cigarette smoking and alcohol abuse. It is important to note that most women with these risk factors do *not* get cervical cancer. Therefore the pattern of oncogenesis is more than a "sexually transmitted disease," which is how this cancer often is depicted. Such a categorization is an undue burden on patients with this disease and is far too simplistic to describe the disease as such. Nor is it a "disease of promiscuity" because women who have only one sexual partner still can get cervical cancer. A burden of causation and censorship is not appropriate to health care givers.

Since the progression of oncogenesis seems to be cumulative in cervical cancer, it is not surprising that a history of cervical intraepithelial neoplasia (CIN) is a risk factor. These lesions need to be thought of as a continuum of disease, not as separate, discrete abnormalities (Fig. 49-1). Clearly, many more women have CIN than invasive cancer, and the progression rate to cervical cancer of untreated CIN varies widely, depending on the grade of CIN and on intrinsic biologic properties of the neoplastic process that are poorly understood at present.

The classic presentation of invasive cancer is bleeding or spotting after intercourse. Rarely is CIN symptomatic. If spotting cannot be explained (e.g., by concurrent infection), malignancy must be highly suspected and the source of the bleeding explained. Bleeding between menses, after menopause, and heavy and unusual discharge or bleeding with menses also can be signs of this disease. Sometimes women describe a watery discharge

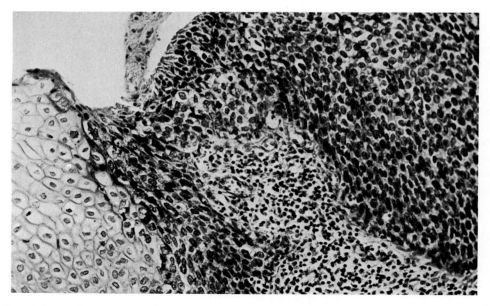

Fig. 49-1. Carcinoma in situ of cervix. Mature cells occur on left with abrupt change to complete loss of maturation on right, with intact basement membrane.

that is blood-tinged. This bleeding generally is painless. Pain occurs only when the tumor has extended far enough to invade the pelvic nerves in the lateral pelvic wall and the nerve roots. Therefore pain usually indicates far-advanced disease.

Most women with cervical cancer remain well nourished, even with advanced disease, because of lack of bowel involvement. Weight loss, then, is a sign of advanced disease.

EVALUATION

Dysplasia and malignant changes of the cervix must be differentiated from normal cervical architecture. The normal cervix undergoes metaplasia throughout a woman's life (Fig. 49-2). This occurs in a transformation zone (TZ), where mucus-secreting glandular cells interact actively with non–mucus-secreting squamous cells. This process is most active during adolescence and pregnancy (which may be related to the higher risk associated with early age of intercourse and exposure to viral material). Furthermore, the by-

products of cigarette smoke are concentrated in cervical mucus and have been associated with a depletion of the cells of Langerhans, which are macrophages that assist in cell-mediated immunity in the TZ.

Benign changes in the cervix such as nabothian cysts, cervical polyps, and ectropion can be quite disturbing to the patient. Differentiation of these from malignancies can be done by colposcopy if not grossly obvious. Nabothian cysts have a characteristic domed, glassy surface and mucus in their internal cavity. Polyps often arise from the endocervix and have a smooth, often friable surface. Ectropion generally is circumferentially equal and uniform in appearance. Colposcopy, however, can additionally identify the fact that the surface is not heaped up or irregular and that there is no abnormality of the blood vessel structure involved. It is important to note that although Pap smears are effective screening methods when the cervix appears normal, the presence of bleeding or inflammation with other pathology decreases the smear's effectiveness. In fact, Pap smears of visible malignant lesions have been read as negative or

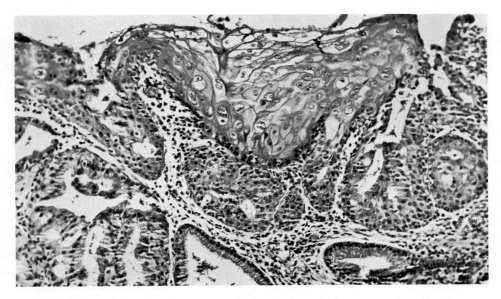

Fig. 49-2. Section showing squamous metaplasia of endocervical mucosa and contiguous crypts (×164).

atypical. If the visible changes are not clearly a normal or infectious condition of the cervix, biopsy is warranted.

Colposcopy is an effective technique to differentiate normal and abnormal epithelial covering of the cervix. This technique involves inspection of the TZ and the squamocolumnar junction under 7.5-power to 30-power magnification after the application of a 3% to 5% acetic acid solution. Findings are based on the increasing metabolic demand of the lesion as developing new capillaries project toward the surface early (punctation) and then consolidate with each other (mosaic) as the metabolic demands increase. Vessels that have an abnormal branching or screw shape reflect an underlying disorganization associated with malignancy. Lesions also can vary in thickness, making them appear white through the colposcope. Abnormal areas are biopsied. An endocervical canal curettage is often performed in conjunction with colposcopy to rule out dysplasia within the canal that might not be seen colposcopically. Obviously only lesions that can be seen are adequately evaluated by this technique. Since the TZ is the most likely area for development of cancerous lesions, the lack of a complete visualization of this area must be noted. Usually, colposcopy and biopsy are done for two sequential "atypical" Pap smears, for any findings consistent with CIN or above on a Pap smear, or for any unusual lesion of the cervix.

TREATMENT

Preinvasive cervical disease

The justification for treating CIN is its potential for progression to invasive disease. Because no tests exist that can differentiate lesions that will or will not progress, treatment is intended to eradicate the lesions. One exception is early CIN I, where progression to higher CINs often is low and regression to normal occurs in up to 40% of cases. If the patient with this lesion is compliant and can be closely evaluated, treatment may be postponed pending further evaluation over time. Also, CIN diagnosed during pregnancy represents a specific situation in which delay until the pregnancy is completed is desired. The TZ usually is easy to identify during pregnancy because the cervical canal is everted and clearly visible. Colposcopic-directed biopsies can be taken, although bleeding is greater than in nonpregnant women. Conization during pregnancy carries a significant risk of hemorrhage and abortion. It is therefore indicated only to exclude an invasive cancer. The extent of the lesion almost always can be determined by colposcopy, eliminating the need for conization in most women.

For all other CIN lesions, the major options are laser vaporization, cryotherapy, or removal of the lesions and a margin. Various means are used, including cervical conization and diathermy loop. Removal with a margin is particularly important if invasive disease is possible or when the suspected lesion cannot be adequately visualized. Cure rates for one treatment range from 85% to 96%. Repeat treatment of an adequately evaluated persistent lesion can effect a cure rate as high as 95%. Posttreatment follow-up is important because risk of recurrent or persistent CIN is at least 5% to 15%. Eighty-five percent are detected within 2 years of the initial treatment. A Pap smear and colposcopy should be done 3 months posttreatment. Repeat Pap smears should be done at least every 6 months and repeat colposcopic exams performed as indicated.

Invasive disease

Early invasive disease is often called "microinvasive." This is a poor term because the definition of this disease differs between institutions and the International Federation of Gynecology and Obstetrics (FIGO) staging system. The FIGO system reports disease that is less than 5 mm deep and less than 7 mm wide as microinvasive. The Society of Gynecologic Oncologists recommends less than 3 mm depth from the basement membrane and no confluent tongues or vascular or lymphatic invasion as its definition of microinvasive disease. This

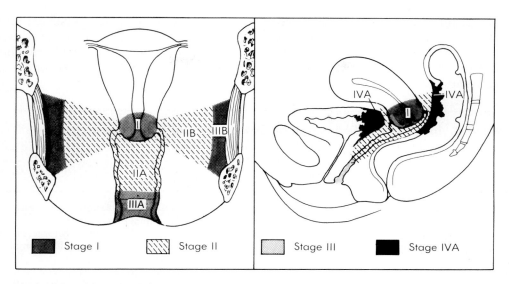

Fig. 49-3. Staging system for carcinoma of cervix uteri according to International Federation of Gynecology and Obstetrics (FIGO).

is the definition that is used to determine treatment, particularly conservative treatment, for this disease. Usually the treatment of microinvasion is hysterectomy. However, in selected cases a cervical conization with clearly negative margins may be adequate for initial therapy if future pregnancy is desired. The need for close observation and evaluation still exists for those managed conservatively.

The extent to which the cervix and its surrounding structures are involved with cancer is referred to as the *clinical stage* of the disease. Because increased involvement influences prognosis (usually measured by a 5-year survival percentage), the stage reflects prognosis. Cervical cancer spreads by direct extension and through the lymphatics. The pelvic lymph nodes, then, are the first echelon of nodes affected. They are involved in 13% of women with stage I lesions, 30% in stage II, 46% in stage III, and 53% in stage IV (Fig. 49-3). Staging is assigned by inspection, vaginal and rectal palpation, and biopsy. Obviously, clinical staging is not always accurate because involved nodes and other extensions of the disease cannot always be recognized. For critical decisions, biopsies of lymph nodes, singly or in greater numbers,

may be appropriate but are not required to stage this disease.

Treatment is predicated on control of the local tumor spread and potential sites of metastases (primarily lymph nodes) (Table 49-1). For early lesions where the entire tumor and nodal tissue can be removed with a margin of normal tissue, radical hysterectomy with lymph node dissection or radiation therapy is appropriate. When tumor has advanced beyond this area, radiation therapy is the mainstay of treatment.

Advanced disease

Little can be done for patients in whom radiation or radical surgical procedures or both have failed to control the cancer. As the disease advances it invades the nerve roots, particularly the sciatic plexus, and constricts the ureters and possibly the rectosigmoid. Continued growth in the cervix itself produces a necrotic crater that may bleed with the slightest irritation. Death usually occurs from uremia caused by ureteral obstruction, infection, hemorrhage, or combinations of the three. Chemotherapy has a limited role in this disease. Cisplatin has activity in squamous cell cancer of the cervix and can be used for metastatic disease. It can provide an objective response in approximately 30% of patients treated but is only palliative in nature.

At this stage, the physician should prescribe whatever medications are needed to relieve pain and keep the patient reasonably comfortable. There is no place for heroic measures simply to prolong life.

Table 49-1. International Federation of Gynecology and Obstetrics stages and treatments

Stage	Description	Treatment
0	In situ	Cryotherapy, laser ablation, cone biopsy
IA$_1$	Microinvasion	Total abdominal hysterectomy
IA$_2$	No greater than 5 mm deep and 7 mm wide	Total abdominal hysterectomy for less than 3 mm deep and without capillary-lymphatic involvement
		Radical hysterectomy, pelvic lymph node dissection for deeper than 3 mm or capillary-lymphatic involvement
IB	Confined to cervix	Radical hysterectomy, pelvic lymph node dissection; bilateral salpingo-oophorectomy optional, depending on age
IIA	Upper ⅔ vagina involved; parametrium free	Radiation therapy preferred; radical hysterectomy for smaller lesions
IIB	Parametrium involved but not to side wall; IVP normal	Radiation therapy
IIIA	Extension to lower ⅓ vagina, not to side wall	Radiation therapy
IIIB	Extension to one or both pelvic side walls or obstructed ureter on IVP	Radiation therapy
IVA	Extension to bladder-rectum	Radiation therapy
IVB	Distant metastases	Chemotherapy, palliative care

IVP, Intravenous pyelogram.

CRITICAL POINTS

- Postcoital bleeding is the hallmark of cervical cancer.
- Risk factors for cervical cancer include increased exposure to HPV, HIV, smoking, and immunosuppressive drugs.
- Biopsy, not Pap smears, provides the appropriate method of evaluation for a visible abnormality of the cervix.
- Colposcopy identifies abnormal areas but does not make a diagnosis.
- Invasive cervical cancer spreads locally and by lymphatic spread.
- Treatment of cervical cancer is either surgical or by radiation therapy.

Questions

1. A 22-year-old gravida I para II is seen for spotting between menses. She is using no birth control and having regular intercourse. She was diagnosed with condylomata of the vulva 1 year previously, but these have not recurred since treatment. On physical examination an ulcerated irregular lesion of the cervix is seen. The next step in management of this lesion is:
   A. Biopsy
   B. Cryotherapy
   C. Pap smear
   D. Darkfield examination
   E. Laser vaporization

2. A 54-year-old woman comes to the physician for a routine evaluation. She is an 80-pack per year smoker. A cervical conization had been performed when she was 49 for CIN III of the cervix. She had menopause 4 years previously and had no bleeding nor pelvic examination since. She was started on estrogen replacement at that time. She has a normal examination, but her Pap smear returns with findings consistent with CIN II. The next step in management of this patient is:
   A. Repeat Pap smear
   B. Perform colposcopy
   C. Cervical conization
   D. Cryotherapy

3. A 25-year-old patient with a question of microinvasive cervical cancer on a biopsy comes to the physician to discuss her options. She has heard that this can sometimes be treated with cryotherapy and would like to try that so she can have children. She has recently married and plans to have children right away. The most appropriate management for this patient is:
   A. Cervical conization
   B. Cryotherapy
   C. Laser ablation
   D. Radical hysterectomy

Answers

1. A
2. B
3. A

50

Uterine leiomyomas

APGO LEARNING OBJECTIVE #50

Joanna M. Cain

Uterine leiomyomas are the most common gyneco-logic neoplasm and often are asymptomatic. Physicians frequently must distinguish myomas from other pelvic masses that may need more urgent management.

The student will demonstrate a knowledge of the following:
A. Symptoms and physical findings of cervicitis and neoplasia
B. Methods to confirm the diagnosis
C. Indications for surgical treatment

Diseases of the uterus are numerous. The therapy of benign conditions of the uterus is predicated on a sound knowledge of the pathophysiology of the disease process. The benign lesions that most often enlarge the uterus are leiomyomas and adenomyosis.

SYMPTOMS AND RISK FACTORS

Leiomyomas—also called myomas, fibromyomas, or fibroids—are found in the uterus in 30% to 50% of all women over age 30. Leiomyomas occur earlier and at a higher frequency in black women. The frequency of adenomyosis is more difficult to estimate, varying from 10% to 90% of women over age 40. Both conditions can present with increasing menstrual abnormalities and flow changes over time. The classic presentation of adenomyosis is increasing colicky pain and menstrual bleeding after age 40. Both conditions can be entirely without symptoms. Leiomyoma is not associated with increased cramping unless the uterus is trying to expel a pediculated myoma. The presence of intermenstrual or postmenopausal symptoms suggests another abnormality, and a diagnosis of leiomyoma or adenomyosis is not adequate to explain the symptom without significant evaluation for a concurrent malignancy.

The presence of pain or pressure suggests either growth in uterine size or potential degeneration of a myoma. Many women experience bladder pressure and frequency of urination as the tumors grow. Occasionally a large tumor in the anterior uterine wall will push the fundus posteriorly into the cul-de-sac and rotate the cervix anteriorly beneath the pubis, where it compresses the vesical neck. As the tumor grows, it becomes progressively more difficult to initiate urination, and obstruction of both the urethra and the ureters can occur. A large posterior fibroid can lead to increasing pressure on the rectum, causing constipation.

The cause of both conditions is unknown, although growth of leiomyomas may be related to stimulation by estrogen. This theory is supported by the fact that the tumors are uncommon before the ovaries have functioned for several years and that their growth usually ceases after menopause. Rapid enlargement of leiomyomas can occur in some women who take oral contraceptives when large doses of estrogen are used, but this effect should be rare with the changes in composition of oral contraceptives.

The relationship of myomas to infertility is difficult to assess because patients with large myomas may have no difficulty with fertility. Therefore the growths cannot be assumed to be a source of infertility, and further work-up is warranted. Myomas are, however, associated with both spontaneous pregnancy loss and early delivery, depending on their location and blood supply.

PHYSICAL FINDINGS AND DIFFERENTIAL DIAGNOSIS

The pathology of these benign conditions is relevant to the physical findings. Leiomyomas develop from immature smooth muscle cells of the uterine wall. These can be made up almost entirely of muscle, but strands of fibrous tissue appear between the bundles of unstriated muscle as the tumor enlarges. Tumors may be single or multiple and may occur in any area of the uterus (Fig. 50-1). They are designated by their position in the uterus, with the submucous fibroid being the most likely to affect pregnancy and bleeding, although it often does not change the uterine size or shape. The classic physical finding of myomas is a smooth, irregularly enlarged uterine shape with normal ovarian structures. Since these myomas can become pediculated, they can mimic enlarged ovaries. They can also become parasitic. Having lost their blood supply from the uterus, they obtain it from such nearby tissues as the colon or small bowel. This is fortunately rare but presents a dilemma in diagnosis that often necessitates additional studies and even surgery to clarify. A painful mass suggests degeneration of fibroids from hemorrhage with necrosis or cystic or carneous (more common during pregnancy) degeneration the result. In postmenopausal women, the mass can feel particularly hard. This is evidence of calcium deposition and is well seen on a flat x-ray film of the abdomen (Fig. 50-2).

Abnormal bleeding is almost always caused by submucous or intramural tumors that enlarge and distort the uterine cavity. The excessive bleeding may simply be caused by the increased endometrial surface in the uterus and possibly by an increase in the number and size of endometrial veins in association with submucous tumors.

Adenomyosis results from the interposition of endometrial glands between the myometrial muscle bundles discontinuous from the endometrial cavity. This is usually a diffuse process throughout the entire thickness of the uterine wall, resulting in a smooth, softly enlarged but regular-shaped uterus. This rarely exceeds a size comparable with a pregnancy of 8 to 10 weeks. As noted previously, this condition needs to be dif-

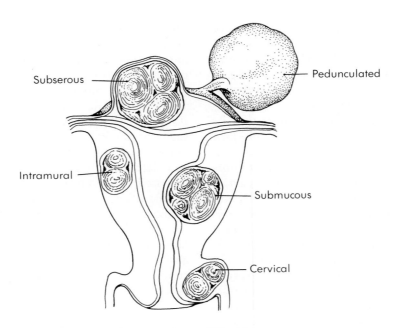

Fig. 50-1. Types of fibroid tumors.

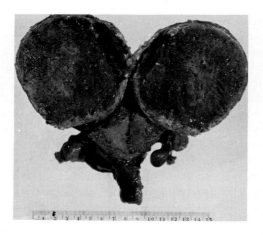

Fig. 50-2. Large, hard, calcified fibroid.

ferentiated from a large submucous fibroid. In general, the uterus is only mildly tender, if at all. The condition is symptomatic only with menses because the confined patches of endometrium grow under the stimulus of the rising estrogen concentration and then disintegrate and bleed as

the stimulus is withdrawn. Excessive bleeding may reflect the expanding endometrial surface as the uterus enlarges.

DIAGNOSIS

Abnormal uterine bleeding in the perimenopausal period warrants sampling of the endometrium to rule out malignancy. Differentiation between benign conditions depends on collaborating the physical findings and symptoms. If this does not present a classic picture, particularly if the ovaries cannot be differentiated from the mass, a pelvic-vaginal ultrasound examination can aid the diagnosis. Hysteroscopy can be helpful if a submucous fibroid is suspected but not confirmed by ultrasound. The use of Ca-125 to screen for malignancy in these patients with uterine abnormalities is not encouraged because of the high frequency of false-positive values in menstruating women and in women with hemorrhage or necrosis of leiomyomas.

THERAPY

Both conditions are significantly improved after menopause. If a patient is near menopause, attempts to wait out the perimenopausal period without surgical or pharmacologic intervention are warranted. These conditions do not rule out replacement estrogen after menopause, however.

Although there are multiple alternative therapies for myomas, the only uniformly successful treatment for adenomyosis is hysterectomy. If dysmenorrhea can be controlled and menopause can be expected soon, surgery should be avoided.

Leiomyomas are treated according to their location and their associated symptoms. If small and symptom-free, observation over time is appropriate. If submucous and symptomatic, hys-

teroscopy with resection of the area is appropriate. Gonadotropin-releasing hormone (GnRH) antagonists can cause significant reductions in size (up to 50%), but rapid growth can occur after cessation. Therefore their use generally is limited to the presurgical reduction in size for proposed myomectomies or rare hysterectomies in which significant increased morbidity might occur if the leiomyoma is not reduced in size. Continuation of the "menopausal" state induced by GnRH agonists carries with it the bone density and cardiac concerns of menopause itself and thus is not indicated as a prolonged medical therapy in young women. Myomectomies allow preservation of the uterus but still necessitate abdominal incisions and exposure to surgical morbidity, including bleeding.

CRITICAL POINTS

- Leiomyomas are more common in black women.
- Postmenopausal and intermenstrual bleeding *are not* characteristic of benign uterine conditions.
- Crampy secondary dysmenorrhea is associated with adenomyosis.
- Inability to differentiate ovaries from the mass warrants further work-up.
- Both adenomyosis and leiomyomas are ameliorated by menopause.

Questions

1. A 46-year-old woman has a history of increasing bladder frequency and slightly increased menstrual flow. She also has had occasional skipped menses and rare hot flushes. On examination a 10-cm smooth fundal mass is palpated in the uterus. Ovaries cannot definitively be felt. The next step in the management of this patient is:
   A. Ca-125
   B. Pelvic ultrasound
   C. Hysteroscopy
   D. Repeat exam in 1 month

2. A 43-year-old gravida II para II comes to her physician because of severe bleeding and increasing cramping with menses. Examination reveals a soft, 10-cm uterus and normal adnexa. An endometrial biopsy shows secretory endometrium. Attempts to treat the dysmenorrhea medically have failed. The most effective next step in management for this patient is:
   A. Laparoscopy

B. Hysteroscopy
C. Gonadotropin-releasing hormone agonist
D. Hysterectomy

3. A 33-year-old gravida IV para III, spontaneous abortion I (6 months previous), comes to the physician because of a crampy feeling unrelated to menses and increased bleeding with menses. On examination a 1-cm smooth mass is seen at the os of a slightly dilated cervix. The woman desires further pregnancies. The best approach to therapy is:

A. Hysteroscopy
B. Hysterectomy
C. Laparoscopy
D. Gonadotropin-releasing hormone agonist therapy

Answers

1. B
2. D
3. A

51
Endometrial carcinoma

APGO LEARNING OBJECTIVE #51

Joanna M. Cain

Endometrial carcinoma is a major concern for women using estrogen replacement therapy.

The student will demonstrate a knowledge of the following:
A. Management of the patient with postmenopausal bleeding
B. Risk factors for endometrial carcinoma
C. Symptoms and physical findings
D. Methods to diagnose endometrial carcinoma
E. International Federation of Gynecology and Obstetrics staging

Carcinoma of the body of the uterus is the most common gynecologic cancer diagnosed in the United States. Approximately 37,000 new cases are diagnosed yearly, and 3000 to 4000 deaths are attributed to endometrial cancer. The most important feature of this disease is the potential for early diagnosis based on its classic presentation as postmenopausal bleeding.

SYMPTOMS AND RISK FACTORS

Carcinoma of the endometrium can occur at any age. However, only 5% occur in women under 40, and 75% occur over the age of 50. Estrogen is implicated in the development of these cancers, but its contribution to the etiology is not known. Estrogen-secreting tumors, polycystic ovarian disease (with its increased estrogen environment), and unopposed estrogen replacement have all been associated with the disease. Obesity is associated with a threefold increase in risk for women who are 20 to 30 lb over their ideal body weight and a ninefold increase for women who are 50 lb over their ideal body weight. Because fat is a major site in which androgenic steroids are converted to estrogen, obese women are subjected to higher levels of estrogen than are those at or below normal weight. Obesity also predisposes to diabetes

467

and hypertension, which is why these medical disorders are likely associated with endometrial cancer.

Cyclic administration of progesterone to women with polycystic ovarian disease, anovulatory bleeding, and during postmenopausal estrogen therapy reduces the incidence of uterine cancer. Regular use of oral contraceptives with subsequent prolonged decreased activity of the endometrium also decreases risk for uterine cancer.

The administration of tamoxifen to patients with breast cancer, or its use for other risk factors for breast cancer such as family history, has been associated with a slight increase in the risk of endometrial cancer (approximately 1.6%). There also is a slight increase in risk for endometrial cancer associated with a diagnosis of breast or ovarian cancer.

The hallmark of aberrations of hormonal stimulation of the endometrium is the presence of hyperplasia. Hyperplasia is a general term that encompasses a variety of proliferative endometrial patterns that often occur with abnormal bleeding. Unless there is cytologic atypia, however, hyperplasias generally are not considered premalignant. Because of the abnormal growth and blood supply of endometrial cancers, they are associated with perimenopausal and menopausal bleeding. In the rare cases in women under age 40, they are associated with abnormal uterine bleeding.

Endometrial cancer often produces early symptoms, the first of which can be a serous, malodorous discharge. Frequently it is not regarded seriously by the patient. The watery leukorrhea soon is replaced by a bloody discharge, intermittent spotting, or steady bleeding that can progress eventually to hemorrhage if ignored.

DIFFERENTIAL DIAGNOSIS

The possibility of carcinoma of the uterus is immediately suggested when irregular uterine bleeding occurs near menopause or when there is post-menopausal bleeding. Although only 20% of postmenopausal bleeding is caused by pelvic carcinoma, the physician cannot afford to disregard this important early sign of the lesion. The possibility of bleeding from other sources such as bladder or rectum also must be considered.

Pap smears are not helpful in the evaluation of endometrial cancer because only 50% are found to be positive in the presence of an abnormality. Glandular abnormalities on Pap smears can, however, be the only sign of endometrial cancer in rare cases. The classic sign of postmenopausal bleeding and irregular bleeding not explained by other causes premenopausally warrants endometrial sampling to differentiate hyperplasias and endometrial cancers. Hyperplasias show a progression from normal-appearing proliferative endometrium to atypical hyperplasia that is thought to be premalignant (Fig. 51-1). The risk of progression from hyperplasias, including atypical hyperplasia, is estimated in the range of 1% to 4%.

Fractional dilatation and curettage (D&C) of the endometrium has been the standard for diagnosis of this disease. However, office endocervical and endometrial biopsy with a diagnosis of cancer is adequate. Further investigation including a D&C is appropriate if the diagnosis does not fit the symptoms. The use of hysteroscopy may be helpful in identifying lesions in patients where diagnoses are not identified by biopsy alone. The important element of diagnosis is the need for sampling of the endocervical and endometrial tissue.

STAGING

The stages of endometrial cancer are outlined in Table 51-1. The metastatic pattern of this disease depends on invasion of the myometrium and access to blood and lymphatic vessels during that invasive process. Spread by access through the lymphatics occurs to the pelvic and periaortic lymph nodes. Spread hematogenously will reach the lungs and liver. Spread across the serosa often

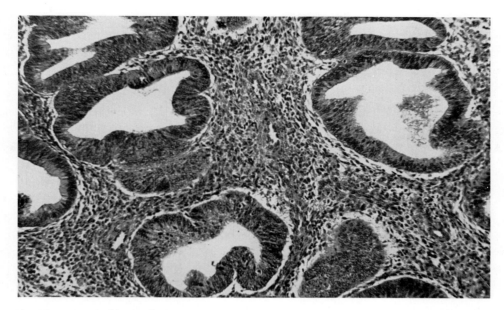

Fig. 51-1. Atypical hyperplasia, or carcinoma in situ, of endometrium. Glands are well formed, show no secretory activity, and have large cells, some cellular disorientation, and disparity in size.

Table 51-1. **International Federation of Gynecology and Obstetrics stages and treatments for uterine cancer**

Stage	Description	Treatment
IA G1, 2, 3	Confined to endometrium	TAH/BSO + RT for G3
IB G1, 2, 3	Less than 50% myometrial invasion	TAH/BSO + RT for G3
IC G1, 2, 3	Greater than 50% myometrial invasion	TAH/BSO + RT
IIA	Endocervical gland involvement	TAH/BSO + RT
IIB	Cervical stromal invasion	TAH/BSO + RT
IIIA	Uterine serosal or adnexal involvement	TAH/BSO + RT
IIIB	Vaginal metastases	Preoperative RT + TAH/BSO
IIIC	Positive pelvic or paraaortic lymph nodes	TAH/BSO + RT
IVA	Extension to rectum or bladder	Preoperative RT + TAH/BSO
IVB	Distant metastatic or inguinal node involvement	TAH/BSO + systemic therapy

G1, Well differentiated; *G2,* moderately differentiated; *G3,* poorly differentiated; *TAH/BSO,* total abdominal hysterectomy/bilateral salpingo-oophorectomy; *RT,* radiation therapy.

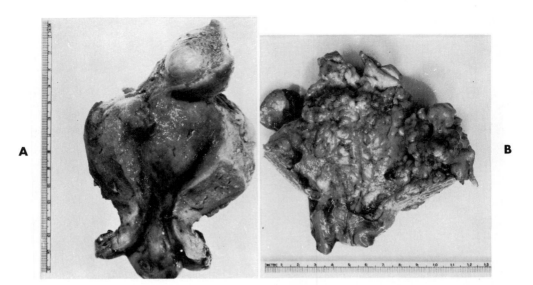

Fig. 51-2. Invasive carcinoma of corpus. **A,** Circumscribed adenocarcinoma: superficial raised area 2.5 cm in diameter is at right cornu. **B,** Diffuse, superficial carcinoma.

presents a picture similar to ovarian cancers. Most endometrial cancers are stage I, probably a function of their characteristic early symptoms, which lead to early diagnosis.

TREATMENT

Abdominal hysterectomy and bilateral salpingo-oophorectomy with pelvic and paraaortic node sampling is the operation most frequently indicated and is the most important part of the treatment of endometrial carcinoma. Vaginal hysterectomy may be preferable to an abdominal operation in extremely obese women, but it may be difficult to evaluate the lymph nodes and to remove the tubes and ovaries if the structures are atrophic.

Primary hysterectomy alone is most appropriate for women with early, well-differentiated, superficially invasive endometrial cancer (Fig. 51-2). Radiation therapy is added postoperatively for high-risk features such as poorly differentiated tumors, deep myometrial invasion, or involved lymph nodes. Radiation may consist of combined external pelvic radiotherapy and vaginal cuff irradiation. In many centers all patients receive at least vaginal cuff irradiation with cesium to decrease the incidence of vaginal cuff recurrence. When cuff irradiation is given preoperatively or postoperatively, the incidence of vaginal cuff recurrence decreases from a reported 10% to 1%.

Results

The prognosis is determined by the clinical stage of the disease when it is diagnosed, the depth of penetration, the histologic pattern, and the degree of differentiation of the tumor. The 5-year survival of women with stage IA grade 1 disease is approximately 95% to 98%; survival decreases to 60% for stage IC grade 3. Treatment failures increase with more advanced lesions. Many failures reflect the condition of the patients, as well as the disease and its treatment. Many women with endometrial cancer are poor risks for any form of treatment; others have disease that is too extensive to eradicate.

CRITICAL POINTS

- Postmenopausal bleeding is the classic symptom of endometrial cancer.
- Endocervical and endometrial sampling is required for diagnosis.
- Endometrial cancers are associated with endogenous and exogenous forms of unopposed estrogen.
- The stage is low and the prognosis excellent for most of these cancers.
- Management of these cancers necessitates removal of the uterus, tubes, and ovaries, and surgical staging in most cases.

Questions

1. A 44-year-old gravida II para II has had increasing menstrual and intermenstrual bleeding for the past 3 months. She had a normal Pap smear 3 months previously. On examination she is 5 feet 3 inches in height and weighs 95 kg. She has no uterine or pelvic abnormalities with the exception of a small amount of blood-tinged mucus in her cervical os. The next step in management of this patient is:
   A. Ultrasound of the pelvis
   B. Endometrial sampling
   C. Hysteroscopy
   D. Endometrial cultures
2. A 71-year-old woman is seen for a routine follow-up evaluation for breast cancer; she is presently on tamoxifen. She reports a watery discharge, occasionally blood-tinged, over the last 2 months. An endometrial biopsy shows necrosis and cystic hyperplasia.

The next step in management is:
   A. Perform a fractional D&C.
   B. Repeat the endometrial biopsy.
   C. Do an ultrasound of the pelvis.
   D. Stop tamoxifen therapy.
3. A 61-year-old gravida V para V has had surgery for grade 2 endometrial adenocarcinoma. She had 10% myometrial invasion and all sampled lymph nodes were negative. The final pathology was read as a grade 1. The stage of this patient is:
   A. IA grade 1
   B. IA grade 2
   C. IB grade 1
   D. IB grade 2

Answers

1. B
2. A
3. B

52

Ovarian neoplasms

APGO LEARNING OBJECTIVE #52

Joanna M. Cain

Adnexal masses are a common finding in both symptomatic and asymptomatic patients. Management is based on determining the origin and character of these tumors.

The student will demonstrate a knowledge of the following:

A. Approach to the patient with an adnexal mass
B. Characteristics of functional cysts and benign neoplasms
C. Other conditions presenting as adnexal mass
D. Clinical issues of carcinoma of the ovary
   1. Symptoms and physical findings
   2. Risk factors
   3. Histologic classification
   4. International Federation of Gynecology and Obstetrics staging

The ovarian mass can be a clinically challenging diagnostic puzzle. The etiology of a mass can range from normal physiologic changes to deadly malignancy. A sense of the range of normal anatomy can aid in determining further evaluation and management.

NORMAL PHYSIOLOGY AND PRESENTATION

The ovarian mass rarely can be differentiated from other adnexal structures, and so *adnexal mass* is a clinically appropriate appellation. This would include the fallopian tube and the surrounding tissues. Normal ovaries in newborn girls contain 1 to 2 million primordial follicles. Many of these degenerate before menarche and continue to be lost even as follicles begin to grow under the stimulus of follicle-stimulating hormone during the preovulatory phase of each menstrual cycle. Functional cysts are a product of this normal cycle. A follicle may reach a maximum size of 4 cm (the ovary may be 5 cm in diameter) before ovulation. If the follicle fails to rupture it may continue to grow, even up to 8 or 10 cm. These are often described histologically as *simple cysts*. A *corpus luteum cyst* may occur when the corpus luteum fails to involute, continues to secrete progesterone, and delays the onset of menses. It also may enlarge and produce pain as it expands or if it ruptures and bleeds intraperitoneally. The persistence of a corpus luteum cyst is rare without a concurrent pregnancy. These cysts are suggested by their relationship to the menstrual cycle, with the follicular cyst occurring before, and the corpus luteum cyst after, menses. Unusual functional cysts include the often bilateral theca-lutein cysts associated with human chorionic gonadotropin (HCG) overstimulation or the usually unilateral luteoma of pregnancy (from overgrowth of luteinized theca cells).

These functional cysts and the benign and malignant neoplasms of the tube and ovary are generally asymptomatic. As a tumor grows, patients may experience pressure, enlargement of the abdomen, and vague gastrointestinal complaints. A fixed tumor may produce painful micturition, painful defecation, tenesmus, or pain during coitus. Menstrual disturbances in women with normal cycles are rare (15%). Acute pain generally represents torsion of the ovary or hemorrhage into an ovary. Torsion occurs most often with tumors of moderate size, 8 to 12 cm in diameter. This pain is different in nature from the pain associated with a tuboovarian abscess, which tends to be chronic rather than of sudden onset.

RISK FACTORS

Risk factors for malignancy of the tube and ovary include multiple factors relating to the length of function of the ovary. For example, early menarche, late menopause, and nulliparity are associated with a higher incidence of epithelial ovarian cancers. In contradistinction, the sustained use of oral contraceptives (with ovarian inactivity) decreases the risk more for each sustained year of use. Likewise, early pregnancies and a greater number of pregnancies (with the concurrent decrease in ovarian function for the duration of pregnancy) are associated with a lesser risk.

DIAGNOSIS

Ovarian neoplasms can be diagnosed by pelvic examination except in early stages, when they are too small to palpate. Vague abdominal symptoms, mild gastrointestinal distress, pelvic discomfort, and increasing abdominal girth are warning signs. An ultrasound examination can confirm a clinical suspicion of adnexal neoplasm when physical examination is unclear. Neoplasms develop in retained ovaries after hysterectomy at least at the same rates as when the uterus is in place; hence, regular examinations are important after hysterectomy. If a mass is palpated, evaluation of the mass with reference to menstrual cycles, age, position, and alternative diagnoses must occur. The differential diagnosis of an adnexal mass includes the gastrointestinal and genitourinary systems, as well as infectious causes and metastatic lesions (e.g., breast and colon). Sometimes, cleansing enemas or reexaminations are warranted because of a suspected nonneoplastic cause of the palpated mass. If, however, a new mass is felt in the adnexa in a postmenopausal woman, this is cancer until proved otherwise.

If ovarian cancer is suspected, further laboratory evaluation is appropriate. Among the diagnostic tests ordered, Ca-125, a marker for epithelial cancers, might be considered in older women. In younger women with solid adnexal masses, germ cell malignances must be considered and α-fetoprotein, β-HCG, lactate dehydrogenase (LDH) also may be appropriate.

OVARIAN NEOPLASMS

Ovarian neoplasms occur less often than do functional cysts, but they are far more important. They may grow to be large, can secrete hormones that alter normal physiologic functions, and may be malignant. Small malignant tumors may not be palpated; by the time they are large enough to be felt, the disease may have spread throughout the peritoneal cavity. Any ovary larger than 5 cm in

Table 52-1. Ovarian classification system

I. Neoplasms of germ cell origin
  A. Dysgerminoma
  B. Embryonal teratoma (embryonal carcinoma)
  C. Partially differentiated teratoma (malignant teratoma, solid teratoma)
  D. Mature teratoma (benign cystic teratoma)
  E. Mixed germ cell neoplasms (teratocarcinoma)
  F. Carcinoma or sarcoma arising in a mature teratoma
II. Neoplasms of celomic (germinal) epithelium and its derivatives
  A. Serous (tubal cell) type
  B. Mucinous (endocervical) type
  C. Endometrioid (endometrial cell) type
  D. Brenner tumors
  E. Mixed and unclassified cell types
III. Neoplasms of specialized gonadal stroma (sex cords and mesenchymal)
  A. Granulosa-theca cell group
    1. Granulosa cell tumor
    2. Theca cell tumor
    3. Granulosa-theca cell tumor
  B. Sertoli-Leydig cell group
    1. Sertoli's cell tumor
    2. Leydig's cell tumor (hilus cell)
    3. Arrhenoblastoma
  C. Luteomas

From Abell MR: Ovarian tumor classification, *Can Med Assoc J* 94:1102, 1966.

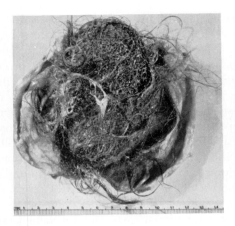

Fig. 52-1. Opened benign cystic teratoma, contents of which are mainly hair and sebaceous material.

diameter at any age may well contain a neoplasm and thus cannot be ignored. The neoplasms of germ cell origin usually occur in women under age 30; those of epithelial origin generally occur after 30. There are many classifications of ovarian neoplasms. A common one is that described by Abell, shown in Table 52-1.

The incidence of carcinoma of the ovaries has been increasing steadily and now accounts for approximately 5% of cancers in women. About 18,000 new cancers of the ovary were diagnosed in 1989, and approximately 12,000 women died of the disease. It is the fourth leading cause of cancer death in women. Cancer of the ovary is unusual before the age of 20 but increases steadily thereafter, with approximately 1.6% of women developing ovarian cancer some time during their lives. The average age at diagnosis is about 50 years. Ovarian cancer occurs somewhat more often in white women than in black women.

Germ cell tumors

A variety of ovarian neoplasms can arise from germ cells. Benign cystic teratomas, or dermoid cysts, which arise from primordial germ cells, comprise approximately 20% of all ovarian neoplasms. They occur at any age and account for about 60% of benign ovarian tumors in girls under age 15. They are the second most common ovarian neoplasm in women of all age groups and are outnumbered only by serous cystadenomas. Benign cystic teratomas usually are between 5 and 10 cm in diameter when diagnosed, but occasionally a dermoid may be 15 cm or larger. Approximately 10% are bilateral.

These tumors are gray, glistening, smooth, and tense. They are cystic, usually a single cavity filled with oily, sebaceous fluid and a mass of matted hair (Fig. 52-1). Usually there is a solid prominence in the tumor wall adjacent to the

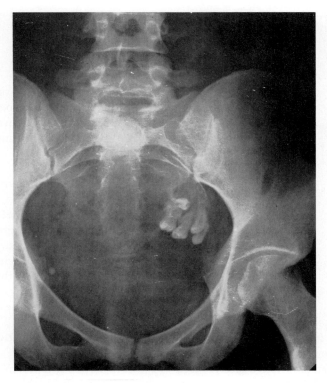

Fig. 52-2. Well-developed teeth within benign cystic teratoma demonstrated by x-ray film examination.

ovary. The prominent tissue is of ectodermal origin, but endodermal and mesodermal structures can be identified. Tissues most often recognized are skin and its appendages, cartilage, and respiratory and neural elements. Importantly, all of the tissues are mature, and occasionally teeth can be seen on flat plate x-ray film examination (Fig. 52-2). Teratomas can give rise to an area of malignancy that develops in an otherwise benign teratoma. It is almost always squamous cell carcinoma.

Immature teratoma

An immature teratoma is a germ cell tumor that contains elements similar to a benign cystic teratoma, but the tissues have undergone a malignant differentiation. The usual tissue is of neural origin. Formerly these tumors were highly malignant and usually fatal, but the advent of multiagent chemotherapy now confers a favorable prognosis.

Dysgerminoma

Dysgerminomas are malignant germ cell tumors, 80% of which are diagnosed during the early reproductive years, usually in teenagers. Usually there are no symptoms except for abdominal enlargement. Although dysgerminomas have no endocrine activity, they may occur in association with ambiguous sexual development. Dysgerminomas usually are unilateral.

The treatment of germ cell malignancies is conservative. Most often a unilateral salpingo-oophorectomy is done, unless widespread me-

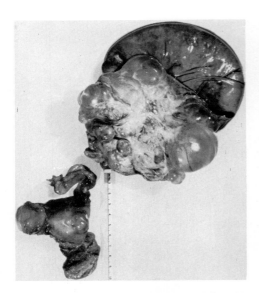

Fig. 52-3. Multilocular serous cystadenoma.

tastases are present, in which case further removal of reproductive organs may be necessary. These tumors have been reported to secrete LDH; when they do so, the LDH often is elevated dramatically to the 10,000 to 15,000 range. These tumors generally are treated with multiagent chemotherapy: cisplatin, bleomycin, and VP-16, for example.

Epithelial tumors

The most common epithelial neoplasms are the serous or mucinous cystadenomas, which account for approximately 50% of all benign ovarian neoplasms. The epithelial neoplasms have a spectrum of differentiation. The cystadenoma is a benign process and is highly treatable by cystectomy or oophorectomy. On the opposite end of the spectrum is a poorly differentiated serous or mucinous cyst, adenocarcinoma. A borderline lesion has been described, sometimes called an ovarian tumor of low malignant potential. This entity, although not completely benign, has a more favorable prognosis and tends to recur late

with an excellent survival in almost all stages of disease.

Serous cystadenoma

Serous cystadenomas occur more frequently than do the mucinous types. They are diagnosed more often in women between the ages of 20 and 50, with a peak incidence during the fourth decade of life (Fig. 52-3).

Mucinous cystadenoma

Differentiating mucinous cystadenomas from serous cystadenomas by gross inspection may be impossible. Mucinous cystadenomas are likely to be larger (Fig. 52-4). Mucinous cysts usually are multilocular and contain thick, straw-colored, viscous fluid. The cells lining the cyst cavity resemble those normally seen in the endocervix.

Malignant epithelial neoplasms

Both serous and mucinous cystadenomas can be malignant from their onset or can undergo malignant change after being present for many years. They account for two thirds of all malignant ovarian tumors; almost all are carcinomas. The endometrioid type is the other common epithelial tumor, and these cells are similar to the endometrial cells that line the uterine cavity. From 30% to 40% of serous tumors are malignant (serous cystadenocarcinoma), compared with only 5% to 10% of the mucinous variety (mucinous cystadenocarcinoma). About half of all ovarian adenocarcinomas are of the serous type, and 15% are mucinous. The remainder are largely of the endometrioid type.

Stromal tumors

Neoplasms of specialized gonadal stroma often secrete either estrogen or an androgen, and the hormone can produce its characteristic effect on the patient.

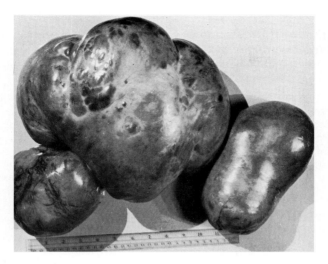

Fig. 52-4.   Bilateral, multilocular mucinous cystadenoma.

Granulosa-theca cell tumors

Granulosa-theca cell tumors may be made predominantly of granulosa cells, theca cells, or a combination of both. Many of these neoplasms secrete estrogen, and thus are called feminizing tumors. The name is not completely accurate, however, as virilization may occur in some women. Granulosa cell tumors are diagnosed most frequently during the climacteric and postmenopausal period, although they may develop in premenarchal girls. The principal symptoms of feminizing tumors are those resulting from estrogen. In young girls, the estrogen stimulates breast and general maturation and uterine bleeding (isosexual precocious puberty). Postmenopausal women with estrogen-secreting tumors may experience postmenopausal bleeding. When this tumor is present, a coexistent endometrial cancer may also exist.

Fibroma

A fibroma occurs most frequently during the fifth and sixth decades of life. Fibromas usually are unilateral and rarely are malignant. Meigs de-

scribed an interesting association of ascites and hydrothorax with ovarian fibromas (Meigs' syndrome). Ascites and hydrothorax also can occur in the presence of other ovarian neoplasms. The physician should consider the possibility of an ovarian neoplasm in anyone with ascites and a pleural effusion.

TREATMENT

The diagnosis and management of ovarian neoplasms usually involves surgery; when malignancy is present, surgery is mandatory for staging (Table 52-2). The benign germ cell and stromal cell tumors should be treated with conservative surgery in the young woman and with at least oophorectomy in the elderly woman. Attention must be paid to future fertility in the young woman, and thus a cystectomy is the usual therapy. In the perimenopausal or postmenopausal patient, a bilateral salpingo-oophorectomy and hysterectomy usually is appropriate, in addition to removal of the benign process. The critical determination is that of malignancy.

Table 52-2. International Federation of Gynecology and Obstetrics stages and treatments for ovarian cancer

Stage	Description	Treatment
IA	Confined to one ovary Capsule intact No tumor on surface	G1, 2: TAH/BSO No further treatment G3: P32 or chemotherapy
IB	Confined to both ovaries	G1, 2: TAH/BSO No further treatment G3: P32 or chemotherapy
IC	Same as IA or IB with positive ascitic fluid or washings, intraoperative rupture and spillage of tumor, extension of tumor through capsule	TAH/BSO P32 or chemotherapy
IIA	Extension to uterus and tubes	TAH/BSO P32 if no residual or chemotherapy
IIB	Extension to other pelvic structures	TAH/BSO P32 if no residual or chemotherapy
IIC	Same as IIA or IIB with positive ascitic fluid or washings, intraoperative rupture and spillage of tumor, extension of tumor through capsule	TAH/BSO Multiagent chemotherapy or whole-abdomen radiation
IIIA	Intraabdominal spread microscopically	TAH/BSO Multiagent chemotherapy or whole-abdomen radiation
IIIB	Intraabdominal spread Macroscopically <2 cm	TAH/BSO Multiagent chemotherapy or whole-abdomen radiation
IIIC	Intraabdominal spread Macroscopically <2 cm Positive retroperitoneal or inguinal nodes	Multiagent chemotherapy
IV	Disease above the diaphragm or intraparenchymal liver metastasis	Multiagent chemotherapy

G1, Well differentiated; *G2,* moderately differentiated; *G3,* poorly differentiated; *TAH/BSO,* total abdominal hysterectomy/bilateral salpingo-oophorectomy.

CRITICAL POINTS

- A mass in the adnexa can be from the ovary, the fallopian tube, or the surrounding tissues.
- Acute pain from an adnexal mass generally represents torsion or hemorrhage of the mass.
- Risk factors for ovarian carcinoma are all related to the length of time of sustained ovulation.
- Germ cell malignancies are more common in younger women.
- Epithelial ovarian cancers are more common in older women.

Questions

1. A 22-year-old woman comes to see her physician because of right lower quadrant pain. She has regular menstrual cycles and uses a diaphragm for contraception, although she has had no sexual intercourse for 6 months. Her last menses was 14 days ago and was normal. The pain was sharp when it began but now is a dull ache. On examination a 4-cm slightly tender mass is palpated in the right adnexa. Pathology of this ovarian mass would most likely show:
   A. Corpus luteum cyst
   B. Ectopic pregnancy
   C. Mucinous cystadenoma
   D. Granulosa cell tumor

2. A 19-year-old woman comes to the emergency room with acute lower abdominal pain she describes as excruciating pain that comes and goes. Her blood pressure is 100/80, her pulse is 96, her respirations are 18 per minute, and her temperature is 37.6° C. She has a soft abdomen with 3+ guarding in the left lower quadrants. She is sexually active and occasionally uses condoms. She states that she has no history of pelvic inflammatory disease. Pelvic examination reveals a tender 8-cm round mass in her left adnexa. Her β-HCG is negative. The next step in management is:
   A. Ultrasound of the pelvis
   B. Intravenous pyelography
   C. Emergency laparotomy
   D. Emergency needle biopsy of the mass

Answers

1. A
2. A

VI

Human sexuality

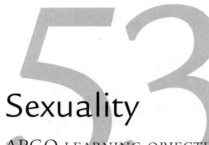

Sexuality

APGO LEARNING OBJECTIVE #53

Melissa Schiff
Lisa M. Fromm
Teresita A. McCarty
Dorothy Kammerer-Doak
Laura Weiss Roberts

All physicians should be able to perform a preliminary assessment of patients with sexual concerns and make referrals when appropriate.

The student will demonstrate a knowledge of the following:

A. Physiologic, emotional, and societal influences on sexuality during the following life events:
   1. Menarche and menses
   2. Initiation of sexual activity
   3. Pregnancy
   4. Postpartum
   5. Menopause
B. Physiology of sexual response
C. Clinical assessment of sexuality
D. Commonly asked questions about sexual function
E. Patterns of sexual dysfunction

Sexuality is an important part of a woman's life, and clinicians should assess sexual health as part of providing complete care. This chapter highlights the impact of life events on female sexuality,
reviews the physiology of the sexual response, and outlines issues of importance in assessing sexual function.

SEXUALITY AND THE FEMALE LIFE CYCLE

Although a woman's sexuality develops and changes during her lifetime, specific life events have an important impact on her sexuality. The onset of menarche, initiation of sexual activity, pregnancy, postpartum, and menopause are each important milestones in the evolution of a woman's sexuality.

Menarche

Onset of menarche represents a transition from childhood and marks the beginning of a number of physical, psychologic, and social changes. Menarche occurs approximately 2 years after secondary sex characteristics begin to develop (e.g., breast tissue, pubic and axillary hair). Although the physical changes happen gradually, changes in a girl's self-perception may occur suddenly and disconcertingly. The average age of menarche is 12 to 13 years (range 10 to 15 years). In recent years, there is evidence that the mean age of menarche has lowered, largely as a result of improved nutrition and living conditions. Menarche is accompanied by increasing awareness of sexual identity, greater concern with personal appearance, and a growing sense of one's future role as an adult.

The menstrual cycle is initiated and maintained by an integrated and complex neuroendocrine rhythm. Certain physical and emotional changes that accompany the cycle are common, usually minor, and are readily assimilated as part of the normal menstrual pattern. A small percentage (3% to 5%) of women will report cyclic emotional or physical symptoms that are severe enough to interfere with usual day-to-day activities. Women are usually over the age of 30 before they bring these problems to a physician. The symptoms commonly reported are depression, irritability, headache, mood swings, fatigue, breast tenderness, edema, and sleep and appetite disturbances. Called premenstrual syndrome, or late luteal phase disorder, debilitating symptoms appear between 4 to 14 days before the onset of menses and usually remit by day 4 of menses. Most women who have had severe premenstrual symptoms will continue to have these symptoms after hysterectomy. Encouraging patients to keep a record documenting which symptoms are most troublesome and how they relate to the menstrual cycle will aid both the physician and patient in identifying target symptoms and devising a treatment strategy.

Initiation of sexual activity

Initiation of sexual activity is another important event in a woman's life. Recent studies suggest that initiation of sexual activity now occurs earlier in life, with 10% of girls having had intercourse by age 13 and 25% by age 15. In addition, overall sexual activity has dramatically increased among adolescents and young adults over the past two decades: reportedly, one quarter of females between 15 and 19 in 1970 were sexually active, but more than one half of females in that age group in 1988 were sexually active. Most adolescents do not consistently use condoms or other forms of contraception. Consequently, during these early years of sexual activity, young women may become pregnant or may become infected with sexually transmitted diseases. Initial sexual experiences may have a lasting impact on the rest of a woman's sexual life, especially if the experiences were traumatic, unwanted, or resulted in medical complications.

Pregnancy and postpartum

Pregnancy is another life event that has an impact on sexuality. A couple's sexual relationship may be affected during pregnancy by numerous physical and psychologic changes. Many couples worry unnecessarily throughout pregnancy that sexual activity may harm the fetus. Many women report decreased sexual interest during the first trimester of pregnancy. During the second trimester, sexual desire and responsiveness are improved; as pregnancy approaches term, sexual interest may again decrease. This decrease may be due to the physical changes and limitations occurring late in pregnancy, and couples may need to find new positions or focus on noncoital sexual activities. Sexual activity can enhance a couple's emotional bond, both to each other and to the pregnancy. Communication, mutual support, and understanding are important in the adaptation to changes in the sexual needs and desires of the individual partners.

Sexual activity is reestablished during the postpartum period. During the initial weeks after delivery, most women are proscribed from any vaginal sexual activity while the vagina is healing. After the first month or two postpartum, most couples resume sexual activity. Some new mothers note temporary discomfort with intercourse (dyspareunia) caused by vaginal trauma from delivery or dryness from altered hormone levels. For some women, dyspareunia persists up to 1 year after delivery. A woman's interest in sexual activity during the postpartum period also may be decreased by the fatigue of caring for a newborn, dissatisfaction with her altered body image, or adjustments in the marital relationship. Usually by 1 year postpartum most women and their partners have settled into a comfortable pattern of sexual activity.

Sexuality and menopause

Menopause is a gradual process that results in a clearly demarcated change in a woman's reproductive life. Occurring around age 51 (range 48 to 55 years), menopause has a relatively predictable course in that over a 2-year or 3-year time span, menses become irregular and ultimately cease altogether. The effect of menopause on a woman's life and sexuality is complex and unique. For some women, it may represent a new phase of improved sexuality, free of worries about contraception, pregnancy, and child-rearing. Many women experience adjustments, both biologically and psychologically, during the menopausal years. Sexual interest and activity tend to decrease with age, although no evidence exists for an abrupt change at the time of menopause. The sexual response cycle remains intact, although it may be slowed for some women. Low estrogen levels may cause vaginal dryness and painful intercourse; appropriate hormone replacement therapy helps alleviate these physical discomforts and is important for preventive health care. Other life events including feeling stressed in marital or family relationships, reentering the work force after children leave home, caring for elderly parents, or losing a spouse can all decrease a menopausal woman's sexual desire and activity. Conscientious attention to these issues may help a woman adapt optimally to this new sexual phase.

SEXUAL PHYSIOLOGY

While sexuality evolves during the course of a woman's life, the basic physiology of sexual response remains the same throughout the years. The sexual response cycle is also the same for all women, regardless of their sexual orientation.

Much of what we know about female sexual physiology can be attributed to the research of Masters and Johnson in the early 1960s. Their work resulted in the description of the four sequential phases of the female response cycle: excitement, plateau, orgasm, and resolution. They observed two basic physiologic changes during the sexual response cycle: vasocongestion and increased neuromuscular tension (myotonia). Vasocongestion occurs in the internal and external genitalia and in the female breasts, whereas myotonia occurs throughout the body in response to sexual arousal. The integration and choreography of these physiologic changes are described in the following text and in Table 53-1.

The breast

In the breast, the first sign of increased sexual excitement is erection of the nipple. Nipple erection is caused by involuntary contraction of the muscle fibers within the structure of the nipple. During the excitement phase, increased blood flow to the breasts results in venous engorgement and increase in breast size. As sexual tension increases during the plateau phase, a pink or red mottling or rash known as the sex flush often appears over the abdomen and breasts. After orgasm, the sex flush rapidly disappears. The nipples and breast engorgement return to their prearousal state more slowly.

Table 53-1. Peripheral manifestations of the female sexual response cycle

	I. Excitement phase (several minutes to hours)	II. Plateau phase (30 sec-3 min)	III. Orgasmic phase (3-15 sec)	IV. Resolution phase (10-15 min; if no orgasm, ½-1 day)
Skin	No change	Sexual flush; inconstant; may appear on abdomen, breasts, neck, face, thighs. May resemble measles rash	No change	Flush disappears in reverse order
Breasts	1. Nipple erection 2. Venous congestion 3. Areolar enlargement	Venous pattern prominent. Size may increase one fourth over resting state. Areolae enlarge, impinge on nipples so they seem to disappear	No change	Return to normal
Clitoris	Glans: glans diameter increased. Shaft: variable increase in diameter. Elongation occurs in only 10% of subjects	Retraction: shaft withdraws deep into swollen prepuce	No change (Shaft movements continue throughout if thrusting maintained)	Shaft returns to normal position in 5-10 sec. Full detumescence in 5-10 min
Labia majora	Nullipara: thin down, flatten against perineum. Multipara: rapid congestion and edema. Increase to 2-3 times normal size	Nullipara: may swell if phase II unduly prolonged. Multipara: become enlarged and edematous	No change	Nullipara: *increase* to normal size in 1-2 min or less. Multipara: *decrease* to normal size in 10-15 min
Labia minora	Color change: bright pink in nullipara and red in multipara. Size: increase 2-3 times over normal	Color change: bright red in nullipara, burgundy red in multipara. Size: enlarged labia form a funnel into vaginal orifice	Proximal areas contract with contractions of lower third	Return to resting state in 5 min

Modified from Sherfey MJ: *The nature and evolution of female sexuality,* New York, 1972, Random House.

Continued

Table 53-1. Peripheral manifestations of the female sexual response cycle—cont'd

	I. Excitement phase (several minutes to hours)	II. Plateau phase (30 sec-3 min)	III. Orgasmic phase (3-15 sec)	IV. Resolution phase (10-15 min; if no orgasm, ½-1 day)
Vagina	Vagina: transudate appears 10-30 sec after onset of arousal. Drops of clear fluid coalesce to form a well lubricated vaginal barrel (aids in buffering acidity of vagina to neutral pH required by sperm)	Copious transudate can continue to form. Quantity of transudate generally increased by prolonging preorgasm stimulation	No change	Some transudate collects on floor of the upper two thirds formed by its posterior wall (in supine position)
Upper two thirds	Balloons: dilates as uterus moves up, pulling anterior vaginal wall with it. Fornices lengthen; rugae flatten	Further ballooning occurs, then wall relaxes in a slow, tensionless manner	No change; fully ballooned out and motionless	Cervix descends to seminal pool in 3-4 min
Lower third	Dilatation of vaginal lumen occurs. Congestion of walls proceeds gradually	Maximum distention reached rapidly; contracts lumen of lower third. Contraction around penis aids thrusting traction on clitoral shaft via labia and prepuce	3-15 contractions of lower third and proximal labia minora at ¾-sec intervals	Congestion disappears in seconds. (If no orgasm, congestion persists for 20-30 min)
Uterus	Ascends into false pelvis in phase I	Contractions: strong sustained contractions begin late in phase II	Contractions strong throughout orgasm. Strongest with pregnancy and masturbation	Slowly returns to normal position
Rectum			Inconstant rhythmic contractions	All reactions cease within a few seconds

The clitoris

During the excitement phase, the clitoris becomes erect and increases in size. Stimulation of the mons pubis close to the clitoris accelerates this response. The clitoris elevates and retracts behind the clitoral hood during the plateau phase. Additional stimulation to the clitoris may be provided by traction on the labia minora with penile thrusting or by direct contact of the mons pubis with the male partner's pelvis. Following orgasm, the clitoris rapidly returns to the prearousal state.

The vulva

The labia majora normally meet in the midline and protect the underlying structures including the labia minora, the vaginal outlet, and the urethral meatus. In the nulliparous woman during the excitement phase, the labia majora thin and flatten against the perineum and move upward and outward away from the vaginal outlet. In the multiparous woman, the labia majora become markedly distended from vasocongestion. The labia majora remain in this position during the plateau and orgasm phase and return rapidly to midline during the resolution phase. The labia minora of both nulliparous and multiparous women expand 2 to 3 times in thickness during the excitement phase. In addition, the labia minora and clitoral hood undergo vivid color changes from vasocongestion. After orgasm, the color changes and vasocongestion resolve quickly.

The vagina

The first physiologic evidence of sexual responsiveness is vaginal lubrication, beginning 10 to 20 seconds after initiation of sexual stimulation. The vaginal secretions are a transudate that forms a smooth, slippery surface over the vaginal walls. As sexual tension increases during the excitement phase, the inner two thirds of the vagina lengthens and distends while the cervix and uterine body are pulled backward and upward into the pelvis. As with the other genital areas, the vaginal walls undergo distinct color changes from pink or red to deep purple due to vasocongestion. The anatomic change associated with the vasocongestion that occurs in the vagina and labia minora is called the *orgasmic platform*. During orgasm, reflex muscular contractions occur at 0.8-second intervals. The subsequent resolution phase is characterized by regression of the vasocongestion as the vagina returns to its preexcitement size and color.

The uterus

During the excitement phase, the uterus and cervix rise in the pelvis, and the vaginal walls expand. This expansion creates a tenting effect and an anatomic basin for the seminal pool. Late in the plateau phase the uterus undergoes strong, sustained contractions that last 2 or more minutes. The contractions continue throughout the orgasm phase. Following orgasm, the uterus descends to its normal resting position.

CLINICAL ASSESSMENT OF SEXUALITY

Assessment of sexual health is integral to the care of every patient. The greatest impediment to the care of the patient's sexual health is the physician's reluctance to explore such sensitive issues. Establishing a routine approach to sexual assessment helps with this barrier. (See Chapter 55, Physicians and Sexuality.) A sexual history can take many forms, but the goal is to understand the patient's unique emotional and experiential sexual development.

A "complete" sexual history is never completed. It begins during the initial evaluation of a new patient (Table 53-2). At the first visit, straightforward questions can be asked about the age of menarche, adaptation to menses, age and nature of first sexual experience, and present sexual activity and interest. Taking a sexual history does not end with the first visit, however. Established pa-

Table 53-2.　Sexual history

GENERAL INFORMATION

Patient	Age, occupation, education, ethnic-cultural-religious background, gender identity, marital status

CHILDHOOD SEXUALITY

Family attitudes about sex	Modesty, nudity, religion, siblings
Learning about sex	Information sources, too soon, too late?
Childhood sexual beliefs	Conception, birth, body parts
Childhood sexual activity	Genital self-stimulation, pleasure, guilt, consequences, peer sexual play, sexual abuse or exploitation by same sex or opposite sex

ADOLESCENT AND ADULT SEXUALITY

Masturbation	Frequency, guilt, orgasm
Necking and petting	Age started, partners, type of activity
Body image	Body habits, gender identity, peer acceptance, self-esteem
Sex practices	Type, frequency, partners, contraception, enjoyment, pain, orgasm
Sex in relationship	Sexual compatibility, mutual and reciprocal satisfaction, enjoyment, masturbation
Pregnancies	Number, result, effect on sex life
Extramarital sex	Partners, attachment, frequency, emotional results, relationship effects
Sexual illnesses	Genital trauma or surgery, mastectomy, hysterectomy, sexually transmitted diseases
Sex after loss of relationship	Sex outlets, family attitudes, personal attitudes, fantasies
Sex trauma	Violence, rape, resultant fears
Sexual variations	Bestiality, pedophilia, voyeurism, exhibitionism, fetishism, transsexualism, transvestism

tients need an alert physician who remembers to ask sexual questions again as conditions change. When a level of comfort has been established with patients, the physician can ask open-ended questions about sexual enjoyment and specific questions about how a new medication or illness has affected sexual activity.

Some patients require more care in the approach to sexual questions than others do. An adolescent, for example, may need a more subtle approach. Volunteering developmentally appropriate sexual information lets adolescents know that sexual issues can be discussed freely, and they are more likely to answer sexual questions honestly. Some sexual questions must be asked directly and specifically because patients often will not disclose certain kinds of information in re-

sponse to open-ended questions. Examples of such sensitive areas are experiences of childhood sexual abuse, rape, violence as a prelude to sex, or any sexual activity that makes the patient physically or psychologically uncomfortable (e.g., heterosexual anal intercourse). Sexual practices that may place the patient at increased risk of infection must also be explored with sensitivity. Patients assume that their physician will be uncomfortable discussing these issues and thus avoid them until asked directly.

With a basic understanding of a patient's sexual history, the physician can address misinformation and gaps in patient understanding about sexuality. Through an ongoing dialogue, physicians can also anticipate new sexual phases and concerns with patients.

SEXUAL DYSFUNCTION

Sexual difficulties represent an important set of clinical problems. In patients presenting for medical evaluations, for example, 10% spontaneously report sexual problems. Physicians who ask patients about their sexual functioning as part of a sexual history find that 50% have an identifiable sexual problem. Dyspareunia (painful intercourse), disorders of sexual desire, disorders of sexual excitement, and inhibition of orgasm—four common areas of sexual dysfunction experienced by women—are described in this section.

Dyspareunia

Patients often report dyspareunia (painful intercourse) as a specific symptom, although it can have many causes. The causes of painful intercourse are divided into those that cause pain in the lower portion of the vagina and those that cause pain deep in the vagina.

Congenital malformations, bladder infections, vaginitis, and injuries during childbirth or assault can cause painful intercourse. Vaginal irritation is sometimes caused by allergies to deodorants in tampons, laundry or hand soaps, spermicides, or the materials used in barrier contraceptives like condoms or diaphragms. Inadequate lubrication, a frequent cause of dyspareunia, can be caused by anxiety and premature vaginal entry or by a decrease in estrogen after menopause. An intact hymen or an episiotomy scar can cause pain. Vaginismus, spasm of the vaginal muscles, also can cause painful intercourse.

When pain occurs deep in the vagina during intercourse, a thorough physical evaluation is required. Such pain can be caused by active pelvic inflammatory disease or the residual effects of scarring. Tumors, cysts, endometriosis, and inflammatory bowel disease also can cause dyspareunia and pelvic pain. Pelvic pain also can be associated with childhood sexual abuse as a somatic or body memory of previously experienced pains. Patients with a history of childhood sexual abuse who also have pelvic pain should have a psychiatric evaluation and psychologic treatment, as well as continuing gynecologic care.

Disorders of sexual desire

A persistent indifference to sexual activity is a disorder of sexual desire. This disorder may be primary, as in a woman who has never had any interest in sex, or secondary, which occurs when previous sexual interest is lost. Secondary losses of desire may be organic, situational, or the result of hidden inhibitions. Many situations such as bereavement, stress, anxiety, or loss of erotic attraction to a partner may cause loss of sexual interest. Treatment of a primary disorder of sexual desire requires psychotherapy and specific sex therapy. A secondary disorder of desire is best treated by identifying and treating the underlying cause.

Vaginismus is a specific syndrome that is defined as a disorder of desire. Psychologic factors cause an involuntary constriction of the vaginal muscles that can prevent penile insertion during intercourse. Vaginismus may be secondary to a medical illness or may be the result of emotional conflict and prior sexual trauma. Vaginismus treatment usually is very successful and simply involves having the patient use graduated dilators in the vagina until she is able to allow penile insertion during intercourse.

Disorders of sexual excitement

Disorders of sexual excitement occur when there is inadequate vasocongestion and lubrication. These problems are often associated with orgasm problems as well. Psychologic causes must be considered once physical problems have been ruled out. Fear of pregnancy, marital discord, or feeling of sexual inadequacy may contribute to disorders of excitement and orgasm. Sex and behavior therapy can be useful in these situations. The overall goals of therapy are to provide accurate information, decrease performance fears, and increase communication between the partners. Usually these goals can be reached within a few weeks of therapy.

Inhibition of orgasm

Inhibition of orgasm represents another significant area of sexual dysfunction. To achieve orgasm, a stimulation threshold during the plateau phase must be reached to trigger this reflex. Primary preorgasmia, in which a woman has never had an orgasm as a result of sexual intercourse or masturbation, is a relatively uncommon problem. Anorgasmia or secondary inhibition of orgasm, in which a woman has experienced orgasm in the past but not currently, is a relatively common problem. Some women fear loss of control during orgasm; others may feel undeserving or ambivalent about sexual pleasure. Primary and secondary inhibition of orgasm can be treated successfully with different types of sex therapy.

Sexual dysfunction associated with illness and medication

Sexual difficulties may arise following illness or medications. Both may affect each phase of the female sexual response cycle (i.e., excitement, plateau, orgasm, and resolution), leading to sexual dysfunction and dissatisfaction. Physiologic factors influencing neurologic, neuromuscular, or endocrine function may cause these problems. Psychologic factors such as lack of interest, arousal, and comfort may accompany the poor

---

Table 53-3. Commonly asked questions about sexuality

1. How does masturbation relate to physical health, psychologic adjustment, and general sexual relations? Is masturbation normal or wrong?
2. Are my genitals normal? Too large (breasts)? Too small (penis)?
3. Is sex during my period safe? Can I get pregnant during my period?
4. What is normal sexual activity in frequency and pattern? Am I or my partner normal, oversexed or undersexed?
5. Does orgasm of the woman affect conception in any way? Pregnancy? Delivery?
6. How does a woman know when she has an orgasm? Why isn't it always clear? How does her partner know?
7. Are there any contraceptives that increase or decrease libido?
8. Will contraceptives like birth control pills or foams prevent transmission of sexually transmitted diseases?
9. Are anal or oral intercourse a part of normal sexual activity?
10. Will pregnancy or childbearing affect sexuality? How?
11. Is sex OK during pregnancy? How long may it continue before delivery? How soon after delivery can sexual activity resume?
12. Will nursing or not nursing my baby affect my sexuality? Will nursing by my partner affect the baby?
13. Will sterilization affect sexual performance or desire?
14. Will hysterectomy affect sexual performance or desire?
15. Will menopause affect sexual performance or desire?
16. What effects on sexual activities are due to aging?
17. Is it OK not to have sex?
18. How might homosexuality affect my or my partner's being a parent?
19. Can withdrawal immediately before ejaculation or douching immediately after sex prevent pregnancy? Can pregnancy occur without "going all the way"?
20. How would you define dyspareunia, impotence, premature ejaculation, and vaginismus? How should these be dealt with?

Adapted from Diamond M: Sex and reproduction: conception and contraception. In Green R, editor: *Human sexuality,* Baltimore, 1979, Williams & Wilkins.

self-esteem, malaise, and pain of certain chronic illnesses as well.

Many commonly prescribed medications cause sexual difficulties. Antihypertensive medications, histamine antagonists, narcotics, barbiturates, lithium, antipsychotics, and others are likely to cause decreased libido, diminished arousal, and impaired orgasm. Rarely certain medications can cause irreversible sexual problems if undiagnosed and untreated, such as priapism and secondary penile erectile damage caused by the antidepressant trazodone. It is important to prepare patients for possible sexual problems associated with illness and medications because patients may not understand or mention these concerns. These issues should be raised during the routine process of obtaining informed consent, a discussion in which the natural history of illness, treatments and alternatives, risks, and benefits are outlined carefully.

SUMMARY

Physicians should have a basic understanding of sexual physiology and sexual dysfunction, as well as an appreciation of the impact of specific life events on a woman's sexuality. Patients need information about the stages of normal sexual development, and they need opportunities to discuss their sexuality as a healthy part of adult life (Table 53-3). Accurate sexual information can prevent unwanted pregnancy and the spread of sexually transmitted diseases. Knowledge of a patient's sexual functioning may uncover problems caused by medications, illness, or injury. This information is necessary so that physicians can educate their patients about sexuality, evaluate their concerns, provide treatment, and refer them for psychologic or sex therapy when appropriate.

CRITICAL POINTS

- Sexuality is an important part of a woman's life from birth to death.
- Specific life events that affect a woman's sexuality include the following:
    Onset of menarche
    Initiation of sexual activity
    Pregnancy and the postpartum period
    Onset of menopause
- The physiology of sexual response remains the same throughout a woman's life and is characterized by four phases:
    Excitement
    Plateau
    Orgasm
    Resolution
- The sexual response cycle is characterized by vasocongestion and myotonia or increased neuromuscular tension.
- A clinical assessment of sexuality should be taken for new as well as established patients.
- Sexual dysfunction is a common problem and may include the following:
    Dyspareunia
    Disorders of sexual desire
    Disorders of sexual excitement
    Inhibition of orgasm

Questions

1. The percentage of teenaged girls 15 to 19 that are sexually active is:
   A. Less than 10%
   B. 25%
   C. Over 50%
   D. 100%
2. Sexual activity for most couples during the second trimester:
   A. Increases
   B. Decreases
   C. Stays the same
3. Sexual activity in the postpartum period may be uncomfortable because:
   A. Breast-feeding causes lowered hormone levels.
   B. The episiotomy site may be painful.
   C. None of the above.
   D. Both A and B.
4. The sequence of events in the female sexual response cycle is:
   A. Excitement, plateau, orgasm, resolution
   B. Excitement, orgasm, plateau, resolution
   C. Orgasm, excitement, plateau, resolution
   D. Plateau, excitement, orgasm, resolution
5. The first physiologic evidence of sexual responsiveness is vaginal lubrication.
   A. True
   B. False
6. Stimulation to the clitoris can be provided by:
   A. Stimulation of the mons pubis
   B. Traction in the labia minora
   C. Direct stimulation by the penis
   D. All of the above
7. In patients having medical evaluations, what percentage spontaneously report sexual problems?
   A. Less than 5%
   B. 10%
   C. 50%
   D. 80%
8. Dyspareunia (painful intercourse) may be caused by all the following *except:*
   A. Vaginitis
   B. Pelvic inflammatory disease
   C. Gastrointestinal viral illness
   D. Endometriosis

Answers

1. C
2. A
3. D
4. A
5. A
6. D
7. B
8. C

54

Modes of sexual expression

APGO LEARNING OBJECTIVE #54

Teresita A. McCarty
Laura Weiss Roberts
Lisa M. Fromm

Expression of adult sexuality is determined by a number of factors. The care of a woman's health problems may be affected by her mode of sexual expression.

The student will demonstrate a knowledge of the following:

A. Human sexual development
B. Sexual behavior patterns and social issues of women who are heterosexual, homosexual, and bisexual
C. Sexual behavior patterns and social issues of people who practice sexual variations, or paraphilias, such as transvestism and transsexualism

Sexual identity is influenced by biologic, social, and psychologic factors. These factors are complex, interdependent, and result in many healthy forms of sexual interest and expression. Clarifying sexual identity, partner choice, and sexual activity pattern is essential in caring for a woman's health needs. In this chapter a foundation for understanding modes of sexual expression is provided by discussing three clinically important areas: (1) aspects of the process of human sexual development; (2) sexual behaviors and related social issues of women who are heterosexual, homosexual, and bisexual; and (3) concerns of women who practice sexual variations, or whose partners practice sexual variations, such as transvestism and transsexualism.

HUMAN SEXUAL DEVELOPMENT

Understanding sexual development involves an appreciation of its biologic complexity and an awareness that environmental, psychologic, behavioral, and cognitive factors all influence the ultimate outcome. Sexual differentiation is determined initially by the pair of sex chromosomes (XX or XY) present at conception. Once the sexual genotype is established, however, the fetal hormonal environment determines whether the dimorphic structure of the developing genitalia and brain assume either a male or a female function and appearance. Normal development of the male sexual organs, for example, requires that the fetus have appropriate receptors for the testicular androgens early in gestation, in addition to the XY genotype. The fetal hormonal environment also affects the structure and organization of the developing brain. The sexual development of the human brain is illustrated somewhat later in gestation when the hypothalamus is differentially organized in a male or female fetus. In turn, the hypothalamus mediates the timing and pattern of gonadotropin release during puberty. Clearly, an anomaly of any of several interdependent, biologic systems (genetics, anatomy, receptors, hormones, or chronology) may greatly influence sexual development.

Although the emphasis is often on prenatal factors that affect sexual development, postnatal factors also influence the developing brain and may not exclusively involve reproductive function or behavior. Overall cognitive abilities do not necessarily differ by sex, for example, but there do tend to be differing patterns of ability. The right cerebral hemisphere remains pliable for a longer time in girls than it does in boys. Girls therefore are relatively protected from the effects of left hemisphere dysfunction, which can result in dyslexia and autism. Another difference is that adult women have less cerebral hemispheric asymmetry than men do, and this can be helpful in recovering from strokes or other neurologic injuries.

Many studies have demonstrated a pattern of cognitive, behavioral, and psychologic differences between men and women and between boys and girls. Although not absolute for all individuals, sex-related differences have been found in five general areas: (1) language and visual-spatial abilities; (2) childhood toy preference and play behavior; (3) tendency toward physical aggression; (4) sexual orientation (preferred partner); and (5) sexual identity (sense of feeling like a man or a woman). In particular, studies suggest that most women tend to have greater verbal fluency, prefer men as their sexual partners, and view themselves

as having a fundamentally female sexual identity. There is also evidence that most girls prefer to play with dolls rather than trucks and are less likely to hit their playmates. Many perfectly normal individuals do not fit into these common patterns of sex differences. Although these studies describe some generally reproducible findings, they also serve as a reminder that much is still unknown about the contribution of culture and individual personality to the differences noted between women and men.

Researchers are looking to see whether the hormonal, anatomic, and behavioral differences that can be found between men and women can also be found between people of the same sex who have differing sexual orientations. For instance, do the hypothalamic nuclei of men who prefer men as sexual partners resemble those of women who prefer men as sexual partners? Very early research has demonstrated some brain anatomic differences between heterosexual and homosexual men, but whether these findings will be substantiated and replicated remains to be seen. Little research has been performed in the area of female homosexuality; consequently, it is poorly understood. Since the factors that determine the development of human sexuality are so complex and since so much of human brain development occurs after birth, it is unlikely that simple microanatomic differences—even if replicated—can provide a complete explanation for the complexity of human sexual behavior.

ISSUES IN THE CLINICAL CARE OF WOMEN

In this section, several issues involved in the clinical care of heterosexual, homosexual, and bisexual women are outlined. The discussion will focus on six areas: (1) the language used to describe modes of sexual expression; (2) the prevalence of heterosexuality, homosexuality, and bisexuality; (3) the process of sexual identity formation; (4) a detailed, research-based description of women's sexual behaviors; (5) objectives in the clinical care of women; and (6) special issues in the care of homosexual and bisexual women.

Language

Efforts to understand the subtleties of sexuality and its modes of expression are reflected in the many terms used to describe these areas of human experience. The concept of *core gender identity* relates to one's internal sense of belonging to the male or female sex. Inclusion of a variety of societally perceived masculine and feminine attributes is compatible with male or female gender identity. In everyday use, *gender* is a term laden with many personal and cultural meanings and is viewed as a social construct atop anatomic sex. *Sexual orientation,* a different idea, places the individual on a continuum reflecting his or her degree of sexual attraction to members of the same or opposite sex or to members of both sexes. The term *heterosexuality* refers to the presence of sexual and emotional attraction to members of the opposite sex, whereas the term *homosexuality* refers to the presence of lasting sexual and emotional attraction to members of one's own sex. *Bisexual* is a designation used to describe individuals who feel aroused and attached to members of both the same and the opposite sex. Finally, *gay* is a word commonly used to describe men and women who are homosexual or bisexual.

Prevalence

The vast majority of individuals maintain a heterosexual orientation and participate in sexual relationships with members of the opposite sex. Current figures on the prevalence of homosexuality and bisexuality are unclear, although estimates suggest that 1% to 3% of women and 3% to 6% of men are exclusively homosexual and that 2% of women and men are bisexual. The number of individuals who have had at least one homosexual experience since adolescence, but who do not have a settled homosexual identity, is perhaps 20% of women and 37% of men.

Sexual orientation and identity formation

The development and origins of sexual orientation are many, diverse, and variable. Heterosexual identity formation involves a sequence of stages that ultimately allow children to have a deep sense of belonging to their anatomic sex, identification with members of the same sex, attraction and attachment to members of the opposite sex, and acquisition of gender identity and role commensurate to anatomic sex. Writings concerning nonheterosexual orientation suggest that there are four stages of homosexual and bisexual identity formation: (1) sensitization, in which a child may feel different and recognize the presence of attraction to the same gender; (2) sexual identity confusion, in which an adolescent attempts to achieve self-understanding and to reconcile internal feelings with negative societal pressures; (3) sexual identity assumption, in which the older adolescent and young adult explores homosexual or bisexual practices and life-style; and (4) integration and commitment, in which the adult accepts his or her orientation. The average time between a homosexual or bisexual person's recognition of his or her sexual orientation and disclosure to others is greater than 4 years, according to one study, and many nonheterosexual individuals never disclose their orientation to others. Through the process of sexual identity formation, people discovering and settling on their sexual orientation—wherever they fit—may experience many feelings, ranging from relief and support to isolation and sadness.

Sexual behaviors of women and their clinical importance

Studies suggest that women, in general, tend to view and value their sexual lives within the context of intimate, lasting relationships. Sexual behavior

---

Table 54-1. Factors contributing to sexual expression

1. Sexual identity (i.e., settled, internal sense of being a man or a woman)
2. Sexual orientation, preferences, and partner choice
3. Quality and character of primary intimate relationship
4. Biologic predisposition (e.g., pattern of arousability, including rate, stimuli, level obtainable)
5. Frequency and character of sexual activity
6. Perceived benefits of sexual practices (e.g., intimacy, satisfaction)
7. Perceived risks of sexual practices (e.g., infection, injury, sexually transmitted illnesses, psychologic harm)
8. Physical and emotional health
9. Timing with respect to developmental life cycle

---

among adult women, for example, is characterized mainly by monogamy and is linked strongly to relationship status. Women typically have fewer sexual partners during their lives than men do. Moreover, heterosexual and homosexual women who are not in stable relationships are more likely to abstain from sex than are men of either group. Factors influencing sexual expression and behaviors are given in Table 54-1. In clinical settings, women may be especially concerned about their sexuality as it connects to and fosters their emotional relationship with a partner.

Knowledge of general trends regarding sexual and reproductive behavior—such as initial and early sexual experiences, contraceptive use, number of sexual partners, unintended pregnancies, specific sexual practices, and abstinence—contribute greatly to an understanding of individual patient experiences. Early first sexual intercourse, for example, is associated in a population level with drug use, sexually transmitted diseases (STDs), increased number of sexual partners, more casual sexual encounters, and cervical cancer. Appreciating how a given patient's personal history fits into larger trends within her culture can help the clinician anticipate the related problems and vulnerabilities she may experience.

Studies of adolescents have yielded several important findings with respect to initiation of sexual activity, condom use, human immunodeficiency virus (HIV), and pregnancy. Approximately 10% of male and female adolescents have had intercourse by age 13, and 25% of female adolescents have had intercourse by age 15. The proportion of female adolescents age 15 to 19 who had intercourse doubled from one fourth in 1970 to one half in 1988. Some cultural differences exist in that 60% of black females, 53% of white females, and 49% of Hispanic females between 15 and 19 years had ever had intercourse, according to one study in 1990. Moreover, 43% of female adolescents in this study used no contraception or used the withdrawal method. Approximately 10% to 20% of adolescents use condoms consistently. There is some evidence that white and Hispanic female adolescents use condoms more commonly than do black female adolescents. It is both disheartening and encouraging to note that this modest level of condom use represents perhaps a threefold increase over the past decade owing to education about STDs. Adolescents represent the largest growing at-risk population for HIV infection. In addition, 3% of female adolescents age 15 to 19 in 1987 were pregnant or had given birth in the previous 2 months. Three quarters of births to teenagers in 1987 derived from unintended pregnancies. Of the teenage pregnancies documented that year, 36% resulted in abortion, 14% in miscarriage, and 50% in live births. To summarize, a growing proportion of female adolescents are sexually active and are at risk for a number of harms, including STDs and unintended pregnancy.

Studies of sexual and reproductive behavior after adolescence suggest that adult women are sexually active, have several partners, and gradually settle into a pattern of monogamy or, in some cases, abstinence over the course of their lives. Most women in young adulthood are sexually active. Many have had two or more partners: Of women age 20 to 34, 70% have had two or more partners in their lives, whereas the percentage of young adult women who have had multiple partners in 1 year is 31%. In adults age 25 and older, predictive factors of having multiple sex partners relate to marital status, gender, age, and race (i.e., a decreased risk if married, female, under 30, and/or have a white cultural background). The vast majority of married women report having sex only with their husbands, and the frequency of intercourse is, on average, 50 times each year. Homosexual women, unlike homosexual men, typically do not have many sexual partners over their lifetimes. Women engage in a number of sexual practices. For example, most heterosexual and homosexual adults engage in oral-genital sex. Heterosexual anal intercourse, important because of greatly increased risk of male-to-female HIV transmission, is practiced regularly by many couples, although seldom discussed in clinical settings. In one study, 19% of college women had had receptive anal intercourse; in another study of nearly 3000 women of all ages, 71% had had anal intercourse, and 26% practiced it routinely. Many studies show decreasing frequency of sexual intercourse with age. In addition, abstinence appears to be a viable sexual alternative for many women. Among unmarried women in one study, 13% of those age 25 to 34, 26% of those 35 to 49, and 60% of those 50 to 64 were abstinent. In one study of homosexual women, 43% had been abstinent for a year or more. Elderly individuals continue to engage in a variety of sexual practices and never cease to have sexual concerns.

The clinical importance of sexual and reproductive behaviors becomes readily apparent when thinking about the sheer numbers of women involved. In 1988, there were 57.9 million women of reproductive age (15 to 44 years) in the United States.

- Estimates concerning the rate of consistent condom use by young, sexually active females in this group of 57.9 million women range from 13% to 40% (i.e., perhaps 25 million women were at some significant risk for contracting STD).
- About 1 million women were pregnant (or had given birth within the previous 2 months) and perhaps another million were seeking pregnancy, representing immense health care needs for this population.
- One third of women in 1988 used reversible methods of contraception.
- For every 1000 women age 15 to 44 in 1987, approximately 109 became pregnant, 61 unintentionally. Of the unintentional pregnancies, 27 resulted in abortion and 8 in miscarriage, with 27 live births.
- In absolute numbers, 4 million women in 1988 were heterosexually active and not using birth control but not seeking pregnancy. Overall, 40% of births were unintended, either mistimed or unwanted, especially in very poor or teenage mothers.

Overall, it is estimated that most of the 57.9 million reproductive-age women in 1988 were potentially fertile, sexually active, at risk for unintended pregnancy, and vulnerable to STDs. If 85% of women using no contraceptive method become pregnant within 1 year, as one study has shown, the number of unintended pregnancies alone is staggering. The risk of HIV transmission is potentially devastating. In summary, the remarkable number of women who were sexually active and inadequately covered for health risks represents a significant clinical challenge in terms of prevention, support, and treatment.

Objectives in the clinical care of women

Caring for the sexual health and well-being of women relates to five primary objectives (Table 54-2). The first is to promote the patient's sense of

---

Table 54-2. Objectives in caring for the sexual health of women

1. Promote in the patient a sense of self-understanding and knowledge with respect to sexual health.
2. Provide appropriate, conscientious, nonjudgmental care regarding reproductive behaviors and choices.
3. Address concerns surrounding satisfaction in intimate relationships and through specific sexual practices.
4. Prevent, detect, and treat illness and reproductive organ pathology.
5. Explore the relationship of sexuality to violence and exploitation in the patient's life.

---

self-understanding and knowledge with respect to sexuality. (See Chapter 53, Sexuality.) The second is to provide appropriate, conscientious care to women regarding their reproductive behaviors and choices. This involves adequate preventive (e.g., contraception, prenatal care) and treatment measures. The third concerns the patient's satisfaction in intimate relationships through specific sexual practices. This is influenced by the patient's own psychology and life cycle. The fourth involves the prevention, detection, and care of physical illness and reproductive organ pathology (e.g., prevention of HIV transmission through safe sex activities; early diagnosis of pelvic infection to eliminate subsequent infertility; treatment of cervical dysplasia to prevent cervical cancer). (See Chapters 34, Pelvic Relaxation, and 49, Cervical Disease and Neoplasia.) The final objective relates to an exploration of the relationship of sexuality to violence and exploitation in the patient's life. (See Chapter 56, Domestic Violence and Sexual Assault.)

Special issues in the care of homosexual and bisexual women

The health care of homosexual and bisexual women requires special attention to both psychiatric and obstetric-gynecologic issues. An initial point is that despite societal prejudices, homosexuality itself is not understood as a symptom of illness or a sign of aberrant development. There is no clear evidence, for example, that homosexual and bisexual women experience more psychiatric

symptoms than heterosexual women. They may undergo more psychologic stresses, however, such as social isolation and ostracism, inadequate family support, and the like. There may be periods in homosexuals' lives that bring greater vulnerability to depression and suicide (e.g., around the time of disclosure of sexual orientation to family and friends). Early studies do suggest that homosexual women have an increased frequency of alcohol dependence and substance abuse. Clinicians should assume responsibility for the exploration and early detection of substance-related illnesses in all patients, but perhaps particularly so in homosexual women. For these reasons, it is important for the clinician to discuss the patient's sources of support and level of comfort surrounding her sexual orientation. Clinicians caring for homosexual and bisexual patients should closely monitor their own assumptions about such issues so that they do not inadvertently act in ways that harm their patients. The experience of being nonheterosexual in a predominantly heterosexual society may alone cause significant suffering. The doctor-patient relationship should offer respite from such stresses.

Two important issues arise with respect to specific obstetric and gynecologic care of homosexual and bisexual women. First, women of any sexual orientation may wish to have and raise children with their partners and, therefore, need reproductive health care. As homosexual and bisexual women may feel particularly unsupported and socially isolated during this process, it is important that clinicians deal sensitively with gay parenting issues. Second, homosexual women are equally or less likely to contract sexually transmitted illnesses when compared with heterosexual women. Homosexual women are not at increased risk for becoming infected with HIV, although homosexual men are. Bisexual women are nevertheless at risk for sexually transmitted diseases and should be cautioned to use safe sex practices, especially those with infected partners.

SEXUAL VARIATIONS

Patients may be distressed by sexual impulses or practices that they recognize to be relatively unusual. Patients may risk talking about their concerns when their level of discomfort overrides their embarrassment about disclosure. Discovery and disapproval by the patient's partner or major changes in the patient's life situation are events that often precipitate a discussion with a physician. Some people feel that unusual sexual behavior is more a social than a medical concept and that most people who practice sexual variations never come to medical attention. Moreover, there are no clear lines dividing one sexual variation from another, and differing sexual behavior patterns may evolve over the course of a person's life, making the clinical issues surrounding sexual variations difficult to categorize. Nevertheless, physicians should be aware of these complex areas of human sexuality because patients who bring these issues to their doctors need informed, compassionate assistance.

Transvestism

Transvestites obtain pleasure from wearing the clothing of the opposite sex (cross-dressing). Transvestites may or may not feel dysphoric about their gender identity and modes of sexual activity. They usually are heterosexual men who initially get sexual pleasure from wearing women's clothing. Over time, the sexual nature of the pleasure may diminish but the enjoyment of

women's clothes often persists. Female transvestites are uncommon and, frankly, less noticeable in the United States, where women have relatively more freedom in their manner of dress in comparison with men. A gynecologist may, however, hear about transvestism from a woman who has just discovered that her partner is cross-dressing. A careful history will often clarify the appropriate recommendations. For example, a woman may feel guilty that she gets excited by her husband's desire to wear her underwear. Reassurance that this can be considered part of the playfulness associated with sexual activity might be all that is needed. In contrast, if the husband is compulsively cross-dressing in public and embarrasses the couple's school-age children, referrals for behavior therapy for the husband and family therapy for the wife and children are necessary. Transvestism may cause conflict in a woman's life or relationships and may necessitate clinical intervention.

Transsexualism

Transsexuals represent a special patient population with a number of difficult medical and psychosocial issues. The term *transsexual* most properly applies to people who have had a sex change operation, although individuals who are in the process of preparing for such surgeries are sometimes referred to as transsexuals as well. Transsexuals are commonly thought to be people who feel that they were "born in the wrong body." They may have a history of transvestism or may be attracted to members of their own sex, but do not consider themselves homosexual. Typically patients explain that they have always felt that some mistake was made—that they should have been born the opposite sex—and request surgery to remedy the error. They often come to physicians seeking sex reassignment after such specific life events as the illness or death of a spouse or the recognition that their children are growing up and developing their own sexuality. Men who ask to become women outnumber women who want to become men by 2 or 3 to 1. In either instance, diagnostic evaluation should include a psychiatric examination. Subsequent treatment involves ongoing psychotherapy while the patient takes hormones and lives and works in the desired gender role for at least 2 years. Many patients are satisfied with the effects of the hormones and superficial cosmetic procedures and do not go on to have genital surgery. There are irreversible consequences of each step of treatment, however, since a woman's voice may be permanently lowered and her body hair permanently increased by a course of hormones. Postsurgical treatment for male-to-female transsexuals typically includes physical procedures such as regular vaginal dilatation. Female-to-male transsexuals face important decisions concerning residual sexual tissues and organs (e.g., uterus, breasts) after the initial sex change operation has been performed. Postsurgery, male-to-female transsexuals have a better genital outcome. Female-to-male transsexuals, however, have a better interpersonal outcome in that they typically are better able to live their societal role as men.

CRITICAL POINTS

- Sexual development is influenced by many biologically based elements, including genetics, anatomy, receptors, hormones, and timing.
- Sexual development is an ongoing process affected by life experiences, attitudes, and social factors.
- Studies have demonstrated a pattern of cognitive, behavioral, and psychologic differences between men and women.
- The origins and expressions of sexuality are many, diverse, and variable.
- Women typically understand and value their sexuality within the context of a primary relationship.
- Sexual behavior of women is clinically important, especially with respect to preventive health care, fertility, pregnancy, and STDs.
- Special issues in the care of homosexual and bisexual women include psychologic stress; comfort with their sexual orientation; coping strategies; and, as with other women, reproductive health care and STDs.
- Care of women who themselves or whose partners reveal sexual variations, such as transvestism or transsexualism, begins with compassionate evaluation and educated recommendations.

Questions

1. Accurate statements concerning sexual variations include all of the following *except:*
   A. Transsexuals are typically comfortable with their birth anatomic sex.
   B. The clinical response to transvestism depends on the degree of discomfort of the patient and its impact on personal, family, and societal function.
   C. Transvestites obtain pleasure from wearing the clothing of the opposite sex.

D. The term *transsexual* most properly applies to people who have had a sex change operation.

2. Homosexual women and men are equally at risk for contracting STDs.
   A. True
   B. False

3. Homosexual women may be at increased risk for alcoholism and substance use.
   A. True
   B. False

4. There is clear evidence that homosexual women show more psychiatric symptoms than heterosexual women.
   A. True
   B. False

5. Human sexual development is influenced biologically by which of the following?
   A. Sex chromosomes (e.g., XX, XY, other)
   B. Hormones (e.g., testosterone)
   C. Cellular hormone receptors
   D. Timing and pattern of hormone release
   E. All of the above

6. Accurate statements about the cognitive, behavioral, and psychologic differences between men and women include:
   A. Sex-related differences surrounding language and visual-spatial abilities are absolutely consistent between individuals.
   B. No sex-related differences have been found with respect to childhood toy preference and play behavior.
   C. Genetics does not influence sexual orientation or sexual identity.

D. Relatively consistent sex-related differences surrounding language and visual-spatial abilities have been found (population studies).
E. No sex-related differences have been found with respect to physical aggressiveness.

7. Factors contributing to sexual expression include:
   A. Biologic predispositions
   B. Pattern of arousability
   C. Frequency and character of sexual activity
   D. Benefits or risks of sexual practices
   E. All of the above

8. The four stages of homosexual identity formation include all of the following *except:*
   A. Sexual identity confusion
   B. Sexual identity assumption
   C. Sensitization
   D. Assimilation
   E. Integration and commitment

Answers

1. A
2. B
3. A
4. B
5. E
6. D
7. E
8. D

55

Physicians and sexuality

APGO LEARNING OBJECTIVE #55

Laura Weiss Roberts
Lisa M. Fromm

A patient's willingness to discuss her sexual concerns with her physician is often a function of several elements within the doctor-patient relationship. Especially important are the physician's comfort level with these issues, ability to communicate with the patient, and informed efforts to address the patient's sexuality in a therapeutic and professional manner.

The student will demonstrate a knowledge of the following:
A. How student attitudes about sexual issues may influence their perceptions and management of patients
B. Skills for managing difficult issues surrounding sexuality that sometimes arise with patients

Creating a trusting and therapeutic context in which patients may discuss their sexual concerns is an essential, if challenging, task in the doctor-patient relationship. In this chapter three elements involved in creating such a context are discussed: (1) the role of the clinician's attitudes and self-understanding in responding to the sexual issues of patients; (2) the importance of the clinician's skill in communicating with patients about such sensitive issues; and (3) the significance of the clinician's ability to provide humane care to patients while maintaining appropriate professional boundaries.

THE CLINICIAN AND SEXUAL ISSUES

A clinician's perceptions, knowledge, and personality influence his or her ability to work with patients about sexual issues. One study of senior medical students showed that they were likely to take inadequate sexual histories if they felt shy socially, held nonsympathetic views of patients' psychosocial problems, believed that the sexual history was unimportant to patient care, or if they felt insecure and poorly trained. A second study involving medical students demonstrated that they were less willing to talk with homosexual patients than with heterosexual patients, irrespective of their health needs. Medical students in this study thought that homosexual patients were more responsible for their illnesses, felt less pain, and were more offensive, inappropriate, and untruthful than heterosexual patients. A significant number of physicians and nurses in a third study felt "more negatively toward homosexuals since the emergence of the AIDS crisis" and believed that "in the hospital, patients with AIDS receive inferior care compared to patients with other illnesses." In this survey, having a close friend or relative who was gay significantly reduced personal anxiety about homosexuals. These studies reflect how attitudes about sexuality may greatly influence clinicians' approach to their work with patients.

Clinicians typically have difficulty dealing with sexual issues in patients whom they perceive to be too different from themselves or, ironically, too similar. Complex interpersonal issues arise as physicians care for patients who appear unlike themselves with respect to gender, sexual orientation and behaviors, culture, religion, or age. For example, a young male physician may feel uncomfortable speaking with an older woman about the changes in her sexuality that accompany menopause, while an older heterosexual physician may be reluctant to ask about the homosexual experiences of an adolescent. When taking care of patients who appear similar to oneself, however, another set of difficulties may emerge. Instead of awkwardly avoiding sexual issues with the apparently dissimilar patient, the clinician may make incorrect assumptions about the concerns and behaviors of the seemingly similar patient. For example,

the young, well-educated female clinician who practices safe sex in her personal life may suppose that the young, well-educated female patient also practices safe sex; thus the clinician may not ask about high-risk behaviors. For these reasons—and because all patients will be both similar to and different from their clinicians in a variety of ways—it is best to have a routine, thorough approach to sexual issues when caring for patients.

Understanding the role that sexuality plays in patients' lives requires that clinicians possess comfort and insight about the sexual issues in their own lives. It is important that physicians make a conscious effort to think about their attitudes and behaviors and consider how such factors may affect their approach to patients. Physicians should attempt to identify potential "blind spots" in their clinical work. Such blind spots may include being shy interpersonally, feeling uncomfortable with patients' sexual behaviors or choices of partners, feeling negatively toward patients with sexually related illnesses, or making assumptions about patients' sexuality. By establishing a routine, thorough approach to sexual matters (see Chapter 53, Sexuality) with patients, consulting with colleagues, and informing themselves accurately about medical issues, clinicians will ensure that they adequately address the health care issues and sexual concerns of their patients.

COMMUNICATION WITH PATIENTS ABOUT SEXUAL ISSUES

Skill in speaking with patients about sexual matters involves two elements: the clinician's attentiveness to the process of communication with patients about the sensitive area of sexuality, and the clinician's knowledge and ability in guiding the content of these discussions. Both elements are important in creating and maintaining a therapeutic dialogue about sexual matters in the doctor-patient relationship.

The clinician can take several steps to help in communicating with patients about sexual issues that are, by definition, personal and intimate. First, the topic should be introduced in an open, nonjudgmental manner (e.g., "One area that is important to discuss with all patients concerns their sexual health . . . "). During the initial assessment, sexual issues should be defined as a subject important to the patient's well-being and as appropriate for discussion with the physician. The clinician should try to anticipate the patient's worries about confidentiality or embarrassment by discussing these matters early and with sensitivity. In addition, the clinician should offer reassurance about the patient's sexuality (e.g., anatomic structures, libido), ask her to raise questions or concerns during future appointments, and revisit the topic from time to time. In these ways, the clinician can demonstrate to the patient that sexual issues can be discussed openly in the context of a therapeutic relationship.

Knowledge and ability in guiding the content of discussions with patients are especially important to effective communication about sensitive sexual issues. To provide necessary and helpful information to patients, however, clinicians must have a solid knowledge base in many areas such as human sexual development, physiologic and psychologic aspects of the human life cycle, patterns of sexual behavior, myths surrounding sexuality, relative risks of certain sexual activities, and the like. (See Chapters 53, Sexuality, and 54, Modes of Sexual Expressions.) Unfortunately, for those early in training, developing this knowledge base may require significant efforts at self-education, since some medical schools and residencies cover sexually related topics very modestly. According to one recent study, for example, although 79% of medical schools discuss the topic of human sexuality in their curricula, the average time spent on the topic of homosexuality is 3 hours and 26 minutes, typically occurring in the preclinical years of training. Moreover, there is concern that medical textbooks are written in ways that underrepresent women's issues and may pathologize women's sexual concerns. For these reasons, it is essential that clinicians take the time to continuously update their knowledge of human sexuality. Such efforts should greatly improve their abilities in communicating with patients.

PROFESSIONAL BOUNDARIES IN THE DOCTOR-PATIENT RELATIONSHIP

Caring for patients requires that clinicians understand their own boundaries and duties in the doctor-patient relationship. In addition to recognizing the potential for sexual and nonsexual exploitation of patients, clinicians should have the skills to address difficult sexual issues that may arise in the doctor-patient relationship.

The doctor-patient relationship is built on trust and professionalism. Such a foundation is crucial because of the vulnerability of the patient who, whether ill or well, relies on the physician for competent clinical care and appropriate emotional support. It is the responsibility of the physician to create a sense of safety, collaboration, and respect within the doctor-patient relationship.

The need to maintain a professional attitude is particularly true when providing obstetric and gynecologic care to patients. One study of 16 women who were sexually abused by a male gynecologist found that he had performed inappropriately lengthy pelvic examinations without having a nurse present, that he had "misused" his hands, and that he had used "excessive" lubricant. These patients felt frightened, thought that something serious was wrong with them medically, or felt powerless to stop the gynecologist during his examinations. This study serves as a reminder that several things may make patients feel less vulnerable, such as explaining the need for procedures and examinations, making sure that a nurse or, if appropriate, spouse or partner is present, and allowing the patient to be clothed or covered as much as possible during clinical encounters.

A major concern in recent years relates to sexual and nonsexual exploitation of patients by physicians. As early as the time of Hippocrates, it was cautioned that having a sexual relationship with a patient (or patient's family member) is countertherapeutic. Such involvement, with either present or past patients, generally exploits emotions derived from treatment and takes advantage of an inherent inequality in the doctor-patient relationship. In fact, in some states it may be a criminal offense to have sex with one's patients. Nonsexual exploitation (e.g., asking favors or accepting large gifts, obtaining unusual gratification or fulfilling inappropriate emotional needs through the doctor-patient relationship, revealing excessive personal details of the physician's life) also is considered nontherapeutic "use" of patients. Analogous to the serious problems that arise when teachers and students, or supervisors and employees, become involved in intimate relationships, exploited patients feel powerless, less trusting and more angry toward others, and experience significantly more physical and psychologic symptoms.

Sexual involvement with patients does occur, however. In one study of 460 family practitioners, internists, obstetrician-gynecologists, psychiatrists, and surgeons, researchers found that 5% to 13% of respondents indicated that they had engaged in erotic behavior with patients, and 5% to 7.2% had had sexual intercourse with patients. Twelve percent of the 460 physicians in this sample believed that erotic behavior destroyed the doctor-patient relationship. In another study involving 164 physicians, researchers found that male physicians were more likely to engage in clearly erotic behaviors and that women (especially those who were young) were more likely to engage in ambiguous though nonerotic physical behaviors (e.g., touching, hugging) with patients. Disturbing were the findings of a third study in which 25% of first-year medical students believed that sexual intercourse with a patient could be appropriate under the "right circumstances" and if the doctor was "genuine." It is essential that medical students and physicians alike recognize the personal and professional risks of becoming sexually involved. Such risks include loss of self-esteem, loss of career, loss of family, and loss of life for both clinician and patient.

Especially difficult are the situations in which sexual attraction arises between clinicians and patients. A recent study of medical students' perceptions of patient-initiated sexual behavior demonstrated that 71% of female students and 29% of male students at one institution had some experience with patient-initiated sexual behaviors during training. Behaviors ranged from "nervous flirtatiousness" to "touching or grabbing the student." At such times, it is important for the clinician to recognize that "things are not as they seem." The physician's feelings and the patient's behavior, intentional or not, should both be viewed as clinical signs in need of interpretation and understanding. It is important for the physician to keep a clinical perspective and attempt to determine what the patient is hoping to communicate through the behavior (e.g., depression, loneliness, hostility, past history of sexual abuse); at the same time, the clinician must remain neutral and manage his or her own sexual impulses. By recognizing these issues early and providing therapeutic interventions to the patient (e.g., support groups, referral for therapy) and perspective-restoring interventions to the clinician (e.g., background information, supervision, or consultation), many serious sexual problems in the doctor-patient relationship can be avoided. Thus clinicians ultimately will provide better care to those patients for whom sexuality may present great difficulty.

CRITICAL POINTS

- Creating a trusting and therapeutic context in which patients may discuss their sexual concerns is an essential task in the doctor-patient relationship.
- Studies have demonstrated clearly that physicians' attitudes, perceptions, and experiences influence their ability to work with patients about sexual issues.
- Physicians should make a conscious effort to think about their attitudes and behavior in communicating with patients about sensitive areas such as sexuality.
- Physicians should also develop a solid knowledge base in the area of human sexuality so that they are well informed as they guide discussions with patients about sexual issues.
- The doctor-patient relationship, based on trust and professionalism, involves clear rules about physician conduct. Exploitation of patients, sexual and otherwise, is a violation of these rules.
- "Sexualized" behavior of patients should be viewed as efforts to communicate clinically important information; in such cases, physicians should recognize these signals, provide therapeutic intervention to their patients, and pursue perspective-restoring intervention for themselves.

Questions

1. Which of the following attitudes and attributes of medical students may interfere with their ability to work with patients about sexual issues?
   A. Feeling shy or embarrassed
   B. Having nonsympathetic views of patients' psychosocial problems
   C. Not feeling confident
   D. Feeling uncomfortable talking with homosexual patients
   E. All of the above

2. Physicians who perceive certain patients to be very dissimilar to themselves may have special difficulties communicating with those patients about sexual issues.
   A. True
   B. False

3. Physicians who perceive certain patients to be very similar to themselves may have special difficulties communicating with those patients about sexual issues.
   A. True
   B. False

4. One study looking at the experience of 16 patients who were sexually abused by a gynecologist indicated all of the following *except:*
   A. The gynecologist performed very lengthy pelvic examinations.
   B. The gynecologist's behavior made some patients fearful that something serious was wrong with them physically.
   C. The patients noticed the absence of a nurse during pelvic exams.
   D. The patients claimed that the gynecologist insisted on sexual intercourse during pelvic exams.
   E. The gynecologist made some patients feel that they could not stop inappropriate behaviors of the physician during pelvic exams.

5. Early studies of erotic and nonerotic physical contact with patients suggest all of the following *except:*

A. Female physicians may engage in more nonerotic touching, and male physicians may engage in more erotic practices with patients.

B. Nonerotic physical contact does occur between physicians and patients.

C. One quarter of physicians acknowledge nonerotic physical contact with patients.

D. A number of physicians believe that erotic physical contact with patients destroys the doctor-patient relationship.

E. Some medical students believe that sexual intercourse with patients could be appropriate.

6. Accurate statements concerning exploitation in the doctor-patient relationship include:

A. Exploited patients may feel powerless, be more mistrustful and angry toward others, and experience more physical and psychologic symptoms.

B. Effects of sexual involvement between physicians and patients are similar to problems that arise when teachers and students or supervisors and employees become intimately involved.

C. It is the clinician's responsibility to prevent sexual involvement with patients.

D. Sexual involvement is one form of patient exploitation; nonsexual exploitation may include practices such as asking favors or accepting large gifts from patients.

E. All of the above.

7. Strategies that medical students can use to become more comfortable with sexual issues in the care of patients include:

A. Learning more about physiologic and psychologic aspects of human sexuality

B. Developing a routine, thorough approach to taking a sexual history that involves addressing the patient's concerns about confidentiality

C. Identifying potential "blind spots" in their clinical work, such as feeling negatively about patients with sexually related illnesses

D. Consulting with supervisors on difficult or confusing cases

E. All of the above

Answers

1. E
2. A
3. A
4. D
5. C
6. E
7. E

Domestic violence and sexual assault

APGO LEARNING OBJECTIVE #56

Laura Weiss Roberts
Teresita A. McCarty
Lisa M. Fromm

Individuals who are the victims of domestic violence and sexual assault often experience significant physical and emotional sequelae. Clinicians should learn to recognize the presence and consequences of domestic violence and sexual assault in order to provide complete care for their patients.

The student will demonstrate a knowledge of the following:
A. Patterns of domestic violence
B. Rape and rape trauma syndrome
C. Evaluation of adult and child victims of sexual assault
D. Long-term physical and psychologic adjustment of victims

The presence of domestic violence and sexual assault in the lives of many women is a sobering reality for most clinicians. Learning to recognize, understand, and address the problems associated with physical and sexual violence is therefore an important, if disquieting, part of medical training. Toward this aim, four areas helpful in caring for victims of domestic violence and sexual assault are described: (1) patterns and consequences of domestic violence for women and families; (2) the experience of rape and the rape trauma syndrome; (3) the assessment of sexual assault victims; and (4) approaches to understanding sexual abuse of children.

DOMESTIC VIOLENCE

Domestic violence is neither trivial nor rare. Between 2 and 6 million women are assaulted by their spouses each year. Forty percent of wives are beaten and 10% of wives are raped by husbands during their marriages. In a study of emergency room visits, one quarter of the women patients identified themselves as victims of domestic abuse. Disturbing is the fact that battering may worsen during pregnancy and often targets the woman's abdomen. In addition, one quarter of homicides occur between family members, and nearly one half of all adult female homicide victims are killed by their spouses. Men are less often the victims of domestic violence; and, if they are injured or killed by wives, studies suggest that this often occurs during the wife's efforts to defend herself from attack. Violence directed at children is also widespread. Each year, 6% of all children in the United States are victims of violence. Annually in the United States 500,000 children experience some form of direct abuse, and another million are seriously neglected. Although little is known about its prevalence, elder abuse has also become increasingly recognized as a significant problem.

The response of social institutions to the problem of domestic violence has been less than adequate. For example, when police respond to domestic abuse reports, arrests occur very infrequently (1% to 3% of calls) although significant injury to women occurs quite commonly (25% to 40% of calls). It has been estimated that for every 200 wife assaults, 28 are reported to the police, 3 arrests are made, 1 conviction occurs, and fewer than 1 abusive spouse serves a jail sentence. Similarly, clinicians have been slow to recognize the phenomenon of domestic violence and to intervene effectively. Studies have shown that battered women often make repeated and fruitless efforts to get help, formally and informally. Many behaviors of abused women are looked upon as "self-defeating" or "enabling" by the health professionals from whom they seek assistance, when these behaviors should in fact be recognized as complex responses to ensure their own survival and that of their children. The helplessness experienced by victims of domestic violence should be viewed as being very real.

Domestic violence has a significant impact on families that goes beyond the immediate injury. These long-term consequences manifest as psychologic suffering and further violence through homicide, suicide, and accidental death. Family violence tends to be repeated and progressive. It usually involves an incident of abuse followed by loving reconciliation and by more frequent violence and less frequent periods of reconciliation as the abuser gains greater control over the victims. Most abusive partners experienced or witnessed a similar pattern of severe violence in childhood. One half of abused women were victims of childhood physical or sexual abuse. One third of abused children become abusive parents. Thus this "cycle of violence" tends to be transmitted across generations. Abused women may develop "battered woman syndrome," a form of posttraumatic stress disorder. The full syndrome is defined by three elements: direct trauma effects, including fear, physical injuries, and somatic symptoms; psychologic difficulties, including anxiety, depression, isolation, hopelessness, and passivity; and compromised coping mechanisms, such as projection, denial, and guilt. A similar constellation of symptoms and signs occurs in children who are victims of violence. Ultimately, a large proportion of abused children develop severe psychiatric problems. In addition, although not true for every child, a vast number of abused children manifest criminal and violent behavior in adulthood. In sum, domestic violence is harmful to women, children, and the society at large.

Intervention strategies should aim to identify the presence of domestic abuse, give immediate safety to victims, prevent future danger, and provide advocacy and support. Assessment strategies for the care of women and children who are victims of sexual assault are described in the next sections. An ability to recognize the clinical signs of domestic abuse and to perform associated triage decisions are skills that should be part of the basic repertoire of every clinician. Treatment may necessitate extensive resources and involvement by psychiatrists, pediatricians, obstetrician-gynecologists, and other health care personnel.

RAPE

Rape is a term used in everyday language to describe the act of forcing a woman to have sexual intercourse against her will. The legal definition of rape is wider in that it involves a range of unwanted sexual activities associated with threats and physical force and may include penetration ("completed rape") or may not ("attempted rape"). The law provides for additional protection and for more severe criminal penalties when sexual assault involves victims from certain age groups (e.g., children) or populations (e.g., psychiatric patients or institutionalized individuals). A violent crime, rape is often thought of as an event involving strangers; but many women are raped by people they know—by husbands, by boyfriends, by acquaintances. Acquaintance rape (sometimes called "date rape") can be devastating and is a form of sexual assault with serious clinical and legal sequelae. Coercive sexuality is a more comprehensive, less pejorative phrase that reflects how violence in the sexual lives of some individuals occurs along a continuum. Irrespective of how certain sexual experiences fit into the various definitions of rape, all coerced sexual events have important physical and psychologic consequences that require sensitive and astute medical attention.

Many personal and social factors make women hesitant to report rape. Consequently, obtaining accurate information about the frequency of rape is very difficult. Women victims fear humiliation and the stigma that accompanies rape disclosure to their family, friends, physicians, and police. When perpetrators are known to the victims (e.g., boyfriend, spouse), women may feel responsible for the assault or fearful of future retaliation. Victims may not recognize some coercive sexual acts as rape, even though they clearly meet the legal definition. Ultimately, fewer than 10% of rapes are reported to the police and only 1% of rapes result in conviction. Thus research may underdocument the presence of rape in women's lives.

Several studies from across the United States suggest that women are at significant risk of rape. An early community study in San Francisco of 930 women showed a lifetime prevalence (i.e., the chance of being raped or a victim of attempted rape in a woman's lifetime) of 44%. Twenty-four percent of the women had experienced a completed rape. A South Carolina study found that 23% of women in their sample had experienced a completed rape and another 13% had experienced a rape attempt, a total prevalence of 36%. A Los Angeles study found a combined rape/attempted rape prevalence rate of 25% in African-American women and of 20% in white women. On college campuses, rape may be even more prevalent. In one large study of 3187 women college students, 53.7% reported sexual victimization, and 27.5% reported attempted or completed rapes. Research on the frequency of sexual assault on university campuses indicates that 25% to 60% of college men acknowledge having perpetrated coercive sexual activity of some form.

Understanding the phenomenon of rape entails an understanding of the behaviors of rapists. Four primary motivations for sexually coercive behavior have been described: (1) opportunistic; (2) pervasively angry; (3) sexualized (nonsadistic and sadistic types); and (4) vindictive (Table 56-1). Opportunistic rapes occur when an impulsive person encounters a situation where sexual exploitation of a woman victim is possible (e.g., acquaintance rape). These men do not plan their attacks. Opportunistic rapists may be impulsive in many areas of their lives or, in contrast, only under special circumstances (e.g., during wartime or while intoxicated) in which temporary suspension of judgment may occur. Opportunistic rapists display little empathy or anger and are unlikely to injure or use force deliberately unless the victim resists.

Pervasively angry rapists experience rage that is nonspecific and inclusive and are likely to assault men, women, and children. They intentionally

Table 56-1. Behaviors and motivations of rapists

Type	Description
Opportunistic	Impulsive act; often suspended judgment; may not physically injure victim; resistance may deter attack
Pervasively angry	Impulsive act; globally enraged; may injure or kill victim; resistance may worsen attack
Sexualized	Obsessive thinking about sex; calculated, ritually planned attacks
Nonsadistic	May not physically injure victim; resistance may deter attack
Sadistic	Derives pleasure from inflicting injury and instilling fear; may seriously injure or kill victim
Vindictive	Impulsive or calculated act; extremely violent and may kill victim; seeks to degrade victim

hurt and even kill their victims, particularly if the victims offer resistance. Predictably, they show anger and impulsiveness in many aspects of their lives, not only in their sexual behavior.

Sexualized rapists differ from opportunistic and pervasively angry rapists in that they think obsessively about sex. They may accumulate items that stimulate their sexual thoughts, such as pornography. They often research and plan their attack ritually in response to intense, unregulated sexual urges. Sexualized rapists are categorized as nonsadistic or sadistic according to their behaviors and forms of gratification. The nonsadistic, sexualized rapist obtains erotic pleasure by enacting his sexual wishes with the coerced victim. Victim resistance may deter the nonsadistic type of sexualized rapist since it may disrupt the careful plan and may not be consistent with the rapist's fantasy. The sadistic rapist, however, experiences sexual arousal and gratification from causing pain and fear in the victim. Such a rapist might encourage resistance to pursue greater violence and heighten the accompanying erotic state.

Vindictive rapists focus their anger specifically on women. Their attacks seem meant to injure and degrade their victims. The hostility displayed ranges from verbal abuse to murder, and the rape is merely part of the larger assault.

Rape trauma syndrome

The rape trauma syndrome, like battered woman syndrome, is a form of posttraumatic stress disorder and follows a predictable course despite differences in victims and the sexual assaults they have survived. Rape trauma syndrome has five phases (Fig. 56-1). It is helpful to think of these phases in terms of the immediate and the enduring psychologic consequences of rape.

Directly following rape, women experience several psychologic and physical difficulties. Women may feel very emotional (frightened, worried, or angry) or excessively restricted (subdued, dazed, or withdrawn). Some may fluctuate from one state to the other. The victim typically feels that her emotional state is beyond her control; that is, she feels different from her usual self and is uncomfortable. Rape victims often develop specific fears that are associated with the circumstances of the rape (e.g., fear of the park or of a room similar to the one where the rape took place). In addition, women who have been raped report feelings of sadness, vulnerability, anxiety, self-blame, and humiliation. Forty percent of sexual assault victims meet the criteria for depression during this acute phase. In addition to psychiatric symptoms, rape victims may experience a variety of physical problems. In

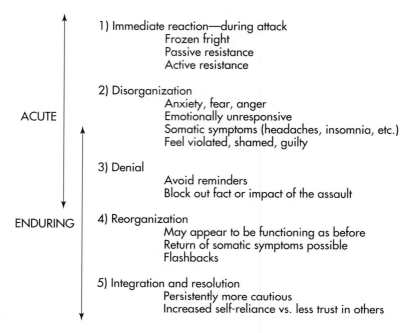

1) Immediate reaction—during attack
        Frozen fright
        Passive resistance
        Active resistance

2) Disorganization
        Anxiety, fear, anger
        Emotionally unresponsive
        Somatic symptoms (headaches, insomnia, etc.)
        Feel violated, shamed, guilty

3) Denial
        Avoid reminders
        Block out fact or impact of the assault

4) Reorganization
        May appear to be functioning as before
        Return of somatic symptoms possible
        Flashbacks

5) Integration and resolution
        Persistently more cautious
        Increased self-reliance vs. less trust in others

ACUTE

ENDURING

Fig. 56-1. Rape trauma syndrome.

the days to weeks after the attack, headache, anorexia, fatigue, startle, insomnia, muscle pain, feeling "edgy," and slow recovery from physical injuries are common complaints.

The immediate effects of rape on relationships are profound. Initially rape victims become socially isolated. They tend to withdraw from their usual friends, family, and work relationships. They may feel inadequate, disconnected, or compromised in their personal lives. Sexual intimacy in particular is disrupted. Over half of women who have been raped will report sexual dysfunction, decreased sexual activity, and diminished pleasure, which may persist for years after the assault. Particularly when women have not fully disclosed the story of the assault, changes in social attachments and sexual intimacy may be misunderstood by others. In the acute period, women who have been assaulted feel that they have lost everything: their sense of being safe and sturdy in the world; their comfort within their own bodies and their

sexuality; and their capacity for closeness with others.

The enduring consequences of sexual assault are especially important to identify because they may lead to an insidious, persistent narrowing of the victim's world. Over a period of time, many women who have been raped limit their lives—they limit their relationships, their expressions of feeling, and their willingness to enter new situations. Women may pretend that the assault never happened and yet avoid all circumstances that remind them of it. Despite such efforts to control their experiences, the memories, intrusive images, startle reflex, and insomnia frequently persist. Victims may think differently about the world, experience a vague sense of rage toward others, and feel a greater degree of self-doubt. Women may not associate the internal changes and the external narrowing of their lives with the assault. Gradually they reorganize their lives. Many aspects of their social adjustment may recover superficially within 4 months; work functioning, however, often takes longer to improve. Somatic symptoms may recur intermittently, and, again, these physical complaints may not seem related to the original assault. Up to 25% of women who have been raped remain depressed for years. A far larger number, if not all women who have been raped, state they feel irreversibly changed by the sexual assault. Many women ultimately feel strengthened by the assault experience; some women feel permanently damaged and unable to recover.

Psychiatric intervention is essential in helping victims of sexual assault, but often it is resisted or refused by the victim. Women who have been raped are reluctant to pursue psychiatric care for a variety of reasons. They may find psychotherapy to be a painful reminder of the assault. They may not recognize or believe that their vague but persistent psychologic and physical symptoms are related to the rape. They may feel further stigmatized by the need for such help. They may feel so altered fundamentally that they doubt the "help" will actually make them feel better. Ironically and sadly, hopelessness and avoidance experienced by rape survivors may prevent them from receiving the help they need.

For these reasons, it is important for clinicians to urge patients who have been assaulted to get psychiatric care, especially if they sense a subtle decline in their patients' well-being. Clinicians should inform their patients that although psychologic and physical symptoms are a natural consequence of sexual assault, they are clearly amenable to treatment. Therapeutic strategies including psychologic support during the disclosure process and subsequent reconstruction of their daily lives, medications such as antidepressants and anxiolytics, and appropriate social interventions greatly benefit traumatized patients. Moreover, psychiatric illnesses that may accompany the rape trauma syndrome (e.g., major depression; posttraumatic stress disorder; generalized anxiety disorder), once established, tend to take on lives of their own beyond the direct sequelae of sexual assault. Consequently,

women who have been raped may ultimately experience other severe psychiatric and psychosocial repercussions, including substance abuse, domestic violence, unemployment, and family dysfunction. Primary clinicians not only play a principal role in identifying victims of sexual assault; they also must make certain that these victims receive the care they need to reestablish healthy lives.

ASSESSMENT OF SEXUAL ASSAULT VICTIMS

The assessment of women who have been sexually assaulted presents several immediate challenges: to ensure safety; to provide emotional support; to give accurate information; and to evaluate the physical and psychologic state of the patient. These are not simple tasks, individually or collectively. Clinicians who remain mindful of their manner in approaching the patient, of the potential for self-blame by the patient, and of the initial goals of emergency care to the patient will be more successful in their efforts to conduct a therapeutic and medically valuable assessment.

The clinician's manner in approaching the victim is crucial in conveying a sense of safety and trust. The victim should be encouraged and allowed to describe the assault in her own way and at her own pace. Appearing to doubt the story by seeming skeptical or by asking questions too early in the interaction is harmful and interferes with the evaluation process. While discomfort may be inevitable for most victims (especially if forensic evidence must be collected), every effort should be made to prevent the assessment from repeating or worsening the trauma associated with the assault experience. Since many women do not seek care after a rape and are frequently reluctant to volunteer information, asking about unwanted sexual activity should be a part of the history gathered during routine obstetrician-gynecologist visits. Clinicians who are nonjudgmental, gentle, and thorough are best able to support their patients, whether the disclosure is of a recent or remote traumatic event.

The clinician's approach is also important while the victim deals with the powerful issue of self-blame. For many reasons, women will blame themselves for some aspect of the assault (e.g., they somehow invited the attack, they could have handled it differently, they should have reported it sooner), although they may not mention this. Every rape situation and every rapist is unique. Given the wide range of rapist motivations and behaviors, it is difficult to second-guess whether a woman should or should not have resisted a rapist. A woman's response will be based on her previous life experiences, her real and perceived abilities in the moment of the attack, and her instantaneous and shifting judgment of what must be done to protect herself and/or others in the situation (e.g., children). It becomes clear, therefore, that reassuring a woman that she made the best decisions possible in a difficult situation is not only helpful but true.

Clinicians should anticipate these issues and explain that sexual assault is always experienced as a life-or-death, terrifying event—even if the perpetrator is familiar to the woman, even if no weapons are involved, and even if the patient escapes without severe physical harm. Reassurance that what happened was not deserved and that she made good choices and conducted herself well, as evidenced by her survival, will greatly help the victim immediately and in the future. The clinician should never suggest that the victim was in any way responsible for the assault.

The goals of emergency clinical care for a woman who has been sexually assaulted include performing a history and physical examination in a sensitive and thorough manner, addressing acute medical needs, clarifying legal issues and collecting forensic evidence, and arranging for treatment. Whenever possible, offering accurate information and allowing the woman to make choices about the context and sequence of the history-taking and physical examination

will put her more at ease. Pressing medical needs should be assessed carefully and treated appropriately. The individual should fully consent to all medical procedures and decisions (e.g., vaginal examination, pregnancy test, and others). Moreover, in nearly all cases, the victim must consent to reporting the assault and to the gathering of evidence for the criminal investigation. The forensic investigation should not be coerced unless there are clear indications involving the law (e.g., homicide in association with the assault). Evidence kits and guidelines for assessment ordinarily are available in emergency room or urgent care settings. Appropriate documentation of information obtained is important (e.g., including direct quotes when possible, not speculating beyond data, not giving personal opinions for or against the victim's story), as it may be used in a police investigation. Efforts to protect the victim's confidentiality despite the need for forensic investigation can be crucial for the woman's privacy and future well-being. Clinicians should disclose only essential information. They should not volunteer information about the woman's history and not give her full medical record carte blanche to the police. Treatment for injuries, pregnancy, and sexually transmitted diseases should be provided to the rape victim. Follow-up for physical and psychiatric sequelae of the assault should be arranged before her departure.

SEXUAL ABUSE OF CHILDREN

Sexual abuse of children is a compelling clinical and societal issue. Conservative estimates of the prevalence of childhood sexual abuse range from 6% for girls and 3% for boys; however, abuse may actually be 10 times greater for both girls and boys. In providing care to families, it is essential that sexual abuse be defined, detected, and addressed. In fulfilling duties as a practitioner, it is imperative that sexual abuse be reported and investigated.

Both of these activities must be handled therapeutically or they may result in greater damage to fragile, ill families and their most vulnerable members, children.

Recognition of sexual abuse involves understanding its definition, knowing about perpetrator attributes, and remaining mindful of clinical signs of abuse. In childhood sexual abuse, three elements must be considered: (1) age difference between child and perpetrator; (2) types of sexual behaviors (e.g., fondling, kissing, penetration, nudity, exhibitionism); and (3) sexual gratification of the perpetrator. Some researchers believe that the experience of dominating the child is also a form of nonsexual gratification for the perpetrator. Incest involves sexual contact between members of the same family (e.g., parents, siblings, stepparents) or those acting in a parental role, such as live-in partners. Proof of coercion is not necessary for sexual abuse of a child, because of the clear power differential between perpetrator and victim and the obvious inability of the victim to choose the sexual activity freely and without fear of ill consequence.

Perpetrators may be of either gender but typically are men who themselves may have been victimized sexually or physically. They may be family members or friends, baby-sitters, teachers, day-care workers, or others. They tend to have multiple victims, including children and adults from within or outside the family. In one study, 49% of incestuous fathers and stepfathers referred for treatment abused both related and nonrelated children. Of these men, 18% also raped adult women during the time they were abusing their own children.

The simple fact of being a child is the major risk factor for becoming a victim of sexual abuse. Clinical signs of childhood abuse include such changes in behavior as worsening school performance, irritability, poor sleep or nightmares, withdrawal, depression, temper tantrums, excessive masturbation; sexually related remarks by children in family and clinical contexts; direct statements reporting sexual molestation; and sexualized play. Medical conditions that lead the clinician to suspect sexual abuse include genital or rectal pain, trauma, dilatation, and infection or unusual physical complaints (e.g., persistent abdominal pain or headaches).

Once sexual abuse is suspected, clinical and forensic issues become extremely important. Assessment of abused children should be done by specialists (pediatrician, family practitioner, gynecologist) who have dealt with these issues. Treatment of children who have been sexually abused is a specialized clinical area; referral to mental health specialists is appropriate and necessary. It is mandatory to report suspicions of abuse to legal authorities who will investigate and, if necessary, intervene on an emergent basis to protect the child from further harm. In many states, a clinician who fails to report suspected abuse may lose his or her medical license. Since sexual abuse investigations can become criminal cases and often involve child custody disputes, following appropriate forensic protocols is imperative. Many problems can arise (e.g., the credibility of the young child, the tendency of children to retract valid allegations in an attempt to preserve the family structure, bias in clinicians who perform assessments, false accusations encouraged by angry, separating parents). Clinicians therefore must be scrupulous in their conduct while caring for abused children.

SUMMARY

The widespread presence of domestic violence and sexual assault is a sobering reality for most clinicians. In the United States, between 2 and 6 million women are assaulted by their spouses annually; 1.5 million children are abused and/or neglected annually; it is unknown how many elderly are victims of domestic violence annually. Between one quarter and one half of women will be victims of sexual assault in their lifetimes.

CRITICAL POINTS

- The response of social institutions to the problems of domestic violence and sexual assault has thus far been inadequate and reinforces the helplessness and hopelessness experienced by victims.
- Clinicians are especially important in identifying domestic violence and sexual assault in their patients. They play a crucial role in providing appropriate medical, psychologic, and social supports for victims. Clinicians are also responsible for reporting suspected abuse in children.
- The outcomes of domestic violence include significant physical injury and psychologic harm (e.g., battered woman syndrome), at times leading to death and perpetration of violence across generations and throughout society.
- Rape trauma syndrome, a form of posttraumatic stress disorder, involves five phases; clinically, it is important to appreciate and provide treatment for the predictable immediate and enduring sequelae of sexual assault.
- Victims of domestic violence and sexual assault should be understood as survivors who have made adaptations under extraordinary difficulties; they should never be blamed or denied treatment because of their postassault symptoms.
- Rapists have been categorized according to their different behaviors and motivations as opportunistic (e.g., acquaintance rape), pervasively angry, sexualized, or vindictive.
- Assessment of sexual assault victims aims to ensure safety, provide emotional support, give accurate information, and evaluate the physical and psychologic state of the patient. Difficult forensic issues often arise; clinicians should follow the guidelines of their institution and state and should seek appropriate consultation when questions occur.
- All children are at risk for sexual abuse. It is a common, though underrecognized, clinical issue and, like physical abuse and neglect, must be reported to legal authorities.
- Signs of child sexual abuse include changes in behavior, verbal statements reporting sexual molestation, and physical indications such as trauma, pain, and infection.

Questions

1. Accurate statements about the definition of sexual abuse of children include all of the following *except:*
   A. An age difference exists between the child and the perpetrator.
   B. Sexual behaviors (e.g., fondling, kissing, penetration, nudity, exhibitionism) are involved.
   C. Sexual gratification of the perpetrator occurs.
   D. Proof of coercion is necessary.
   E. Some believe that domination of the child represents a form of nonsexual gratification for the perpetrator.

2. During the assessment of a woman who has been the victim of sexual assault, efforts to ensure that the evaluation process is therapeutic and not retraumatizing include all of the following *except:*
   A. Reassuring the patient that she was not at fault for the assault
   B. When possible, allowing the patient to control the context and sequence of the evaluation process

C. Insisting on the presence of the police during the evaluation for the patient's sense of safety

D. Assuming a nonjudgmental attitude when speaking with the patient

E. Encouraging the patient to tell her story of the assault in her own way and at her own pace

3. A patient being examined immediately after being raped might display:
   A. Emotional outbursts
   B. Calm demeanor
   C. Concern for the rapist
   D. Reluctance to inform family or police
   E. Doubt about how she responded to the rapist
   F. All of the above

4. Indications of sexual abuse in children include:
   A. Irritability and poor sleep or nightmares
   B. Temper tantrums
   C. Excessive masturbation
   D. Sexually related remarks by children in family and clinical contexts and/or sexualized play
   E. All of the above

5. Rapists have been described as:
   A. Pervasively angry
   B. Vindictive
   C. Opportunistic
   D. Sexualized—sadistic and nonsadistic types
   E. All of the above

6. Accurate statements about the battered woman syndrome include all of the following *except:*
   A. It is a form of posttraumatic stress disorder.

B. All women who are victims of domestic violence develop the syndrome.

C. Direct effects of trauma include fear, anxiety, physical injury, and somatic symptoms.

D. Women may develop depression, isolation, hopelessness, and passivity.

E. Compromised coping mechanisms include projection, denial, and guilt.

7. Research-based statements about domestic violence include:
   A. Between 2 and 6 million women are assaulted by their husbands each year, and between one third and one half of women homicide victims are killed by their spouses.
   B. Battering may worsen during pregnancy, and battering during pregnancy often targets the woman's abdomen.
   C. Forty percent of wives are beaten, and 10% of wives are raped during the course of their marriages.
   D. One quarter of the women patients seen in a study of emergency room visits identified themselves as victims of domestic abuse.
   E. All of the above.

Answers

1. D
2. C
3. F
4. E
5. E
6. B
7. E

VII

Professional behavior, ethics, and legal issues

57

Personal interaction and communication skills

APGO LEARNING OBJECTIVE #57

Joseph B. Buxer

> *The ability to interact cooperatively with all members of a health care team and with a patient is a hallmark of professional medical care.*

The student will demonstrate the ability to:
A. Establish rapport with patients
B. Work cooperatively and dependably with patients and other members of the health care team
C. Recognize personal limitations

ESTABLISH RAPPORT WITH PATIENTS

The traditional approach to patient interactions that medical schools teach a physician involves three steps: (1) gathering data by listening to the patient's complaint and noting any pertinent medical history; (2) examining anatomy, testing physiology, and developing a diagnosis; and (3) prescribing treatment. Although this approach is eminently logical and quite effective for detective work, it is not designed to establish rapport with patients. As the physician meticulously explains the treatment plan, hoping to enlist compliance, the patient is not necessarily thinking about health care in the same way as the physician and probably will not comply. Research shows that only about 30% of patients actually fill a prescription and take a medication exactly as directed.

For a successful physician-patient encounter to occur, there must be bonding on a person-to-person basis, however brief. An exchange of information and of understanding can take place only if both the patient and the physician are actively engaged in the process—together. The physician, as the consulted professional, is responsible for making this happen. Steps to take and attitudes to adopt are explored here.

Approach to the patient

Always greet a new patient while she is fully clothed. This would also be good to do for all subsequent patient visits if possible. Introduce yourself and your helpers to every new patient, communicating welcome with body language, facial expression, and words. Express interest in the patient as a person, not just as a medical problem, acknowledging her value as an individual. Try to sit or stand so that your head is at approximately the same height as the patient's because unequal height conveys dominance.

Next, use common experiences or background situations to establish familiarity. Familiarity creates comfort, and comfort engenders trust. Listen to your patient's use of language and consider trying to say things the way she says them to enhance her understanding and comfort level. Listen to her words and use them in conversation with her as appropriate.

Recognize that your thoughts and your speech differ from those of your patient. In addition, your unique thought process is always dominated by the decision tree. The patient is the only one who can tell you the story of her illness. It is unreasonable to expect her to tell it in case presentation format. She is much more likely to talk in terms of expected life consequences and fear of being forced to change her role either at work or at home. Encourage your patient to tell her story in her own words. Protect the first 3 minutes of each interview as the patient's *time to tell her story* without interruption. Research recently indicated that the average physician interrupts a patient's narrative after only 18 seconds.

Search for and listen to all complaints. The average patient comes to an office visit with three complaints or worries, and the first one mentioned usually is not the most important. Once all complaints are voiced, you must prioritize them. If all issues clearly cannot be addressed in one visit, you should ask, "What were you hoping we could accomplish today?" The patient can then join in deciding with you what is most important for that day. Without this process, major complaints surely will be "doorknob" complaints, mentioned as the patient is about to leave the office: "By the way, doctor, . . . "

When the patient is done, acknowledge that you have heard her story by using responses that communicate interest, such as, "That must have

been very uncomfortable." You can use body language to encourage her, perhaps by leaning toward her. Always look at the patient. Use open-ended questions, such as, "Tell me more about . . . " At least at first, avoid questions that can be answered with one word.

Do not assume that you now know why the patient has come. Ask, "What else has been happening?" "Is there something else you were worried about?" Sometimes a visit is simply to get a form signed. More frequently, all the patient wants is reassurance about a situation. If you find that the patient's concerns are clearly too extensive to cover in one visit, ask her to return for a second visit.

Always express empathy. Although everyone wants you to be technically excellent, each individual patient also needs you to present yourself as a human being. Luckily, empathy is not an inherited trait but can be learned. It involves an active concern for and a curiosity about the emotions, values, and experiences of others. This includes demonstrating an awareness that the patient has feelings and values. Notice and comment on what she says. See and hear her, and let her know that she has been seen and heard. Help her see that not only are her feelings and values understood, they are both acceptable and valuable to you, her physician. Sometimes just a word about yourself as a person can communicate to your patient that her feelings and values are appropriate topics for discussion.

Empathy means that you are attentive to and engaged with the patient. Remaining distant and distracted cannot achieve your goal of a successful physician-patient encounter. You must express attentiveness, curiosity, and sincere interest in her world. Do not write in the chart and pretend to listen at the same time. It is preferable not to write at all; if you must write, you may alternate writing and listening. In addition, do not read the chart while the patient is talking. Give her your full attention.

Acknowledge the patient's thoughts, but do not evaluate them. A good approach would be, "I understand that you're scared at the thought of surgery. Let's talk about it." It is never effective to tell her that "There's no reason to be scared." She won't believe it.

Notice facial expressions. They always communicate feelings, but they don't do it very well. When you comment on her facial expression, you give the patient permission to express her feelings; for example, "I see you frown when I say the word *diet*." It is helpful at times to share your own experience with a similar problem if you believe it will facilitate your patient's well-being.

Patient education

Patient education is a complex process, not only because patients have different desires and different needs for information, but also because of your need to obtain truly informed consent. A few patients want to know about diagnosis, etiology, treatment, prognosis, and functional consequences. These should be easy subjects for you because they are part of your natural thought processes.

Many patients think they already have the information they need because of previous conversations about their condition with friends, relatives, and workmates. Their residual questions may have nothing to do with what the physician thinks is important.

You may need to prompt the patient to ask questions, even if they are important to her. Examples include, "Am I doing the right thing?" "Do I have to stop working the night shift?" You should ask, "Is there anything else that you have been wondering about?" and maintain an interested, nonrushed expression.

Most patients do want to know what happened to them and why it happened. They may also ask, "What's going to happen to me in the short run? What about long term? What are you going to do to me? Why are you doing this instead of something else? Will it hurt? How much? For how long? When will you know what all these tests mean? When and how will I know?"

Patient education is more than providing information. It doesn't work until your patient is able to use the information you provide effectively. Therefore you should ask open-ended questions that are clear invitations for the patient to express her fears and frustrations, such as "Are there other answers that you need? What information would be useful to you at this time?"

To evaluate whether the patient understands what you have said, a good approach is, "I know that I forget to mention things at times. Tell me what you understand so far. I may have forgotten something important."

Failure to establish rapport

From time to time you meet patients who are unable to respond to your efforts. They may be too frustrated and angry about their condition, too frightened for constructive engagement, or simply rude and demanding for no obvious reason. Others may be emotionally disturbed. Whatever the reason, if you have made the effort to bond with the patient and it has not been successful, it does not reflect on your competence. An unexpected and unwanted response should not be interpreted as personal rejection. Understand that it would have happened with anyone at that particular time, and do not react negatively. Try to understand the situation.

WORK COOPERATIVELY AND DEPENDABLY WITH OTHER MEMBERS OF THE HEALTH CARE TEAM

Unreasonable responses must not occur between members of the health care team. Each is a professional whose role is clearly defined, and each understands that the team's ultimate goal of excellence in patient care can be achieved only through the smooth cooperation of its members, much like the frictionless meshing of gears in a precision instrument. But even the best machine may need lubrication from time to time, so an interesting process has evolved to avoid misunderstandings or to manage them should they occur. If anyone perceives a problem, each team member involved is asked to recognize the problem. Each person's role is then redefined in light of the problem, and therapeutic measures are devised that are acceptable to all. In the process, each member of the team is asked to recognize the other members' discomfort.

For example, assume a third-year medical student rotating through clinical clerkships in obstetrics and gynecology at a teaching hospital complains that a few nurses treat her badly. The nurses may communicate clearly through body language and facial expression, as well as verbally, that a student is underfoot, in the way, nearly useless technically, and sure to say something inappropriate to patients. In this situation, the nurses do not understand the role of medical students or their 36-hour work shifts, endless study, texts, lectures, and constant house officer and faculty evaluations, so they are unsympathetic. The medical student does not understand the nurse's role, duties, responsibilities, pressures, and frustrations, so she feels rejected. As a result, communication freezes.

A very successful preemptive solution to this problem is called "the shadow program." Each medical student, on the first working day of a rotation, "shadows" an experienced labor room nurse. The student does everything with the nurse for the entire shift, learning the nurse's duties and responsibilities and experiencing her professional pressures and frustrations. The student "walks in the nurse's shoes." An originally unexpected, but very welcome, side benefit of the program is that the shadowed nurse learns the student's role and becomes a committed teacher. As a result, communication flourishes.

The steps used in solving communications problems between a physician and other members of the health care team are as follows:

1. Each person involved must admit there is a problem.

2. Each person's role must be defined.
3. Appropriate therapeutic goals must be agreed upon.
4. Each person must understand the other's defensiveness.
5. The program must be repeated with each new student group.

Working cooperatively and dependably with colleagues is a similar, and actually simpler, issue, necessitating only the courtesy of direct physician-to-physician communication. When physicians make the effort and take the time to talk to each other, patient care always improves. When physicians find they haven't the time for courtesies, patient care suffers.

Assume that a patient has entered an emergency room because she is ill and doesn't know where else to go. Her chart identifies her as a member of the hospital's gynecology clinic. The emergency room physician, knowing that "her doctor" (the gynecology resident on call) is always in house, pages her. A nurse answers the page and says that the resident is about to scrub for surgery. The nurse asks the nature of the problem and is told that the patient is having trouble breathing and that her wheezing can be heard across the room. The nurse replies that this is obviously a medical problem and the internal medicine resident should be called.

The emergency room physician reaches the internal medicine resident and describes the patient's respiratory distress. The resident, who is also quite busy, asks who the attending physician is and, when told, immediately considers the patient a "dump"—a bundle of work transferred without permission by a lazy colleague. Although the internal medicine resident insists he is too busy to see the patient, within an hour he reaches the emergency room and successfully treats the patient.

The results of this brief three-physician encounter are as follows:

1. The patient suffered respiratory distress for an hour longer than necessary.

2. The emergency room physician wasted valuable time attempting to "sell" a patient to two colleagues instead of attending to other patients who were waiting.

3. The gynecology resident infuriated both the emergency room physician and her internal medicine colleague without saying a word to either one and without even knowing that anything was wrong.

4. The emergency room physician planned never again to talk to either resident.

5. The internal medicine resident, feeling abused and resenting both the emergency room physician and the gynecology resident, risked doing an angry and superficial evaluation of the patient's problem; without saying anything to either the emergency room physician or the gynecology resident, the internal medicine resident discharged the patient with instructions to appear at the gynecology clinic the next morning. The gynecology clinic, of course, was unprepared to see the patient when she arrived.

This problem with communication among colleagues is all too common. Although its resolution is both simple and intuitively obvious, it necessitates direct communication.

1. Each physician must agree that there is a problem. (This is not difficult in this case because everyone is angry.)

2. Each physician's role must be defined. (The emergency room physician could have evaluated the patient, reported his evaluation and acute treatment to the gynecology resident, and suggested follow-up the next day at the clinic. The gynecology resident could then alert the clinic staff to prepare for the patient's arrival. Reevaluation at the clinic would determine the need for specialty consultation, and, if needed, the gynecology resident would personally call the internal medicine resident requesting his help.)

3. Appropriate goals must be agreed upon. (The ultimate appropriate goal, of course, is for physicians to communicate directly with physicians, not through intermediaries. Had the gynecology resident explained to the emergency room physician that her surgery patient had a ruptured ectopic pregnancy and was unstable, the emergency room physician might well have volunteered to treat the patient until the surgery was done. Failing that, the gynecology resident must deal with two simultaneous emergencies. She must personally call the internal medicine resident, acknowledge responsibility for the patient in the emergency room, and ask for emergency help for her patient's respiratory distress. This would not be perceived as a "dump," but rather as an urgent request from one physician to another for emergency consultation for the benefit of a patient. The gynecology resident has not withdrawn from her ultimate responsibility for the patient and remains involved.)

4. Each individual must understand why the others feel put upon. (If the emergency room physician understood why the gynecology resident could not respond, he would be far less critical. If the gynecology resident knew how the internal medicine resident perceived the call from the emergency room physician and how badly the case was presented, she would have called the internal medicine resident just as soon as she broke scrub to explain her temporary absence. Had the internal medicine resident been consulted by either physician as a specialist colleague instead of simply summoned to do "scut work," a thorough evaluation and a helpful consultation report would have resulted, with recommendations for further care. In the end, the patient would have been better served.)

5. The program requires constant reinforcement.

House staff, always overworked and under pressure, are constantly rotating to other services. Each new group must be instructed that courteous, direct communication among colleagues saves both time and tempers and always results in improved patient care.

RECOGNIZE PERSONAL LIMITATIONS

I believe that the most important personal limitation physicians work with on a daily basis is the normal human emotional response to being challenged. Statements to support this view include, "The patient is totally unreasonable in her endless demands, and I know she will eventually consult a lawyer." "The nurse doesn't follow my orders as written, and then she writes incident reports." "I wrote an order on the chart 3 days ago to get the ethics committee involved in this case, but they never came." Each of these problems is certainly unwanted, probably unnecessary, and possibly amenable to solution. Try to understand why the patient is unreasonable. Once you understand her underlying problem, you may be able to find a way to help her. Talk with the nurse to discover why she objects to the way you write your orders. Once you understand her objection, you may find a change beneficial to both of you. Talk with the colleague whose help you need, one on one. Explain the problem. If your colleague can help, he or she will do so immediately. If not, the colleague may be able to guide you to those who can, in one brief conversation, without the need for endless daily chart notes to each other.

CRITICAL POINTS

- To foster a patient's understanding of and compliance with her care, she must be engaged by the physician to become an active partner in that care.
- To avoid misunderstandings among members of a health care team, all potential problems must be acknowledged by each member and addressed together by those directly involved.
- To enhance patient care, colleagues must always communicate directly, one-on-one, and not through intermediaries.

Questions

1. A patient tells a member of the office staff that her physician seemed inattentive during her last visit. As the physician talks to this patient during her next visit, actions that would help to improve her impression include:

A. Looking directly at her when she speaks
B. Repeatedly reassuring her that her worries are really worrisome
C. Answering her questions in the simplest terms possible
D. Allowing her interview to be interrupted only by telephone calls, lab results, and nurse's questions

E. Writing down everything she says while she is saying it
2. Problem solving within the health care team includes all of the following *except:*
    A. Each team member must understand what is bothering other team members.
    B. Each team member must realize that a problem exists.
    C. All problem solving should be done by whoever is in charge of the team that day.
    D. Each team member's role must be restated for the others.
    E. All potential problems must be restated with the arrival of every new team member.
3. An attending physician recognizes that her hospitalized patient may be developing a medical problem beyond her expertise. A reasonable and convenient way to handle this issue would be to:

A. Discharge the patient early so that she can see her primary care physician
B. Order for the patient whatever she says helped this symptom in the past
C. Write an order in the chart for "Dr. Jones to see pt."
D. Ask her office receptionist to call Dr. Jones' office receptionist to arrange for a hospital consultation.
E. Find Dr. Jones in the doctor's lounge the same day and discuss the question over coffee.

Answers

1. A
2. C
3. E

58

Legal issues in obstetrics and gynecology

APGO LEARNING OBJECTIVE #58

Joseph B. Buxer

Legal obligations describe minimal obligations to protect patients' interests and are effective only when understood and applied.

The student will demonstrate a knowledge of the following:

A. Informed consent
   1. Right to refuse care
   2. Outcomes
   3. Options and alternatives
   4. Capacity to choose
   5. Surrogate decision makers
B. Advance directives for health care
C. Confidentiality
D. Abandonment
E. Contractual nature of medical care
F. Fraud

So many laws govern the practice of medicine that lawyers have found it necessary to develop a separate specialty for health care law to manage these matters adequately for physicians, hospitals, insurance companies, and government. Although these laws concern all aspects of the physician's professional life, this chapter is limited to defining and briefly explaining a few of those that involve the physician-patient relationship.

INFORMED CONSENT

"Informed consent" is a legal doctrine that requires a physician to obtain consent for *any* treatment, whether medical or surgical. It also includes ancillary services such as laboratory, radiology, or physical therapy. Without informed consent the physician may be held liable for violating a patient's rights, regardless of whether the treatment was appropriate and rendered with due care.

Without consent any treatment may be considered *battery,* which is the unauthorized and offensive touching of one person by another. Battery can be broadly defined as physical contact of any type with a patient who has not consented to the contact.

Consent may be either expressed, as in signing a consent form, or implied, as in entering an examining room specifically for an annual Pap smear. A separate signature on a form is not required for the examination if obtaining a Pap smear is the purpose for which the patient made the appointment. However, should the physician see cervicitis during the examination and wish to perform cultures for sexually transmitted diseases, the physician is required to explain his or her intent to the patient and ask her permission, although she does not have to sign a form.

Informed consent, then, is a process, not just a signature on a form. It is an exchange of information between a physician and a patient that culminates in the patient's accepting a specific test, procedure, or treatment. Nevertheless, a document is needed to record the process. For surgery, the document may be a specific form citing a specific procedure. For an office visit the document is the medical record, which should state "Mrs. Jones entered for her annual well-woman visit and Pap test."

A patient must be fully informed to give valid consent. The physician supplies information and recommendations and then allows time for the patient to think about what was said. It takes time for a patient to think of questions, and the physician should encourage questions as a way to determine how well the patient understands what was said. When nonemergent surgery is discussed, it is useful for the patient to return with her partner or a trusted friend for an "informed consent briefing" during which all of her questions may be discussed.

The physician must provide sufficient information to allow the patient to make a rational and voluntary decision about receiving or not receiving treatment. The patient should understand, when there is another way to treat the condition, why the physician has suggested a particular treatment and what will happen if there is no treatment.

The patient also should be educated about complications that may occur with treatment, as well as what may happen with alternative therapy or with no treatment, so that she may weigh the relative risks. The physician should be comfortable in answering valid questions, such as whether the procedure is experimental, what the physician's experience with the procedure is, and what the expected failure rate is. This extensive exchange of information is best accomplished in the consultation room of the physician's office, with the patient fully clothed, and is best documented in the patient's office medical record.

The informed consent process is intended to educate a patient so that she may participate more fully in making difficult decisions, and nothing more. Even the finest informed consent document cannot excuse negligence.

Informed consent is *not* necessary when a patient's life is at risk in an emergency and the patient is not conscious to give consent or is incompetent for some other reason. It is expected that a physician will try to stop a hemorrhage or establish an airway. However, the physician must discuss the patient's treatment with the next-of-kin as soon as possible, even as it happens, and the effort to do so must be documented concurrently in the medical record. Notes written days later are less reliable and therefore less helpful when defending a claim.

Informed refusal

Sometimes a patient may refuse needed, even lifesaving, treatment for herself or for her fetus. This refusal must be documented in the medical record at the time of refusal. As with informed consent, refusal of treatment must be truly informed. The patient is told why a treatment has been proposed and what may happen if she refuses. This, too, should be recorded in the chart calmly, precisely, and without editorial comment.

A "good faith effort" should be made to enlist others' help in obtaining consent. People such as a husband, close relatives, clergy, medical colleagues, and an ethics committee may be consulted and their opinions noted. However, should all of these efforts fail, the final refusal of a competent patient will prevail out of respect for her autonomy. We advise physicians to restrain the natural impulse to force a competent patient to "do the right thing" against her will by seeking a court order. The American College of Obstetricians and Gynecologists stated in its Committee Opinion on Patient Choice, "The use of the courts to resolve these conflicts is almost never warranted."

The doctrine of *assumption of risk* means that the patient understands the possibility of untoward results of treatment or no treatment and knowingly consents to the course selected. However, if all of the risks that, in fact, occur have not been carefully explained to the patient, as a matter of law the doctrine of assumption of risk is not applicable. Once again the law insists on documentation at the time the risk is assumed.

Outcomes

The outcome of any medical or surgical therapy for any individual patient depends on too many variables to be absolutely predictable. No outcome of a practice of medicine can be guaranteed. This critical concept is difficult to explain during the informed consent process because this is precisely when the patient needs reliable options from which to choose. How can she be asked to choose a treatment if the physician is unable to promise a specific result? Unfortunately, too often what she is really asked to choose is the least onerous of several poor options.

Physicians must resist the very human impulse to give the patient blanket reassurance. Patients frequently have unreasonable expectations of what medical science can accomplish, even under ideal circumstances, and physicians must not indulge fantasies. Should the results be less than the patient expects, she will express her disappointment and is likely to ask others to find out what went wrong, even if, in reality, nothing went wrong.

The physician must tell the patient what could happen, as well as what is hoped will happen, with the treatment proposed. If the surgery involves prolonged urethral catheterization, for example, the patient should be prepared to expect a urinary tract infection. Honesty in discussing how patients have fared in the past may avoid surprise and disappointment, the feelings that may lead to legal inquiry. Patients have a right to know what to expect and must be given the best information available—gently perhaps, but always honestly.

Options and alternatives

Reasonable alternative treatments or procedures, including no treatment, must be part of the informed consent discussion and should include a description of their material risks and possible complications. Of course, it is not necessary to know Chinese folk medicine or the ways of the Navajo shaman, but it is necessary to be able to describe the natural history of the condition in question with no treatment, with alternative treatment, and with the proposed treatment so that the patient may choose.

Physicians may have a preference for what they propose but should acknowledge that not all conditions will be fatal without their preferred methods. Family planning choices, for example, differ in effectiveness, convenience, cost, and side effects, and none is best for all women. Gynecologists have no difficulty explaining a dozen different methods for birth control, so they should have no difficulty explaining half a dozen different treatments for stress urinary incontinence, even though they may prefer one. This is precisely what is meant by options and alternatives in the informed consent process. The patient has a right to know so that she may choose. The law insists that she express her preference.

This does not mean, however, that a patient has a right to demand a form of treatment that you think is substandard or contraindicated. You are never obliged to do anything that you think may harm your patient.

Capacity to choose

A valid consent must be informed, competent, and voluntary. *Informed* and *voluntary* have been discussed, but what if the patient is not competent and does not have the capacity to make an informed and voluntary choice? The determination of competency depends on whether the patient can understand the nature of her condition and her choices for care. A competent patient, of course, always decides what may be done. But some patients are very young children and some are unconscious or under anesthesia. Others may be in a coma or simply incapable of making a decision. None of these people has the capacity to give informed consent to anything, so "surrogate decision makers" are needed. Most situations are easy. Decisions are made for young children by parents and for people incapable of making a decision by husbands, wives, or adult children. When the decisions are agreed to by the attending physician, they may be carried out without difficulty as long as they are not expressly forbidden by state law or hospital policy. When there is disagreement, however, only a court may determine incompetency, and the court will appoint a guardian to speak for the patient.

Surrogate decision makers

The law says that an incompetent person does not lose the right to self-determination or to accept or refuse treatment merely because of incompetence. Instead the right is exercised by a surrogate using "substituted judgment." The state expects the surrogate to make the choice the patient would have made.

The Durable Power of Attorney for Health Care is a legal document through which a competent adult appoints a surrogate decision maker, in advance, for future health care decisions should the patient no longer be competent. Unlike a "living will," the durable power of attorney is enforceable, making the holder the primary surrogate decision maker.

Next powerful, perhaps, is the court-appointed guardian, a legally frustrating, time-consuming and cumbersome entity best avoided when possible and used only if there is conflict among decision makers. When there is no conflict between the physician and the parents of a child, or the spouse or children of an incompetent adult, these loved ones always act as surrogate decision makers because the state expects them to act in the best interests of the patient.

ADVANCE DIRECTIVES FOR HEALTH CARE

The Federal Patient Self-Determination Act of 1991 requires all hospitals, as well as other health care entities, to provide information to all patients regarding advance medical directives and their right to accept or refuse medical treatment. Generally, the term "advance directive" includes both the living will and the health care power of attorney. Both are supposed to control decisions relating to the acceptance or refusal of care.

The holder of a health care power of attorney, the *agent* or *appointed surrogate,* is an adult who has the authority to make health care treatment decisions for another person. This authority is granted by the patient while still competent to make a decision or by a court should a guardian be needed. The *living will* is a directive created in advance, describing in detail which treatments the patient intends to allow when she is no longer able to express an opinion.

Although these goals are laudable, the wishes of the no longer competent patient still may not prevail. The surrogate she or the court has appointed may not make decisions that the patient would have made. Or the family or attending physician may describe the patient's condition in terms not precisely covered by the living will, and unwanted treatment may be given in spite of efforts made well in advance by the thoughtful patient.

It is incumbent upon care givers to follow the intent of the patient, even when the letter of the directive is faulty. Usually, it is obvious what an individual had in mind. Should the attending physician or other professional be unable to follow the intent of the directive because of personal, ethical, or religious constraints, the professional must find a substitute to continue care as directed. The professional may not leave the patient until the substitute has accepted responsibility for providing continuing care. Withdrawing prematurely is called *abandonment* (see later discussion).

CONFIDENTIALITY

Confidentiality is defined as the patient's right to peace of mind regarding the revelation of her medical information. Broadly, it is the patient's right to privacy, recognized by the Supreme Court as a constitutional right and thus as a legal duty of the physician. Narrowly, it is the principle giving a patient the right to know a medical student's or house officer's identity and role in the management of her condition.

No state allows unauthorized breach of confidentiality, and differences in laws only address differences in punishment, sometimes including loss of license to practice. There are exceptions, of course. Information must be given when required by law (e.g., the required reporting of various contagious diseases, gunshot wounds, or child abuse).

All members of the health care team have access to patients and their information. Members include students, chaplains, and many others, in addition to physicians and nurses. The patient must be informed of each person's involvement and given an opportunity to accept or reject him or her. Students should be identified as student physicians and house officers as resident physicians. Unauthorized persons are not permitted to observe procedures, for example, without the patient's consent.

It is wise for a physician to obtain permission from any patient able to give permission, even to discuss the details of the patient's care with relatives as close as a husband or a parent. The patient must always be consulted. Written information may be transferred only with the patient's written consent or under a court order signed by a judge. Information may not be transferred if the court order is signed by a clerk of the court, a common legal ploy. These principles must never be violated.

ABANDONMENT

Termination of a physician-patient relationship by the physician, without reasonable notice and without an opportunity for the patient to acquire adequate replacement medical care, is termed abandonment. Although civil law usually is invoked only if there is some form of damage, it is medically unethical to abandon a patient, even if no harm comes of it. In short, although the patient may fire the physician at any time, the physician may not fire her.

Should the patient be noncompliant with treatment, in keeping appointments, in paying bills, or even in being so psychologically "difficult" that the physician cannot cope, the physician may dismiss the patient in writing (certified mail, return receipt requested), but only under very special circumstances. First, there must be no acute emergency or treatment under way. Then, sufficient time must be allowed for the patient to find another physician. Six weeks, in a metropolitan area with many doctors, may be enough time if the patient is not acutely ill.

If the physician can expedite the transfer of care by finding another, equally competent physician who will accept responsibility, the problem is solved. If no substitute is anywhere around, the patient may not be dismissed. For example, an obstetrician may wish to terminate care of a pregnant patient for very good reason. His or her letter of termination is received by the patient, the receipt signed and returned, and the 6 weeks specified in the letter long expired. The patient then enters the labor area in active labor and says that the obstetrician is her doctor. The obstetrician is obliged to respond and deliver the patient. Worse, should anything go wrong during the process, the obstetrician can be blamed for not providing prenatal care in the interim to prevent whatever went wrong. Ultimately, the physician is responsible.

The physician must respond to his or her established patient in any emergency. The difficult patient will certainly identify the physician as her doctor when she reaches the local emergency room, and the physician must respond. If another physician has agreed to provide ongoing care, there is no abandonment. But transferring the patient to another hospital so that the index physician does not have to treat her is expressly forbidden by federal law, with attendant enormous fines.

CONTRACTUAL NATURE OF MEDICAL CARE

If a physician specifically promises any result from his or her treatment, a specific "contract of warranty" is created. Reassurances, hopefulness, and positiveness must not be confused by the patient with specific promises, or there may be a claim for breach of contract warranty.

The physician-patient relationship, however, even without any promises, is one of an implied contract. The theory of medical malpractice rests on that contract because there can be no malpractice without a contractual duty to provide proper care. The four elements necessary for the successful prosecution of a claim for medical negligence are duty, breach of duty, causation, and damages.

The *duty* that a physician owes to a patient is based on the physician-patient relationship. The obligation begins when the physician offers to treat the patient and the patient accepts the physician's services. Although quite simple, this agreement is undoubtedly a contract. If the patient's condition is nonemergent, the physician may refuse the contract. But in an emergency, refusal is not an option. In addition, the physician's duty to a patient is to provide that degree of care ordinarily exercised by physicians practicing in the same specialty, and all must practice in accordance with the "standard of care." Unfortunately, house officers are now held to the same standard of care as their fully trained, board certified, specialist counterparts.

Breach of duty is simply breach of the physician-patient contract and occurs when a physician fails to meet the standard of care in treating a patient. Duty means contract, and breach of duty means breach of contract.

CAUSATION AND DAMAGES

Causation is the most difficult element to prove in a lawsuit for negligence. A patient cannot recover damages unless she can prove that the breach of the physician's duty—the violation of the standard of care—directly caused her injuries.

Expert testimony is essential in proving the existence of the element of causation. A plaintiff's expert witness must be able to state that the violation of the standard of care resulted in the patient's injuries to a reasonable degree of medical probability. In legal terms, medical probability means that the injury was "more likely than not" caused by the physician's breach of the standard of care.

Damages are the final element that must be proved to sustain a medical malpractice cause of action. *Damages* in a medical malpractice case are defined as the sum of money a court or jury awards as compensation to a patient for an injury that has been proved by expert testimony to be the result of a physician's negligence. To recover damages, a plaintiff must establish that she suffered physical, financial, or emotional injury caused by a physician's violation of the standard of care.

Special damages are awarded to a plaintiff for expenses that are directly related to, and are an actual consequence of, the injury suffered. These may include medical expenses, lost wages, and the cost of rehabilitation.

General damages are awarded for intangibles such as physical pain, emotional suffering, disfigurement, and interference with the ordinary enjoyment of life.

The purpose of punitive damages is to punish wrongdoing that is outrageous in character, exhibiting reckless disregard for a patient's wellbeing. These may include treatment by the physician who is under the influence of alcohol or drugs, or who fails to respond to repeated calls for help from his patient.

Many aspects of the physician-patient relationship are clearly contractual, including payment for services rendered. Under the fee-for-service model, a specified fee is charged for a specified service, which is a contract usually agreed to in advance. Managed care or salaried positions merely complicate the contract but do not change the fact that money is paid for service.

Indeed, the Association of Professors of Gynecology and Obstetrics educational objectives for this chapter are all elements of a contract, elements that one would insist an attorney include in any contract he might draw up for any reason. The elements include consent to proceed, the right to refuse a product, the expected outcome, options in design, the authority of management, definitions of terms, confidentiality, failure to complete the contract, and fraud.

FRAUD

Although Congress has passed numerous laws concerning fraud in medicine—such as the Medicare and Medicaid Fraud and Abuse Act, which authorizes the Inspector General to ferret out "kickbacks" and other prohibited practices—the word *fraud* generally takes two forms in the physician-patient relationship. The first is deception by the physician in any matter discussed in this chapter. The second concerns insurance fraud.

Deception is the deliberate misrepresentation of facts. It includes explicit lying, as well as deception by implication or by omission of information needed by patients to make decisions. Deception for economic advantage is unethical.

It is also unethical for a physician to misstate facts about his or her credentials and experience or facts about specific treatment, complications, and success rates. It is deceptive to cite national experience and imply that the same data apply locally when they do not. It is equally deceptive to alarm a patient by implication about abnormal but relatively innocuous conditions, thereby promoting diagnostic procedures, unnecessary surgery, and general overtreatment.

It is unethical to deceive by omission of information, such as omitting description of an alternative but equal treatment that is less advantageous to the physician. It is equally unethical for financial arrangements to result in undertreatment, as when professionals profit from inappropriately limiting care. Conflict of interest must be avoided or disclosed and resolved without deception.

Insurance fraud involves the deliberate miscoding of conditions and treatments to enhance reimbursement. Inappropriate "unbundling" of services, the separating out of portions of a procedure usually covered by a global fee, may be considered fraudulent activity. It is inappropriate to submit a claim for payment for an exploratory laparotomy in addition to a claim for payment for removal of an ectopic pregnancy when they are really the same procedure. It is equally illegal to submit a claim for tests and services not performed. Furthermore, it is fraudulent to claim that a patient is seen for a pain that her insurance will pay for when she really is seen for a noninsured reason; it also is fraudulent to not record a complaint in the record until her insurance is in force and any waiting period has expired. Patients frequently ask for such favors, perhaps not knowing that they are asking physicians to commit insurance fraud. Physicians must resist these temptations to be "helpful."

CRITICAL POINTS

- Informed consent is the process of exchanging information to allow the patient to make appropriate decisions.
- Competent patients have the right to refuse any care.
- Advance directives are designed to direct a patient's care after the patient is no longer competent.
- Patients' medical information is strictly confidential except under very limited and specific circumstances.
- Abandonment is walking away from a patient without providing a suitable substitute care giver.
- The physician-patient relationship is an implied contract.
- Fraud in dealing with patients is unethical, immoral, and illegal.

Questions

1. An unknown woman in labor at home finds a physician's name in the phone book and calls asking the physician for help with her home delivery. The physician refuses. She sues for negligence. The physician's valid defense is:
   A. Labor is not a disease, so attendance is not necessary.
   B. The woman had no prenatal care, so she does not deserve a physician.
   C. The baby was born healthy so no harm was done.
   D. Since the physician never accepted the woman as a patient, no physician-patient relationship existed.
   E. The woman was contributorily negligent in not calling well in advance.

2. A physician has a longstanding relationship with a gynecology patient who becomes pregnant. When the patient calls to complain of morning sickness she finds that the physician is on vacation and no one is covering her practice. Three months later the patient delivers prematurely and the baby dies. The physician's valid defense against the suit that follows is:
   A. No physician-patient relationship existed.
   B. The physician did not breach any duty owed to the patient.
   C. The physician's negligence was not the proximate cause of the premature birth.
   D. A premature infant is not a viable human being.
   E. The patient has not been injured.

3. A patient brings her 15-year-old daughter for examination because of a vaginal discharge. The introitus is marital and the discharge contains *Trichomonas vaginalis*. The physician asks the mother to leave the room and then asks the child if she is using contraception. The child answers that a friend told her that she cannot get pregnant and then begs that her mother not be told anything. The physician should legally do all of the following *except*:
   A. Tell the mother that the child is sexually active and has a venereal disease.
   B. Give the child the prescription for the vaginal discharge and say nothing to her mother.

C. Tell the child that she has a venereal disease, that her partner must be treated too, and that she will get pregnant.
D. Arrange for two weekly follow-up visits alone with the child so that she may be counseled without betraying confidentiality.
E. Give the child Planned Parenthood's address in case she would feel more comfortable there.

4. A physician receives a phone call from someone who says she is a paralegal for an attorney and tells the physician to send her a copy of a patient's medical record. "If you don't," she adds, "I will issue a subpoena for the records." The physician should do all of the following *except:*

A. Call his or her medical liability insurance company to report the conversation.
B. Call the patient to ask her if she wants her records sent.
C. If the patient wants her records sent, tell her she must sign a records release form.
D. Review the record in question to refresh his or her memory.
E. Copy the record and send it to avoid the subpoena.

Answers

1. D
2. C
3. A
4. E

59

Ethics in obstetrics and gynecology

APGO LEARNING OBJECTIVE #59

Joseph B. Buxer

Recognizing and understanding the basis of ethical conflicts in obstetrics and gynecology will allow better patient care and prevent critical errors in treatment planning.

The student will demonstrate a knowledge of the following:

A. A systematic approach to ethical problems
B. The basis of ethical conflict in maternal-fetal medicine
C. Issues of justice relating to access to obstetric and gynecologic care
D. Ethical issues raised by induced abortion
E. Ethical issues raised by reproductive technology

A chapter on bioethics must start with the statement, "First, do no harm," because those words have been spoken by physicians for thousands of years, and the modern medical student is unlikely to disagree with what seems so intuitively obvious. Why, then, an entire separate chapter devoted to the principles of bioethics? Is not "do no harm" sufficient? No, it is no longer sufficient because in our present pluralistic society readers probably will have their own system of values with their own definition for the word *harm*.

Bioethics, studied and discussed as a code of behavior, the right way to act, and the right thing to do, is fundamental to the meaning of the word *professional*. For example, a professional may not apply technologic expertise without considering the ethical consequences. But, with even greater urgency, bioethical principles are studied and discussed to develop a method for making decisions, a way to find answers to ethical dilemmas involving individuals who may have very different viewpoints.

The problem is particularly acute in the field of obstetrics and gynecology because no medical specialty has undergone more changes in technology, and some of these changes have had revolutionary implications. In addition, no medical specialty has been more involved with the legal system than obstetrics and gynecology. Obstetrician-gynecologists are sometimes plaintiffs, frequently defendants, and very frequently expert witnesses. Occasionally they even seek a court order to force a woman to do something against her will for a perceived benefit to her unborn child. Each disagreement presents a dilemma, a conflict between people who live with different values, view issues from different points, and thus reach different conclusions—each individual absolutely certain of his or her position. When untrained, physicians usually are unable to cope with ethical dilemmas.

A SYSTEMATIC APPROACH TO ETHICAL PROBLEMS

To deal effectively with a seemingly endless list of constantly evolving ethical dilemmas, students of ethics have developed a systematic approach or discipline that permits individuals from many different professions, who have no personal stake in a dilemma, to discuss the problem, identify ethical alternatives, and offer a reasoned solution.

Sometimes parties to a conflict will request the service of a single ethicist, someone trained specifically for the task. Sometimes the issue will be referred to a hospital ethics committee, not for arbitration but for consultation that binds neither party in the dispute to the committee's conclusion.

The following seven steps comprise the systematic approach to ethical problems. They should be considered in the context of a patient who is unable to make a medical decision for herself.

1. Identify the decision makers—usually the physician, the nurses, the family of the patient, and/or the hospital administrator. Decide who should be involved in the decision. The ultimate power rests with the competent patient. But for those assessed incapable of making a decision, other interested parties are heard. Disputes about competence are decided only by a court. A pregnant woman is almost always considered the appropriate decision maker for the fetus she is carrying.

2. Gather all the medical data—history, present condition, and prognosis. Remember that decisions about what may or may not be relevant or important to a case are based on personal values, and the presenter must always maintain objectivity.

3. Gather the values data from decision makers in the conflict. Try to get a sense of the perspective each party is bringing to the discussion so that values held in common can be identified.

4. Identify the options, including those deemed unacceptable. Decide whether any option violates an ethical principle that all agree is important. Reexamine those options remaining and their ethical consequences.

5. State the conflicts and prioritize them. Define conflicts in terms of ethical principles and determine which are most important to the decision makers. Review ethics decisions from the past as they relate to the present issue.

6. Reach a solution that is justified by ethical principles. A rational solution should be justifiable to others in terms of ethical principles with universal appeal.

7. Discuss the solution with the involved parties. The decision makers frequently reject an ethics committee's solution at first but realize its value in time.

A hospital bioethics committee gathers interested individuals from various occupations and professions. Together they examine ethical issues, arguments, and principles to offer help in conflict resolution. Their goal is to learn to use this systematic approach so that decisions are not based on emotion or intuition. During the committee's discussions, three general theories, or ethical systems, are frequently debated:

1. *Teleology.* Consequence-based; right depends upon good, with "the greatest good for the greatest number."

2. *Deontology*. Because all consequences cannot be known, certain truths and duties must be fulfilled regardless of consequences.
3. *Virtue*. Character-based, the question becomes, "What would a virtuous person do?"

Four general principles of ethics are always used as the basis for each case analysis:

1. *Autonomy*. A duty to respect self-determination.
2. *Beneficence*. A duty to do good.
3. *Nonmaleficence*. A duty to refrain from causing harm.
4. *Justice*. A duty to treat fairly and honestly.

Autonomy

The principle of autonomy, most simply stated, is self-rule. In medicine it means that the patient makes the final decision about what to do with her body. Her decisions are based on consistent, self-imposed principles that are meaningful to her, so the physician must regard the patient's judgment as valid even when disagreeing with it. The physician must not impede the actions the patient undertakes in accordance with her principles.

If the patient is deemed competent, the physician is required to honor her autonomous decision, even if it does not promote health, because the patient may have values to which life and health are subordinate. The well-informed patient must even be allowed to make tragic decisions. The issue of autonomy always arises when there is conflict caused by refusal of treatment, even life-saving treatment, or attempted suicide.

Beneficence

The principle of beneficence covers the physician's duty to benefit his or her patient. Although beneficence may be accompanied, at first, by ill effect, it eventually should produce a positive result. For example, surgery might destroy a valued function, such as fertility, to achieve a perceived greater value, such as removing a malig-

nancy. But even this example requires that both patient and physician rank these values in the same order.

Beneficence, as a duty, also may arise in the physician's relationship with society. Whereas a passerby may not be duty-bound to aid an accident victim, ethically—although usually not legally—a medical professional would be expected to help because of his or her chosen role in society.

Nonmaleficence

The principle of nonmaleficence is where this discussion started: *Primum non nocere*—"First and foremost, do no harm." Although there can be no argument about avoiding intentional harm, there is much discussion concerning the duty to guard a patient against "unnecessary" risk; to exercise "sufficient" care; or to be as knowledgeable as one is "reasonably" expected to be, or as one claims to be. Courts use their version of the principle of nonmaleficence, for example, in cases of wrongful birth when a parent is not advised of a genetic hazard because a physician either lacked the knowledge or failed to disclose the information.

Paradoxically, always ensuring that one will do no harm may result in a violation of the duty of beneficence. Therapies offering great promise for patients also may have harmful side effects. Thus a fair disclosure of the risk/benefit ratio is required to obtain an autonomous informed consent.

Justice

The principle of justice, stated most simply, is that people must be treated equally. If isolettes are in shortage in an intensive care unit, clearly prematurity would be an ethically relevant matter and race and sex would not. National allocation of resources may some day force physicians to make choices about care delivery. Yet society may still expect an individual physician to act as if no shortage exists when dealing with an individual patient. This untenable situation is now under great debate.

ETHICAL CONFLICT IN MATERNAL-FETAL MEDICINE

Ethical dilemmas unique to obstetrics frequently involve conflicts between the pregnant woman and her fetus, with the physician being deemed incidental. In pregnancy the mother and fetus are separate beings, each with individual rights; but they are joined so that treating one may inflict risk of great harm to the other. Occasionally a mother may be asked to sacrifice her fetus because her own life is threatened. For example, she may require pelvic radiation treatment for cancer during the first half of pregnancy.

More often, conflict arises because access to the fetus is through the mother. A fetus may be at great risk and in need of immediate abdominal delivery, but the mother can refuse to undergo surgery. Questions to consider in this case include the following:

1. What is the law with regard to fetal rights in this state?
2. Under what circumstances may a physician be allowed to perform a surgical delivery without maternal consent?
3. Is the physician's patient the mother, the fetus, or both?
4. What are the societal implications of compelling a pregnant woman to submit to medical treatment?

Ethical issues to consider include the following:

1. Patient autonomy: Is the mother allowed to refuse care?
2. Justice in maternal-fetal conflict: Are the two equal?
3. Beneficence: Whom does one benefit?
4. Nonmaleficence: Whom does one hurt?
5. Physician autonomy: Does one have any rights?

Although the aim of medicine is to foster the greatest benefit with the least risk, risks and benefits may be valued differently by the pregnant woman and her obstetrician. Refusing cesarean section is the most dramatic example, but less dramatic problems also pose major ethical dilemmas. A woman's behavior with regard to a compli-cating illness or her life-style may jeopardize her fetus. For example, her failure to take insulin for her diabetes, to follow a proper diet in phenylketonuria, or even to discontinue substance abuse will cause great risk to the fetus.

The physician's response to her refusal to comply must be to explain the reasons for the current recommendations and encourage responsible behavior through education and counseling. Acknowledging that medical judgments have limitations and fallibility, the obstetrician must continue to assign clinical risks and benefits in order to advise patients, being careful to present a balanced evaluation of maternal and fetal expectations. Actions of coercion to obtain consent or to force a course of action limit maternal freedom of choice and violate the principles underlying the informed consent process.

The obstetrician should make every reasonable effort to protect the fetus, but the pregnant woman's autonomy must be respected. The physician should act as informed educator and counselor and should encourage consultation with others, including the institutional ethics committee, which may be able to help resolve the conflict. These efforts may maintain the physician-patient relationship. Use of the courts in conflict resolution is almost never warranted and destroys the physician-patient relationship.

ISSUES OF JUSTICE RELATING TO ACCESS TO OBSTETRIC AND GYNECOLOGIC CARE

Justice, as it pertains to access to health care, is the ethical principle underlying a person's claim for service to be rendered by another. The second party is obligated to provide the service requested. The right to make this claim for service has been acknowledged by our society for many things, such as elementary and secondary education, basic nutrition, protection from fire, and protection from violent crime. Indeed, the right to medical care for people who are indigent is as old as the first city and county charity hospitals.

Justice demands that the care provided for one individual in need be the same as the care provided any equal individual in need. The ethical dilemma is in the definition of the word *equal*. Does it mean that all tax-paying, married men under the age of 50 should get the same treatment, or does *equal* mean that all humans of any means, sex, or age should get the same consideration? If the latter is meant, then basic medical care becomes a fundamental right of all individuals in our society.

The principle of justice acknowledges that resources are insufficient for unlimited care for all. So it asks society what criteria it will use for a just and fair distribution of health care resources. Society must ask in return if justice dictates that a physician's obligation to benefit a patient must be subordinate to the economic constraints on the delivery of care. An example of the questions raised is *Do people who are illegal aliens have a claim to health care?* All humans in need merit basic care from fellow humans (beneficence). Might one justify denying the claim of an alien because aliens are not members of an eligible community (distributive justice) or because individuals have a right to choose whom to serve (autonomy)?

Discussing the principle of justice in the doctor-patient relationship is quite simple. The physician must treat all of his or her patients' equal needs equally and honestly. Discussing the principle of justice at a societal level is vastly more complicated. Although certain truths are self-evident and have inherent merit (deontology), it may be argued that ethical principles must not be allowed to demand societal suicide *(reductio ad absurdum)*. Another great debate continues.

ETHICAL ISSUES RAISED BY INDUCED ABORTION

The systematic approach to ethical problems has not dealt effectively with the dilemmas of induced abortion because the usual approach requires reasonable people and disciplined negotiation. Un-

fortunately, some people at both extremes of this issue are unreasonable, and each group bases its arguments on absolutely nonnegotiable dicta. One group argues that the taking of fetal life is always wrong (deontology) and thus is not negotiable. The other group argues that personal autonomy and reproductive choice are absolute (also deontology) and may not be restricted in any way. Two opposing deontologic arguments cannot be resolved.

For the overwhelming majority of people whose beliefs rest somewhere in the middle there is ample room for negotiation with a clear expectation of conflict resolution. Reasoning that what is right for society depends on what is good (teleology), the question becomes, "What do we want to accomplish?" If it is undesirable to allow repeated abortion as a method of birth control (deny autonomy), is it more desirable to allow abortion only for specified indications? Should first trimester abortion on demand be allowed once or twice but not allowed for repeaters (deny justice)? What should the list of allowable indications include?

Approaching the issue from the practitioner's point of view, should the individual gynecologist be allowed to refuse to perform any abortions (autonomy) or be allowed to decide for himself or herself which abortions to perform and which to refuse (deny justice)? Physicians, like other members of society, have values and viewpoints of their own. They may not impose those values on their patients (nonmaleficence), but they retain their right of self-determination (autonomy).

Assume, for a moment, that a physician is willing to perform some abortions under certain circumstances. Consider the following patients who request termination:

1. A 40-year-old woman whose fetus has trisomy 18
2. A 12-year-old child who did not know it could happen
3. A 32-year-old executive who just received a promotion
4. A 22-year-old single mother of two whose rhythm method failed

5. A 33-year-old secretary whose fetus is seen to be missing a leg
6. A 15-year-old student who was gang-raped
7. A 39-year-old woman who wanted a girl and it is a boy

Which will the physician do? Which will he or she refuse? Conflicting obligations may include the following needs:

1. To benefit the woman (beneficence)
2. To respect her reproductive choice (autonomy)
3. To maintain one's own status as a moral agent (nonmaleficence)
4. To limit patient choice for some (justice)

ETHICAL ISSUES RAISED BY REPRODUCTIVE TECHNOLOGY

Teleologically, sexual tension is the driving force that must exist to demand sexual intercourse, which must result in reproduction, the purpose of which is to maintain the species. In nature there is much intercourse to produce many babies so that enough will survive to maintain a population. But in the natural order of things it is not expected that every coupling will succeed. Man has interfered with this natural order in many wonderful ways, only one of which is the treatment of couples who do not succeed in conceiving. Reproductive technology today offers a wide variety of treatments from the very simple to what just a few years ago would have been thought science fiction. But along with the incredible advances in the ability to assist the infertile couple have come some very perplexing legal and ethical questions.

Consider, for example, donor insemination, perhaps the simplest of the assisted reproduction technologies. A couple consults the reproductive endocrinologist because the husband is known to be azoospermic, and all agree that donor insemination is an appropriate treatment. The couple are informed and they consent. The semen is from a sperm bank and is anonymous. There are no problems. Yet simple questions may be asked: Does the husband need to adopt the child after

birth? Will there be inheritance issues? In the event of divorce, is the husband responsible for child support?

Less orthodox consultations raise more difficult issues. May a single woman receive donor insemination? Should a married woman receive donor insemination without the knowledge of her husband? Should a woman be able to choose her donor, perhaps an old friend? Should a gay woman be denied insemination? Does the donor have any parental rights? Does he have any parental responsibilities, such as child support? May the physician decide who deserves this help and who does not? How is this decision reached? And who is responsible if the donor has a communicable disease for which there is no known test?

All of these questions may be answered by reasonable people reasoning together. But without a systematic approach any answer may appear arbitrary.

Ovulation induction is a more complicated technology that may result in multiple gestations. Should selective termination be encouraged? Can society afford a technology that fills newborn intensive care nurseries with premature triplets and quadruplets?

Gamete intrafallopian transfer (GIFT), zygote intrafallopian transfer (ZIFT), and in vitro fertilization (IVF) and embryo transfer are even more complicated. Think of the scientist who must choose which eggs to fertilize and which to discard, and which living embryos to transfer, which to freeze for later use, which to save for investigation, and which to discard.

When dealing with defective sperm the scientist must choose which sperm from among those incapable of independently fertilizing an egg to inject directly through a zona pellucida to form a zygote, a new life. Another choice to be made is which cell to remove from an eight-cell embryo to check for chromosome and gene content before transferring the remaining embryo to a waiting uterus. If the wrong gene is present, the scientist may choose to discard the embryo.

Finally, consider the questions that may be raised by sperm donation, egg donation, and/or uterine donation (surrogate motherhood) in any combination. Would prohibition of surrogate motherhood be paternalistic? Does surrogacy violate any ethical principle? Does surrogacy exploit the birth mother or the infertile couple? May the gestational mother choose to terminate the pregnancy or decide to parent the child? If so, should she expect child support from the infertile couple? If the adopting couple doesn't like the child, may they refuse to take it? Which gamete donor has primacy in the disposition of frozen embryos? Is it ethical for a couple who no longer need the preserved embryos to sell them to another couple or to a single woman? Which ethical principles would be violated if they did? Would it be illegal, like selling a baby? May a judge decide to give embryos to an infertile couple against the will of one or both of the gamete donors?

In less than a generation's time the marvelous advances in reproductive technology have brought joy and fulfillment to many thousands of infertile couples. But the questions that accompany these advances, for the most part, remain unanswered. Rational debate based on the principles of bioethics offers the best hope for solving these dilemmas.

SUMMARY

The ethics of medicine is too complex to be managed by a menu of do's and don'ts. Modern treatment allows some people to survive catastrophic events, but not all survive intact. Resources will be even more limited in the future. Physicians will ask the dual questions of whether they will be allowed to treat all problems with current resources and whether they ought to treat some problems at all. Concurrent answers are hard to find. Which conditions are to be treated? Which conditions are hopeless? When does one admit failure and discontinue futile therapy? In an effort to help their house officers cope with these universal ethical dilemmas, the Optimum Care Committee of the Massachusetts General Hospital discussed, agreed to, and posted the following guidelines in their intensive care units:

1. Life is not the absolute good nor death the absolute evil.
2. Clinical decisions to stop "heroics" apply only to irreversibly moribund patients.
3. The will of the patient, not the health of the patient, is the supreme law.

CRITICAL POINTS

- The seven steps in ethical decision making are as follows:
  Identify decision makers.
  Gather medical data.
  Gather values data.
  Identify options.
  Identify conflicts.
  Reach resolution.
  Discuss resolution with decision makers.
- The four general principles in bioethics are autonomy, beneficence, nonmaleficence, and justice.
- Bioethics is both a code of professional behavior and a way of finding answers to ethical dilemmas.

4. Treatments that cannot reverse illness in a moribund patient are not necessary and, when they will cause more suffering than benefit, are contraindicated.
5. Stopping treatment is ethically no different from never starting it.

Questions

1. A 23-year-old gravida V, para V is a Jehovah's Witness. She is hemorrhaging 3 hours after a cesarean delivery. She and her family refuse blood transfusions. The patient says she would rather die than receive blood or blood products. The physician finds her beliefs unacceptable. The ethical choice of action should be to:
   A. Accede to the patient's demands against transfusion.
   B. Separate the patient from her family and change her mind.
   C. Transfuse forcibly.
   D. Seek a court order for transfusion.
2. The ruling ethical principle in the dilemma above is:

   A. Do not allow harm to happen (nonmaleficence).
   B. Don't let her children become orphans (justice).
   C. Listen to her decision (autonomy).
   D. Give her what she needs anyway (paternalism).
3. Once the patient loses consciousness, is unable to continue her protestations, and is deemed incompetent:
   A. Transfusion becomes acceptable.
   B. It is all right to leave her because she rejected the physician's advice and he or she does not want to watch the patient die.
   C. The physician is bound by her advance directive prohibiting transfusion.
   D. The physician may do anything he or she can to save the patient's life without fear of a charge of assault and battery.

Answers

1. A
2. C
3. C

VIII

Preventive care and health maintenance

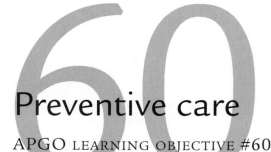

Preventive care

APGO LEARNING OBJECTIVE #60

Joseph B. Buxer

The student will recognize the value of routine health surveillance as part of health promotion and disease prevention.

The student will demonstrate a knowledge of the following:

A. Screening procedures and recommended time intervals for the following:
   1. Pap smear
   2. Mammogram
   3. Blood pressure monitoring
   4. Blood lipid profiles
B. Patient education for the following topics:
   1. Contraception
   2. Prevention of sexually transmitted diseases
   3. Diet
   4. Exercise
   5. Stress management
   6. Smoking
   7. Immunization
C. Costs and benefits of routine health surveillance

OVERVIEW

Clinical medicine in the United States historically has tended to focus predominantly on the management of illness by an individual practitioner or a small group of practitioners. Although the value of preventive care has long been recognized, it has received no uniform direction from federally funded programs and national medical organizations nor from those on regional levels. Yet few examples of the success of preventive care are more dramatic than the reduction of polio after vaccine was available and the virtual elimination of rubella and the sequelae of congenital rubella syndrome. Similar impressive results have been obtained in the significant reduction of cervical cancer by use of the Papanicolaou smear. As the United States struggles to use health care dollars in the most appropriate, cost-effective manner, the perceived value of preventive care is increasing.

The report of the U.S. Preventive Services Task Force, *Guide to Clinical Preventive Services,* ed 2, 1996, gives the health care provider a solid approach to preventive care. Likewise, the American College of Obstetricians and Gynecologists published an abbreviated document in 1994 that deals with periodic health screening and preventive care in women.

Although somewhat determined by the size of the community where the individual practices, the obstetrician/gynecologist often functions as a primary care physician. This dual role has important ramifications: women serve as the securers of health care for their families and therefore are a major conduit to care for their spouses and children. Often the obstetrician/gynecologist is the only physician that women in the reproductive age range, 18 to 45 years, will see. In the role of primary care physician the provider is responsible not only for performing annual examinations, but also for educating about disease prevention; providing appropriate screening for disease detection, early recognition, and therapy; counseling; providing immunization services; and coordinating appropriate referrals.

Preventive services must fulfill certain criteria to be effective. A screening test must be accurate and capable of early detection of medical problems without excessive error. Likewise, treating people with early disease should improve the health outcome as compared with waiting until more serious illness is present.

Pap smear

In 1941, Drs. Papanicolaou and Traut demonstrated that exfoliative cytology could be used to detect changes to the hormone milieu in the cervical and vaginal epithelium and later to detect preinvasive cancer of the cervix. The acceptance of the "Pap smear" as *screening test* by both patients and physicians is undoubtedly the reason for the significant decline in the incidence in and deaths from invasive cervical cancer.

The test is noninvasive, easy to perform, and inexpensive; early detection of abnormal cells can avert major disease because of the relatively well-defined time frames for the development of invasive cancer. Excellent collection technique increases the reliability of the test. False-negative results should occur in under 10%; false-positive results also should occur in under 10%. These low percentages are dependent on the adequacy of the smear and the quality of the interpretation. If an abnormal smear is identified, the response should be to make a more definitive diagnosis, usually through the use of colposcopy.

National organizations have disagreed on the frequency of the test but recommend that women should begin pelvic examinations and Pap smears when they become sexually active or by the age of 18 years. After a woman has had three or more consecutive satisfactory normal examinations, a Pap smear may be performed less frequently, at the discretion of the physician, with the time interval ranging up to 3 years and provided that the patient is compliant and there are no additional risk factors present. Increased risk factors for cervical intraepithelial neoplasia include infection with human papillomavirus (HPV) and other sexually transmitted diseases (STDs), multiple sexual partners, cigarette smoking, and use of birth control pills; there is a slight increase in adenocarcinoma of the cervix in women who use birth control pills.

Mammogram

In 1995 there were an estimated 182,000 new cases of breast cancer and 46,000 deaths from this disease. The current *lifetime risk* in the United States is *1 in 9 women.* Annual mammography in conjunction with self-examination of the breast (SBE) is recommended for women after the age of 50. The evidence and supporting recommendations for women between the ages of 40 and 49 years was for some time inconclusive, but national agencies now recommend that a baseline mammogram be performed after the age of 40, with repeat examinations every 2 to 3 years. The frequency of screening should increase if there are risk factors such as a breast biopsy showing atypia, a family history and a first-degree relative with breast cancer, and detection of a mass.

Again the quality of the screening depends on a high level of technical expertise and interpretation. One should distinguish between a *screening mammography* and a more diagnostic assessment of the breast, which could include not only more detailed examinations with x-ray but also the use of ultrasound. It should be clearly understood that mammography and the SBE are complementary screens and do not substitute for one another. *A negative mammogram does not eliminate the risk of cancer if a palpable breast mass is present.* Approximately 10% of palpable breast masses do not show up on a mammogram.

There is conflicting evidence regarding the benefit of mammography for women between the ages of 70 and 74; there is no evidence for the benefit of screening for women over 75. Although there is insufficient evidence to determine if SBE should be taught routinely, clinical prudence suggests this is a valuable exercise and every woman should be given instruction at the time of her annual examination.

Hypertension

Hypertension is defined as a systolic blood pressure of 140 mm Hg or higher or a diastolic pressure of 90 mm or greater. It is the most significant risk factor for coronary artery disease, congestive heart failure, stroke, aortic aneurysms, renal disease related to vascular problems, and retinopathy. Heart disease is the leading cause of death in the United States. It accounts for nearly 740,000 deaths annually. Controlling hypertension, lowering cholesterol levels, and ceasing to smoke, as well as making life-style modifications, have all been shown to reduce the death rate. Screening for hypertension is noninvasive, inexpensive, and very easy to perform. Therefore potential lethal disease may be detected and treated at an early stage.

One of the most vexing problems is "white coat hypertension." If during the initial office visit the blood pressure is elevated, the patient should be encouraged to relax for 10 or 15 minutes and the blood pressure taken again. The current recommendation for screening for hypertension is to evaluate all children and adults. Most offices determine the blood pressure as part of the vital signs at each visit.

Blood lipid profiles

Elevated blood cholesterol is an easily determined and a treatable risk factor for coronary artery disease. Although more complicated than checking the blood pressure, it is justified. Screening should begin at 18 years of age; if the nonfasting, total cholesterol remains below 200 mg/dl, the test is repeated every 5 years. More commonly, physicians tend to order the lipid profile, which includes HDL-C (high density lipoprotein) and LDL-C (low density lipoprotein).

As women age, the risk of elevated blood lipids increases with the subsequent increased risk for coronary heart disease. Levels between 200 and 239 mg/dl are considered borderline, and levels of more than 240 are considered high. There are other significant factors that should be addressed when interpreting cholesterol levels, such as age at menopause, estrogen replacement therapy, family history, smoking, hypertension, and diabetes, as well as the familial dyslipidemias. Birth control pills are known to elevate triglycerides, which should probably be monitored if there is a history of hypertriglyceridemia. Growing evidence suggests that elevated triglycerides may also pose a risk for heart disease. Should elevation in cholesterol be found, appropriate life-style and diet modifications, as well as medication to lower the levels to a safer range, are recommended.

Other tests

In the interest of brevity and focusing on more common issues related to preventive health care in women, further descriptions of additional important tests are not included; however, the *Guide to Clinical Preventive Services* should be a ready reference in the office of every practicing physician.

PATIENT EDUCATION

In the practice of medicine, nothing is more frustrating than trying to modify adverse health behavior in patients. Most practitioners conclude that until the individual expresses a desire for change, the recommendations for health improvement will go unheeded. One has only to look at current job environments to understand that there is excessive work and stress; dietary habits also need improvement. Regular exercise and lifestyle modifications that exclude the use of tobacco and alcohol would probably reduce the current level of illness in the United States by an estimated 50%. What is apparent, though, is that without a thorough educational program and an attempt to engage patients by providing them with accurate, timely, and consistent information, no changes will occur.

Unfortunately, the current practice of medicine in the United States relies strongly on fewer ambulatory visits and a reduction in time designated for teaching. Many patients are sent home with a handful of brochures, with the hope that, in their free time, women will study them and subsequently present the provider with a series of questions. In a clinical setting, a valuable tool for the physician is to encourage the patient to record notes while giving her instructions. This is one way for her to involve herself in the educational milieu.

Contraception

Over half of the 6.4 million pregnancies each year are unplanned. It is estimated that approximately 10% of the 40 million women at risk for pregnancy use no method of contraception. Unplanned pregnancy among the teenage popula-tion has become an epidemic in the United States; the percentage of teenage pregnancies is higher than in any other country in the developed world. Therefore contraceptive counseling for women in the reproductive age range is a critical part of preventive care.

The educational information must be concise and tailored to a woman's age, reproductive wishes, social attitudes, and religious convictions. A woman should determine the number of children that she desires. The task of the physician is to provide sufficient information so that she may avoid a pregnancy she does not want.

Any physician whose practice involves women between the ages of 16 and 45 should develop significant expertise in the use and discussion of all contraceptive methods. One should be able to explain clearly the mechanism and action, the advantages and disadvantages, and the failure rates and cost. The different methods are discussed in detail in Chapter 29, Contraception. It is not unusual for a woman to be noncontracepted and state clearly that she is "not trying to get pregnant." Sometimes a provocative question such as, "When was the last time you had unprotected intercourse?" can open a discussion about contraceptive methodologies. The use of condoms can serve a dual purpose of providing contraception and significant protection against STDs. All agencies in the community, including Planned Parenthood clinics, should be known to the provider, and lists of resources should be made available to the patient. Liberal distribution of pamphlets and handouts and the availability of video recordings in the office setting, along with time taken to instruct the patient in contraception, are necessary; those efforts will be rewarded. Younger women in particular may feel more at ease with a female provider, and the role of the nurse practitioner as a major conduit for information cannot be underestimated. One must remember that the maternal mortality rate is second only to the mortality rate for automobile accidents. Therefore contraceptive counseling is important preventive care.

Sexually transmitted diseases

The exact prevalence of STDs is unknown. The current estimates are that there are 12 million new cases annually in the United States. Approximately one third of these cases are from chlamydia, but there are a significant number of cases of gonorrhea, syphilis, trichomonas, nonspecific urethritis, HPV, genital herpes, and human immunodeficiency virus. High-risk behaviors include multiple sexual partners, intravenous drug use, and a promiscuous life-style. Sexually transmitted diseases have a disproportionate impact on women, and an estimated 12% to 24% of women have had multiple sexual partners. When STDs occur in pregnancy, some can be transferred to the fetus with serious sequelae.

Although there are methods to reduce risk (e.g., counseling, condoms, spermicides), there are few well-designed controlled studies showing the efficacy of counseling per se. In some developed countries young women are encouraged to carry condoms, and the prevalence of condom usage is much higher in these countries. This approach has not been well accepted in the United States.

Historically counseling has been focused more on adolescents. Young women, specifically teenagers, should be urged to consider abstinence and avoid using alcohol and drugs, which is associated with high-risk sexual behavior. Thorough instruction about the use and application of condoms should be included in counseling. Many individuals are unaware that only latex condoms should be used because lubricants can cause other condom materials to disintegrate quickly. Health care providers must be vigilant in their roles as educators for individual patients. However, they should also be working in every venue possible to provide information to community organizations, schools, and churches when possible.

Diet

Diet is related to the risk of heart disease, hypertension, obesity, and probably many forms of cancer. Diets rich in fruits, vegetables, potatoes, and whole grain cereals are associated with lower rates of coronary heart disease and cancers of the lung, colon, esophagus, and stomach. Although the use of vitamin supplements is a multibillion dollar a year industry, there have not been adequately controlled studies demonstrating that vitamin supplements are helpful for the general population. However, through the National Institutes of Health, there are studies in the preliminary stage, and one hopes there will be more information concerning the use of vitamin supplements to prevent disease. Carefully inquiring about the patient's diet, particularly what has been ingested in the last 24 hours, or asking her to keep a diary for a week are helpful tools. There are no adequate tests for determining low vitamin levels, and by the time systemic symptoms occur, there are significant sequelae in other areas.

The subject of weight control should be gently introduced at each visit. Very few patients are completely satisfied with their weight. Most women wish to lose weight, but some women should increase their body mass. The Committee on Diet and Health of the National Research Council recommends (1) a total fat intake of less than 30% of calories, saturated fat intake of less than 10% of calories, and cholesterol intake of less than 300 mg/day; (2) five servings of vegetables and fruits and six servings of bread, cereal, and potatoes daily ("strive for five"); (3) a protein intake of 1.6 g per kilogram of body weight; (4) an alcohol intake for a person of legal age of less than 1 oz/day (2 cans of beer, 2 glasses of wine, or 2 cocktails); and (5) a total salt intake of less than 6 g/day. Again, the health care provider should be thoroughly familiar with the available resources in the community. There are reliable weight loss programs and regimens that use a type of 12-step approach and can provide a safe environment for patients. In an active ambulatory setting there is usually not sufficient time to pay attention to the details for those women who are seriously motivated about lowering their weight.

Exercise

Those individuals who engage in a regular exercise program, 3 to 4 times per week for approximately 30 minutes, generally "feel better." Whether this is related to the production of endogenous opioids or just a general increase in self-esteem relating to taking better care of themselves is unclear. Exercises have different components, from aerobic conditioning to muscle stretching to increasing bone density with weight bearing exercise. Varied exercise programs are sometimes more tolerable than doing a repetitive workout over and over. Women should be instructed that they will experience less primary dysmenorrhea, have less fatigue, and probably experience improved sleep patterns with regular exercise. Exercise is also a regular component of a well-balanced weight control program. It is important to encourage patients to develop the habit of exercise early because as individuals age, this becomes a critical part of their health maintenance. An 80-year-old woman who can no longer ambulate satisfactorily is facing a life-threatening situation.

Exercise can be rather simplistic and conducted in the home. It can involve friends and thereby develop a social interaction component, or it can be more formalized in a health club setting.

Stress management

Most individuals in the United States live at a very frenetic pace, with significant stresses arising from the workplace, families, and financial responsibilities. One should think of stress management as an attempt to strengthen the coping mechanisms of functional people. Physiologic, psychologic, and sociologic balance are maintained by minor adjustments and rest periods that improve biochemical, cellular, and organ system function. Although all of these processes are not yet clearly understood, they are thought to involve central and peripheral cortisol secretion, adrenergic responses that increase arousal, vigilance, and attention in preparation for action. These actually are defense mechanisms that occur automatically and result in behavioral responses that are judged by others to be good or bad (coping well or poorly). Stress implies that an individual's threshold for comfort has been exceeded.

There are many techniques for managing stress, and an individual should seek out the method that is suitable for her. Relaxation methodologies include deep breathing, stretching, visual imagery, meditation, prayer, yoga, biofeedback, massage, music, and self-help groups. It is important for the patient to understand when stress is excessive, and how the undesirable responses can be reduced or the interval can be altered.

General health maintenance to manage stress always includes exercise, advice regarding nutrition, cessation of smoking, reduction of alcohol, and elimination of substance abuse. Preventive care, in fact, requires identifying the patient who wants help, helping her to accept her stress as normal, and guiding her to the proper environment for health.

Smoking

The reduction of cigarette smoking and all other forms of tobacco usage should be encouraged by all health care professionals. Cigarette smoking is the greatest cause of preventable morbidity and mortality among American women. It is responsible for 55% of the cardiovascular deaths in women under the age of 65 years, and women smokers are 12 times more likely to die of lung cancer than women who have never smoked. The number of lung cancer deaths now exceeds the number of breast cancer deaths each year. Lung cancer and other diseases are largely preventable.

Thirty percent of American women still smoke and are less likely than men to have attempted to quit. They can be influenced, however, through counseling and smoking cessation guidance. Although the list of the deleterious effects of smoking is quite long, it is encouraging that 10 years after smoking cessation, a former smoker's risk of lung cancer drops to that of a nonsmoker.

One should begin by asking the patient if she smokes and by assessing her motivation to stop. The physician should clearly advise the patient to stop smoking, emphasizing the benefits of cessation, but also keeping in mind that it is an addiction. The patient should set a firm date to stop, and the physician should suggest cessation strategies and insist on close follow-up. If the patient does not want to stop, she will not. However, if she really wants to quit, the support of the health care provider may be just enough to make it work.

Immunizations

Children's immunizations are a routine part, mandated by the health department, of normal pediatric preventive care. Most people, however, are unaware that adults require immunizations. The American College of Obstetricians and Gynecologists has compiled a list of recommended immunizations, by patient age, to be given by the generalist obstetrician/gynecologist as part of the routine primary care function. They are divided into periodic and high-risk groups; the recommendations are as follows:

Age 13-18   Periodic: tetanus-diphtheria booster once at 14-16
High risk: measles-mumps-rubella, hepatitis B, hepatitis A

Age 19-39   Periodic: tetanus-diphtheria booster every 10 years
High risk: measles-mumps-rubella, hepatitis B, influenza, pneumococcal vaccine, hepatitis A

Age 40-64   Periodic: tetanus-diptheria every 10 years, influenza annually beginning at age 55
High risk: measles-mumps-rubella, hepatitis B, influenza, pneumococcal vaccine, hepatitis A

Age 65 and up   Periodic: tetanus-diptheria booster every 10 years, influenza vaccine annually, pneumococcal vaccine once
High risk: hepatitis B and A vaccine

BENEFITS OF PREVENTIVE CARE

In this limited discussion there are areas that should be considered, depending on the age of the patient presenting for her periodic health screen, that are not covered. There should be counseling regarding prevention of motor vehicle injuries, household and recreational injuries, domestic violence, back pain, dental periodontal disease, and unintended pregnancies, and about postmenopausal hormone prophylaxis, antibiotic prophylaxis for infectious disease, and the use of aspirin prophylaxis in pregnancy. The reader is again referred to the *Guide to Clinical Preventive Services,* ed 2, 1996.

While virtually no one disagrees with the desirability of preventive care, review of the government document, *Healthy People 2000,* shows that numerous goals that are relatively conservative have been set to improve the health of the people in the United States. Sometimes it is difficult for any one practitioner to see the impact that he or she might make on the health care of populations; however, there are data accumulated that show the value of a public health approach to prevention. In 1954 there were 18,300 cases of polio in the United States, whereas only three cases were reported in 1993. The 11,000 fetal losses and 20,000 infants born with congenital rubella in 1964 have been reduced by 99%. Smoking cigarettes alone accounts for 1 out of every 5 deaths in the United States, and this can be reduced. Because of the use of safety belts the number of vehicle fatalities has diminished substantially, although still accounting for 41,000 deaths in 1992.

It should be evident to all health care providers that the timely, thorough, and complete periodic health screen that pays attention to those conditions for which the patient is at risk, points out to her any life-style modifications that would help her, makes her aware of all of the community resources, and conveys a strong interest in her personal welfare is probably one of the most significant things that can be accomplished in the practice of medicine.

CRITICAL POINTS

- The generalist obstetrician/gynecologist is the primary care physician for women and is responsible for preventive care.
- The Pap smear and the mammogram are not definitive diagnostic tests but are population screening tests necessitating appropriate follow-up, usually biopsy, for a diagnosis.
- All preventive care starts with patient education that is provided by the physician or her or his surrogate.
- Preventive care is cost-effective for populations over the long term.
- The goal of preventive care is to decrease suffering while increasing longevity.

Questions

1. A properly performed Pap smear is not:
   A. A cost-effective test
   B. A diagnostic test for cervical cancer
   C. Recommended in a 16-year-old sexually active female
   D. As cost-effective as a colposcopy
   E. Recommended annually in women who are at risk for cervical neoplasia
2. All of the following statements concerning mammography are true *except:*
   A. A baseline mammogram should be acquired in women 40 years and older.
   B. Mammography and SBE complement each other as screening tests for breast cancer.
   C. A mammogram should be ordered in a woman less than 40 if she is at increased risk for breast cancer.
   D. A mammogram is not indicated if a breast mass is palpated.

E. A negative mammogram reduces the chance of cancer to less than 10% (the false-negative rate).
3. When using screening tests in women, one should recall that:
   A. Cardiovascular disease is not a major cause of death.
   B. Serum cholesterol screening should be determined in a fasting state.
   C. "White coat hypertension" predisposes women to stroke.
   D. A serum cholesterol above 200 mg/dl necessitates additional evaluation.
   E. Birth control pills can elevate serum triglycerides to levels placing a woman at risk for myocardial infarction.

Answers

1. B
2. D
3. D

abortion

    elective (induced) Termination of a pregnancy by medical or surgical intervention.

    spontaneous Termination of a pregnancy before the twentieth week of gestation, when the fetus weighs less than 500 g.

        complete Expulsion of the entire products of conception.

        incomplete Expulsion of the entire products of conception retained in the uterus.

        inevitable Bleeding or rupture of the membranes accompanied by pain and dilatation of the internal cervical os.

        missed Intrauterine retention of the dead products of conception.

        recurrent Three or more consecutive first-trimester abortions.

        septic A threatened, inevitable, or incomplete abortion complicated by infection.

        threatened Vaginal bleeding in the presence of a closed cervix during pregnancy.

abruptio placentae Separation of the normally located placenta from its uterine attachment between the twentieth week of pregnancy and the birth of the infant. It occurs mainly in the third trimester.

acromegaly Overgrowth of the terminal parts of the skeletal system after epiphyseal fusion as a result of overproduction of growth hormone.

From Association of Professors of Gynecology and Obstetrics (APGO): *Medical student educational objectives,* ed 6, Washington, DC 1993, The Association.

adenomyosis presence of endometrial tissue within the myometrium as a result of direct extension.

adnexa The uterine appendages, including the fallopian tubes, ovaries, and associated ligaments.

adrenal hyperplasia A congenital or acquired increase in the number of cells of the adrenal cortex, occurring bilaterally and resulting in excessive excretion of 17-ketosteroids with signs of virilization.

amenorrhea Absence or cessation of menstruation.

    postpill Failure of menstruation to return after oral contraceptives have been discontinued.

    primary Failure of menarche to occur by the sixteenth year of life.

    psychogenic Failure of menstruation to occur because of emotional disturbances.

    secondary Absence of menses for 3 or more months after menarche.

amniocentesis Aspiration of amniotic fluid, usually transabdominally, for diagnostic or therapeutic purposes.

amniotic fluid The fluid confined by the amnion.

anemia, megaloblastic Anemia with an excessive number of megaloblasts in circulation, caused primarily by deficiency of folic acid, vitamin B_{12}, or both.

anorexia nervosa Marked reduction in the intake of food, caused by psychogenic factors and leading to malnutrition and amenorrhea.

anovulatory bleeding   Periodic uterine bleeding without ovulation.

antepartum   Before labor or delivery.

Apgar score   A physical assessment of the newborn usually performed at 1 and 5 minutes after birth.

arrhenoblastoma   An uncommon ovarian neoplasm that is associated with androgen production and causes amenorrhea, defeminization, and virilization.

ascites   An abnormal accumulation of fluid in the peritoneal cavity.

atony, uterine   Loss of uterine muscular tonicity, which may result in failure of labor to progress or in postpartum hemorrhage.

autonomy   In medicine, a patient's right to determine what health care she will accept.

Barr bodies   Sex chromatin masses on the nuclear membrane. The number of Barr bodies is one fewer than the number of X chromosomes in that cell.

Bartholin cyst   Cystic swelling of a Bartholin gland caused by obstruction of its duct.

Bartholin glands   A pair of glands located at the 4 o'clock and 8 o'clock positions on the vulvovaginal rim. They are homologs of the bulbourethral glands in the male.

basal body temperature   The temperature reading at rest, which is used for detection of ovulation.

basophilic adenoma   A benign tumor of the pituitary, composed of basophilic cells.

benign cystic teratoma   The most common germ cell tumor, consisting of mature elements of all three germ layers (often called dermoid cyst).

biophysical profile   A physical assessment of the fetus, including ultrasound evaluation of fetal movement, breathing movements, fetal tone, amniotic fluid volume, and electronic fetal heart monitoring.

biphasic temperature curve   A graph showing a basal body temperature in the luteal phase that is 0.3 to 1° F higher than that of the follicular phase and indicates that ovulation has occurred.

blood flow, uteroplacental   The circulation by which the fetus exchanges nutrients and waste products with the mother.

breakthrough bleeding   Nonorganic endometrial bleeding during the use of oral contraceptives.

breech   The buttocks (often refers to a fetal presentation).

cancer staging   The clinical evaluation of the extent of cancer.

carcinoma in situ   A neoplasm in which the tumor cells are confined by the basement membrane to the epithelium of origin.

cesarean delivery   Birth of the fetus through incisions made in the abdomen and uterine wall.

chloasma (mask of pregnancy)   Irregular brownish patches of various sizes that may appear on the face during pregnancy and sometimes during the use of oral contraceptives.

chorioamnionitis   Inflammation of the fetal membranes.

choriocarcinoma   A malignant tumor composed of sheets of cellular and syncytial trophoblast.

chorionic villus sampling   The transcervical or transabdominal sampling of the chorionic villi for cytogenic evaluation of the fetus.

chromophobe adenoma   An adenoma of the pituitary gland, consisting of cells that are neither acidophilic nor basophilic.

climacteric   The period of life or the syndrome of endocrine, somatic, and psychic changes that occur in a woman during the transition from the reproductive to the nonreproductive state.

clomiphene A synthetic nonsteroidal compound that stimulates the maturation of follicles and thereby ovulation as a result of its antiestrogenic effect on the hypothalamus.

coitus interruptus Withdrawal of the penis during coitus before ejaculation.

colpocytogram The tabulation of various types of cells observed in a smear taken from the vaginal mucosa.

colporrhaphy

   anterior A surgical procedure used to repair cystocele.

   posterior A surgical procedure used to repair rectocele.

colposcopy Examination of the vagina and cervix by means of an instrument that provides low magnification.

condyloma acuminatum A benign, cauliflower-like growth on the genitalia, thought to be caused by human papillomavirus.

cone biopsy A cone of cervical tissue excised for histologic examination.

contraception Prevention of conception.

corpus luteum The yellow endocrine structure formed in the ovary at the site of a ruptured ovarian follicle.

cryptomenorrhea A condition in which menses occurs without external bleeding, as with an imperforate hymen.

cul-de-sac The pouchlike cavity between the rectum and the uterus, formed by a fold of peritoneum.

culdocentesis Needle aspiration of intraperitoneal fluid or blood through a puncture of the posterior vaginal fornix into the cul-de-sac.

culdoscopy Visual examination of the female pelvic viscera by means of an endoscope introduced into the pelvic cavity through the posterior vaginal fornix.

curettage Scraping of the interior of a cavity or other surface with a curet.

   fractional Separate curettage of the endometrium and the endocervix for diagnostic evaluation. Specimens are submitted separately for pathologic examination.

Cushing syndrome A symptom complex caused by hypersecretion of glucocorticoids, mineralocorticoids, and sex hormones of the adrenal cortex.

cystocele Protrusion of the urinary bladder that creates a downward bulging of the anterior vaginal wall as a result of weakening of the pubocervical fascia.

cystogram A radiogram of the urinary bladder after the injection of a contrast medium.

cystometry Measurement of the function and capacity of the urinary bladder by pressure-volume studies.

cystoscopy Direct instrumental inspection of the interior of the urinary bladder.

D immunoglobulin [Rh0(D) immunoglobulin] An immunoprotein that prevents D sensitization.

decidua Identifiable changes in the endometrium and other tissues in response to the hormonal effects of progesterone.

dermoid cyst *See* benign cystic teratoma.

dilatation The physiologic or instrumental opening of the cervix.

disseminated intravascular coagulation (DIC) A coagulopathy occurring more readily in the presence of pregnancy, fetal death, hemorrhage, and sepsis.

double set-up   The simultaneous availability of two sterile set-ups for both vaginal and abdominal operations.

dysgerminoma   A solid germ cell tumor of the ovary.

dysmaturity   Intrauterine growth retardation leading to a small-for-dates baby, associated with placental insufficiency.

dysmenorrhea   Painful menstruation.

dysontogenetic tumor   A neoplasm caused by defective embryonal development.

dyspareunia   Difficult or painful intercourse.

dystocia   Abnormal or difficult labor.

dysuria   Painful urination.

eclampsia   The convulsive form of preeclampsia-eclampsia syndrome.

ectropion   The growth of the columnar epithelium of the endocervix into the ectocervix.

effacement   Taking up, or shortening, of the cervix.

embryo   The conceptus from the blastocyst stage to the end of the eighth week.

endometrial biopsy   The procedure of obtaining endometrial tissue for diagnostic purposes.

endometriosis   The presence of endometrial implants outside the normal intrauterine location.

endoscopy   Instrumental visualization of the interior of a hollow viscus.

enterocele   A herniation of the small intestine into the cul-de-sac, usually accompanied by (and sometimes confused with) rectocele.

episiotomy   An incision made into the perineum to facilitate delivery and prevent laceration.

estrogen replacement   The exogenous administration of estrogen or estrogenic substances to overcome a deficiency or absence of the natural hormone.

estrogen, unopposed   The continuous and prolonged effect of estrogen on the endometrium, resulting from a lack of progesterone.

eversion   *See* ectropion.

exenteration, pelvic   The removal of all pelvic viscera, including the urinary bladder, the rectum, or both.

fern (ferning)   The microscopic pattern of dried cervical mucus caused by estrogen and associated with the ovulatory period or the microscopic appearance of dried amniotic fluid, often used to diagnose premature rupture of membranes or amniotic fluid leakage.

fetus   The conceptus from 8 weeks until birth.

fibrocystic changes (breast)   Mammary disease characterized by fibrosis and formation of cysts in the fibrous stroma.

foreplay   The preliminary stages of sexual relations, in which the partners usually stimulate each other by kissing, touching, and caressing.

frigidity   An imprecise term, usually used in reference to women, indicating sexual disinterest, unresponsiveness, or aversion.

functional ovarian cyst   A physiologic cyst arising from the graafian follicle or the corpus luteum.

functioning ovarian tumor   A hormone-producing ovarian neoplasm.

fundal dominance   A condition in which uterine contractions are strongest at the top of the uterus and weakest in the lower uterine segment.

galactorrhea   The spontaneous flow of breast milk in the absence of a recent pregnancy.

gender (sex) role An individual's understanding and feeling of the activity and behavior appropriate to the male or female sex.

gonadal agenesis The congenital absence of ovarian tissue, or its presence only as a rudimentary streak.

gonadal dysgenesis The congenitally defective development of the gonads.

gonadotropin

> **human chorionic (HCG)** A glycoprotein hormone that is produced by the syncytiotrophoblast and is immunologically similar to luteinizing hormone (LH).

> **human menopausal (HMG)** A preparation isolated from the urine of postmenopausal women, consisting primarily of follicle-stimulating hormone (FSH) with variable amounts of LH.

> **pituitary** The gonad-stimulating anterior pituitary hormones (FSH and LH).

granulosa cell tumor A feminizing, estrogen-producing ovarian tumor.

gravida A pregnant woman.

gravidity The pregnant state, or the total number of pregnancies a woman has had, including the current pregnancy.

hemoperitoneum Blood in the peritoneal cavity.

hermaphrodite A person who exhibits a variance from chromosomal sex in one or more of the following criteria: (1) gonadal structure, (2) structure of the internal or external genitalia, (3) hormonal status, and (4) sex of rearing (gender or sex role). A true hermaphrodite may exhibit any of these anomalies but is characterized by the presence of both ovarian and testicular tissue.

hilus cell tumor An uncommon ovarian tumor that is usually associated with defeminization or virilization and has a low incidence of malignancy.

hirsutism The development of various degrees of hair growth of male type and distribution in a woman.

hormone replacement therapy (HRT) *See* estrogen replacement.

hot flashes A vasomotor symptom characterized by transient hot sensations that involve chiefly the upper part of the thorax, neck, and head, are frequently followed by sweats, and are associated with cessation or diminution in the ovarian secretion of estrogen.

hydatidiform mole A pathologic condition of pregnancy characterized by the hydropic degeneration of the chorionic villi and variable degrees of trophoblastic proliferation.

hydramnios Excessive amounts (more than 2 L) of amniotic fluid at term.

hyperplasia, endometrial The abnormal proliferation of the endometrium with a marked increase in the number of glands or cystic dilatation of glands. These changes may be related to prolonged unopposed estrogen stimulation. Atypical adenomatous hyperplasia is sometimes a precursor to carcinoma of the endometrium.

hyperthecosis (cortical hyperplasia, thecomatosis) Proliferation of the ovarian cortical stroma, usually in the postmenopausal state. It may be associated with increased estrogen and androgen production.

hypertonic intraamniotic saline or urea Hypertonic saline (usually a 20% solution) or urea injected into the amniotic cavity by amniocentesis, which usually initiates the onset of labor with death of the fetus. It has been used to induce abortion in pregnancies of 15 to 20 weeks of gestation.

hypoestrogenism A condition of subnormal estrogen production with resultant atrophy or failure of development of estrogen-dependent tissues.

hypofibrinogenemia   A deficiency (usually < 100 mg/ml) of circulating fibrinogen that may be seen in conditions such as abruptio placentae, amniotic fluid embolism, fetal death, and occasionally intraamniotic instillation of hypertonic saline, in which the fibrinogen is consumed by disseminated intravascular coagulation.

hypogonadism   The subnormal production of hormones by the gonads.

hysterectomy

  abdominal   The removal of the uterine corpus and cervix through an incision made in the abdominal wall.

  radical   The removal of the uterine corpus, cervix, and parametrium, with dissection of the ureters; usually combined with pelvic lymphadenectomy.

  subtotal (supracervical)   The removal of the uterine corpus, leaving the cervix in situ.

  total   The removal of the uterine corpus and cervix (without regard to tubes or ovaries).

  vaginal   The removal of the uterus through the vagina.

hysterosalpingography   Roentgenography of the uterus and tubes after injection of radiopaque contrast medium through the cervix. It is useful in ascertaining irregularities of the uterine cavity and patency of the fallopian tubes.

hysteroscopy   The transcervical endoscopic visualization of the endometrial cavity.

hysterotomy   Surgical incision of the wall of the uterus.

immaturity   The condition of a fetus weighing 500 to 999 g at birth.

imperforate hymen   Failure of a lumen to develop at a point where the budding vagina arises from the urogenital sinus.

impotence   The inability to achieve or sustain penile erection.

incoordinate uterine activity   Lack of a synchronous contraction pattern from the fundus toward the cervix, resulting in ineffective labor.

infertility   The inability to achieve pregnancy with regular intercourse and no contraception within a stipulated period of time, often considered to be 1 to 2 years.

intervillous space   The space in the placenta in which maternal blood bathes chorionic villi, thus allowing the exchange of materials between the fetal and maternal circulations.

intraductal papilloma   A benign mammary tumor, often multiple, occurring predominantly in parous women at or shortly before menopause. It is typically located beneath the areola and is often associated with bleeding from the nipple.

intrauterine device (IUD)   A device inserted into the uterine cavity for contraception.

intrauterine growth retardation (IUGR)   *See* dysmaturity.

intromission   Introduction of the penis into the vagina.

justice   Ensuring or maintaining what is considered to be just or fair according to predetermined criteria.

karyotype   A photographic reproduction of the chromosomes of a cell in metaphase, arranged according to a standard classification.

labor   The process of expulsion of the fetus from the uterus.

  induced   Labor that is initiated artificially.

  stimulated   Labor that is stimulated, usually with oxytocin.

lactogen, human placental (HPL)   A polypeptide hormone that is produced by the syncytiotrophoblast, is similar to prolactin and somatotropin from the pituitary, and is involved in carbohydrate metabolism by the mother and fetus.

laparoscopy The transabdominal endoscopic examination of the peritoneal cavity and its contents after inducing pneumoperitoneum.

leiomyoma A benign tumor derived from smooth muscle; colloquially referred to as a fibroid.

leiomyosarcoma An uncommon malignant tumor of smooth muscle.

leukoplakia An imprecise clinical term usually referring to white lesions of the vulva.

levator muscle The muscular sheet, consisting of the iliococcygeus pubococcygeus, and puborectalis muscles, that forms most of the pelvic floor (pelvic diaphragm) and supports the pelvic viscera.

libido Sexual desire or urge.

lie *See* presentation.

ligament

    cardinal The dense connective tissue that represents the union of the base of the broad ligament to the supravaginal portion of the cervix and laterally to the sides of the pelvis. It is considered to be the primary support of the uterus.

    uterosacral The peritoneal folds containing connective tissue, autonomic nerves, and involuntary muscle, arising on each side of the posterior wall of the uterus at about the level of the internal cervical os and passing backward toward the rectum, around which they extend to their insertion on the sacral wall. They are considered to play an important part in axial support of the uterus.

ligation, tubal The surgical or mechanical interruption of the continuity of the fallopian tubes for the purpose of permanent contraception.

LMP Last menstrual period.

LNMP Last normal menstrual period.

mastitis Inflammation of the breast.

masturbation Sexual stimulation by manipulation of the genitals.

maturation index The ratio of parabasal to intermediate to superficial vaginal epithelial cells (e.g., 0/20/80).

maturity The condition of a fetus weighing 2500 g or more.

membranes, premature rupture of (PROM) Rupture of the amniotic membranes before the onset of labor.

menarche The onset of menses.

menopause The permanent cessation of menses, naturally caused by ovarian failure.

menorrhagia Excessive or prolonged uterine bleeding occurring at regular intervals.

metaplasia A reversible change in which one adult cell type is replaced by another cell type. The most common type of epithelial metaplasia is the replacement of columnar cells by stratified epithelium (squamous metaplasia).

metrorrhagia Uterine bleeding occurring at times other than the expected menses; for example, intermenstrual bleeding.

midpelvis An imaginary plane that passes through the pelvis and is defined by three points: the inferior margin of the symphysis pubis and the tips of the ischial spines on either side. This plane usually includes the smallest dimensions of the pelvis.

mortality A fatal outcome.

    fetal Death of the conceptus between 8 weeks of gestation and birth.

    maternal Death of the mother.

    neonatal Death of the infant in the first 28 days of life.

perinatal   Death of the fetus or neonate between 20 weeks of gestation and 28 days after birth.

mosaicism   The presence in an individual of cells of different chromosomal constitutions.

mucus, cervical   The secretion of the cervical mucous glands; its quality and quantity are influenced by estrogen and progesterone. Estrogen makes it abundant and clear, with spinnbarkeit and a fern pattern on drying. Progesterone makes it scant, opaque, and cellular without a fern pattern on microscopic examination.

neonatal   Referring to the first 28 days of life.

nonstress test (NST)   Evaluation of the fetus by electronic fetal heart monitoring, not in labor.

oligomenorrhea   Infrequent menstruation.

orgasm   The climax of sexual excitement.

osteoporosis   Atrophy of bone caused by demineralization.

ovulation, induction of   Stimulation of ovulation by artificial means.

oxytocin   An octapeptide formed in the hypothalamus and stored in the posterior lobe of the pituitary. It has stimulant effects on the smooth muscle of the uterus and the mammary glands.

Papanicolaou smear (Pap smear)   A cytologic smear of exfoliated cells (e.g., from the cervix, endometrial cavity, or vagina) used in the early detection of cancer or for evaluation of a patient's hormonal status.

parity   The number of pregnancies of a particular woman in which the fetus has reached viability.

pelvic floor   The floor or sling for the pelvic structures, located at the level of the pelvic outlet. The most important structures are the levator ani muscle and fascial sheaths.

pelvic inflammatory disease (PID)   An infection of the pelvic viscera, usually by ascending routes. The likely etiologic pathogens include: *Neisseria gonorrhoeae, Chlamydia trachomatis,* and other polymicrobic organisms, both anaerobic and aerobic.

pelvic inlet   An imaginary plane passing through the pelvis that represents the upper boundary of the true pelvis. It is bounded posteriorly by the promontory and alae of the sacrum, laterally by the linea terminalis, and anteriorly by the horizontal rami of the pubic bones and the upper margin of the symphysis pubis.

perinatal   Pertaining to the combination of fetal and neonatal periods, considered to begin after 20 weeks of gestation and to end 28 days after birth.

perineorrhaphy   Plastic repair of the perineum.

perineum   The pelvic floor and associated structures occupying the pelvic outlet.

pessary   A device placed in the vagina or uterus to support the uterus.

placenta previa   A condition in which the placenta is located in the lower portion of the uterus and extends to, or covers part or all of, the internal os.

PMP   Previous menstrual period.

pneumoperitoneum   The presence of air in the peritoneal cavity.

polycystic ovary syndrome (Stein-Leventhal syndrome)   A syndrome of secondary oligomenorrhea and infertility associated with multiple follicle cysts of the ovary and failure to ovulate.

polymenorrhea   Cyclic uterine bleeding that is normal in amount but occurs at too-frequent intervals.

position   The relationship of a designated point on the presenting part of the fetus to the anterior, transverse, or posterior portion of the maternal pelvis (e.g., occiput left anterior [OLA]).

postmenopausal bleeding   Bleeding from the uterus, cervix, or vagina that occurs after menopause.

postpartum   After delivery or childbirth.

postterm pregnancy   Pregnancy prolonged beyond the end of the forty-second week of gestation.

preeclampsia   A specific hypertensive disorder of pregnancy, with the diagnosis made on the basis of hypertension with proteinuria, edema, or both. It occurs after the twentieth week of pregnancy.

pregnancy, ectopic   A pregnancy located outside the usual sites in the corpus uteri.

prematurity   The condition of a fetus weighing 1000 to 2499 g.

premenstrual syndrome (PMS)   A complex of symptoms occurring in the progestational phase of the menstrual cycle.

presentation   The relationship of the long axis of the fetus to the long axis of the mother. A presentation is either longitudinal (head or breech) or transverse.

presenting part   The portion of the fetus that is felt through the cervix on vaginal examination. The presenting part determines the presentation.

primigravida   A woman who is pregnant for the first time.

prolapse

   cord   A condition in which the umbilical cord precedes the presenting part.

   uterine   Prolapse of the uterus, usually due to the loss of supporting structures. It is related to injuries of childbirth, advanced age, or congenital weakness.

pseudocyesis   False pregnancy, in which some of the signs and symptoms of pregnancy are present, although no conception has taken place.

puberty   The period between the beginning of the development of secondary sexual characteristics and the completion of somatic growth.

   delayed   The lack of appearance of secondary sexual characteristics by age 14.

   precocious   The appearance of secondary sexual characteristics before 7.5 years of age.

puerperium   The period after delivery in which the reproductive tract returns to its normal, nonpregnant condition, generally 6 to 8 weeks.

quality of life   In medicine, the experience of the worth of living as a patient-centered moral criterion.

quickening   The first perception by the mother of fetal movement, usually around the twentieth week of gestation.

rectocele   Protrusion of the rectum through the supporting structures of the posterior vaginal wall.

reflux, tubal   The retrograde flow of uterine or tubal contents into the abdominal cavity.

resection, tubal   Surgical removal of a segment of fallopian tube for the purpose of permanent contraception.

rhythm   A method of contraception in which coitus is avoided when ovulation is likely.

rubella (German measles)   An acute exanthematous viral disease that may cause fetal malformation if contracted during the first trimester of pregnancy.

salpingectomy   Surgical removal of a fallopian tube.

salpingo-oophorectomy   Surgical removal of a fallopian tube and ovary.

Schiller test   The application of a solution of iodine to the cervix. The iodine is taken up by the glycogen in normal vaginal epithelium, giving it a brown appearance. Areas lacking in glycogen are white or whitish yellow, as in leukoplakia or cancer. Although nonstaining areas are not diagnostic of cancer, they aid in choosing the spot to which a biopsy should be directed.

secondary sexual characteristics   The physical changes that have occurred in response to endocrine changes during puberty.

semen analysis   The evaluation of the components of semen, especially spermatozoa, as a means of evaluating male fertility.

sexuality   The physiologic and psychologic expression of sexual behavior. The periods of infancy, adolescence, and adulthood and the postclimacteric state each have characteristic manifestations of sexuality.

Sims-Huhner test   A test for infertility in which cervical mucus is aspirated after coitus and examined for quality and presence or absence of infection. The motility, normality, and number of sperm are noted.

Skene glands   The vestibular glands that open into and around the urethra.

somatomammotropin, chorionic   *See* lactogen, human placental.

sonography (ultrasonography, ultrasound)   In obstetrics and gynecology, a diagnostic aid in which high-frequency sound waves are used to detect the presence of normal and abnormal pregnancies and pelvic tumors. It is used also to locate the placenta and to measure the fetal biparietal diameter.

spinnbarkeit   The ability of the cervical mucus to be drawn out into a thread, characteristically greater in the preovulatory and ovulatory phases of the menstrual cycle.

station   The position of the fetal presenting part (leading bony point) relative to the level of the ischial spines. Station +2 means the presenting part is 2 cm below the ischial spines. Station −1 means the presenting part is 1 cm above the ischial spines.

sterility   The absolute inability to procreate.

stress incontinence   The involuntary leakage of urine during an increase in intraabdominal pressure as a result of weakness of the supports of the internal vesical sphincter and bladder neck.

striae gravidarum   Streaks or lines seen on the abdominal skin of a pregnant woman.

supine hypotensive syndrome   A hypotensive syndrome often characterized by sweating, nausea, and tachycardia. It occurs in some pregnant women in the supine position when the pregnant uterus obstructs venous return.

teratogen   An agent or factor that produces physical defects in the developing embryo.

testicular feminization   A syndrome of androgen insensitivity characterized by primary amenorrhea, a female phenotype, testes (abdominal or inguinal) instead of ovaries, the absence of a uterus, and a male genotype.

thecoma   A functioning ovarian tumor composed of theca cells.

thelarche   The onset of development of breasts.

trimester   A period of 3 months. The period of gestation is divided into three units of 3 calendar months each. Some important obstetric events may be conveniently categorized by trimesters.

trophoblast   The epithelium of the chorion, including the covering of the placental villi. It comprises a cellular layer (cytotrophoblast) and syncytium (syncytiotrophoblast).

tubercles, Montgomery   The enlarged sebaceous glands of the areolae of the mammary glands during late pregnancy and lactation.

ultrasonography   *See* sonography.

ultrasound   *See* sonography.

urethrocele   Protrusion of the urethra through the supporting structure of the anterior wall.

vasectomy   The surgical interruption of the ductus (vas) deferens for permanent contraception.

VBAC   Vaginal birth after cesarean delivery.

viability   The condition of a fetus weighing 500 g or more; the ability to live independently outside of the uterus.

virilization   The development of masculine traits in a female.

withdrawal bleeding   Uterine bleeding after the interruption of hormonal support of the endometrium.

A page number followed by *f* indicates figure; *t* indicates table.